Atlas of Robotic Upper Gastrointestinal Surgery

Omar Yusef Kudsi • Peter P. Grimminger
Editors

Atlas of Robotic Upper Gastrointestinal Surgery

Springer

Editors
Omar Yusef Kudsi
Department of Surgery
Tufts University School of Medicine
Boston, MA, USA

Peter P. Grimminger
Department of General, Visceral and Transplant Surgery
University Medical Center Mainz
Mainz, Rheinland-Pfalz, Germany

ISBN 978-3-030-86577-1 ISBN 978-3-030-86578-8 (eBook)
https://doi.org/10.1007/978-3-030-86578-8

This Springer imprint is published by the registered company Springer Nature Switzerland AG
The registered company address is: Gewerbestrasse 11, 6330 Cham, Switzerland

To my family, I share this publishing achievement with you with love and gratitude. —Omar Yusef Kudsi

This atlas is dedicated to all robotic surgeons in the field of upper-GI surgery as well as students and medical staff at the OR. —Peter P. Grimminger

Preface

> Advancing from novice to amateur can break the rethinking cycle. As we gain experience, we lose some of our humility. We take pride in making rapid progress, which promotes a false sense of mastery. That jump-starts an overconfidence cycle, preventing us from doubting what we know and being curious about what we don't. We get trapped in a beginner's bubble of flawed assumptions, where we're ignorant of our own ignorance. — Excerpt from Adam Grant, "Think Again."

Over the last decade, there has been an increase in robotic surgery adoption among general surgeons worldwide. Robotics has become the hot topic of most surgical meetings and social media surgical platforms such as robotic surgery collaboration with thousands of surgeons debating the value and discussing the outcomes.

The Atlas of Robotic Upper Gastrointestinal Surgery draws on the expertise of world-class surgeons to share their pearls of wisdom. The main focus of this atlas is to demonstrate visually how to perform the most common upper-GI procedures. This is possible via a set of beautiful high-quality annotated images showing step-by-step guidance on "how to do it." With a total of 25 chapters and 50 contributors, this atlas is surely the preeminent source for the newest techniques by capturing the key points of the procedures, written by experts in the field actively involved in robotic upper GI surgery education and hands-on training. Editors Dr. Kudsi (USA) and Dr. Grimminger (Germany) have hosted and taught hundreds of surgeons and performed over 3000 robotic surgeries. They have traveled and collaborated with surgeons in the USA, Europe, South America, and Asia to perform live robotic surgeries.

Boston, MA, USA — Omar Yusef Kudsi

Acknowledgments

I would not have been able to edit this book without the inspiration of my mentors Daniel Jones at Harvard Medical School; Barry Mann, John Marks, and John Gefen at Lankenau; and Michael Tarnoff at Tufts. I have had the privilege of working alongside clinical and research robotic surgery fellows Fahri Gokcal, Naseem Bou-Ayash, Sara Lagrange, Karen Chang, and Alexandra Chudner. Special thanks to Peter Dion, Susan Michaud, and the staff at Good Samaritan Medical Center who have helped establish a world-class robotic epicenter and being a role model for developing one of the most efficient robotic programs in the nation.

Lastly, I would also like to thank my co-editor Dr. Grimminger of Germany, a world-class surgeon. —Omar Yusef Kudsi

Many thanks to Lee Klein from Springer for the great support and communications.

Special thanks to UGIRA (UGIRA.org) for all the support, especially the UGIRA President: Richard van Hillegersberg. Thank you. —Peter P. Grimminger

Contents

Contributors

Abubaker A. Ali, MD Department of General Surgery, Wayne State University, Detroit, MI, USA

Michael M. Awad, MD, PhD, FACS Section of Minimally Invasive Surgery, Washington University School of Medicine, St Louis, MO, USA

Dirk Bausch, MD Department of Surgery, Marien Hospital Herne, Universitätsklinikum der Ruhr-Universität Bochum, Herne, Germany

Jan Henrik Beckmann, MD UKSH Department of General, Visceral-, Thoracic-, Transplantation-, and Pediatric Surgery, University Medical Center Schleswig-Holstein, Kiel, Germany

Felix Berlth, MD Department of General, Visceral and Transplant Surgery, University Medical Center of the Johannes Gutenberg University, Mainz, Germany

Matthias Biebl Department of Surgery, Campus Charité Mitte|Campus Virchow Klinikum, Charité – Universitätsmedizin Berlin, Corporate Member of Freie Universität Berlin, Humboldt-Universität zu Berlin, and Berlin Institute of Health, Berlin, Germany

Adrian Billeter, MD, PhD Department for General, Visceral and Transplantation Surgery, Division for Minimally Invasive and Robot-Assisted Surgery, Division for Upper Gastrointestinal Surgery, Heidelberg University Hospital, Heidelberg, Germany

Alberto Biondi, MD Fondazione Policlinico Universitario A. Gemelli IRCCS, Catholic University of the Sacred Heart, Rome, Italy

Marco Augusto Bonino, MD Division of Digestive Surgery, Department of Surgery, Geneva University Hospital and Faculty of Medicine, Geneva, Switzerland

Ivo A. M. J. Broeders, MD, PhD Department of Surgery, Meander Medical Center, Amersfoort, The Netherlands

University of Twente, Robotics and Mechatronics, Enschede, The Netherlands

Manuela Capek, MD Department for General, Visceral and Transplantation Surgery, Division for Minimally Invasive and Robot-Assisted Surgery, Division for Upper Gastrointestinal Surgery, Heidelberg University Hospital, Heidelberg, Germany

Giovanni Capovilla, MD Department of General-, Visceral- and Transplant Surgery, University Medical Center Mainz, Mainz, Germany

Mickael Chevallay, MD Division of Digestive Surgery, Department of Surgery, Geneva University Hospital and Faculty of Medicine, Geneva, Switzerland

Christian Denecke, MD Department of Surgery, Campus Charité Mitte|Campus Virchow Klinikum, Charité – Universitätsmedizin Berlin, Corporate Member of Freie Universität Berlin, Humboldt-Universität zu Berlin, and Berlin Institute of Health, Berlin, Germany

Domenico D'Ugo, MD Fondazione Policlinico Universitario A. Gemelli IRCCS, Catholic University of the Sacred Heart, Rome, Italy

Tomasz Dziodzio, MD Department of Surgery, Campus Charité Mitte|Campus Virchow Klinikum, Charité – Universitätsmedizin Berlin, Corporate Member of Freie Universität Berlin, Humboldt-Universität zu Berlin, and Berlin Institute of Health, Berlin, Germany

Jan-Henrik Egberts, MD Department for Surgery, Israelitisches Krankenhaus Hamburg, Hamburg, Germany

Kevin El-Hayek, MD, FACS Department of Surgery, The MetroHealth System, Cleveland, OH, USA

Katherine Fay, MD Department of Surgery, Emory University School of Medicine, Atlanta, GA, USA

Carolina Froiio, MD Department of General-, Visceral- and Transplant Surgery, University Medical Center Mainz, Mainz, Germany

Carlos A. Galvani, MD Division of Minimally Invasive Surgery. Department of Surgery, Tulane University School of Medicine, New Orleans, LA, USA

Prakash Gatta, MD, FACS Department of Surgery, Multicare Health System, Tacoma, WA, USA

Torben Glatz, MD Department of Surgery, Marien Hospital Herne, Universitätsklinikum der Ruhr-Universität Bochum, Herne, Germany

Augustus Gleason, MD Surgical Simulation and Education Research Fellow, Lahey Hospital and Medical Center Department of Surgery, Burlington, MA, USA

Peter P. Grimminger Department of General-, Visceral- and Transplant Surgery, University Medical Center Mainz, Mainz, Germany

Eline de Groot, MD Department of Surgery, University Medical Center Utrecht, Utrecht, The Netherlands

Richard van Hillegersberg Department of Surgery, University Medical Center Utrecht, Utrecht, The Netherlands

Torjborg Holtestaul, MD Department of Surgery, Multicare Health System, Tacoma, WA, USA

Caitlin Houghton, MD Department of Surgery, Keck School of Medicine, University of Southern California, Los Angeles, CA, USA

Minoa Karin Jung, MD Division of Digestive Surgery, Department of Surgery, Geneva University Hospital and Faculty of Medicine, Geneva, Switzerland

Jan-Niclas Kersebaum, MD UKSH Department of General, Visceral-, Thoracic-, Transplantation-, and Pediatric Surgery, University Medical Center Schleswig-Holstein, Kiel, Germany

Danuel Laan, MD Division of Minimally Invasive Surgery. Department of Surgery, Tulane University School of Medicine, New Orleans, LA, USA

Laura Lorenzon, MD General Surgery Unit, Fondazione Policlinico Universitario A. Gemelli IRCCS, Catholic University of the Sacred Heart, Rome, Italy

Fazaldin Moghul, MD Department of General Surgery, Wayne State University, Detroit, MI, USA

Stefan Paul Mönig, FEBS, MHBA Division of Digestive Surgery, Department of Surgery, Geneva University Hospital and Faculty of Medicine, Geneva, Switzerland

Beat Peter Müller-Stich, MD Department for General, Visceral and Transplantation Surgery, Division for Minimally Invasive and Robot-Assisted Surgery, Division for Upper Gastrointestinal Surgery, Heidelberg University Hospital, Heidelberg, Germany

Robert Öllinger, MD, Prof. Department of Surgery, Campus Charité Mitte|Campus Virchow Klinikum, Charité – Universitätsmedizin Berlin, Corporate Member of Freie Universität Berlin, Humboldt-Universität zu Berlin, and Berlin Institute of Health, Berlin, Germany

Ankit D. Patel, MD Department of Surgery, Emory University School of Medicine, Atlanta, GA, USA

Curtis Peery, MD, FACS, FASMBS Department of Surgery, Sanford School of Medicine University of South Dakota, Sioux Falls, SD, USA

Ashwini S. Poola, MD Department of Surgery, Multicare Health System, Tacoma, WA, USA

Johann Pratschke, MD, Prof. Department of Surgery, Campus Charité Mitte|Campus Virchow Klinikum, Charité – Universitätsmedizin Berlin, Corporate Member of Freie Universität Berlin, Humboldt-Universität zu Berlin, and Berlin Institute of Health, Berlin, Germany

Laila Rashidi, MD MultiCare Colon and Rectal Surgery – Tacoma Clinic, Tacoma, WA, USA

Benedikt Reichert, MD Department of General, Abdominal, Thoracic, Transplantation and Pediatric Surgery, University Hospital Schleswig-Holstein, Kiel, Germany

Jelle P. Ruurda, MD, PhD Department of Gastro-intestinal and Oncologic Surgery, University Medical Center, Utrecht, The Netherlands

Pietro Santocchi, MD Fondazione Policlinico Universitario A. Gemelli IRCCS, Catholic University of the Sacred Heart, Rome, Italy

William C. Sherrill III, MD Section of Minimally Invasive Surgery, Washington University School of Medicine, St Louis, MO, USA

Hubert Stein Department of Clinical Development Engineering, Intuitive Surgical Inc, Sunnyvale, CA, USA

Evangelos Tagkalos, MD Department of General-, Visceral- and Transplant Surgery, University Medical Center Mainz, Mainz, Germany

Hany Takla, MD, FACS, FASMBS Departments of General and Bariatric Surgery, Beth Israel Lahey Health Winchester Hospital, Winchester, MA, USA

Frank J. Voskens, MD Department of Surgery, Meander Medical Center, Amersfoort, The Netherlands

University of Twente, Robotics and Mechatronics, Enschede, The Netherlands

Martin Wagner, MD Department for General, Visceral and Transplantation Surgery, Division for Minimally Invasive and Robot-Assisted Surgery, Division for Upper Gastrointestinal Surgery, Heidelberg University Hospital, Heidelberg, Germany

Han-Kwang Yang, MD Department of Surgery, Seoul National University College of Medicine, Seoul, South Korea

Robotic Median Arcuate Ligament Release

1

Kevin El-Hayek

Introduction

Median arcuate ligament syndrome (MALS) is a rare pain disorder characterized by postprandial abdominal pain, nausea, and weight loss. Because these symptoms overlap with common gastrointestinal orders, patients with MALS often present after an extensive work-up and multiple prior interventions. Median arcuate ligament compression is confirmed by a combination of dynamic elevated celiac artery velocities on mesenteric duplex ultrasonography and a celiac artery stenosis on computed tomography angiography (CTA) or magnetic resonance angiography (MRA). While median arcuate ligament compression is a relatively normal variant in human anatomy, in a select group of patients, this finding may induce irritation of the celiac ganglion and neurogenic pain. MALS is further suspected when patients have a favorable response to a diagnostic celiac plexus block.

Traditional laparotomy with median arcuate ligament release and celiac ganglionectomy was the standard of care until the first laparoscopic approach was described in 2000 [1]. An early series of minimally invasive cases cautioned against the use of the robot due to the loss of tactile feedback in a case which resulted in an aortic injury and conversion [2]. Since this early experience with the robotic platform, multiple centers have demonstrated improved safety and efficacy [3]. A stable high-definition image, precise surgical movements around the aorta and celiac artery, and the addition of real-time augmented image guidance (ultrasound and indocyanine green angiography) may create a more favorable platform to complete this operation robotically.

Approaching a patient with MALS begins with a careful review of the preoperative CTA or MRA, paying special attention to arterial and venous anatomy near the median arcuate ligament. Specifically, small phrenic arteries or the left gastric vein may be in close proximity to the ligament and celiac ganglion. After docking the robot, the left hepatic lobe is retracted with a laparoscopic liver retractor or a liver hammock suture. The gastrohepatic ligament is then divided to the level of the right crus. Pre-release ultrasound is performed to identify the median arcuate ligament and the takeoff of the celiac artery under the right crus. Next, the right crus is divided longitudinally to expose the supraceliac aorta. The median arcuate ligament is then carefully dissected free with a partial celiac ganglion resection to expose the takeoffs of the left gastric artery, splenic artery, and common hepatic artery for 180 degrees. To ensure adequate release, intraoperative indocyanine green angiography and ultrasound are performed after dissection.

Procedure: Illustrated Steps

Figures 1.1, 1.2, 1.3, 1.4, 1.5, 1.6, 1.7, 1.8, 1.9, 1.10, 1.11, 1.12, 1.13, 1.14, 1.15, 1.16, 1.17, 1.18, 1.19, 1.20, 1.21, 1.22, 1.23, 1.24, 1.25, 1.26, 1.27, 1.28, 1.29, 1.30, 1.31, 1.32, 1.33,

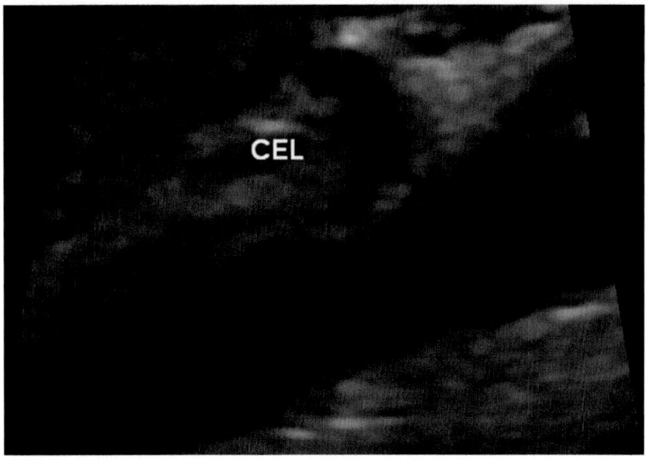

Fig. 1.1 Mesenteric duplex sonography showing celiac artery (CEL) with median arcuate ligament compression

K. El-Hayek (✉)
Department of Surgery, The MetroHealth System, Cleveland, OH, USA
e-mail: kelhayek@metrohealth.org

O. Y. Kudsi, P. P. Grimminger (eds.), *Atlas of Robotic Upper Gastrointestinal Surgery*,
https://doi.org/10.1007/978-3-030-86578-8_1

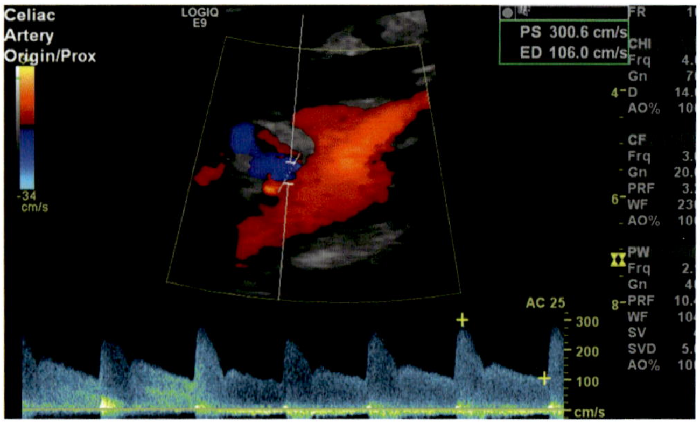

Fig. 1.2 Mesenteric duplex sonography showing dynamic elevated velocities of the celiac artery (300 cm/s) consistent with median arcuate ligament compression

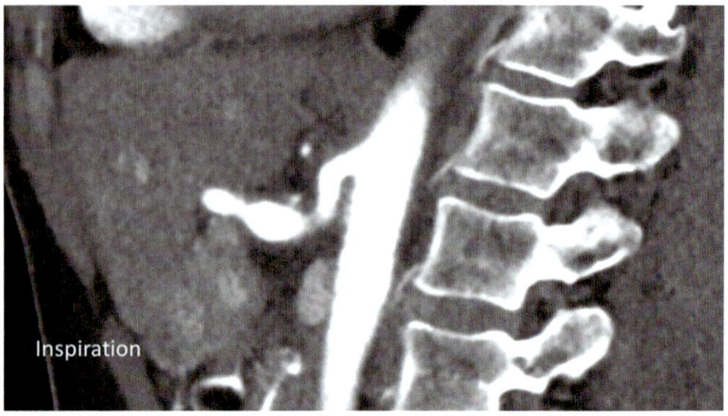

Fig. 1.3 Coronal view of CTA of patient during inspiration demonstrating compression of mid-celiac artery

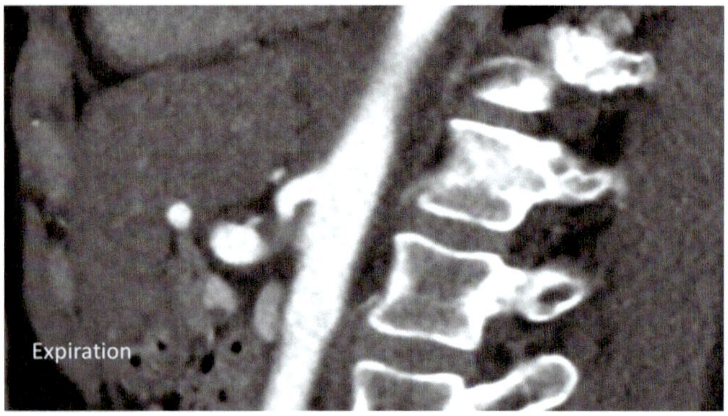

Fig. 1.4 Coronal view of CTA of patient during expiration, with increase in post-stenotic dilation

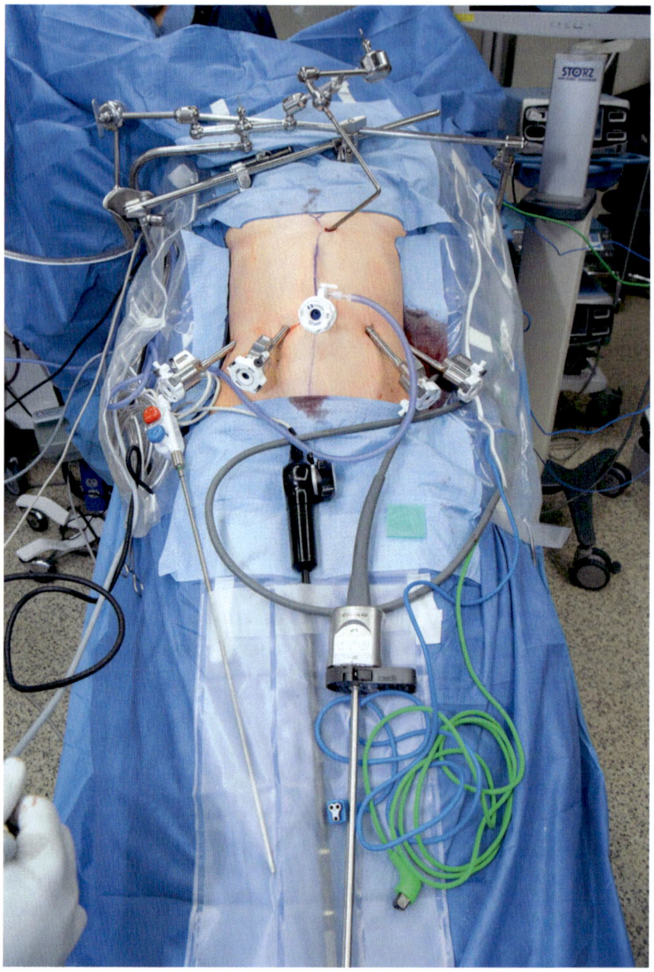

Fig. 1.5 Operative setup including trocar placement, liver retractor, and open retractor connected to bed for preparation should conversion to open be required

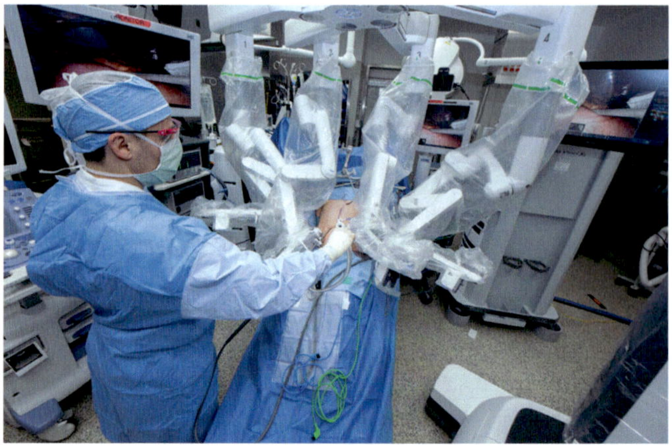

Fig. 1.6 Operative setup with robot docked, showing position of bedside assistant who provides downward retraction with suction/irrigator and passes ultrasound probe, sutures, and sponges

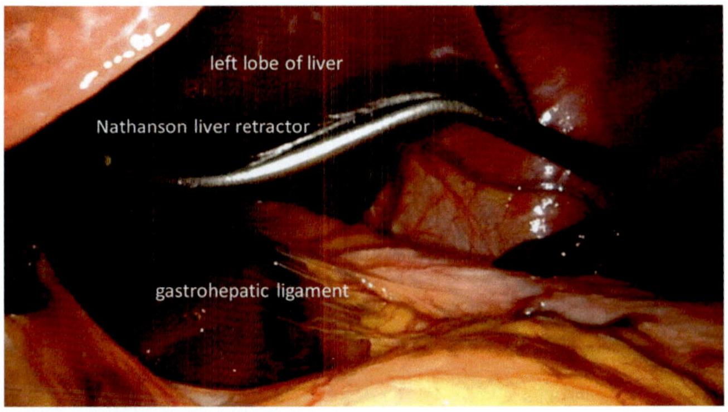

Fig. 1.7 After placement of trocars and instruments, a Nathanson liver retractor can be placed under the left lobe of the liver

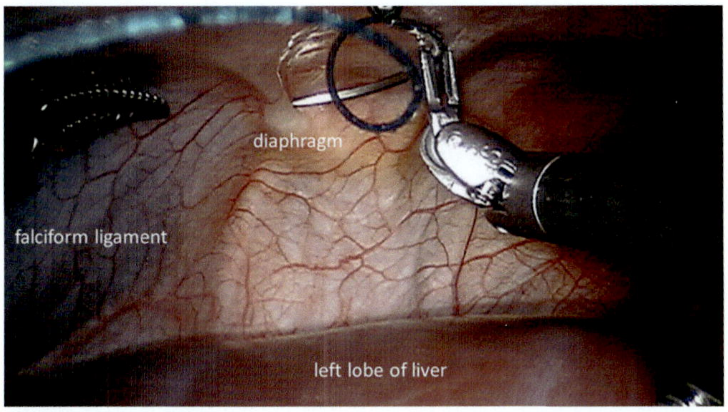

Fig. 1.8 To eliminate the liver retractor incision, a liver hammock suture can be placed. This figure shows the first step, using a 12-inch, 0 barbed suture bite to the left side of the falciform ligament above the left lobe of the liver

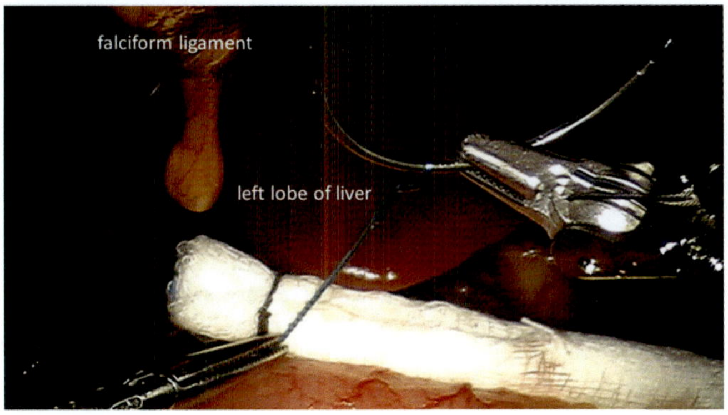

Fig. 1.9 The suture is then taken through the pre-formed loop, pulling it tight

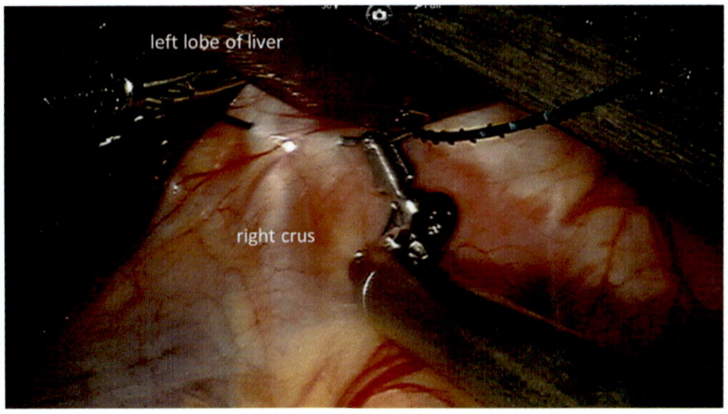

Fig. 1.10 The next bite is along the superior aspect of the right crus

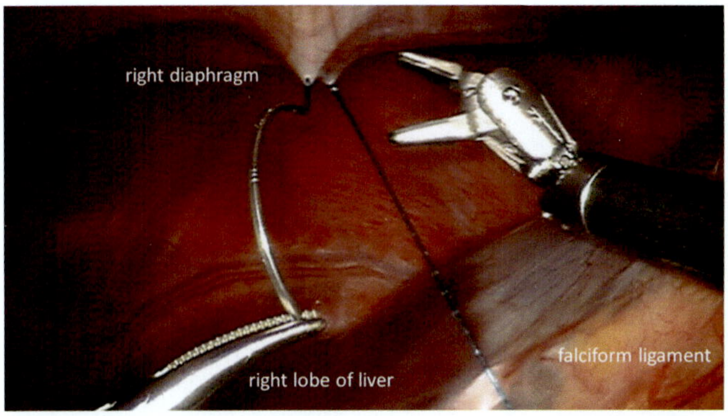

Fig. 1.11 The following bite is to the right of the falciform ligament, high along the right diaphragm

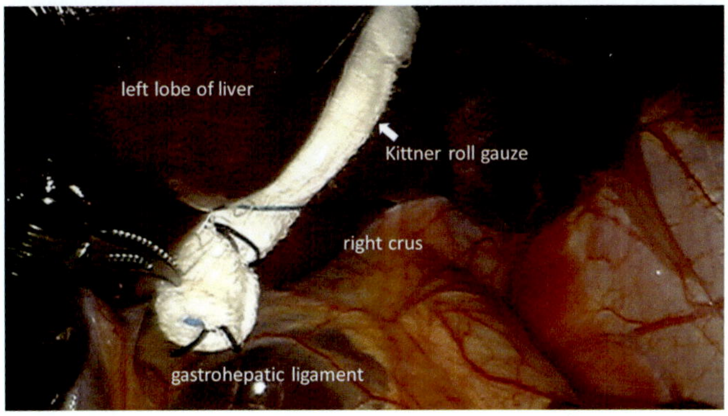

Fig. 1.12 The final appearance of the liver hammock stitch with a Kittner roll gauze (Carefree Surgical Specialties, Inc. New Castle, CA) under the suture to protect the liver parenchyma

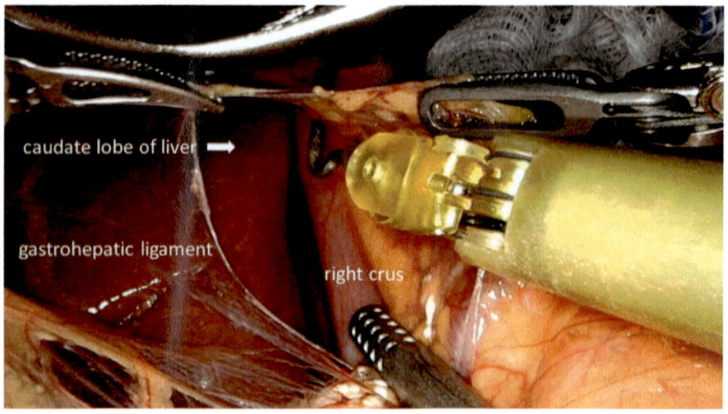

Fig. 1.13 Division of the gastrohepatic ligament to the level of the right crus

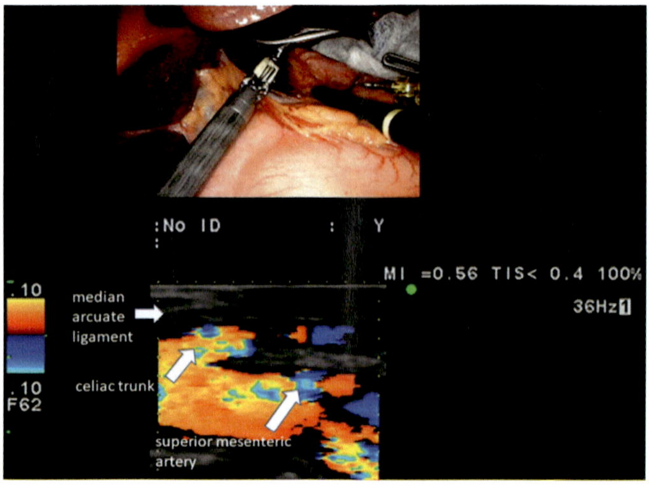

Fig. 1.14 Bedside assistant laparoscopic flexible tip ultrasound probe placement to identify the median arcuate ligament, celiac trunk, and superior mesenteric artery takeoff. Ultrasound image is seen in real time at the robotic console with TilePro™ (Intuitive Surgical, Sunnyvale CA) adjunct

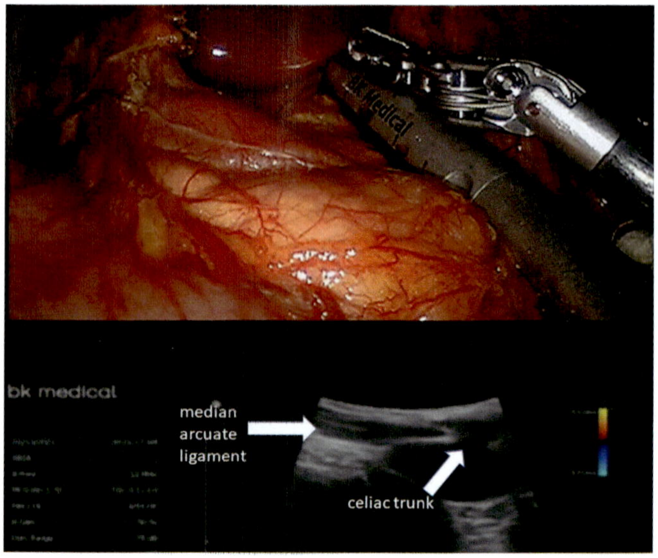

Fig. 1.15 A drop-in ultrasound probe can also be used and controlled by the console surgeon to identify the median arcuate ligament and celiac trunk, again using the TilePro™ (Intuitive Surgical, Sunnyvale CA) adjunct

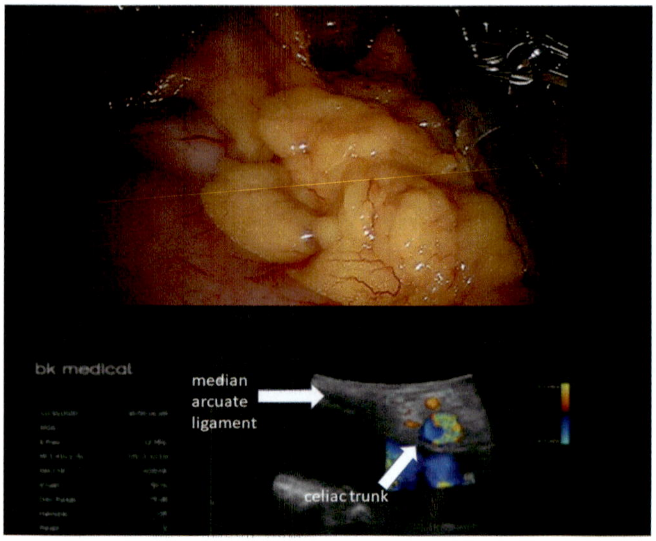

Fig. 1.16 The color/flow option on the ultrasound machine can be helpful to identify the celiac trunk and adjacent median arcuate ligament prior to release. The celiac takeoff diameter can also be measured before and after release to ensure that the compression is adequately relieved

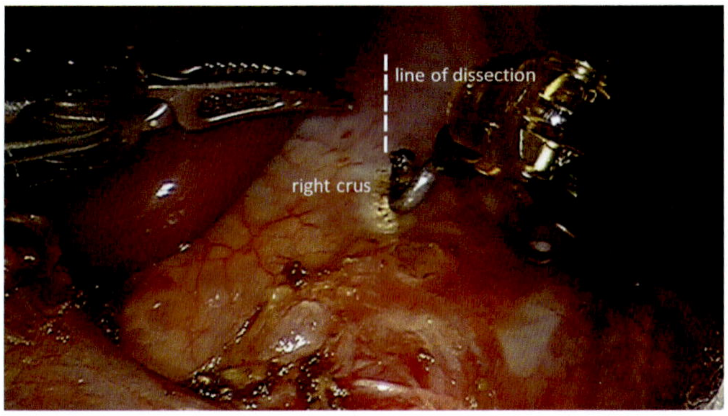

Fig. 1.17 After confirmation of the location of the median arcuate ligament by ultrasound. The right crus is divided longitudinally from the base of the crus toward the anterior portion. Approaching the median arcuate ligament with this approach allows for the esophageal hiatus to remain intact

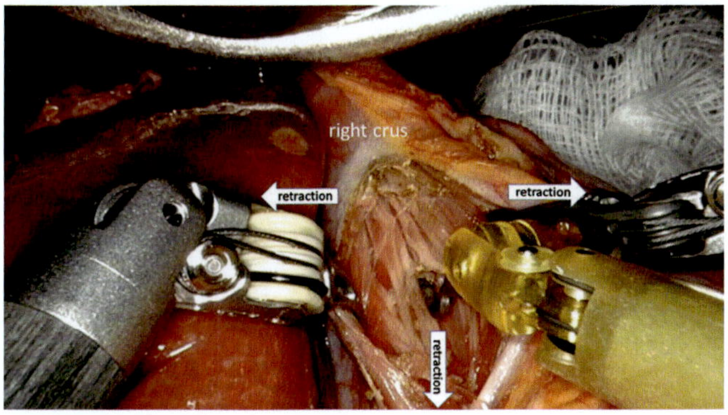

Fig. 1.18 Further division of the right crus should target the supraceliac aorta prior to dissecting the median arcuate ligament. The crural incision is extended roughly 4–6 cm longitudinally. The three most common robotic instruments for this operation include the Maryland tip bipolar, hook cautery, and ProGrasp forceps. Retraction of the crus should proceed using traction and countertraction, with the bedside assistant providing caudal retraction of the celiac artery (white arrows)

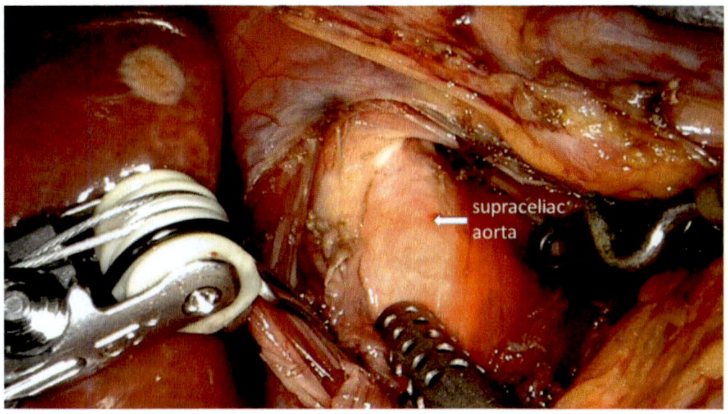

Fig. 1.19 Exposure of the supraceliac aorta after complete division of the right crus

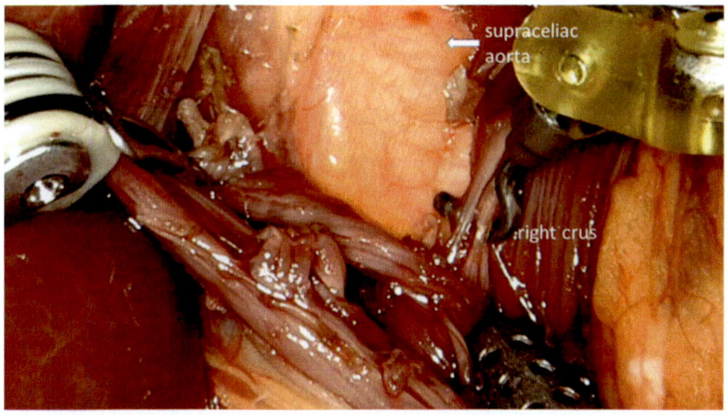

Fig. 1.20 Additional right crural fibers are dissected until the base of the celiac artery is encountered

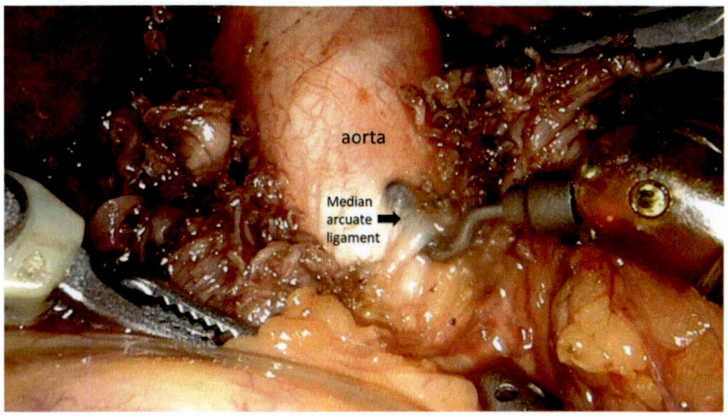

Fig. 1.21 After complete division of the right crus, the fibrous bands of the median arcuate ligament become apparent. These fibers are white and eventually will contain the celiac ganglion more distally along the celiac artery. Dissection proceeds distally to the takeoffs of the left gastric artery, splenic artery, and common hepatic artery

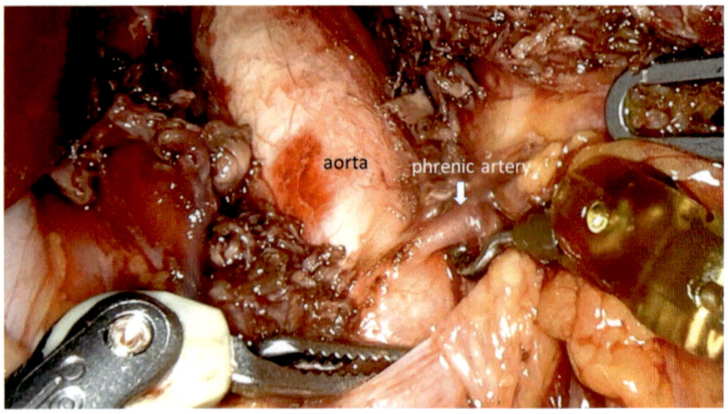

Fig. 1.22 Often, the first branches of the celiac trunk are phrenic arteries, which can be paired or single. These may be divided if this would aid in full dissection of the celiac artery

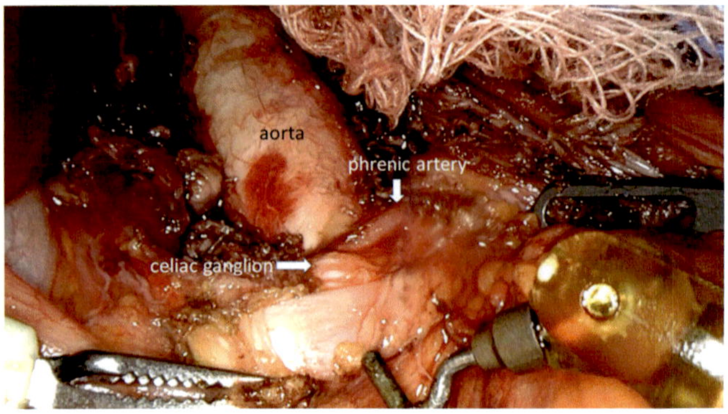

Fig. 1.23 While the phrenic arteries will often take off from the lateral aspect of the celiac artery, the white-appearing celiac ganglia cross over the celiac artery and make up a portion of the median arcuate ligament complex. These fibers must be completely divided or resected to expose the celiac artery and to ensure a complete neurolysis

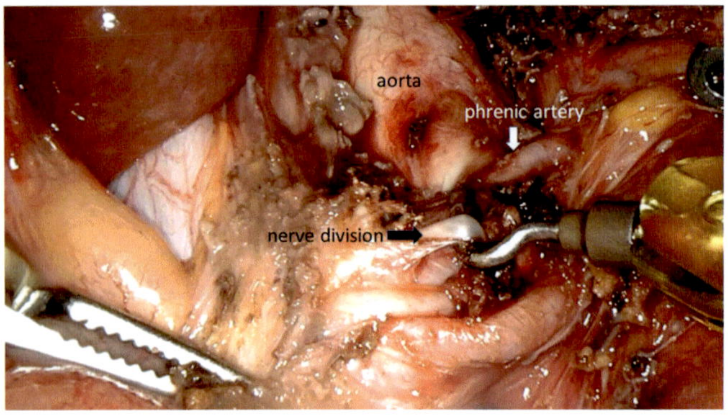

Fig. 1.24 Using the electrocautery hook in an oblique fashion, each individual nerve fiber of the celiac ganglion can be dissected free from the underlying artery and divided safely. Care must be taken to avoid an arterial injury with the heel of the hook. This can be kept in view prior to applying energy by orienting the hook as depicted here

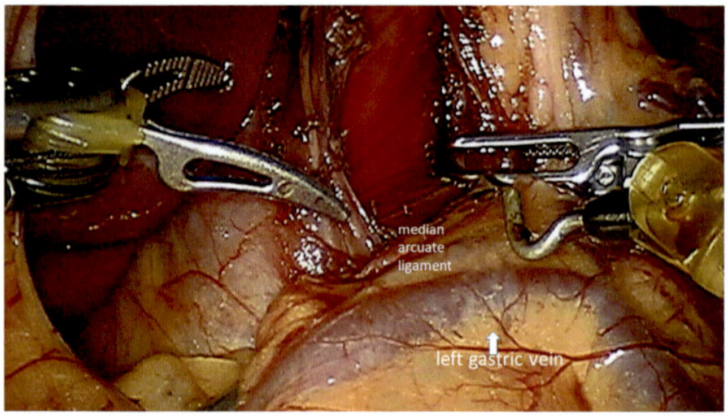

Fig. 1.25 Left gastric vein crossing the median arcuate ligament

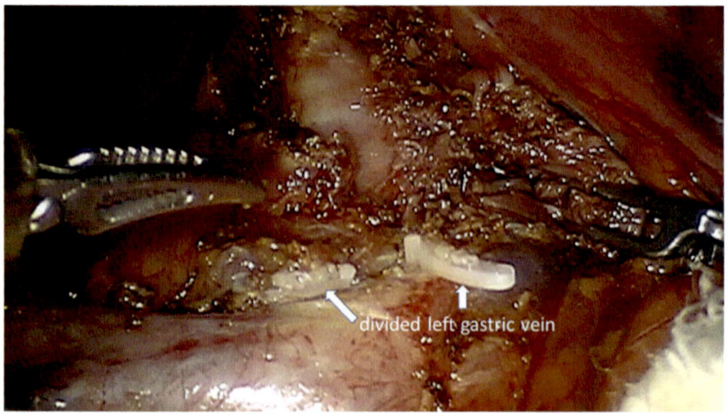

Fig. 1.26 Divided left gastric vein

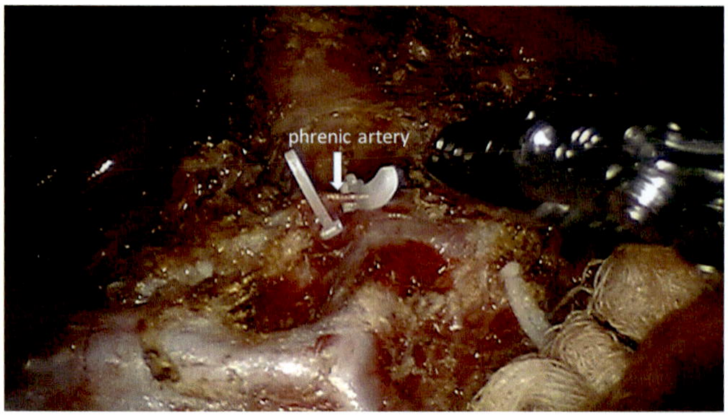

Fig. 1.27 Ligated phrenic artery

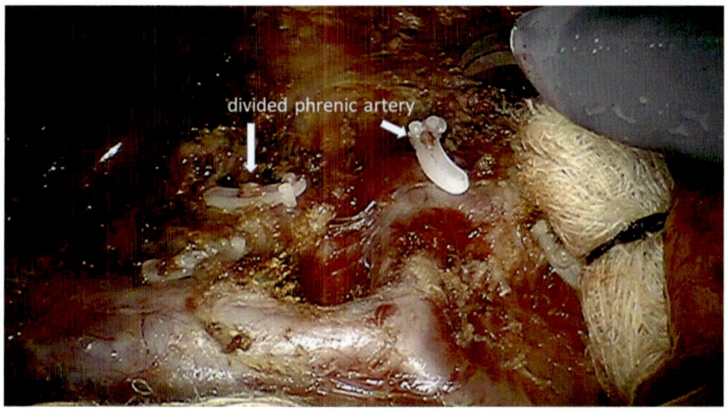

Fig. 1.28 Divided phrenic artery

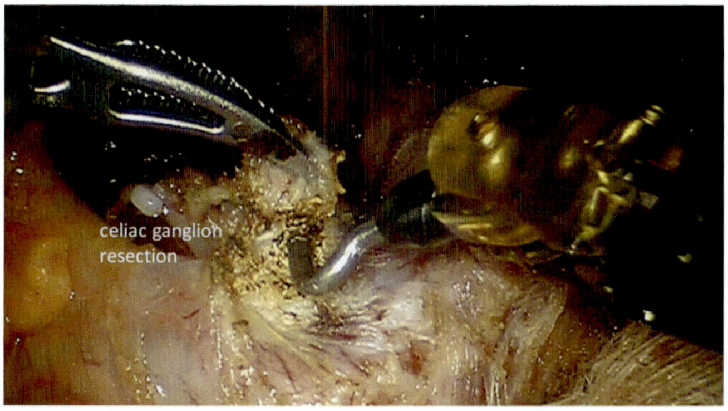

Fig. 1.29 Partial celiac ganglion resection

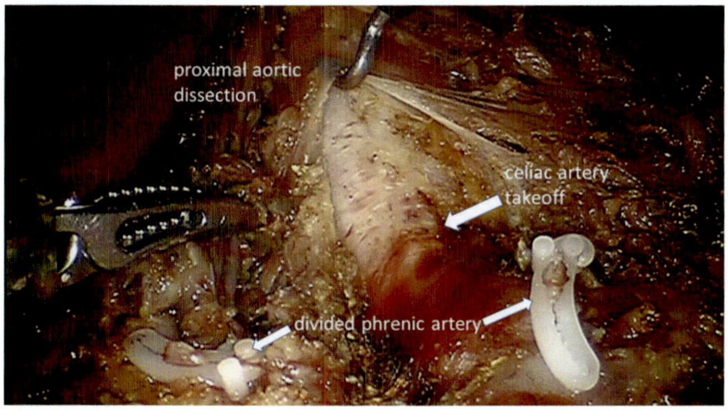

Fig. 1.30 Proximal aortic dissection, celiac takeoff, and divided phrenic artery

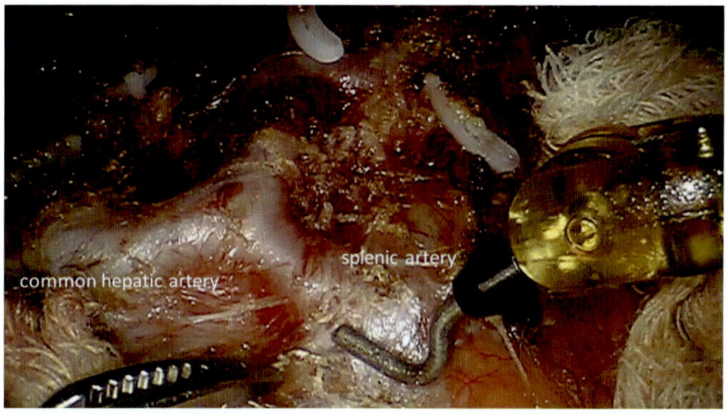

Fig. 1.31 Distal dissection exposing 180° of splenic artery, common hepatic artery

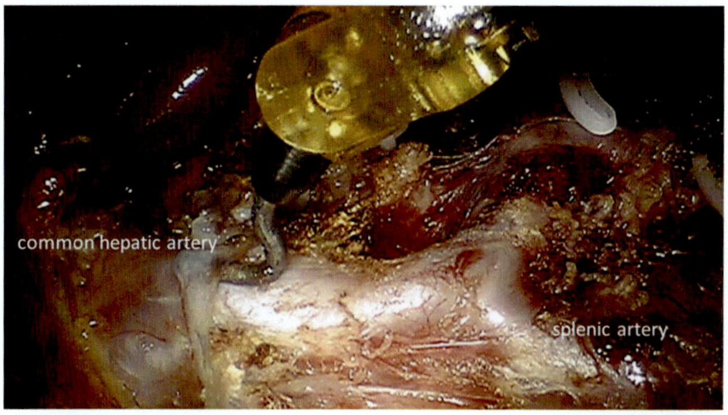

Fig. 1.32 Continued distal dissection of the common hepatic artery

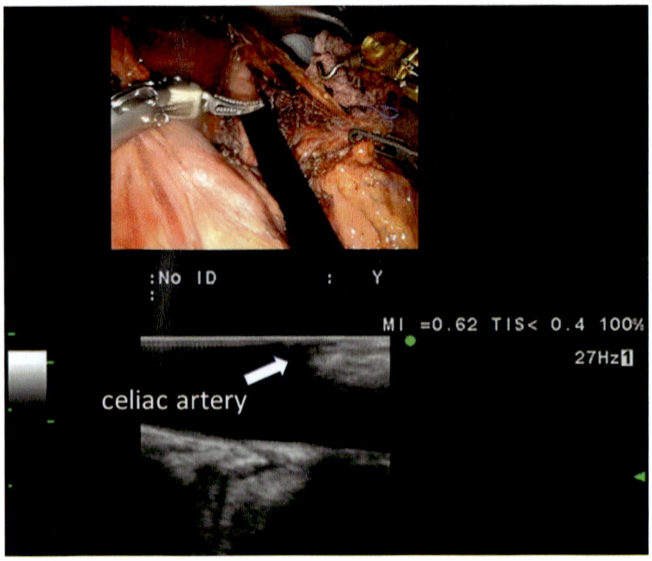

Fig. 1.33 Post-release ultrasound confirms no additional median arcuate ligament tissue above the celiac artery

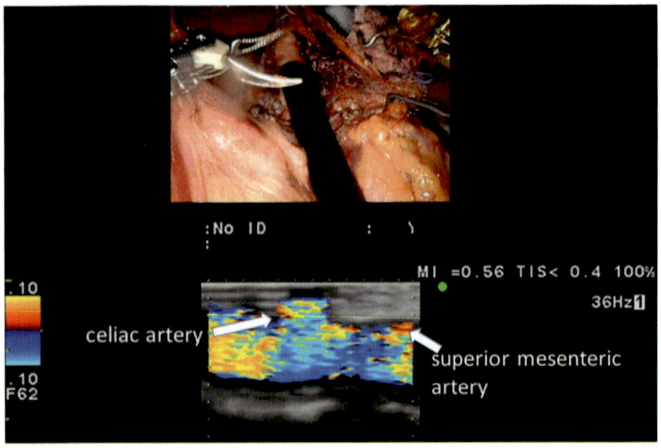

Fig. 1.34 Post-release ultrasound with color Doppler highlights excellent celiac artery and superior mesenteric artery flow

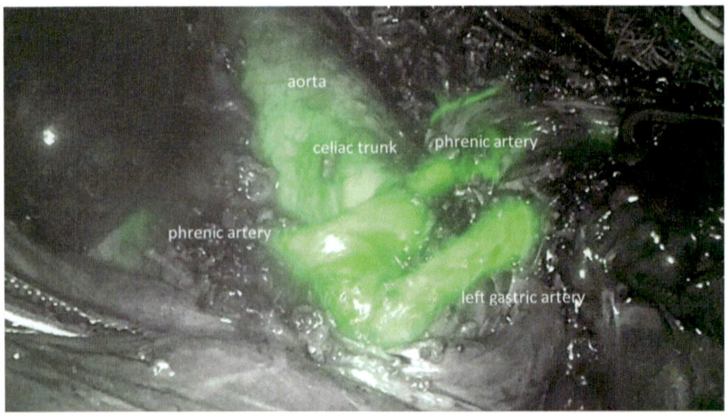

Fig. 1.35 Indocyanine green with FireFly™ (Intuitive Surgical, Sunnyvale, CA) fluorescence angiography to confirm complete release

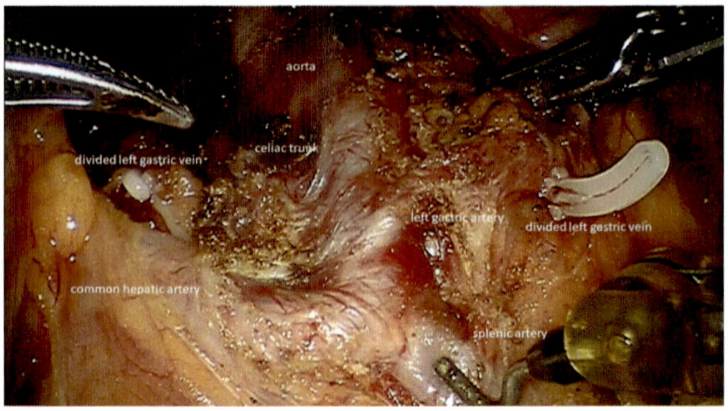

Fig. 1.36 Completed median arcuate ligament release with celiac ganglionectomy highlighting aorta, celiac trunk, left gastric artery, splenic artery, common hepatic artery, and divided left gastric vein

1.34, 1.35, and 1.36 illustrate the technical aspects of robotic median arcuate ligament release with celiac ganglionectomy.

References

1. Roayaie S, Jossart G, Gitlitz D, Lamparello P, Hollier L, Gagner M. Laparoscopic release of celiac artery compression syndrome facilitated by laparoscopic ultrasound scanning to confirm restoration of flow. J Vasc Surg. 2000;32:814–7.
2. El-Hayek KM, Titus J, Bui A, Mastracci T, Kroh M. Laparoscopic median arcuate ligament release: are we improving symptoms? J Am Coll Surg. 2013;2:272–9.
3. Fernstrum C, Pryor M, Wright GP, Wolf AM. Robotic surgery for median arcuate ligament syndrome. JSLS. 2020;24(2):e2020.0014.

Robotic Esophageal Diverticulectomy

2

William C. Sherrill III and Michael M. Awad

Introduction

Esophageal diverticula present in a variety of ways from asymptomatic to debilitating symptoms such as dysphagia, regurgitation, and aspiration events. Proper workup is targeted at evaluating not only the anatomy of the diverticula but also its underlying cause. Epiphrenic and Zenker's diverticula (pulsion type) are usually due to inherent dysmotility diseases or anatomical obstruction of the lower and upper esophageal sphincters, respectively. Midbody diverticula (traction type) tend to be due to factors external to the esophagus such as mediastinal or pleural inflammatory or neoplastic processes [1]. Toward this end, our diagnostic workup includes upper endoscopy, contrast esophagram, and high-resolution esophageal manometry. While small, symptomatic diverticula may be treated with esophageal myotomy alone, larger ones are generally treated with surgical resection of the diverticulum, especially if food or fluid trapping occurs [2].

We have found the robotic approach to esophageal diverticulectomy to be advantageous due to the greater reach and added dexterity afforded by the robotic instrumentation, particularly when working in the mediastinum. In this chapter, we describe our technical approach to robotic esophageal diverticulectomy. Shown is a patient that has both a midbody esophageal diverticulum and two epiphrenic diverticula, presumably due to a prior 360° fundoplication resulting in esophagogastric junction outflow obstruction (EGJOO). Lysis of adhesions is first performed, followed by mediastinal dissection and exposure. The diverticula are isolated at their base from the surrounding normal esophageal tissue and, under endoscopic visualization, are transected using a surgical stapler. A contralateral esophagogastric myotomy is performed, followed by a partial fundoplication to minimize GERD [3].

Our post-operative protocol involves an aqueous followed by barium esophagram on post-operative day 1. The patient is then placed on a pureed diet for 2 weeks followed by a mechanical soft diet for an additional 2 weeks before regular diet is resumed (Figs. 2.1, 2.2, 2.3, 2.4, 2.5, 2.6, 2.7, 2.8, 2.9, 2.10, 2.11, 2.12, 2.13, 2.14, 2.15, 2.16, 2.17, 2.18, 2.19, 2.20, 2.21, 2.22, 2.23, and 2.24).

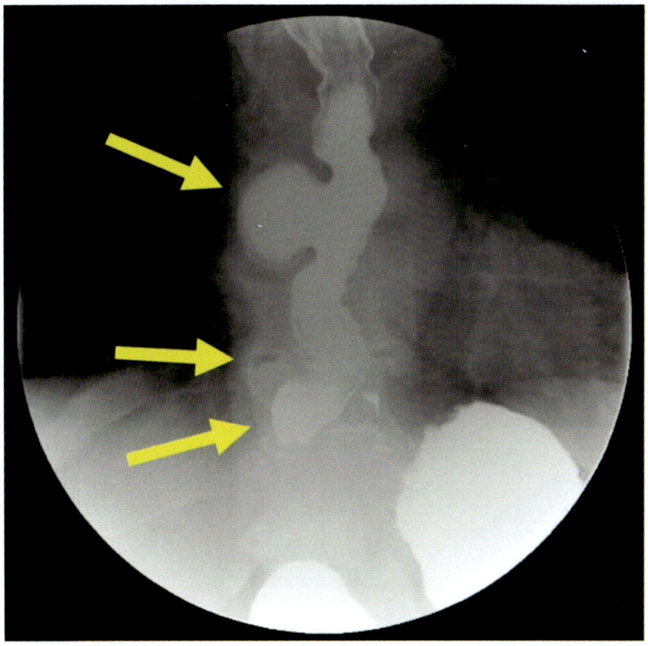

Fig. 2.1 Preoperative barium esophagram showing the presence of two epiphrenic diverticula just above the diaphragm and the mid-body diverticulum

W. C. Sherrill III · M. M. Awad (✉)
Section of Minimally Invasive Surgery, Washington University School of Medicine, St Louis, MO, USA
e-mail: awadm@wustl.edu

O. Y. Kudsi, P. P. Grimminger (eds.), *Atlas of Robotic Upper Gastrointestinal Surgery*,
https://doi.org/10.1007/978-3-030-86578-8_2

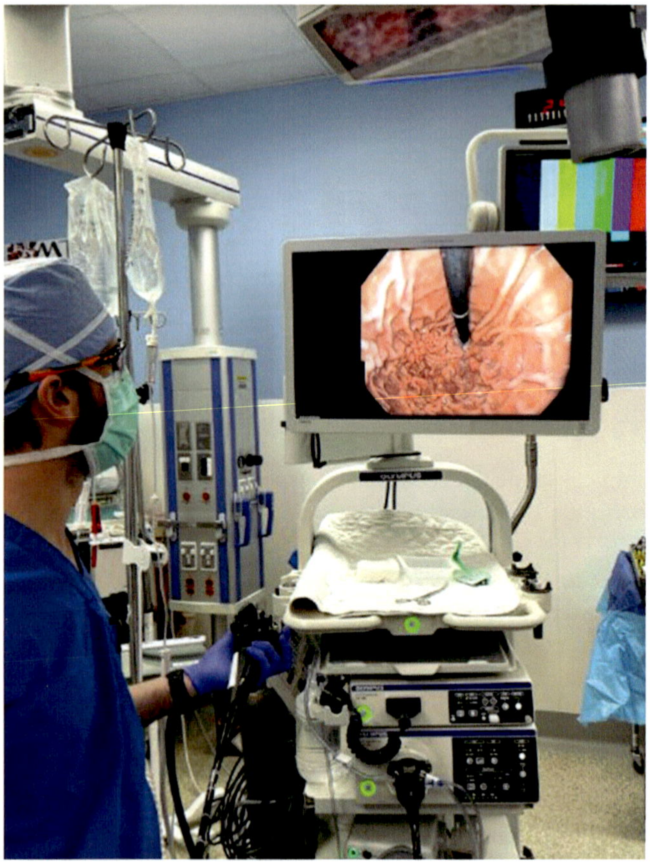

Fig. 2.2 Upper endoscopy is performed to evaluate the diverticula to confirm they do not contain retained food matter, evaluate for the presence of esophagitis or candidiasis, and document the preoperative Hill grade of the gastroesophageal junction

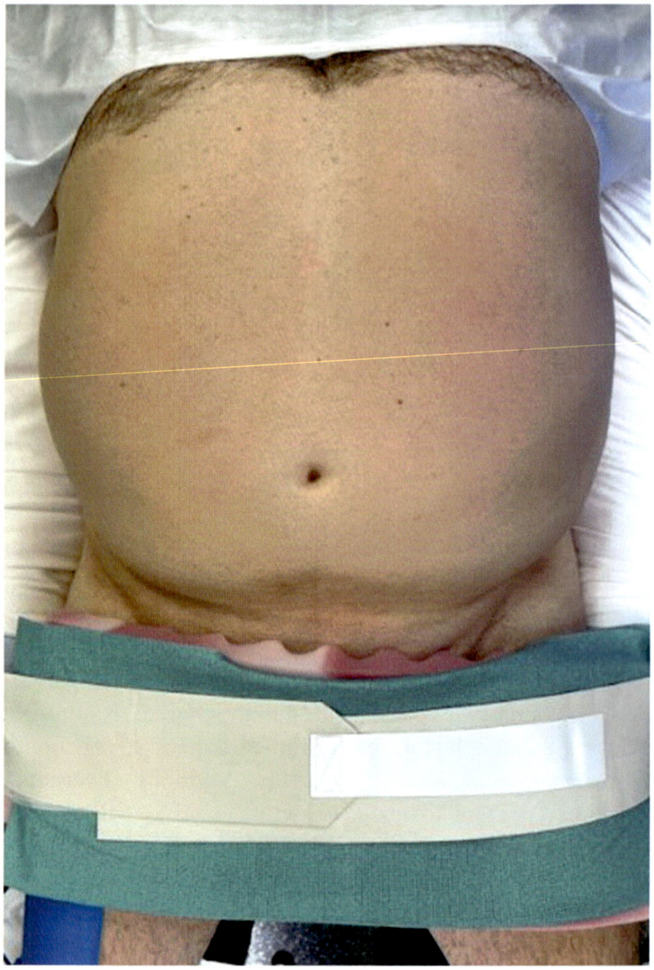

Fig. 2.3 The patient is placed on the operating room table with both arms tucked and heavily padded. Legs are split to allow the bedside assistant to assist from between the patient legs

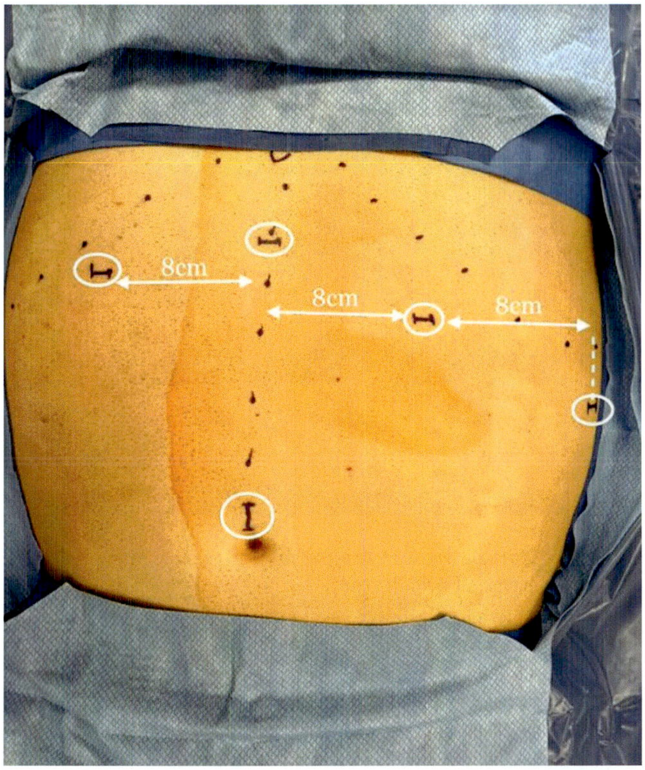

Fig. 2.4 The patient is then prepped and draped. Port placement is shown, with a minimum of 8 cm between every port. A non-robotic assistant port is placed in the supra- or infra-umbilical region depending on patient's body habitus

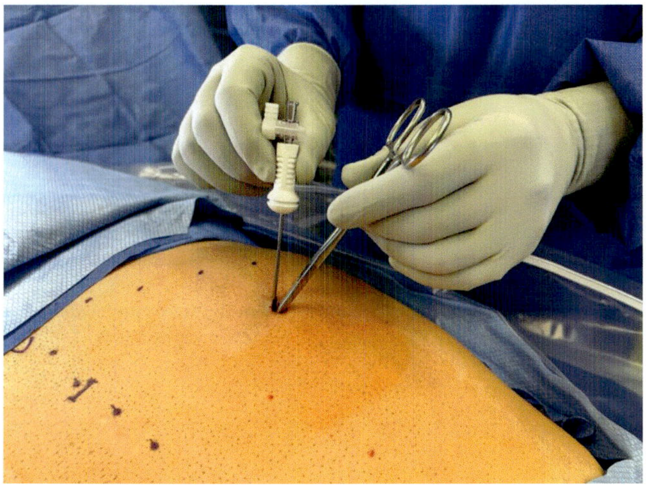

Fig. 2.5 An 8 mm incision is made in the left upper quadrant. The anterior fascia is grasped and elevated during Veress needle insertion

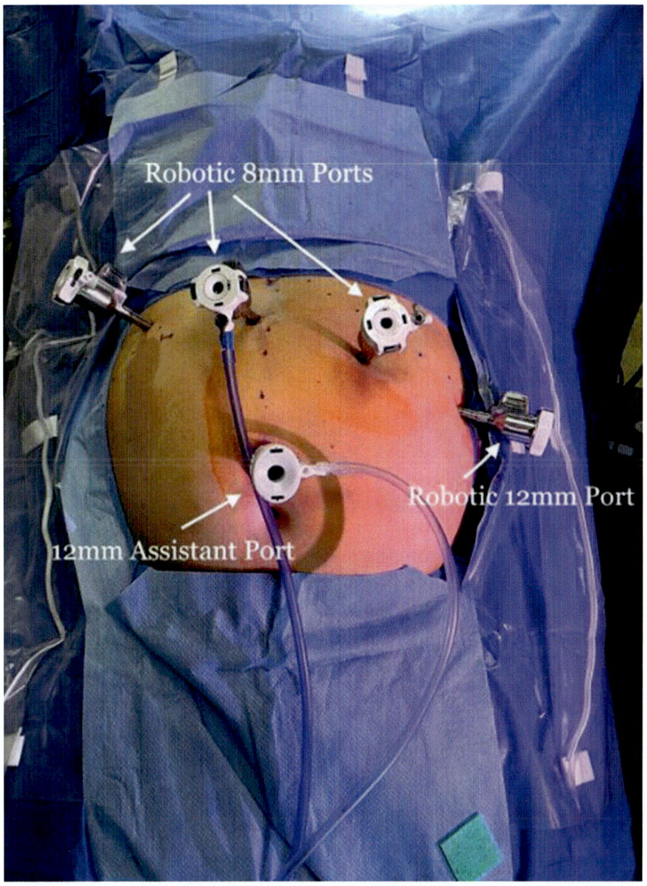

Fig. 2.6 Once the abdomen is insufflated, an 8.5 mm robotic trocar is placed. The robotic camera is then inserted, and the abdomen is inspected. The patient is then placed in 30° reverse Trendelenburg position, and the remaining trocars are placed under direct visualization. The robot is then docked

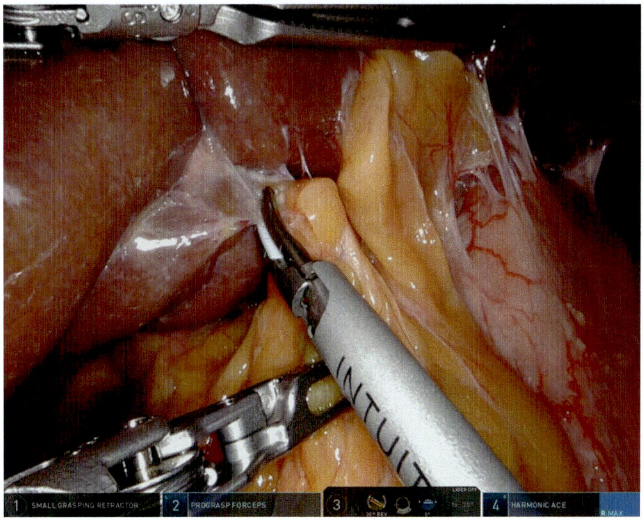

Fig. 2.7 Adhesions from the previous fundoplication procedure are noted. Adhesiolysis begins where the lesser curve of the stomach is adhered to the left lateral liver and to the hiatus

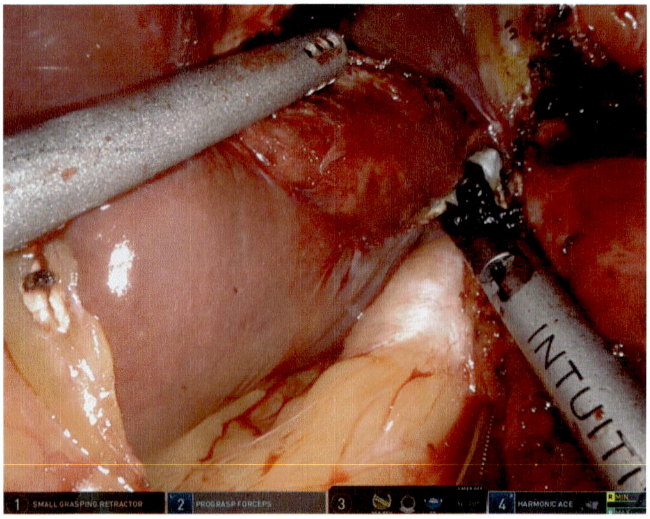

Fig. 2.8 The gastrohepatic ligament is divided up to the apex of the right crus. If an accessory or replaced left hepatic artery is present, an attempt is made to preserve it. As this was a re-operative procedure, the gastrohepatic ligament had previously been sufficiently divided

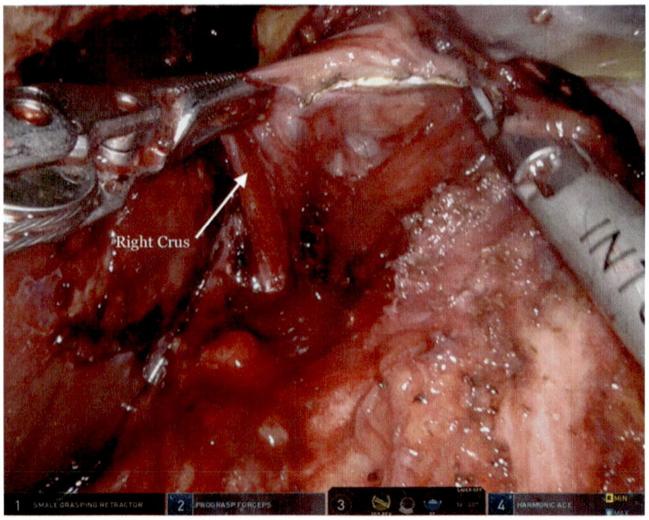

Fig. 2.9 In re-operative foregut cases, we begin the circumferential hiatal dissection toward the base of the right or left crus to minimize injury to the anterior esophagus and anterior vagus (In primary procedures, we begin the hiatal dissection at the 12 o'clock position)

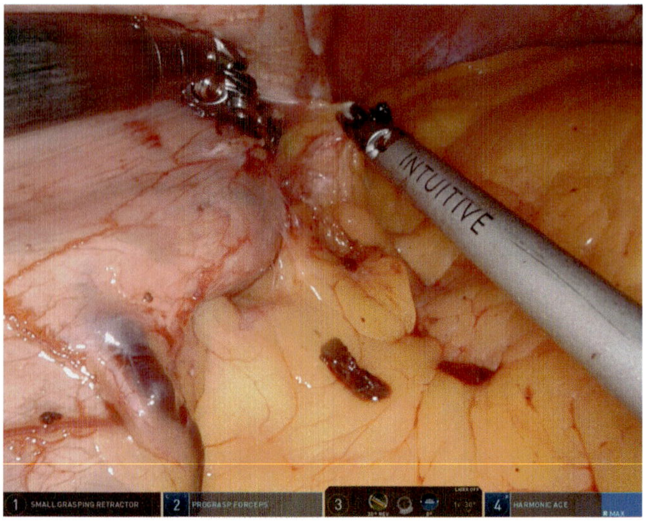

Fig. 2.10 Short gastric vessels are divided to facilitate remaining dissection at the base of the left crus

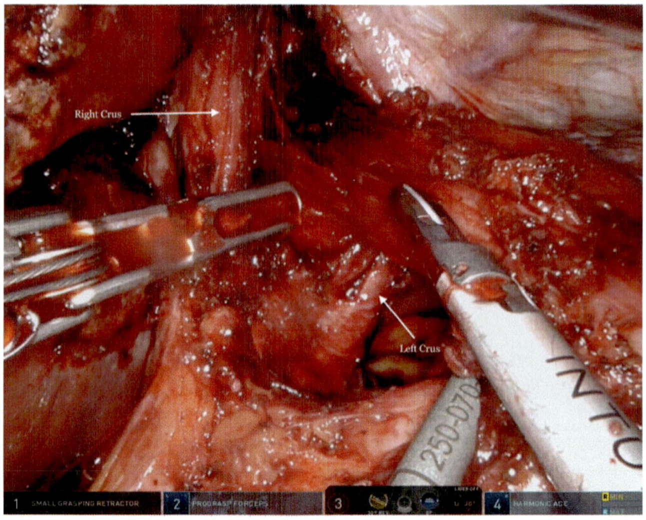

Fig. 2.11 The dissection continues through the retroesophageal window. Care is taken here to preserve the posterior vagus nerve

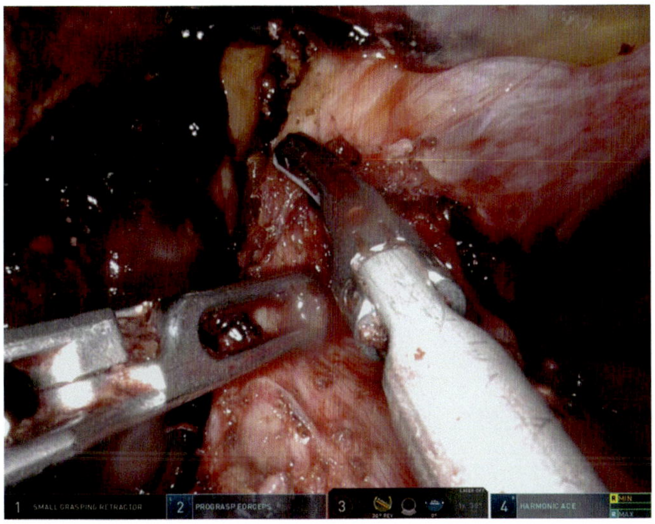

Fig. 2.12 Circumferential dissection of the esophagus is then completed at the 12 o'clock position once the anterior vagus nerve is safely identified

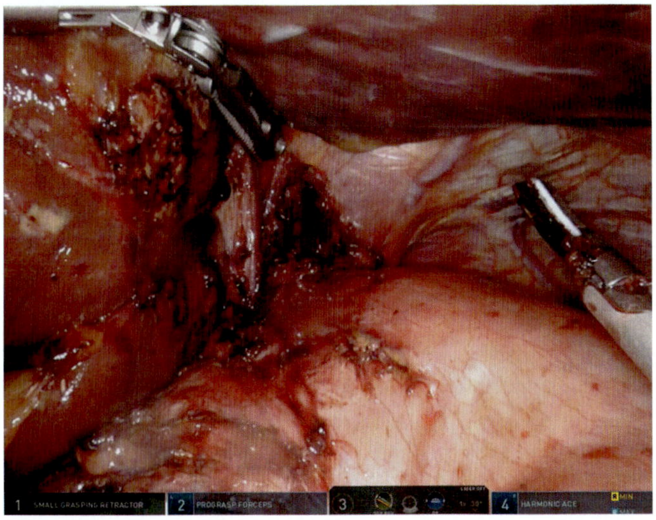

Fig. 2.13 Further dissection is performed to completely reverse unwrap the previous fundoplication. The fundus is returned to its normal anatomical position near the spleen. Repeat intra-operative endoscopy is then performed to ensure there is adequate intra-abdominal esophageal length, to confirm that the previous fundoplication is completely undone, and to perform a leak test to assess for esophageal or gastric mucosal full-thickness injuries. The robotic TilePro feature can be used to facilitate simultaneous visualization of the laparoscopic and endoscopic views

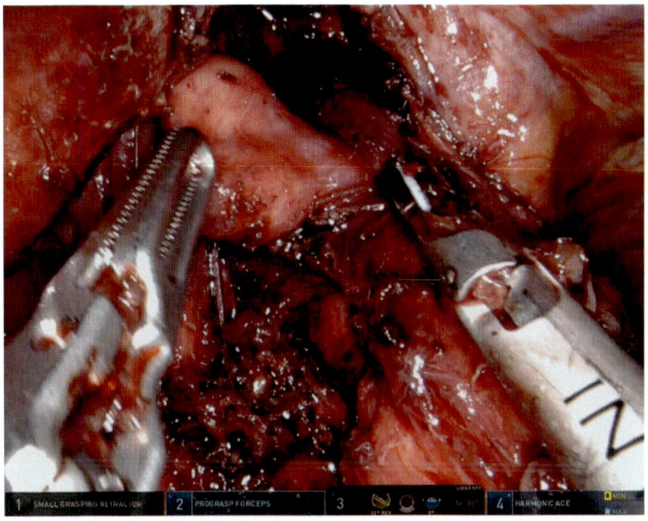

Fig. 2.14 The esophagus is then circumferentially mobilized in the mediastinum. The first epiphrenic diverticulum is encountered. The neck of the diverticulum is carefully dissected to isolate it from the normal surrounding esophageal tissue

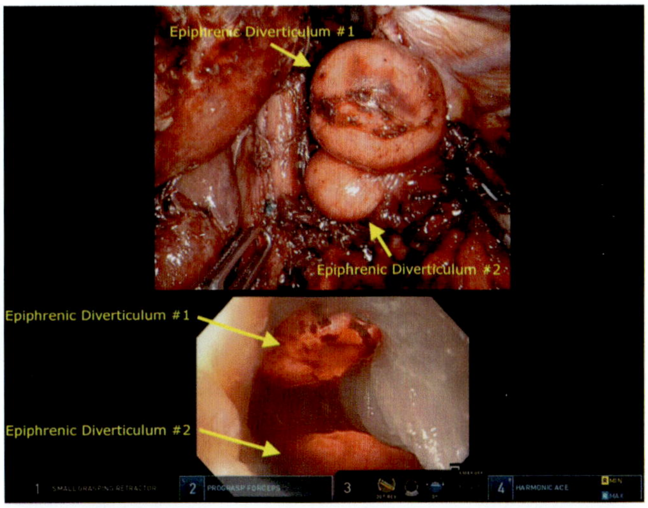

Fig. 2.15 A second nearby epiphrenic diverticulum is identified, separated by a thin strip of esophageal muscle. TilePro is again used to facilitate visualization

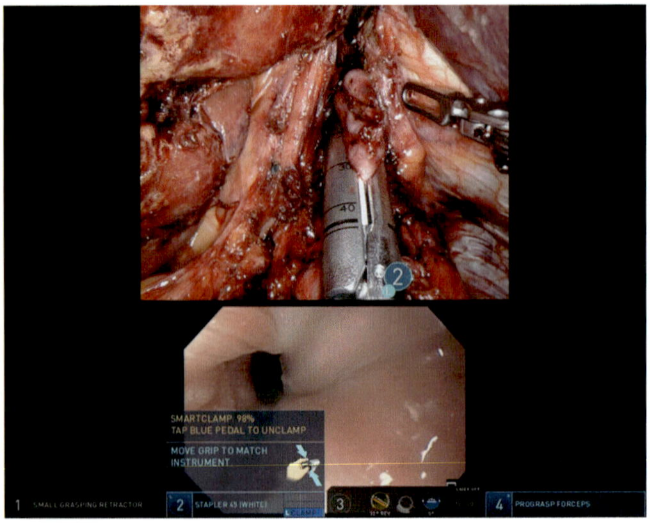

Fig. 2.16 A robotic stapler with vascular load is placed across the base of both diverticula and closed. Prior to firing the stapler, endoscopy is again used not only to confirm complete encapsulation of both diverticula but also to ensure the esophageal lumen is not narrowed

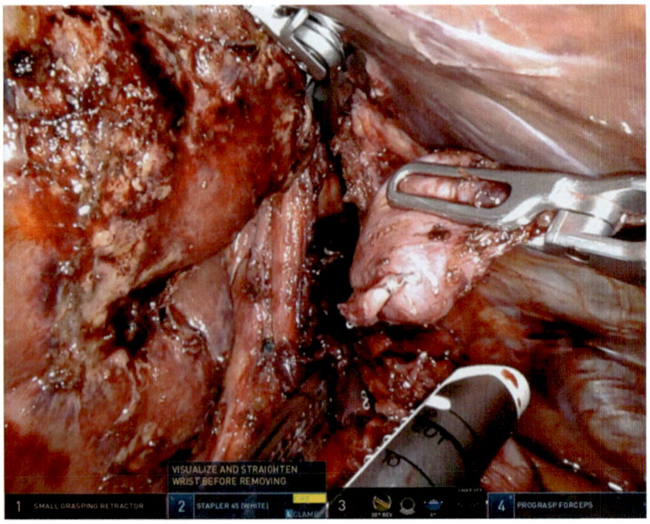

Fig. 2.17 The diverticula are then removed via the assistant port, and the staple line is carefully inspected for bleeding. Noted is the use of the third robotic arm to elevate the apex of the hiatus to facilitate mediastinal exposure

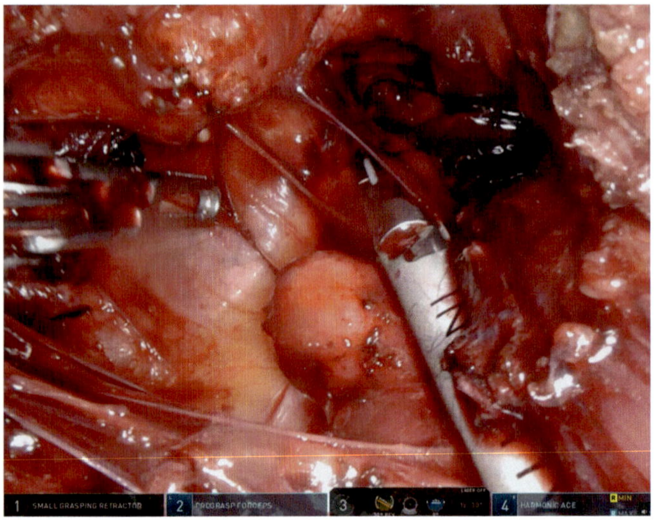

Fig. 2.18 Proximal mediastinal dissection of the esophagus is continued in order to isolate the mid-body diverticulum

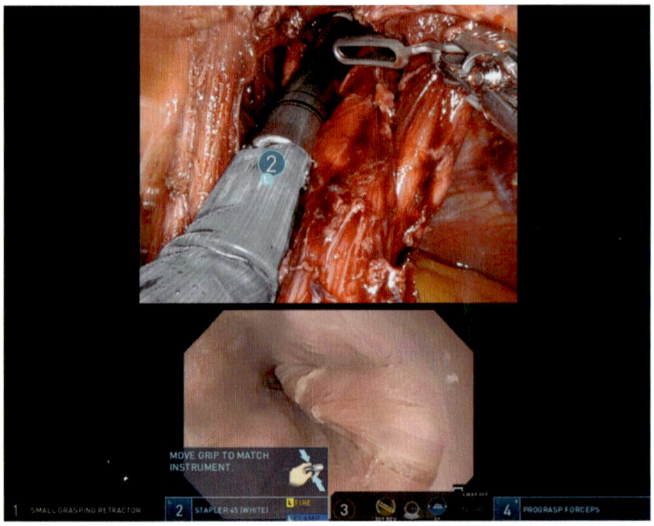

Fig. 2.19 The process is repeated, and the diverticulum is stapled under direct endoscopic visualization

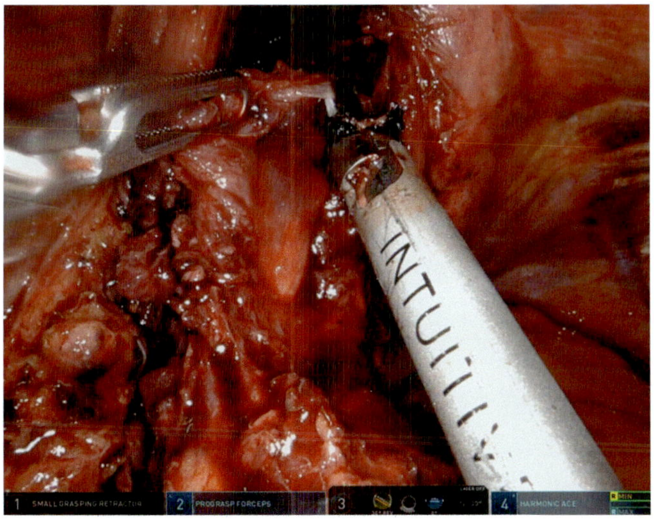

Fig. 2.20 Esophagogastric myotomy is then performed on the contralateral side of the esophagus from the diverticula. The myotomy is begun 2 cm above the GE junction and continued to a point above the proximal-most extent of the midbody diverticulum. The myotomy is then extended distally 3 cm onto the anterior stomach wall. Care is taken to perverse the anterior vagus by tunneling the myotomy beneath the nerve

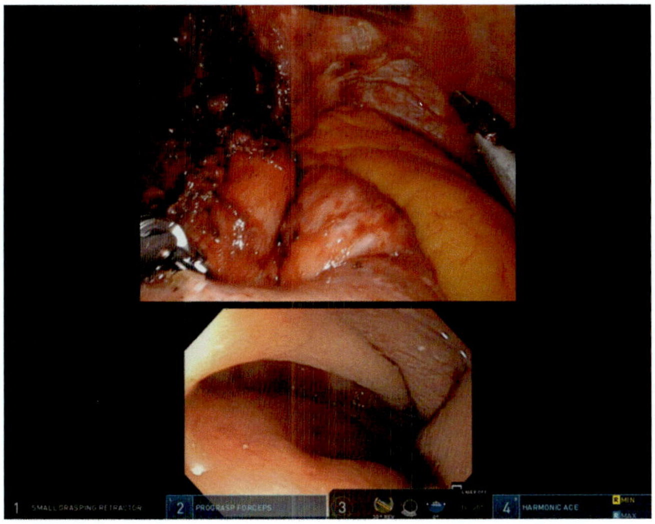

Fig. 2.21 The myotomy is carefully inspected to ensure there are no mucosal injuries and all muscle fibers are complete divided. Endoscopy is again performed to ensure adequate gastric length of myotomy and to perform leak test

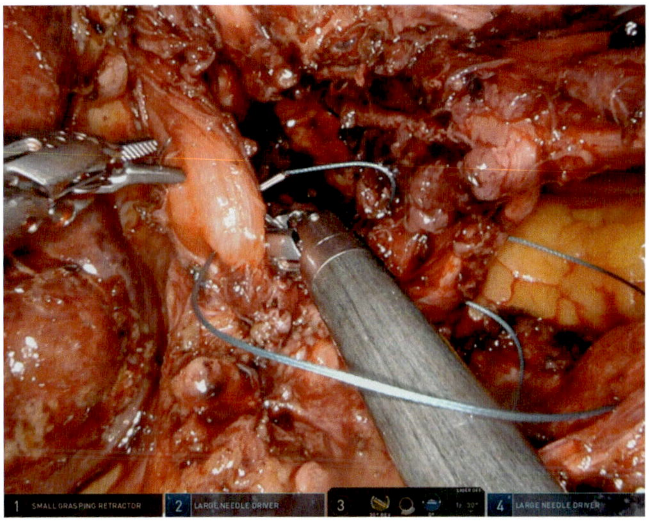

Fig. 2.22 The posterior crura are re-approximated with non-absorbable suture in a figure of eight fashion

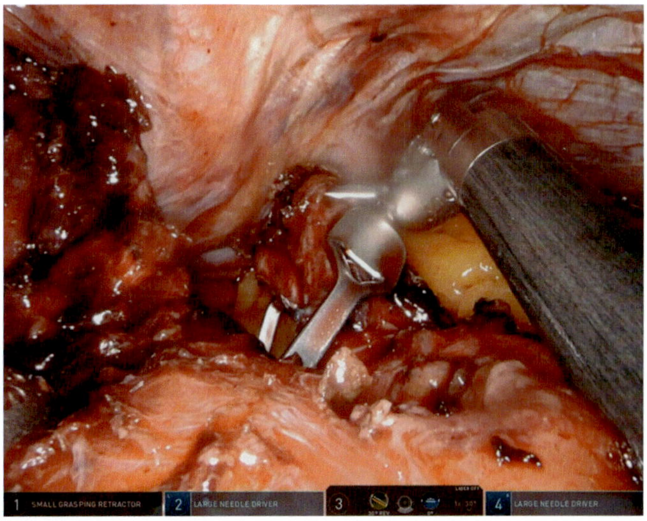

Fig. 2.23 The fundus is grasped and brought through the retroesophageal window to create a partial posterior 270° fundoplication

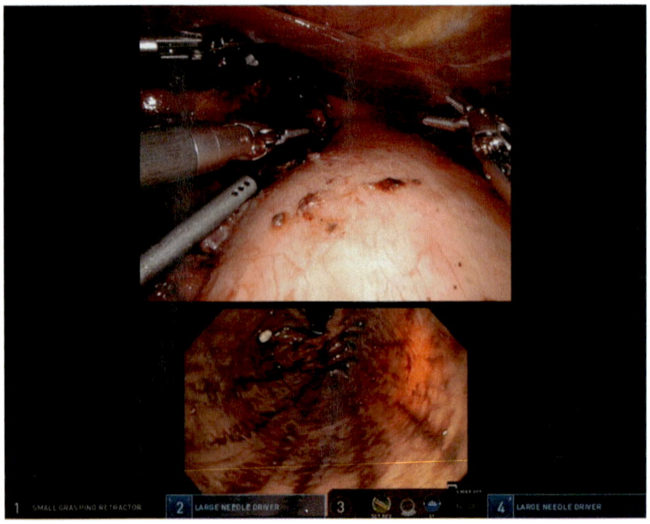

Fig. 2.24 Once the fundoplication is completed, intraoperative endoscopy is once again performed to document the presence of a Hill grade I valve

References

1. Kao AM, Arnold MR, Schlosser KA, et al. Epiphrenic diverticulum: 20-year single institution experience. Am Surg. 2018;84(7):1158–63.
2. Soares R, Herbella FA, Prachand VN. Epiphrenic diverticulum of the esophagus. From pathophysiology to treatment. J Gastrointest Surg. 2010;14(12):2009–15.
3. Achim V, Aye RW, Farivar AS. A combined thoracoscopic and laparoscopic approach for high epiphrenic diverticula and the importance of complete myotomy. Surg Endosc. 2017;31:788–94.

Robotic Esophagus Leiomyomectomy

3

Benedikt Reichert and Jan-Hendrik Egberts

Introduction

Intramural, submucosally localized tumors of the esophagus are usually benign, so that enucleation is an adequate therapy. However, these tumors are a special challenge for the surgeon. If the tumor is larger as expected, the mucosa tube is injured, or the esophagus cannot be mobilized sufficiently, esophageal resection is still necessary. The anastomosis performed during esophageal resection increases the risk of insufficiency with frequently serious consequences. Dysphagia and regurgitation are long-term problems after esophageal resection [1].

Esophageal resections like esophagectomy or enucleation are safely performed robotically in larger centers. Compared to the laparoscopic technique, the robotic approach offers angled instruments with 6 degrees of freedom, tremor correction, and an excellent 3D camera, which allow a finest dissection in a technically highly demanding procedure [2].

Esophageal resections are performed from the right thoracic side in single-lung ventilation. The patient is placed in left sided, modified prone position to allow a thoracotomy in case of an emergency conversion. The lung is ventilated via a double lumen tube. Four ports are inserted intercostal, as described previously [3]. In contrast to the described technique, Port 4 is placed more ventrally in the axilla.

Procedure: Illustrated Steps

Figures 3.1, 3.2, 3.3, 3.4, 3.5, 3.6, 3.7, 3.8, 3.9, 3.10, 3.11, 3.12, 3.13, 3.14, 3.15, 3.16, 3.17, 3.18, 3.19, 3.20, 3.21, 3.22, 3.23, 3.24, 3.25, 3.26, and 3.27 illustrate the technical aspects of robotic enucleation of an intramural esophageal tumor.

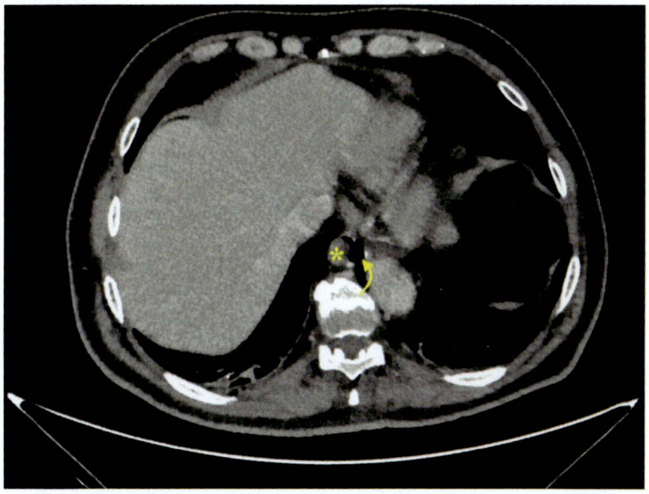

Fig. 3.1 CT scan: The tumor (*) is localized in the distal esophagus, anterior to the esophageal-gastric junction. The lumen is significantly obstructed (→)

B. Reichert
Department of General, Abdominal, Thoracic, Transplantation and Pediatric Surgery, University Hospital Schleswig-Holstein, Kiel, Germany

J.-H. Egberts (✉)
Department for Surgery, Israelitisches Krankenhaus Hamburg, Hamburg, Germany
e-mail: J.Egberts@Ik-H.De

O. Y. Kudsi, P. P. Grimminger (eds.), *Atlas of Robotic Upper Gastrointestinal Surgery*,
https://doi.org/10.1007/978-3-030-86578-8_3

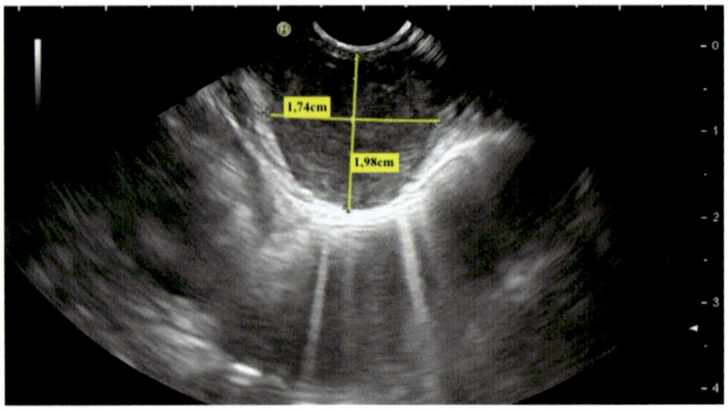

Fig. 3.2 Endoscopic ultrasound: The tumor is localized 39–41 cm from incisor teeth and has a spread of 1.98 cm × 1.78 cm in longitudinal view

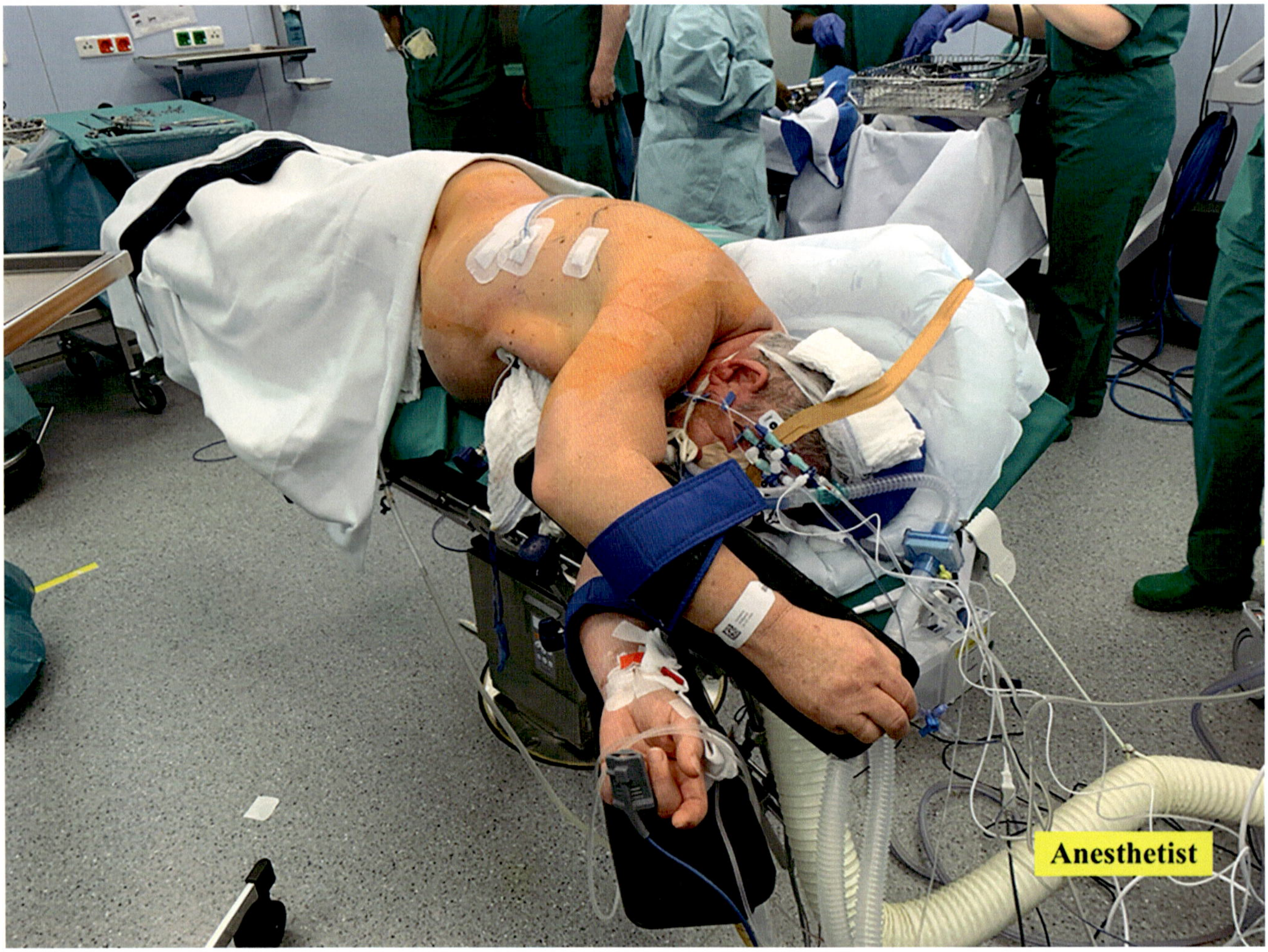

Fig. 3.3 The anesthetist is positioned at the head. It is important that all catheters are easily reachable, as repositioning is not possible during the operation

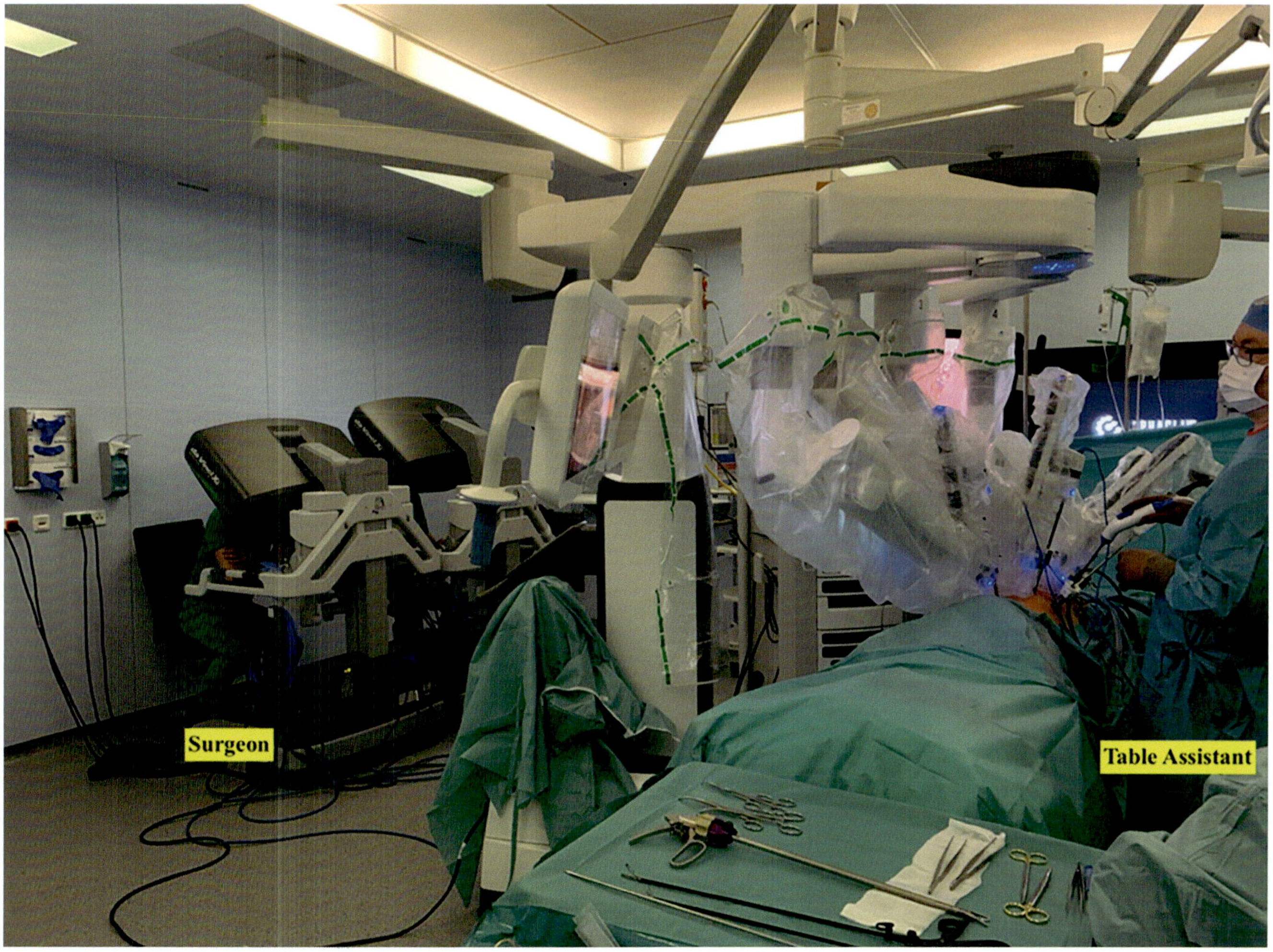

Fig. 3.4 The surgeon sits at the console, the table assistant stands ventral to the patient. The table assistant guides the docking of the robot, sucks and removes the specimen via the assistant's access. This access also serves as an emergency access in case of intrathoracic bleeding

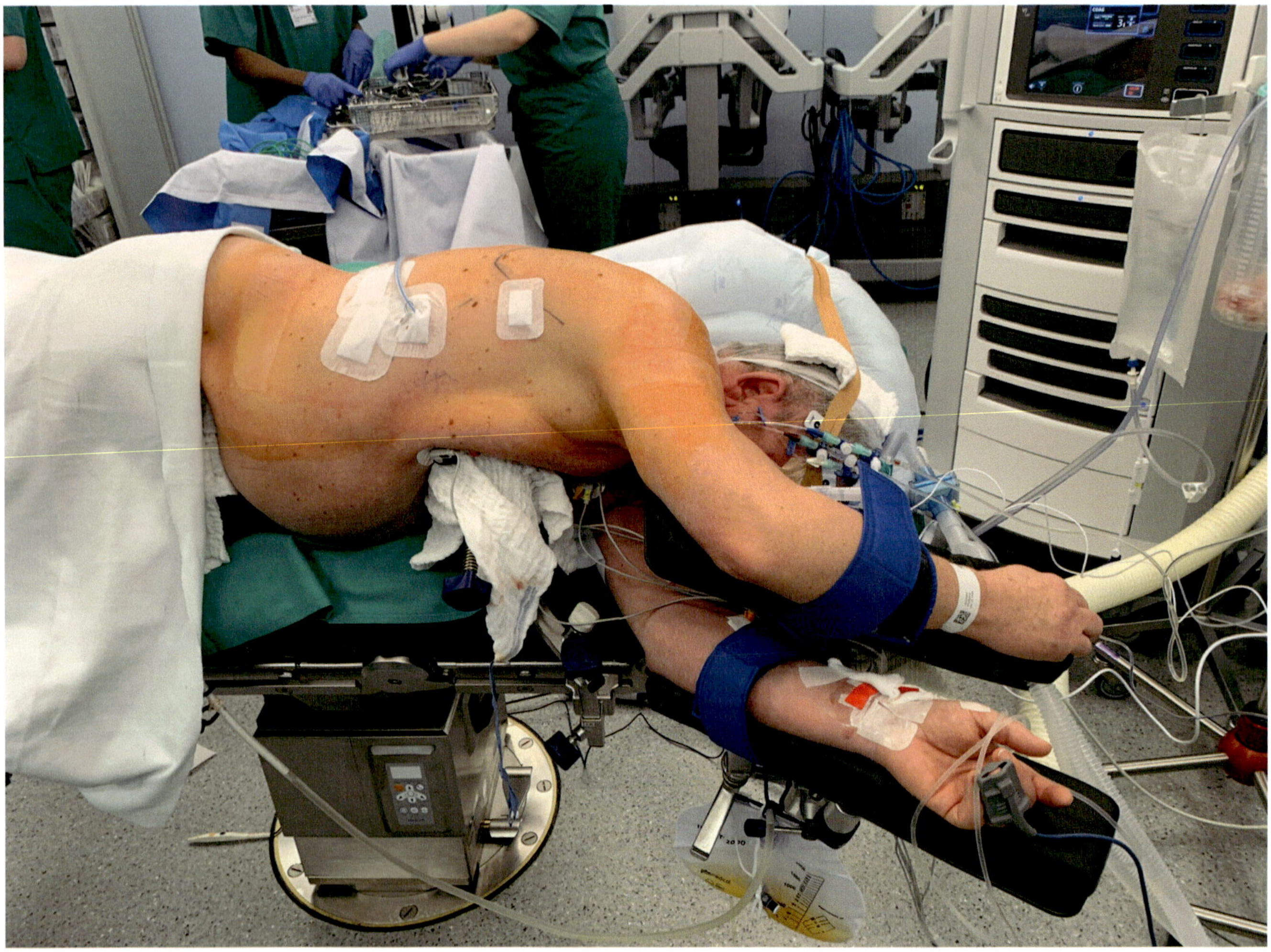

Fig. 3.5 The patient lies on the left side in a modified prone position (~45°-rotation). To prevent the robot arm 1 from colliding with the patient, the patient's right arm is brought to its maximum cranial position and only minimally extended outwards (This figure was taken at the end of the procedure)

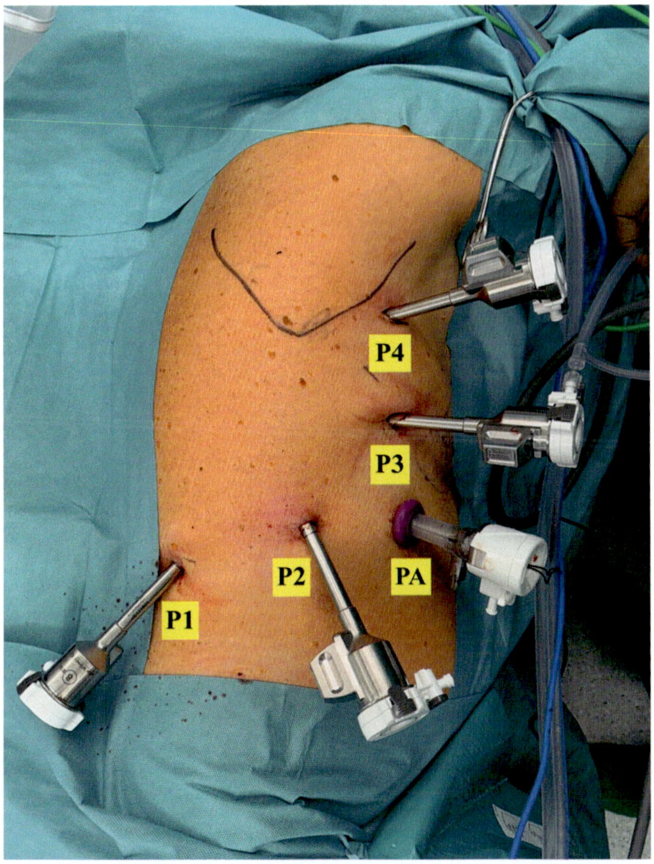

Fig. 3.6 The ports are placed as described below. The first port placed is P3 to insert the camera. The further placement of the ports is done under view. P1, laterally, in the 8th or 9th ICR; P2, posterior axillary line in the 8th ICR; P3, 6th ICR in the mid-axillary line (for camera); P4, ~2 cm away from the medial edge of the scapula in the 4th ICR; PA, the assistant port in the mid-axillary line in the 7th ICR

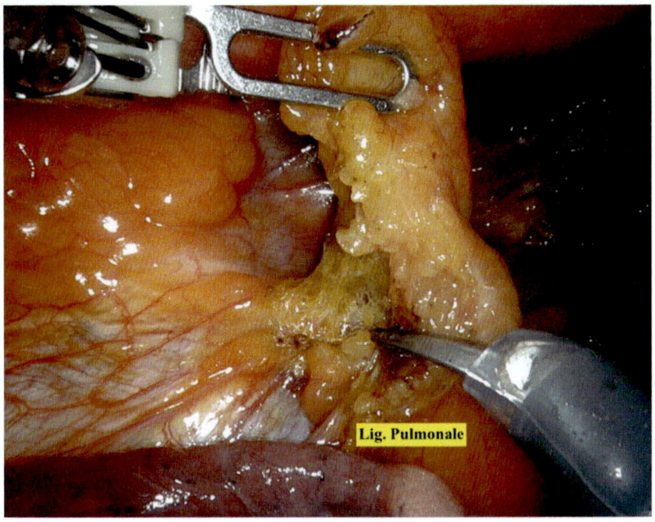

Fig. 3.7 Single-lung ventilation is started, and CO_2 insufflation of 8 mmHg intrathoracic is established. The pleura is inspected for irregularities. If there are none, an esophageal bougie is inserted by the anesthetist. Now the ligamentum pulmonale is mobilized, and lymphadenectomy of level 9 is performed

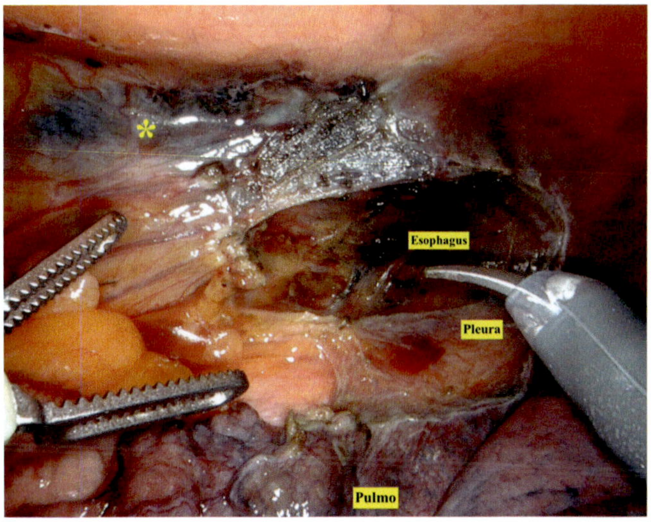

Fig. 3.8 After incision of the pleura parietalis, the preoperative ink marking of the tumor is visible (*). As described in the endosonography, the tumor has an extension of ~ 2 cm

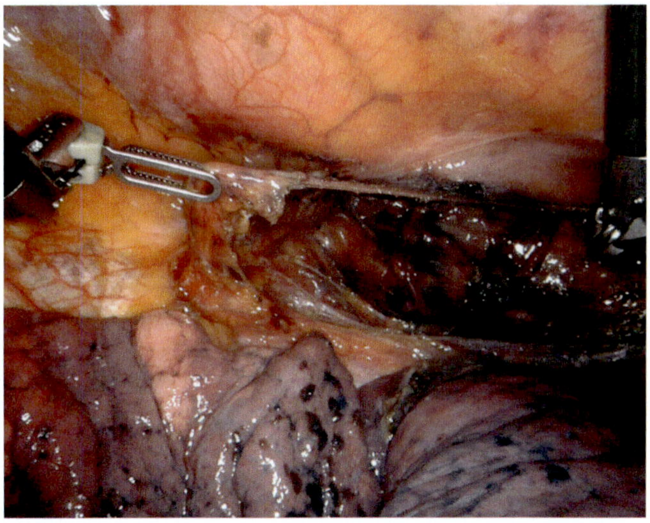

Fig. 3.9 The esophagus is mobilized, and the pleura is opened over the entire distance until the tumor can be exposed cranially and caudally

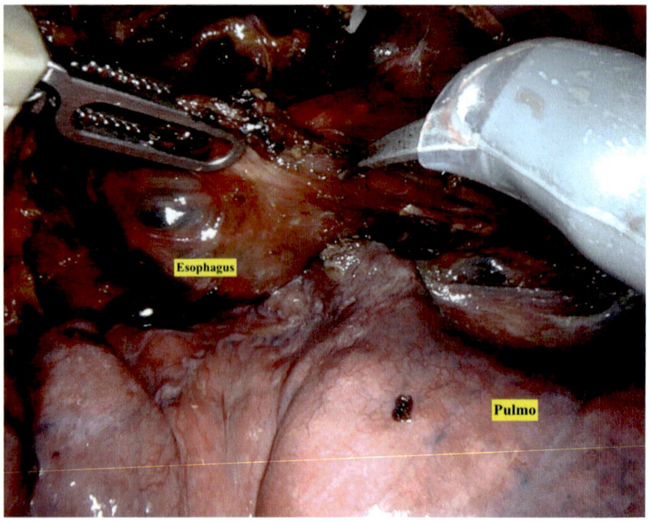

Fig. 3.10 Directly above the tumor, the adventitia is opened and carefully preparated onto the muscle layer

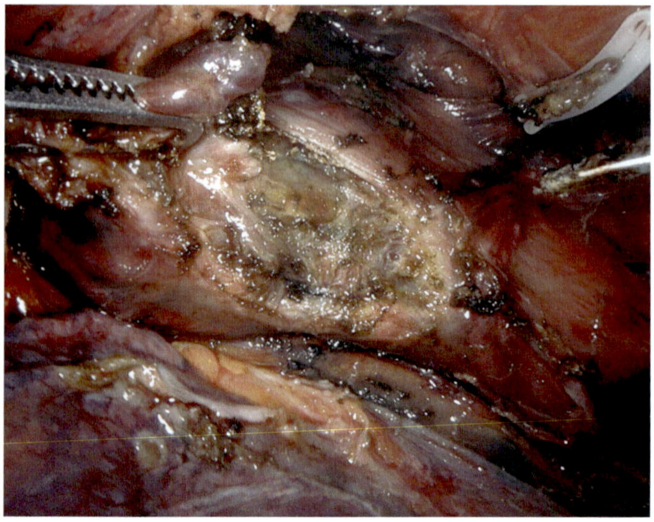

Fig. 3.12 The muscle layer is opened in a semilunar pattern so that the tumor is visible underneath

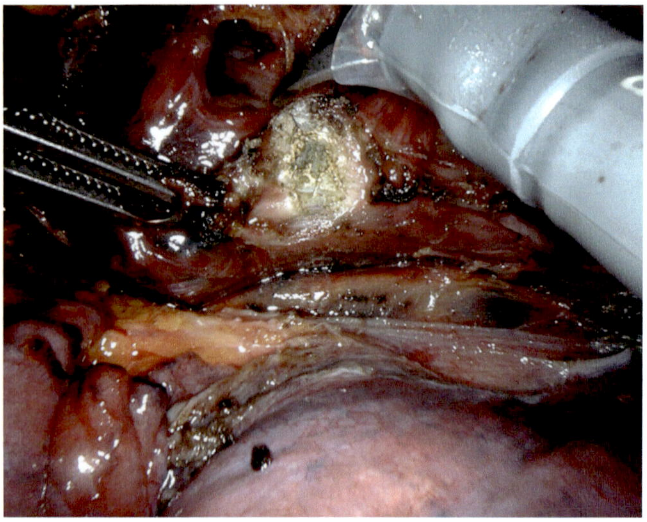

Fig. 3.11 The muscle layer is first carefully coagulated electrically and then opened in this area

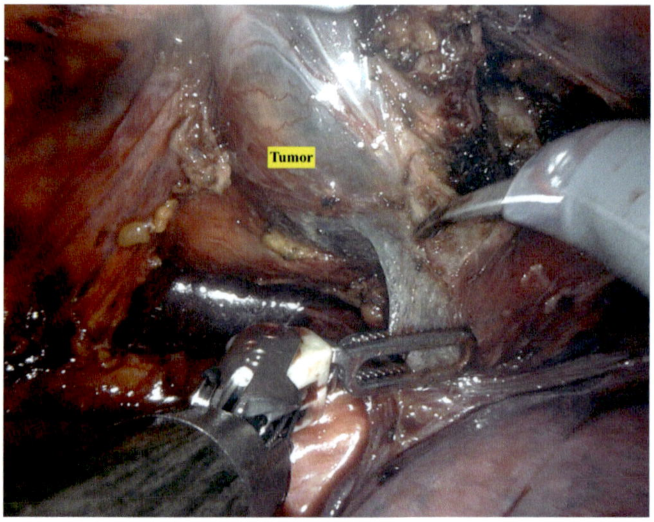

Fig. 3.13 Grasping the tumor: protrusion of the tumor, beginning of transection of the lateral layers with severing of the surrounding muscle fibers

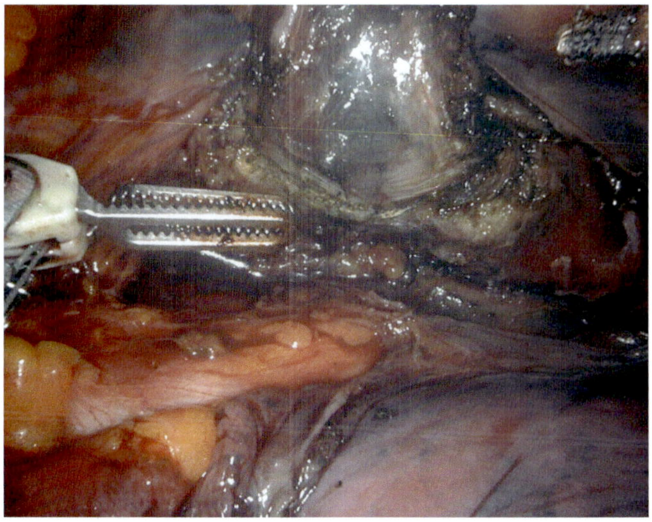

Fig. 3.14 The tumor can be carefully dissected and removed from the surrounding layers

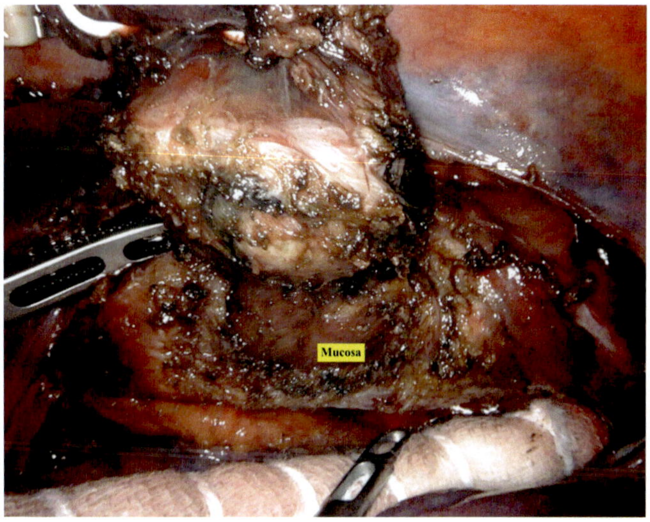

Fig. 3.16 When preparing in depth, care should be taken not to injure the mucosa

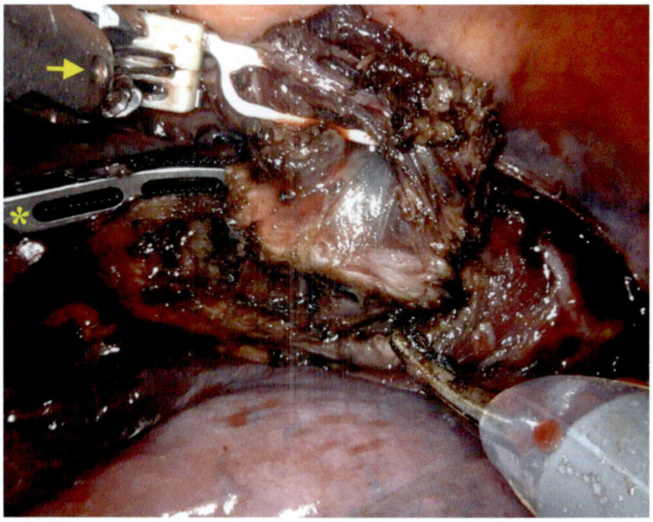

Fig. 3.15 The tumor is held with fenestrated bipolar forceps (→). A Tip-Up fenestrated grasper (*) tightens the surrounding layers, and with the use of the electric scissors, the coagulation and following separation of the layers is performed

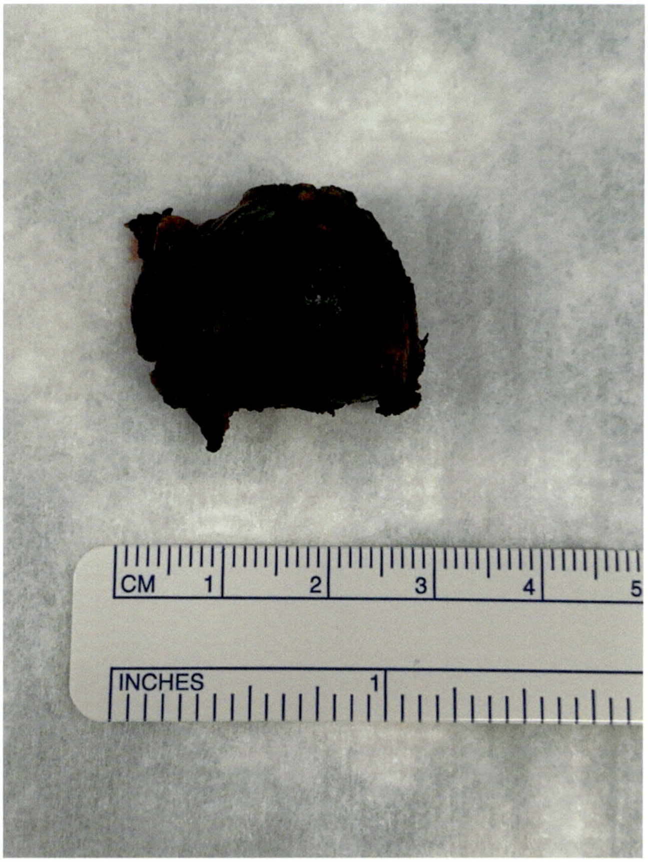

Fig. 3.17 The resected tumor is removed in a salvage bag by the table assistant via the assistant port. The tumor shows clear margins and is submitted for histological examination

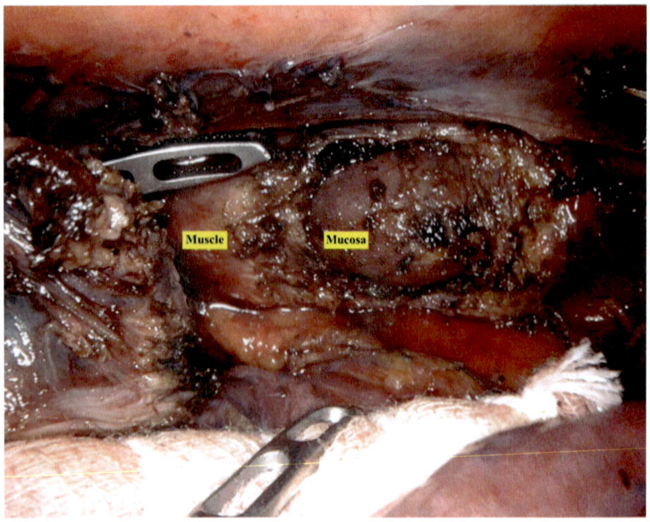

Fig. 3.18 After removal of the tumor, the mucosal tube is visible in depth and appears intact

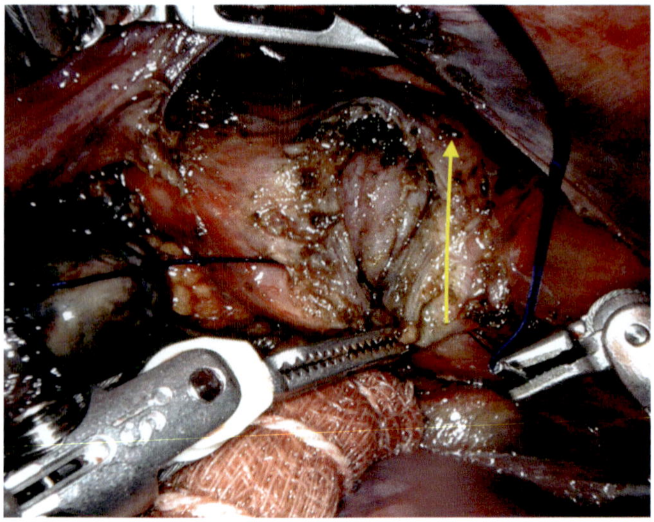

Fig. 3.20 The muscle layers can be adapted without tension so that a direct suture is possible. The muscular defect is then closed in a transverse fashion to avoid postoperative stenosis (>)

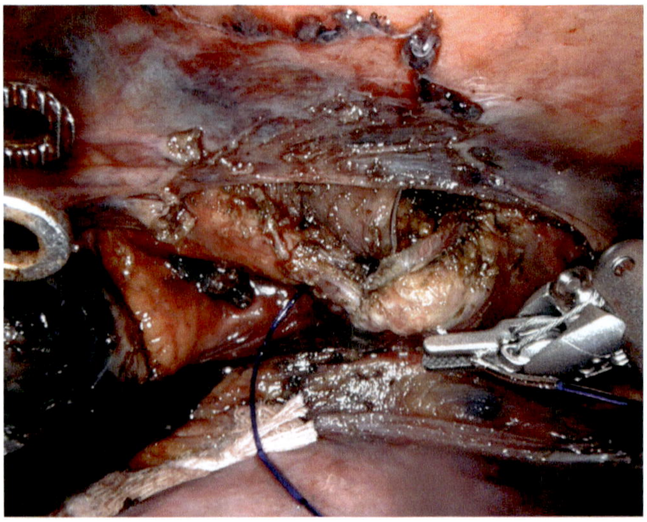

Fig. 3.19 A requirement for direct suturing of the esophagus is that the esophagus can be mobilized sufficiently and that there is no tension on the suture

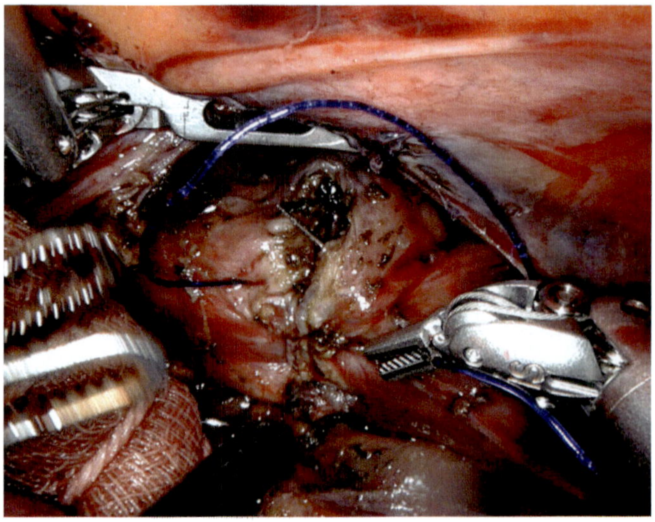

Fig. 3.21 The musculature is sutured continuously with STRATAFIX strength 3.0

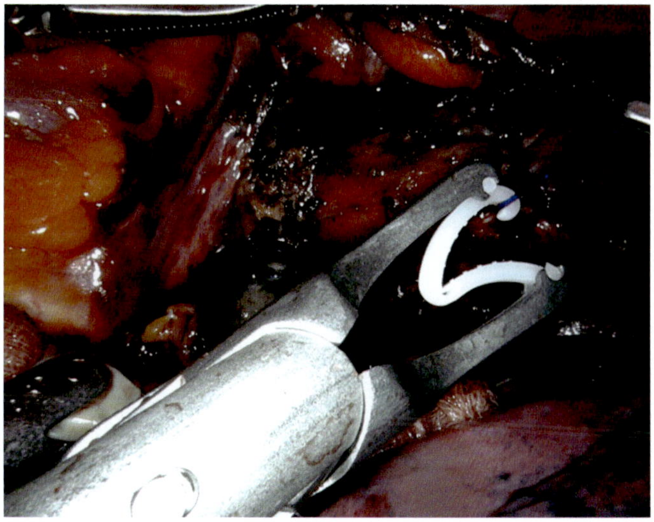

Fig. 3.22 The suture is fixed with a clip and protected from loosening

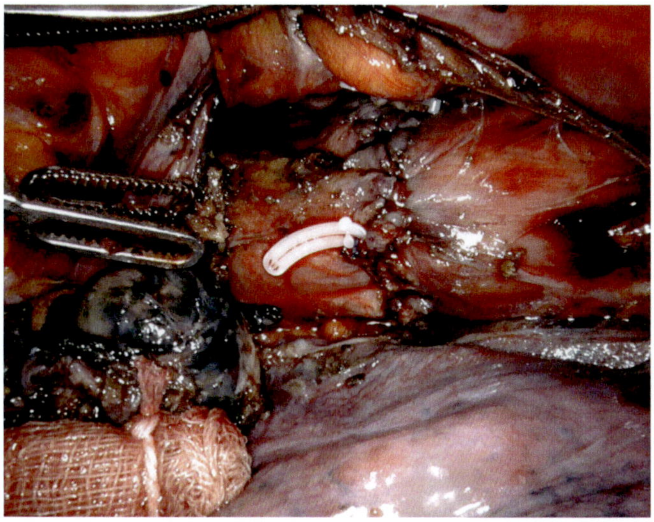

Fig. 3.23 The esophagus is closed sufficiently. The clip secures the suture. The suture is without tension

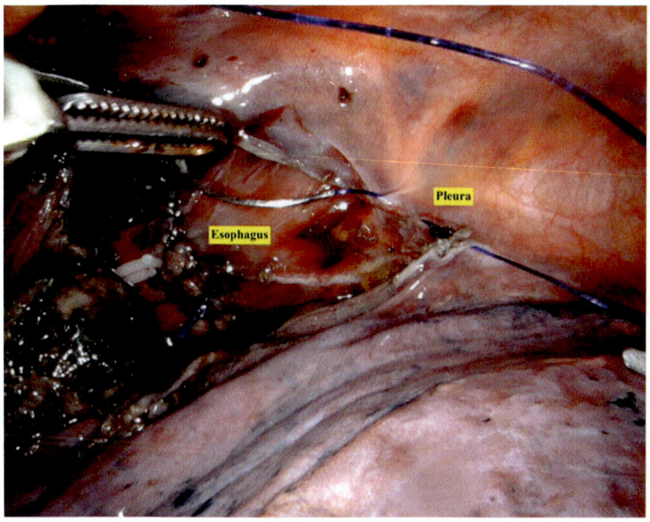

Fig. 3.24 The closure of the parietal pleura begins with continuous with STRATAFIX strength 3.0

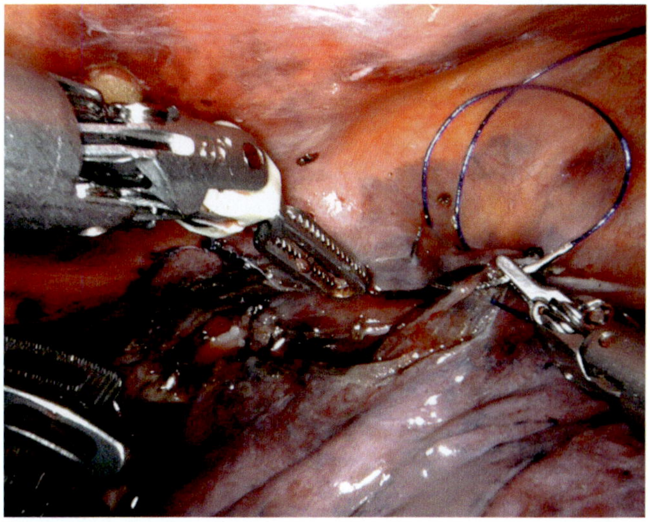

Fig. 3.25 The pleura parietalis closure is continued

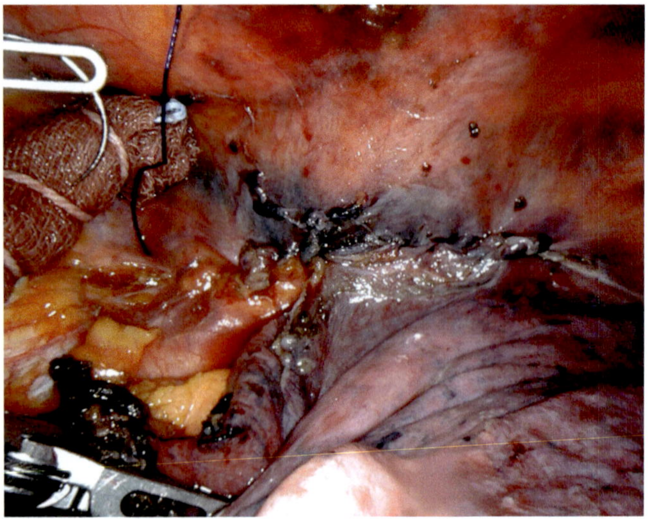

Fig. 3.26 The pleura suture is closed sufficiently. The thorax is inspected for bleeding and injuries to the lungs

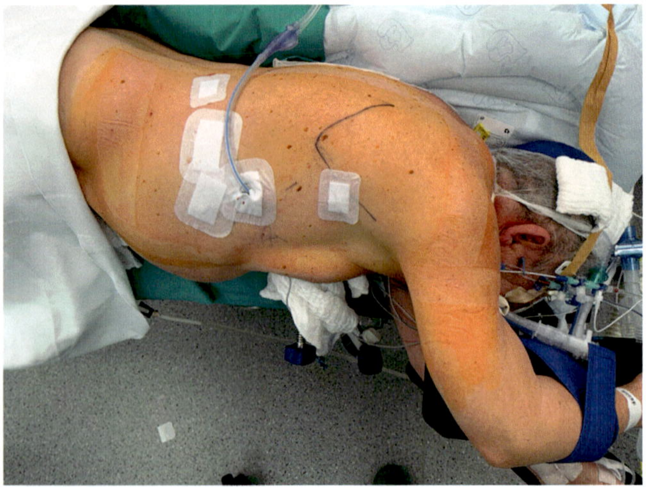

Fig. 3.27 A 24-Charriere chest drain is placed via the camera port. The right lung is ventilated again, the remaining ports removed and the thorax closed. The patient is transferred to the regular ward via the recovery room

References

1. van der Sluis PC, van der Horst S, May AM, Schippers C, Brosens LAA, Joore HCA, et al. Robot-assisted minimally invasive thoracolaparoscopic esophagectomy versus open transthoracic esophagectomy for resectable esophageal cancer: a randomized controlled trial. Ann Surg. 2019;269(4):621–30.
2. van der Sluis PC, Tagkalos E, Hadzijusufovic E, Babic B, Uzun E, van Hillegersberg R, et al. Robot-assisted minimally invasive esophagectomy with intrathoracic anastomosis (Ivor Lewis): promising results in 100 consecutive patients (the European experience). J Gastrointest Surg. 2021;25(1):1–8.
3. Franke F, Moeller T, Mehdorn A-S, Beckmann JH, Becker T, Egberts J-H. Ivor-Lewis oesophagectomy: a standardized operative technique in 11 steps. Int J Med Robot. 2021;17(1):1–10.

4 Robotic Heller Myotomy with Dor Fundoplication

Laura Lorenzon, Alberto Biondi, Pietro Santocchi, and Domenico D'Ugo

Introduction

Oesophageal achalasia is a motility disorder of unknown cause, due to the selective loss of inhibitory neurons of the myenteric plexus. It is characterized by aperistalsis of the oesophageal body and impaired LES relaxation, and the typical symptoms include dysphagia for solids and liquids, regurgitation, gradual weight loss, and retrosternal pain. Specific tests performed to confirm diagnosis are gastroscopy, a barium XR or CT scan swallow (Figs. 4.1 and 4.2) and high-resolution manometry. This latter exam is mandatory to classify the oesophageal motility disorders on the basis of objective metrics (specifically, the integrated relaxation pressure (IRP) and the presence/absence of peristalsis) using the Chicago Classification (CC). Using these features, the CC version 3.0 distinguishes achalasia into three forms, namely, Type I (IRP greater than the upper limit of normal values and absence of oesophageal contractility), Type II (IRP greater than the upper limit of normal values and absence of peristalsis/pan-oesophageal pressurization with >20% of swallows) and Type III (IRP greater than the upper limit of normal values and absence of peristalsis/premature contractions with >20% of swallows) [1]. Although several endoscopic treatments are currently available [2], the mini-invasive myotomy is recommended for Type I and Type II achalasia and – when associated with Dor fundoplication – it has the advantage of resulting in less post-operative reflux symptoms at 2 years of follow-up [3].

The robotic approach for achalasia was first described in 2001 [4], and current experiences report lower rates of intra-operative oesophageal perforations comparing laparoscopy, although more powered studies are advocated to confirm this positive trend [5].

Procedure: Illustrated Steps

Figures 4.1, 4.2, 4.3, 4.4, 4.5, 4.6, 4.7, 4.8, 4.9, 4.10, 4.11, 4.12, 4.13,4.14, 4.15, 4.16, 4.17, 4.18, 4.19, 4.20, 4.21, 4.22, 4.23, and 4.24 illustrate typical imaging, operating room set-up and the technical aspects of a robotic Heller myotomy with Dor fundoplication for oesophageal achalasia using XI Da Vinci system as standardized at our Institution.

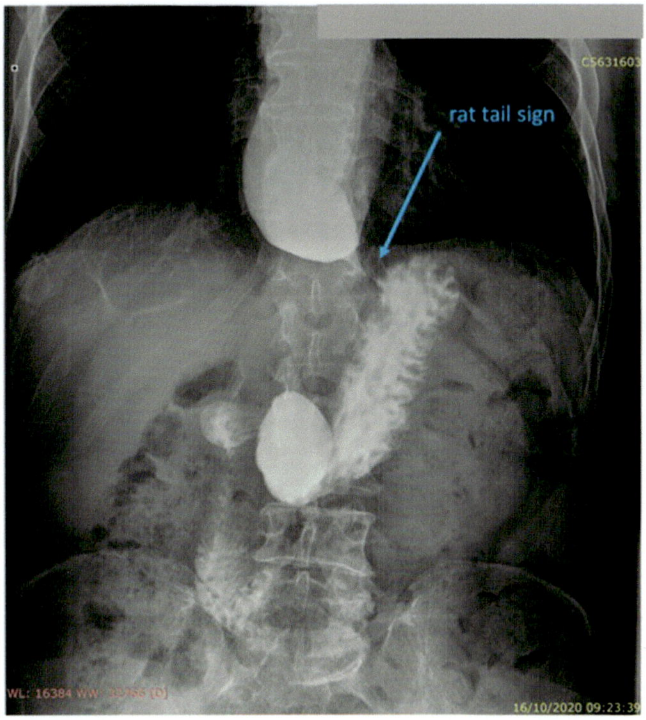

Fig. 4.1 XR swallow with barium documenting a typical oesophageal dilatation with rat tail sign at the cardia level in a patient with Type II achalasia

L. Lorenzon
General Surgery Unit, Fondazione Policlinico Universitario A. Gemelli IRCCS, Catholic University of the Sacred Heart, Rome, Italy

A. Biondi · P. Santocchi · D. D'Ugo (✉)
Fondazione Policlinico Universitario A. Gemelli IRCCS, Catholic University of the Sacred Heart, Rome, Italy
e-mail: domenico.dugo@policlinicogemelli.it

O. Y. Kudsi, P. P. Grimminger (eds.), *Atlas of Robotic Upper Gastrointestinal Surgery*,
https://doi.org/10.1007/978-3-030-86578-8_4

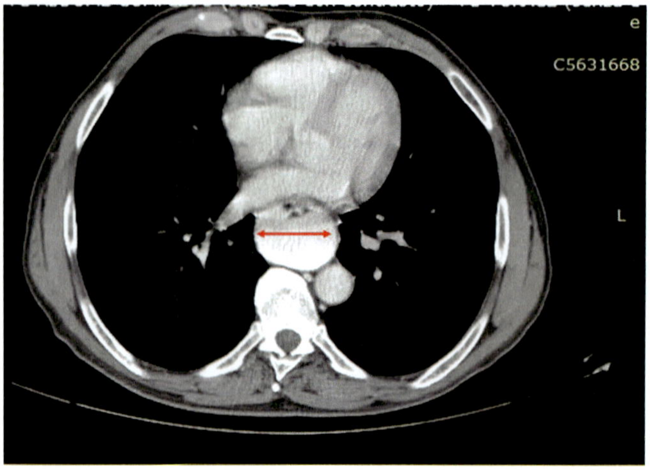

Fig. 4.2 CT scan showing a dilatated oesophagus filled with ingest (same patient as above). Red arrow showing oesophageal diameter

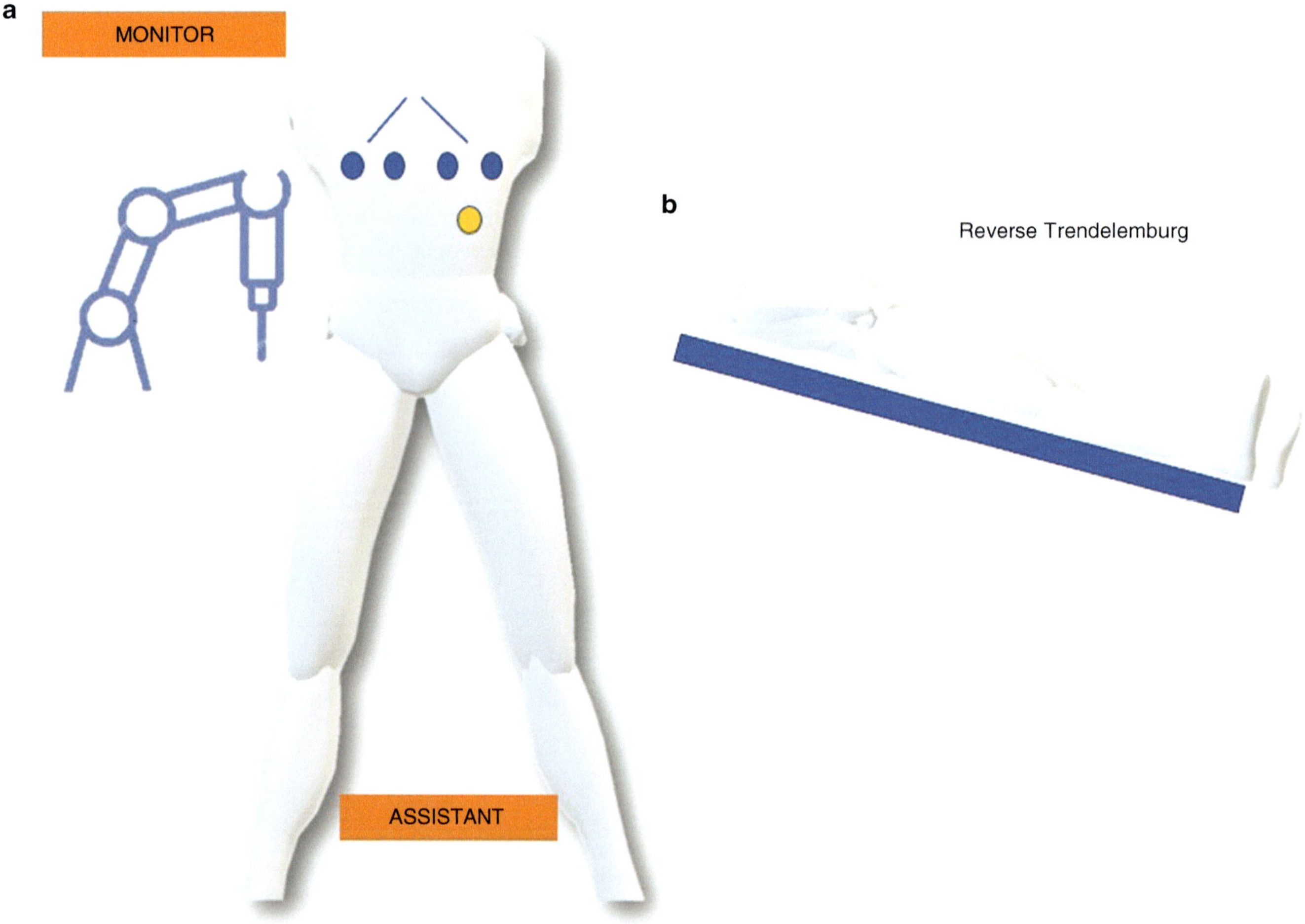

Fig. 4.3 Operating room setting. (**a**) The patient is positioned with abducted legs, the monitor is placed on the right shoulder and the assistant operates between the legs of the patient. The robot (Da Vinci Xi) enters from the patient's right side. Pneumoperitoneum is induced using a Veress needle in the left hypochondrium. After insufflating the abdomen with CO_2 (target pressure 14 mmHg), four robotic trocars (8 mm) are placed, all of them above the umbilicus: two in the right quadrant (one below the costal arch margin and one lateral to the rectus abdominis), one left to the midline and one in the left quadrant. A further 12 mm trocar for the assistant is placed in the left iliac fossa. (**b**) Finally, the patient is placed in reverse Trendelenburg position before starting the docking

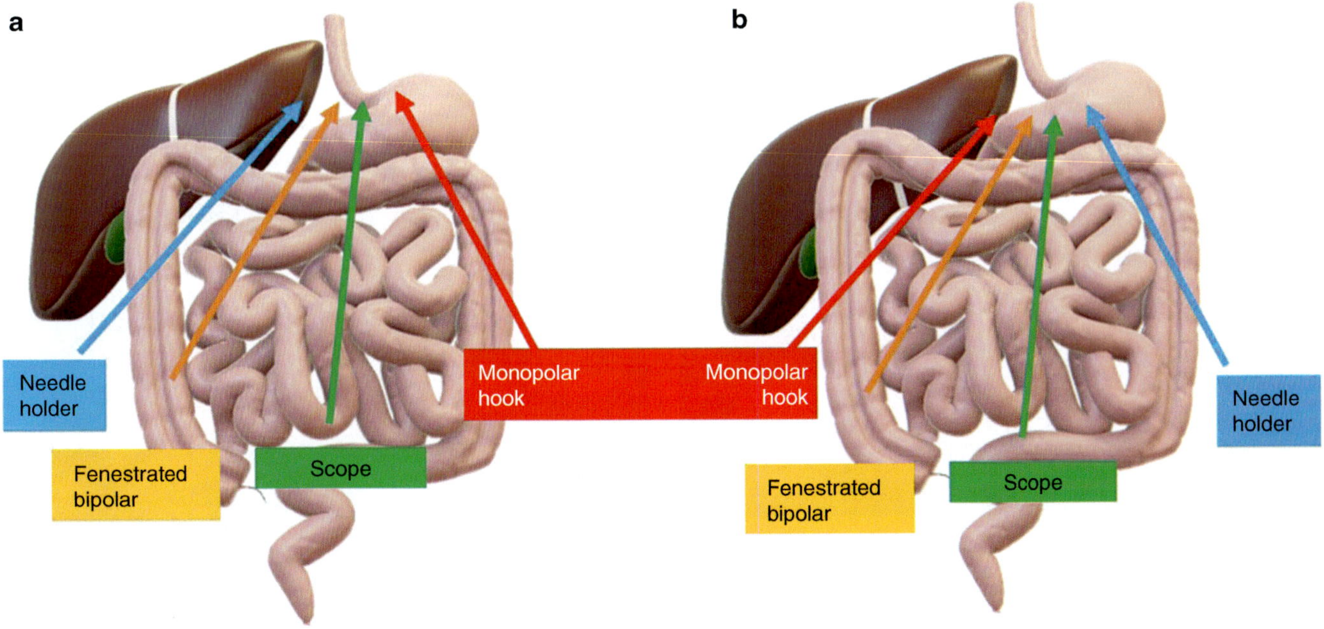

Fig. 4.4 Docking is performed using four robotic arms. (**a**) At the beginning of the procedure, in order to perform the Heller myotomy, the needle holder is introduced in the right lateral trocar and used to suspend the left liver lobe; the other robotic trocars are used to introduce (right to left): a fenestrated bipolar grasper, the robotic scope and a monopolar hook. (**b**) After completing the myotomy, the Dor fundoplication is performed inverting the position of the hook (now used to suspend the liver) and the needle holder (now placed in the trocar in the left hypochondrium)

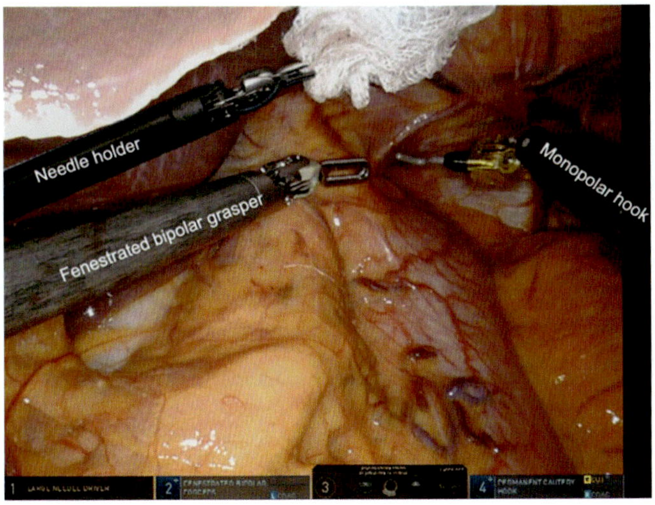

Fig. 4.5 Left lobe liver suspension using a swab and the needle holder to expose the operating field (the needle holder has been added to the picture to illustrate positioning of the robotic instruments to expose the surgical field and to start the procedure)

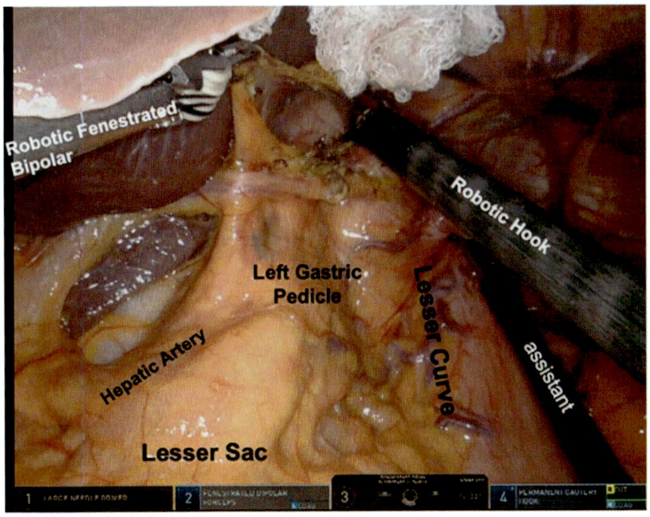

Fig. 4.6 Opening of the lesser sac. While the assistant helps divaricating the stomach to the left quadrant using a laparoscopic grasper, the surgeon opens the lesser sac using a monopolar hook and the fenestrated bipolar. In patients with low BMI, the left gastric pedicle and the hepatic artery may be visualized through the omental bursa

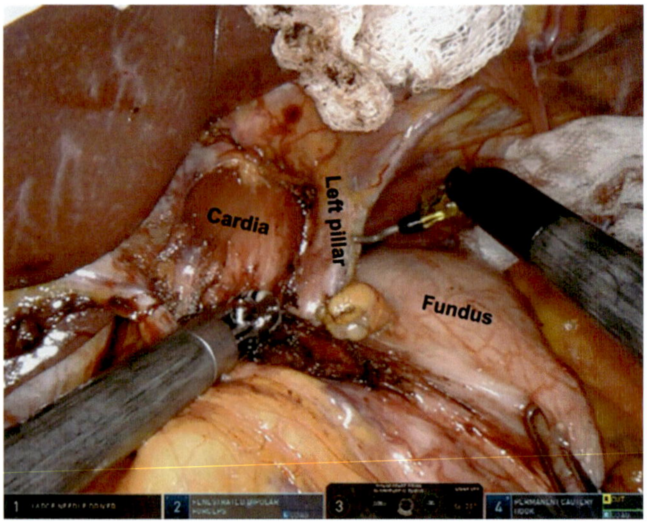

Fig. 4.7 The cardia region is then exposed by dissection of the right and left diaphragmatic pillars. The dissection should include the phreno-oesophageal and gastrophrenic ligaments. The anterior vagus nerve should be identified and preserved

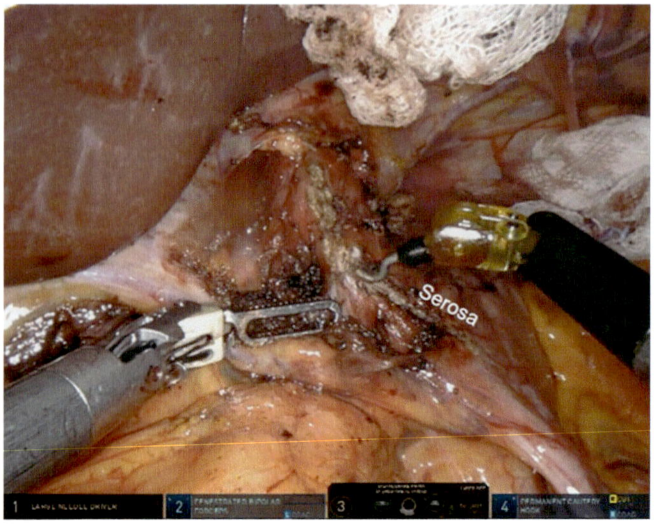

Fig. 4.9 The serosal layer is dissected to expose the muscular fibres

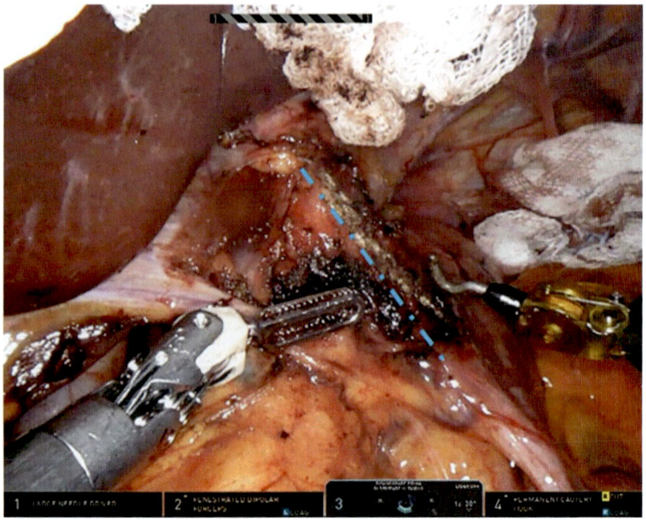

Fig. 4.8 After completing the exposure of cardia region, the myotomy extension is marked using the monopolar hook on the serosa of the oesophago-gastric junction (EGJ), usually starting 5 cm above the EGJ to 2 cm onto the gastric wall

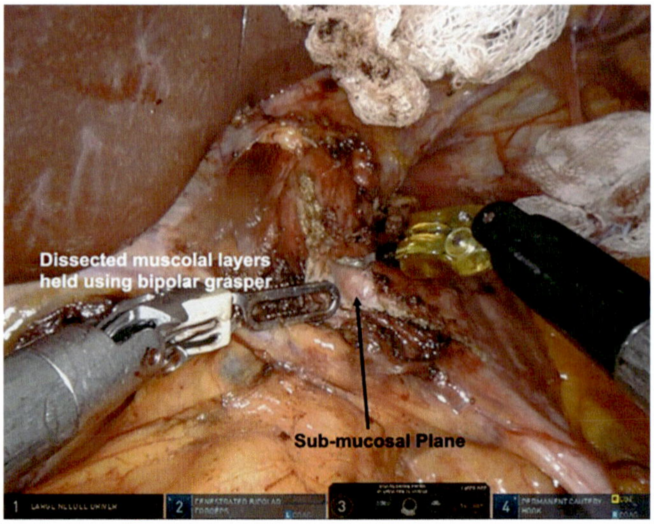

Fig. 4.10 The submucosal plane is reached, and the myotomy is performed cutting both circular and longitudinal fibres, using a smooth dissection with the robotic hook

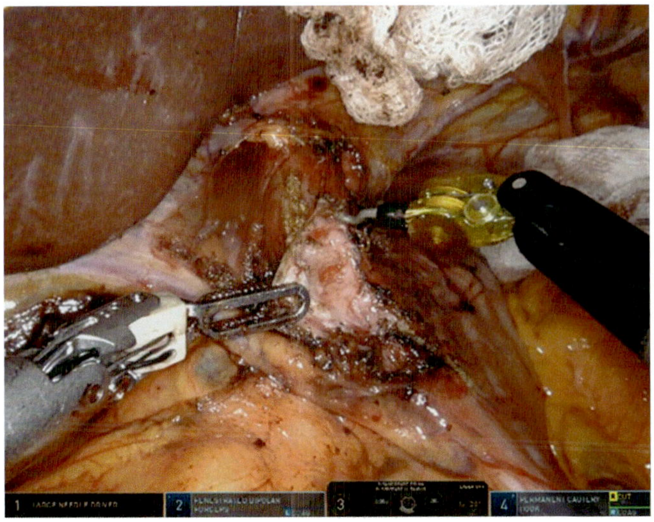

Fig. 4.11 The dissection proceeds to reach the proximal and distal extension using the robotic hook but avoiding cauterization

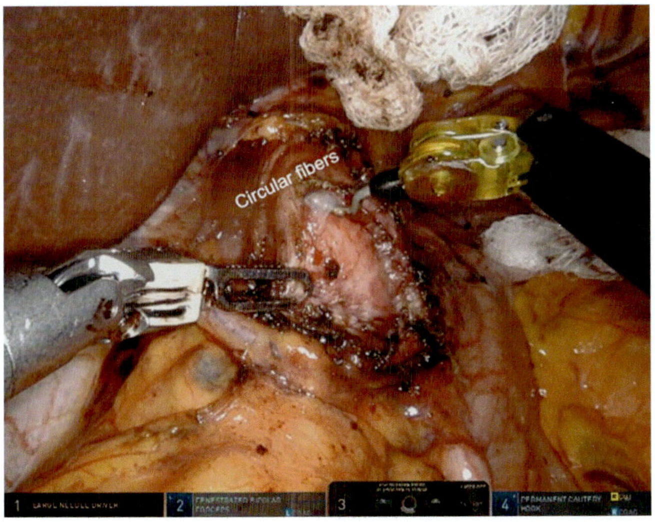

Fig. 4.12 Dissection of the circular oesophageal fibres

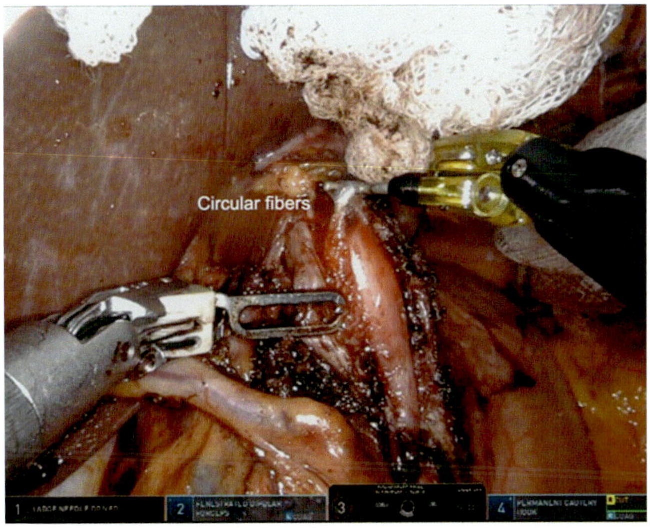

Fig. 4.13 Another image showing dissection of the circular oesophageal fibres: note how the robotic hook is used to dissect smoothly the muscular layer

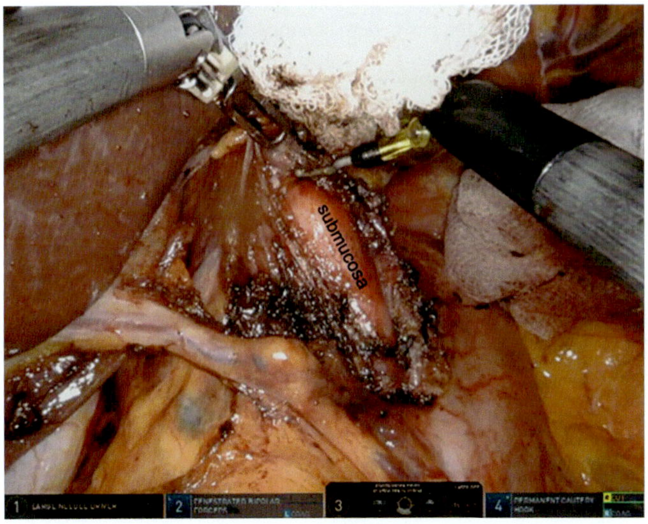

Fig. 4.14 Final view of myotomy showing exposure of the submucosal plane

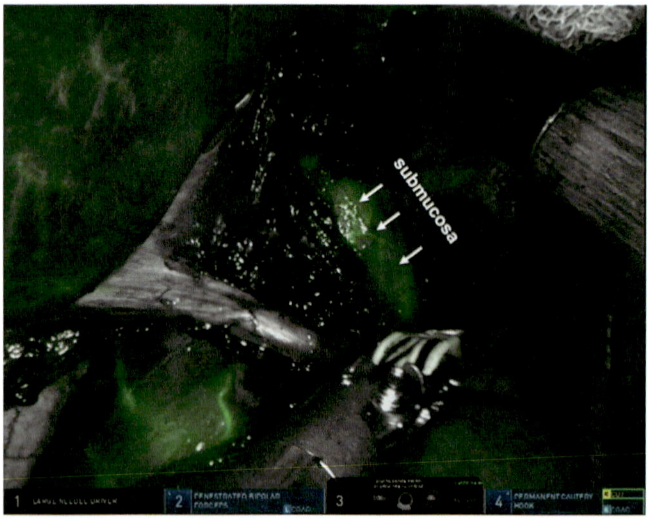

Fig. 4.15 The most worrisome complication during myotomy is a perforation of the oesophagus. In order to rule out any intra-operative problems, after the completion of myotomy, a near-infrared (NIR) indocyanine green (ICG)-induced fluorescence angiography (FA) is performed to check the integrity of the submucosal layer. NIR-ICG-induced FA is conducted administering IV a bolus of 3.75–7.5 mg of ICG and evaluated using the Da Vinci Fluorescence Imaging System. This image shows the early view obtained few seconds after the ICG injection

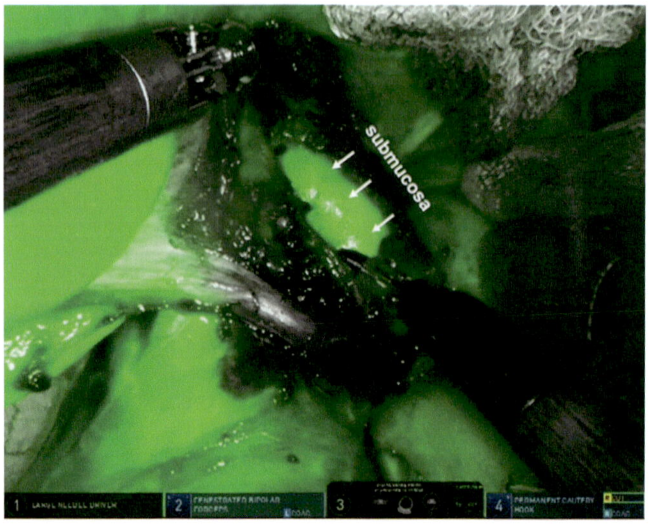

Fig. 4.16 NIR-ICG-induced FA showing the integrity of the oesophageal submucosal layer

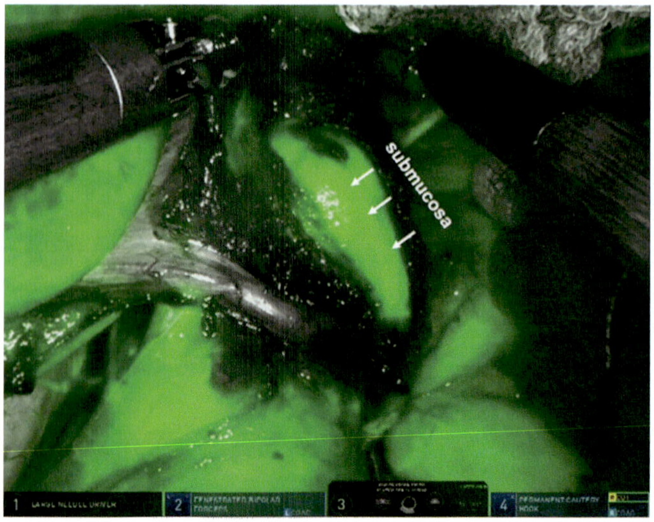

Fig. 4.17 NIR-ICG-induced FA final view

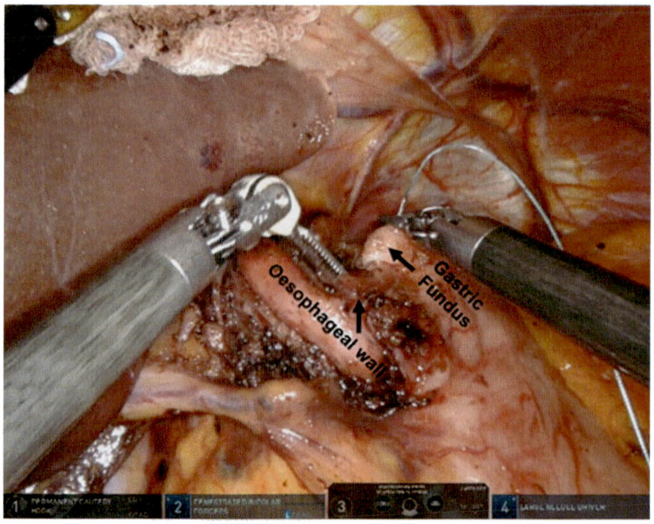

Fig. 4.18 Anterior partial fundoplication: Dor procedure. As explained before, the position of robotic instruments is changed. The hook is now used to suspend the liver, and the needle holder is positioned in its place. Sometimes, in order to avoid any tension, it can be useful to take down the short gastric vessels. A polyester fibre suture of the ideal length of 15–18 cm (MERSILENE® 0, Ethicon) is used for suturing. The first stitch incorporates the gastric fundus and the oesophageal wall

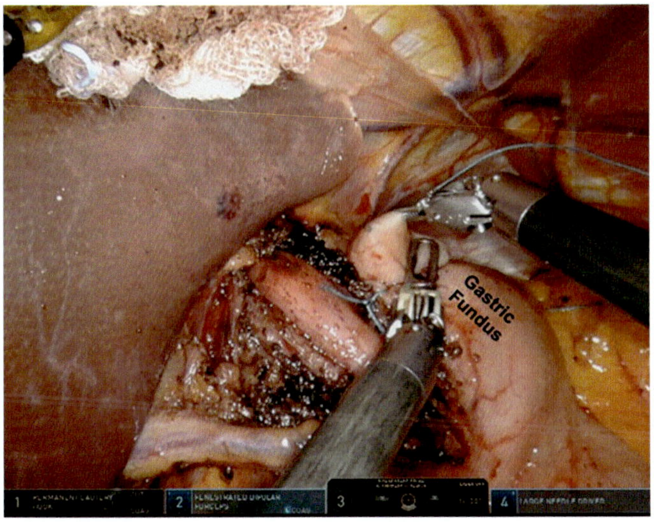

Fig. 4.19 Final view of the first stitch to show the attachment of the gastric fundus at the oesophageal wall. The needle holder is pointing at the level where the second stitch will be placed

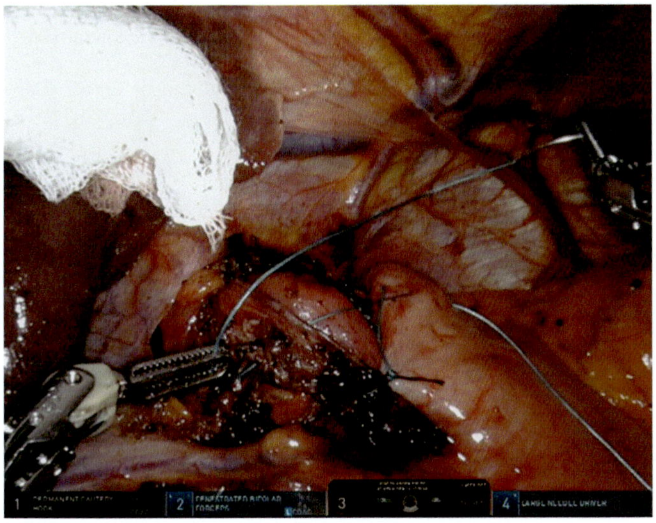

Fig. 4.20 A second stitch is placed cranial to the first one

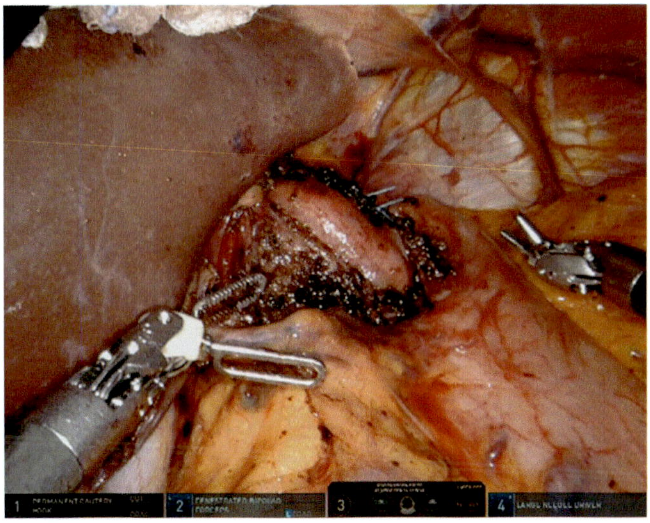

Fig. 4.21 View of the second stich. The gastric fundus is now fixed to the oesophageal wall

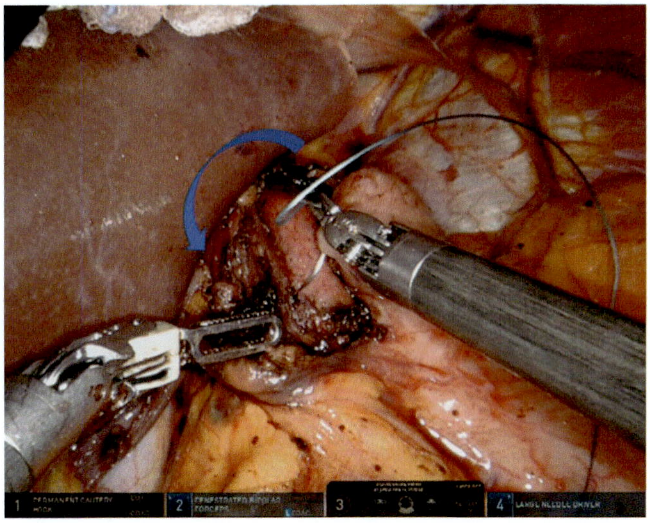

Fig. 4.22 Second row of suture. The gastric fundus is folded over the myotomy, to attach the fundus to the opposite oesophageal wall

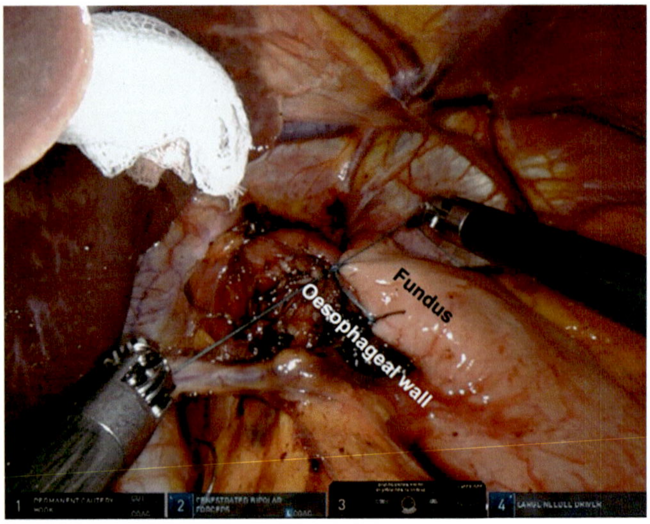

Fig. 4.23 The gastric fundus is folded over the myotomy to cover the sub-mucosa of the oesophagus

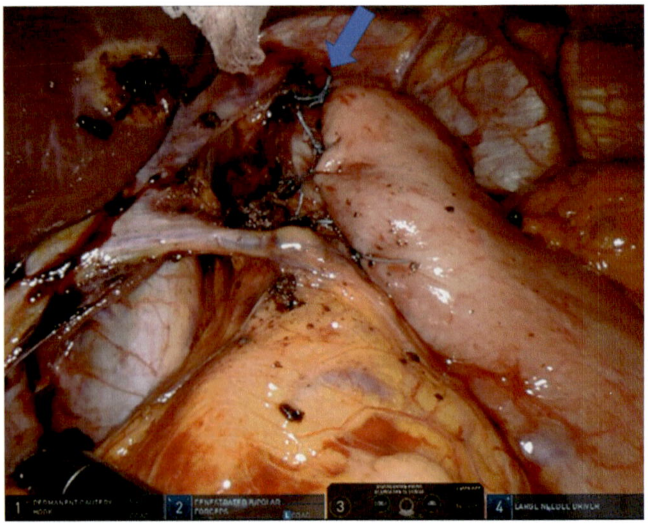

Fig. 4.24 Final view of the Dor fundoplication. The arrow is pointing to the stitch used to fix the fundus to the left pillar of the crus

References

1. Kahrilas PJ, Bredenoord AJ, Fox M, Gyawali CP, Roman S, Smout AJ, Pandolfino JE, International High Resolution Manometry Working Group. The Chicago classification of esophageal motility disorders, v3.0. Neurogastroenterol Motil. 2015;27(2):160–74. https://doi.org/10.1111/nmo.12477.
2. Kahrilas PJ, Bredenoord AJ, Fox M, Gyawali CP, Roman S, Smout AJPM, Pandolfino JE, International Working Group for Disorders of Gastrointestinal Motility and Function. Expert consensus document: advances in the management of esophageal motility disorders in the era of high-resolution manometry: a focus on achalasia syndromes. Nat Rev Gastroenterol Hepatol. 2017;14(11):677–88. https://doi.org/10.1038/nrgastro.2017.132.
3. Schlottmann F, Luckett DJ, Fine J, Shaheen NJ, Patti MG. Laparoscopic Heller myotomy versus peroral endoscopic myotomy (POEM) for achalasia: a systematic review and meta-analysis. Ann Surg. 2018;267(3):451–60. https://doi.org/10.1097/SLA.0000000000002311.
4. Melvin WS, Needleman BJ, Krause KR, Wolf RK, Michler RE, Ellison EC. Computer-assisted robotic Heller myotomy: initial case report. J Laparoendosc Adv Surg Tech A. 2001;11(4):251–3. https://doi.org/10.1089/109264201750539790.
5. Milone M, Manigrasso M, Vertaldi S, Velotti N, Aprea G, Maione F, Gennarelli N, De Simone G, De Conno B, Pesce M, Sarnelli G, De Palma GD. Robotic versus laparoscopic approach to treat symptomatic achalasia: systematic review with meta-analysis. Dis Esophagus. 2019;32(10):1–8. https://doi.org/10.1093/dote/doz062.

Robotic Gastric Neurostimulator Placement

5

William C. Sherrill III and Michael M. Awad

Introduction

Gastroparesis is a complex disease that can be severely debilitating. Patient outcomes are optimized when a multidisciplinary treatment plan is employed, utilizing a combination of dietary, behavioral, and medical management strategies and occasionally surgical therapy. One of these surgical options is gastric electrical stimulation which, when employed with proper workup and strict protocols, has been shown to provide significant relief [1].

Our preferred diagnostic workup for these patients involves a 4-hour solid-phase gastric emptying study. It is important that the test is conducted for the full 4-hour duration, and off all opioids and THC-/marijuana-containing products, as these can interfere with gastric emptying times. It is essential to rule out concomitant mechanical gastrointestinal obstruction with upper endoscopy and imaging studies such as cross-section imaging or contrast radiography.

Once the diagnosis of gastroparesis has been established, conservative therapy includes dietary and behavioral modifications as well as medical management. Carbohydrates and insoluble fiber should be minimized as these delay gastric emptying. Meal volumes should be small, and consistency should be soft. Liberal liquid intake may help to prevent food bolus formation in the stomach. Carbonated beverages, alcohol, and smoking are to be avoided and glycemic control optimized [2]. The mainstays of medication management involve antiemetic and prokinetic agents, as well as elimination of opioids and other agents that reduce GI motility. The Gastroparesis Cardinal Symptom Index (GCSI) is recorded prior to the onset of therapy and throughout the management course to monitor treatment efficacy [3].

Surgical therapy is generally reserved for patients that fail or have inadequate relief from conservative management. In addition to pylorus-relaxing procedures (e.g., pyloroplasty and endoscopic pyloromyotomy), feeding tubes, and near total gastrectomy, we have utilized gastric neurostimulation (Enterra; Medtronic, Minneapolis, MN) with high levels of success. Proper patient selection is key. Candidates must be compliant with frequent initial follow-up visits, as often several adjustments are required before an optimal level of therapy is reached. They must also have no metal allergies, be nonsmokers, and cannot be dependent on MRI for other conditions.

Our technical approach is described in this chapter. We utilize robotic technology to facilitate a minimally invasive placement of the neurostimulator leads in the gastric wall. They must be placed precisely in the muscle layer – too deep and the mucosa is traversed; too superficial and the leads are serosal or exposed to the peritoneal cavity resulting in high impedance. The robotic instrumentation allows for this level of precision while maintaining a laparoscopic approach.

Postoperatively, patients are seen initially at 1 month in the outpatient setting where the first adjustment is made using a handheld programming device. Patients are then seen back every 6–8 weeks for further adjustments. On average, most patients take approximately 4–6 months to reach an optimal level of symptom control. We strongly encourage them to continue to see their gastroenterologist during this time as their medication therapy can often be changed, reduced, or even eliminated as their symptoms improve. Following this initial period, we see patients at regular 1-year intervals to monitor the generator function as the battery life can last anywhere from 5 to 10 years depending on the neurostimulator settings (Figs. 5.1, 5.2, 5.3, 5.4, 5.5, 5.6, 5.7, 5.8, 5.9, 5.10, 5.11, 5.12, 5.13, 5.14, 5.15, 5.16, 5.17, 5.18, 5.19, 5.20, 5.21, 5.22, 5.23, 5.24, 5.25, 5.26, 5.27, 5.28, 5.29, 5.30, 5.31, 5.32, 5.33, 5.34, 5.35, 5.36, 5.37, 5.38, 5.39, 5.40, 5.41, 5.42, 5.43, 5.44, 5.45, 5.46, 5.47, and 5.48).

W. C. Sherrill III · M. M. Awad (✉)
Section of Minimally Invasive Surgery, Washington University School of Medicine, St Louis, MO, USA
e-mail: awadm@wustl.edu

O. Y. Kudsi, P. P. Grimminger (eds.), *Atlas of Robotic Upper Gastrointestinal Surgery*,
https://doi.org/10.1007/978-3-030-86578-8_5

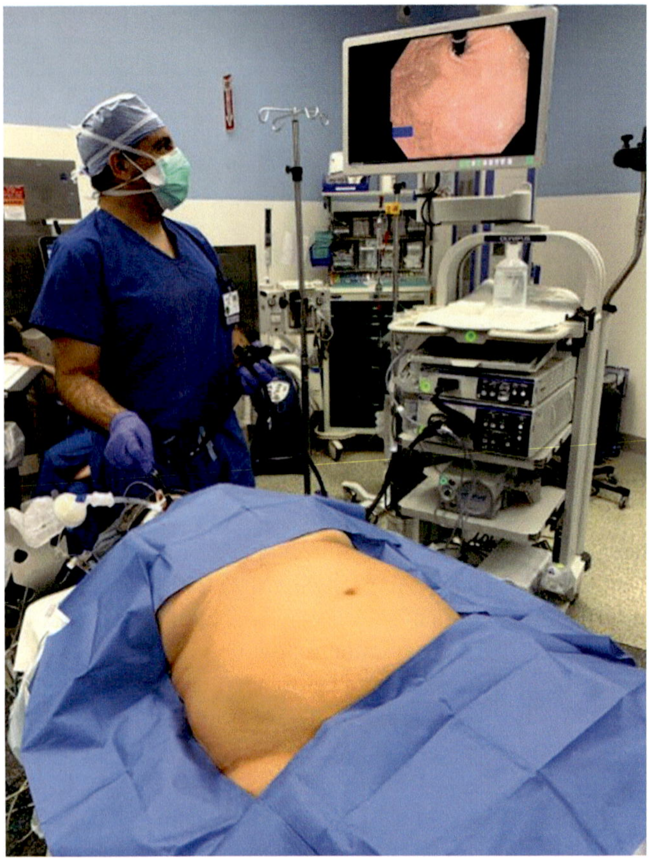

Fig. 5.1 Upper endoscopy is initially performed to confirm the absence of gastric ulcers, neoplasms, or bezoars which would preclude device placement

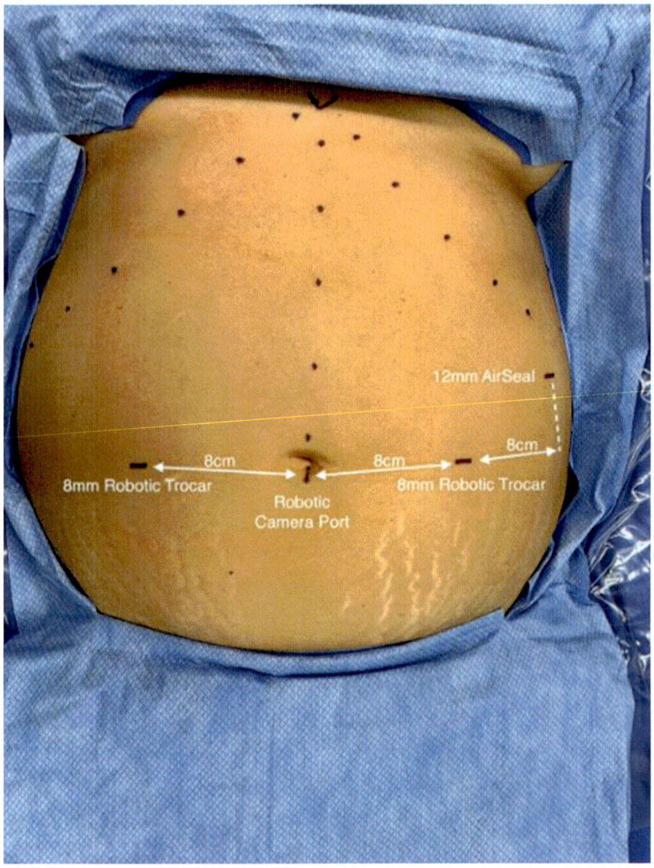

Fig. 5.2 Patient external landmarks are shown. Robotic trocars should be separated by at least 8 cm to allow for optimal working space

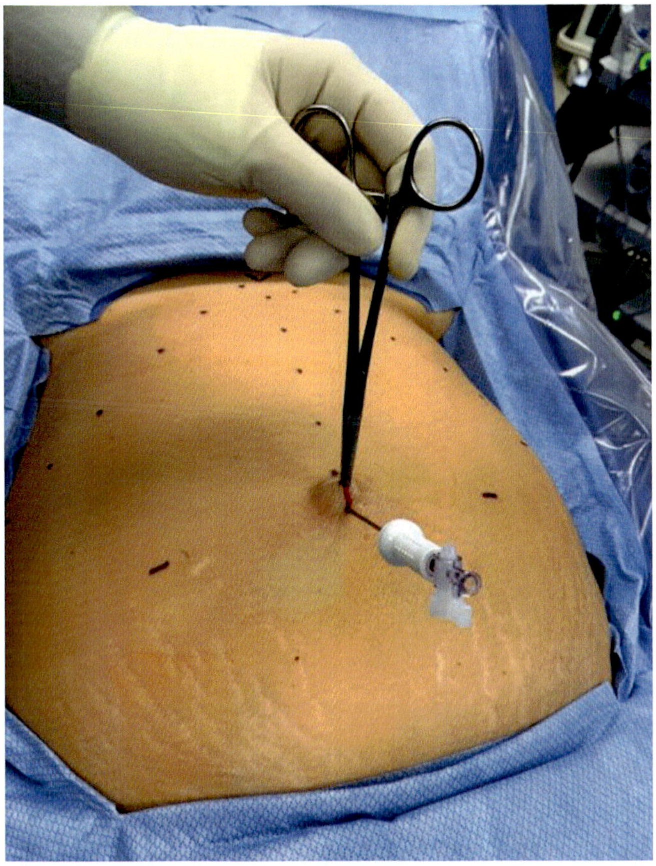

Fig. 5.3 An 8 mm incision is made in the periumbilical region. The fascia is retracted, and a Veress needle is inserted into the peritoneal cavity. Insufflation is started while intra-abdominal pressure is carefully monitored

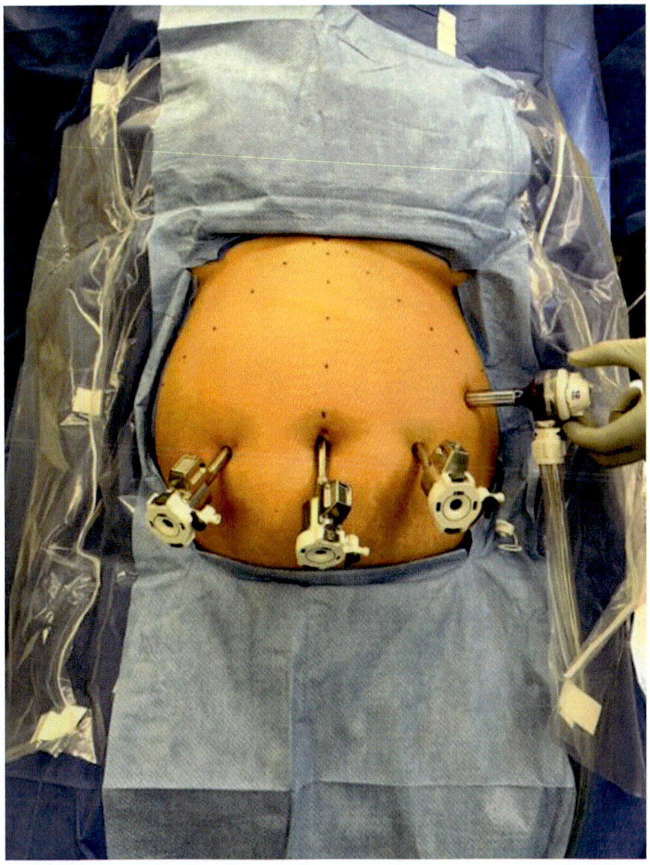

Fig. 5.4 An initial 8.5 mm robotic trocar is placed at the periumbilical incision with fascial countertraction. The robotic camera is introduced and the abdominal cavity is inspected. Two additional 8.5 mm robotic trocars are placed on either side of the umbilicus, 8 cm away from the initial port. A 12 mm AirSeal™ trocar is placed in the left upper quadrant/left flank as a non-robotic assistant port and where the leads will eventually traverse the abdominal wall

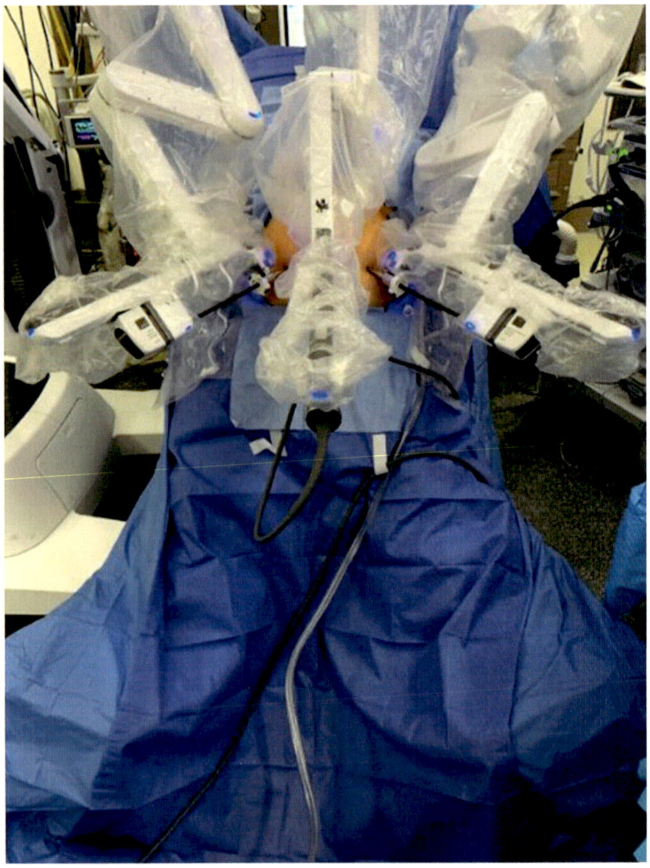

Fig. 5.5 The patient is placed in reverse Trendelenburg position at 30 degrees, and the robot is docked from the patient's right side

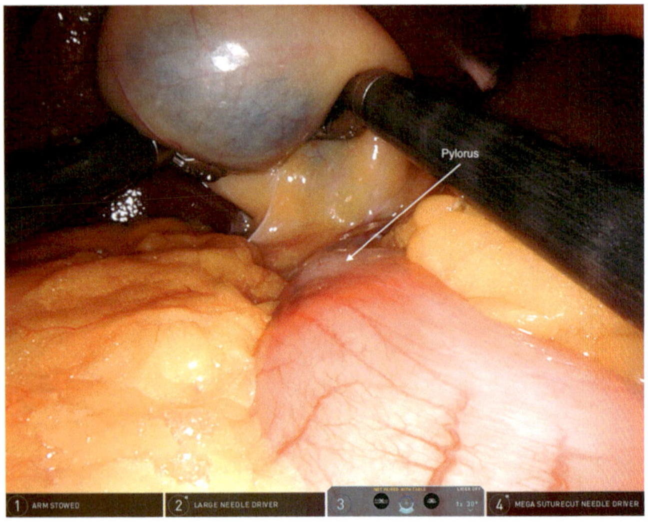

Fig. 5.6 The upper abdomen is again carefully inspected for any unexpected pathology. The distal stomach and pylorus are identified

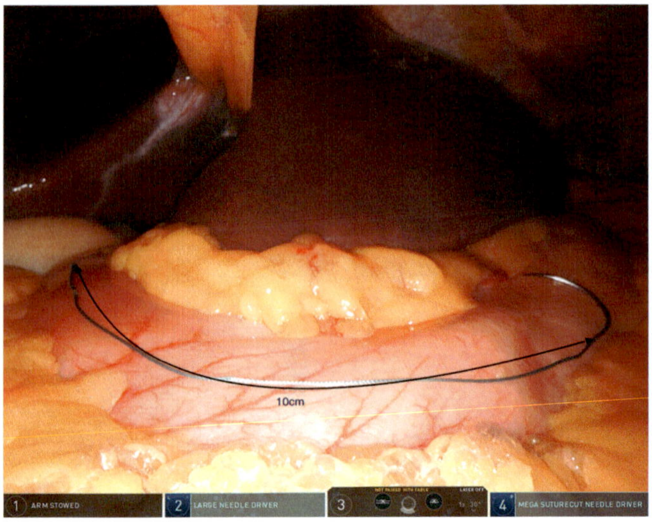

Fig. 5.7 A position on the anterior wall of the antrum, precisely 10 cm proximal to the pylorus is identified. We use a 2-0 Ethibond™ suture pre-cut to 10 cm to facilitate measurement and for use as our first stitch

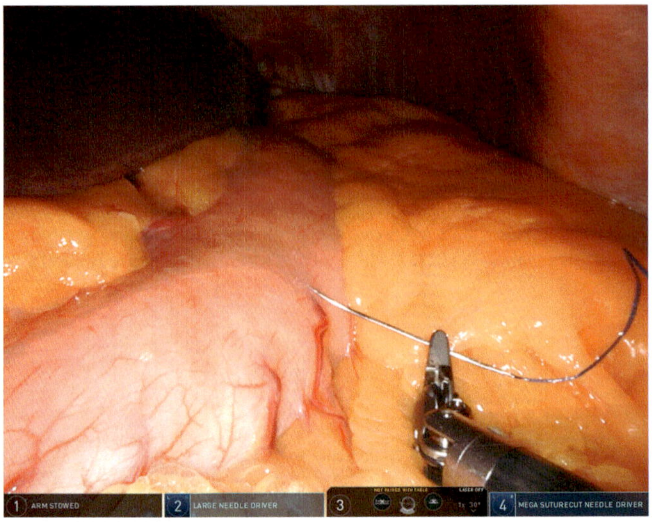

Fig. 5.8 The ski needle on the first neurostimulator lead is grasped. Care must be taken not to grasp the lead itself as it may become damaged

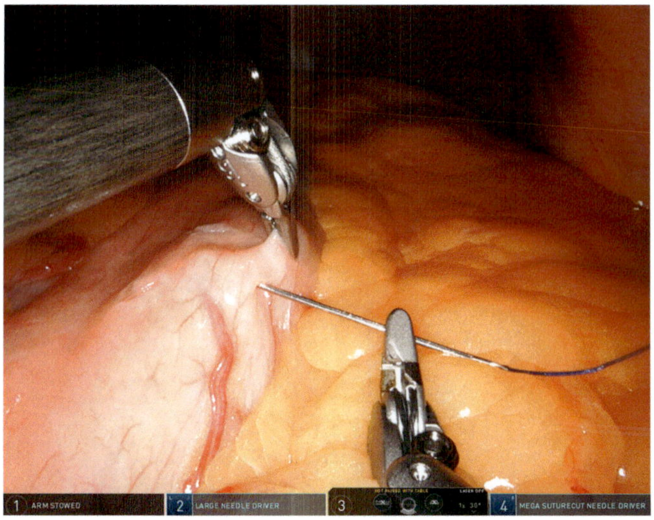

Fig. 5.9 The needle is then tunneled through the muscularis layer of the stomach, taking care to avoid the larger vessels on the greater curvature of the stomach. The lead must be placed precisely so as not to enter the gastric lumen or be visible under the serosa

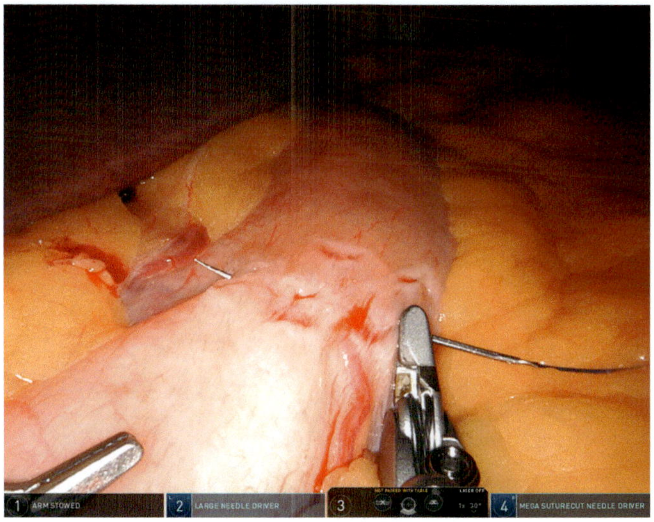

Fig. 5.10 The needle direction is perpendicular to the major axis of the stomach and traverses the muscularis layer

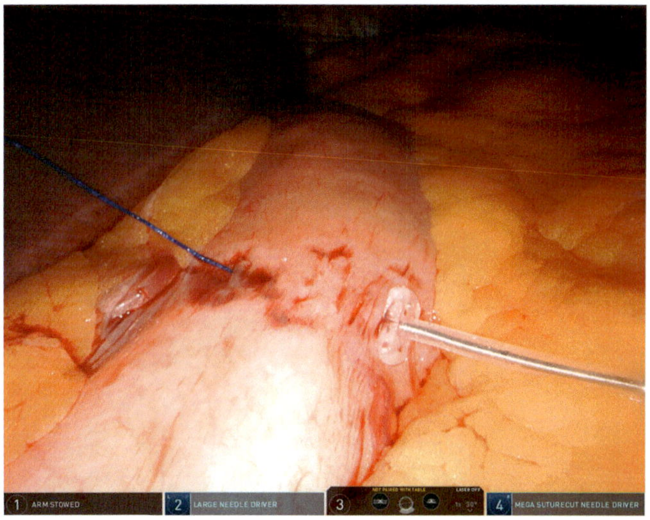

Fig. 5.11 After a minimum of 1 cm of gastric wall tunneling, the needle may be resurfaced and exit the serosa. It is then grasped again and pulled through until the bare metal of the neurostimulator lead enters the tunnel and the provided silicone flange is flush with the stomach wall

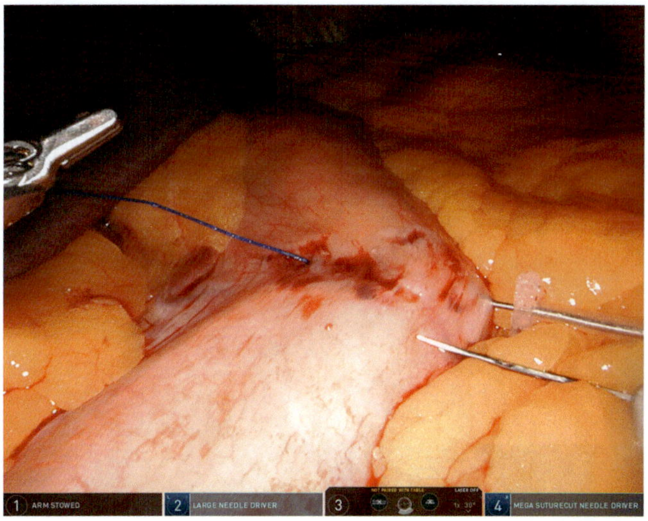

Fig. 5.12 The second neurostimulator lead is similarly placed in the stomach wall, 1 cm away from the first lead in parallel fashion

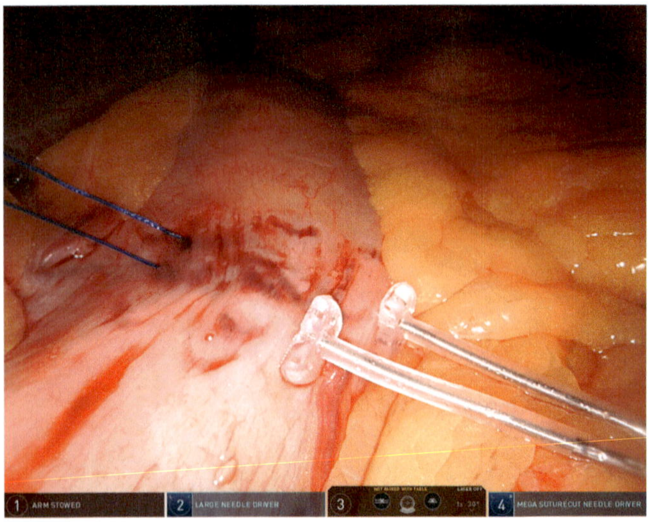

Fig. 5.13 Neurostimulator lead placement checks are performed before the leads are secured to the stomach wall. The robotic instruments can be used to stabilize the leads in position while the placement checks are performed

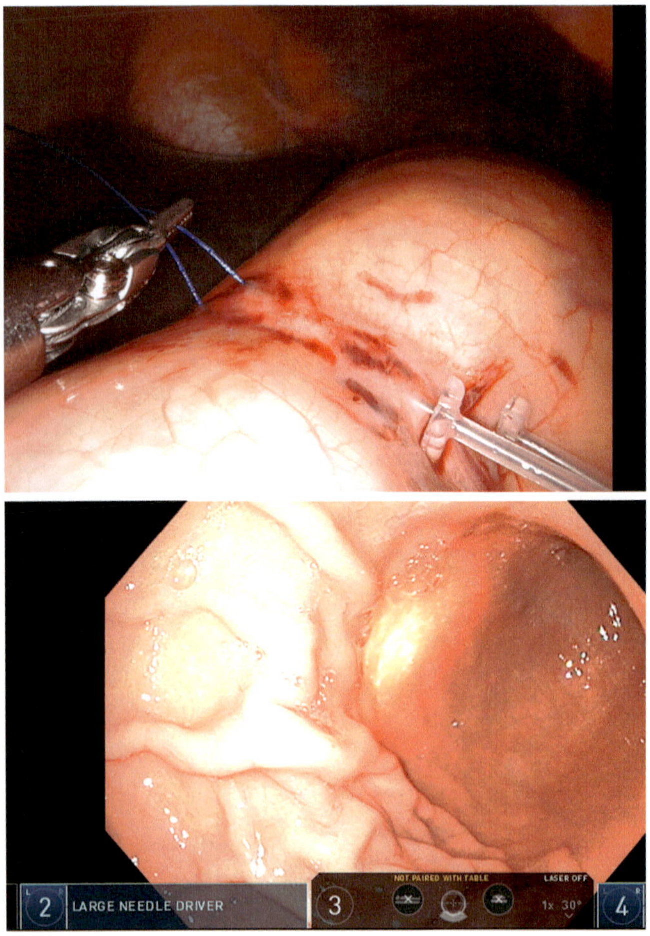

Fig. 5.14 The first placement check is performed endoscopically. The upper endoscope is used to ensure no metal from the neurostimulator leads are visible within the gastric lumen. The robotic TilePro feature can be used to simultaneously view the robotic and endoscopic fields during this step

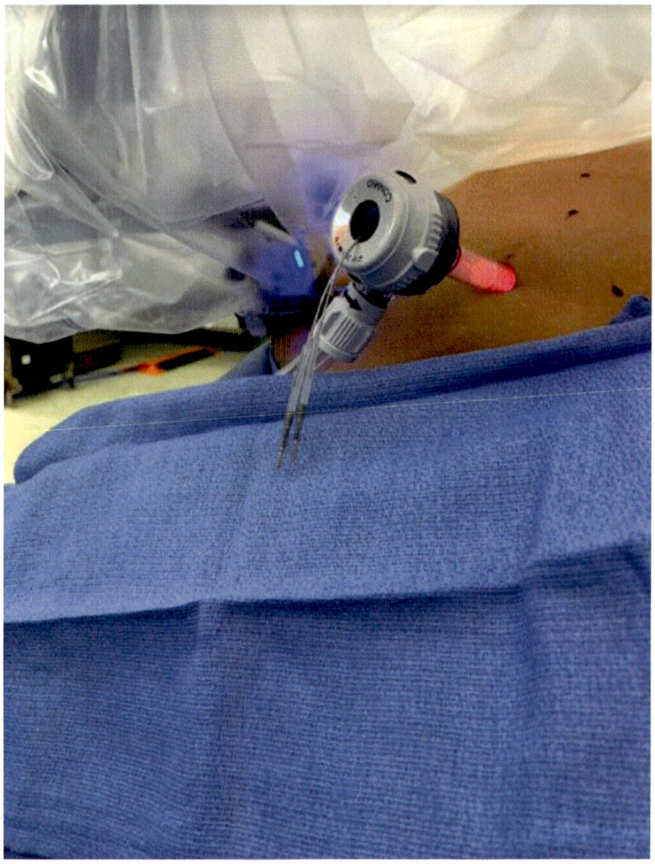

Fig. 5.15 The other end of the leads are gently held outside of the 12 mm assistant port to prevent them from being inadvertently pulled into the abdomen

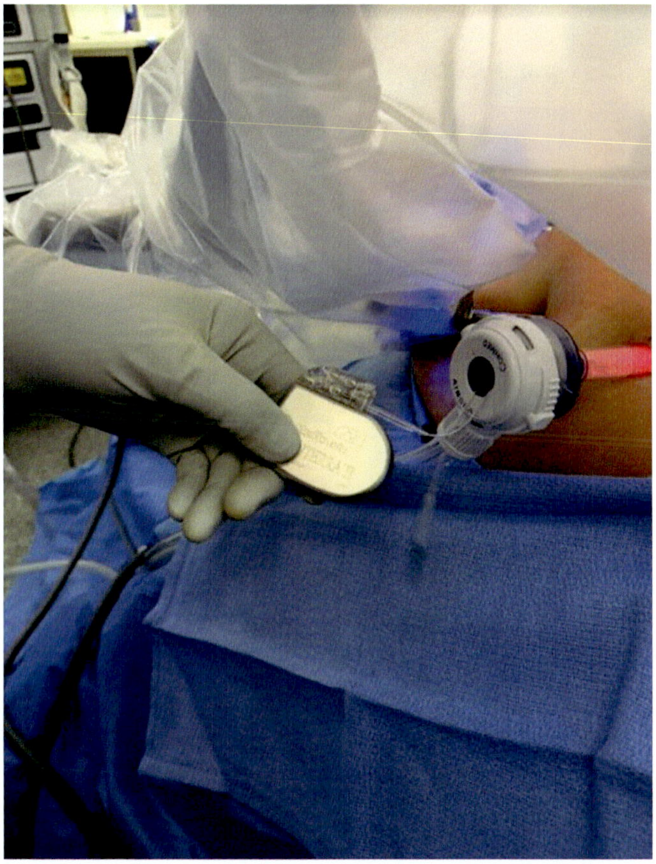

Fig. 5.16 The second lead placement check is then performed by confirming an appropriate current through the circuit. First, the two neurostimulator leads are inserted into the gastric neurostimulator in the provided slots. Either lead can be placed in either slot

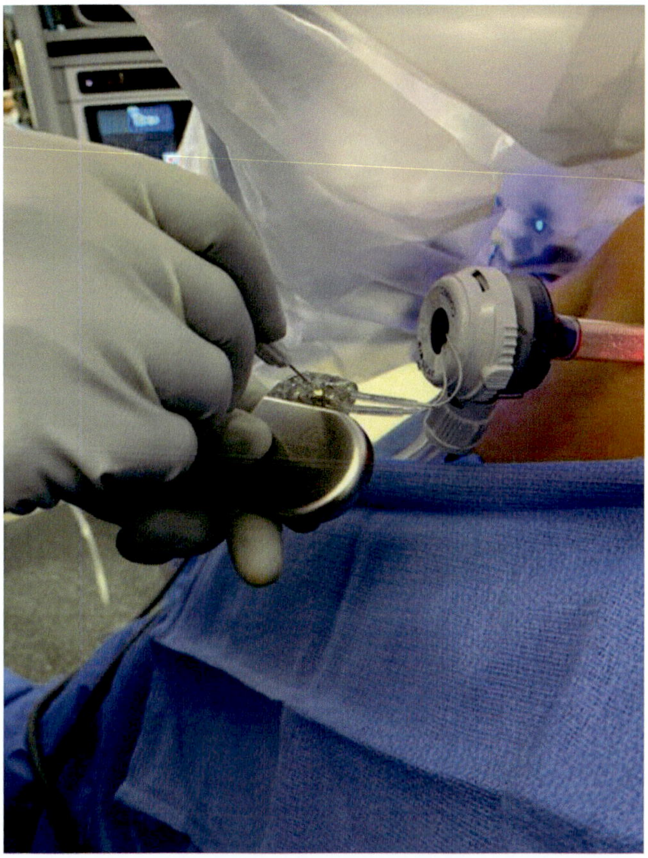

Fig. 5.17 Leads are then secured in place using the provided torque wrench. All four screws are tightened through the holes in the plastic generator housing. The torque wrench prevents overtightening of the screws

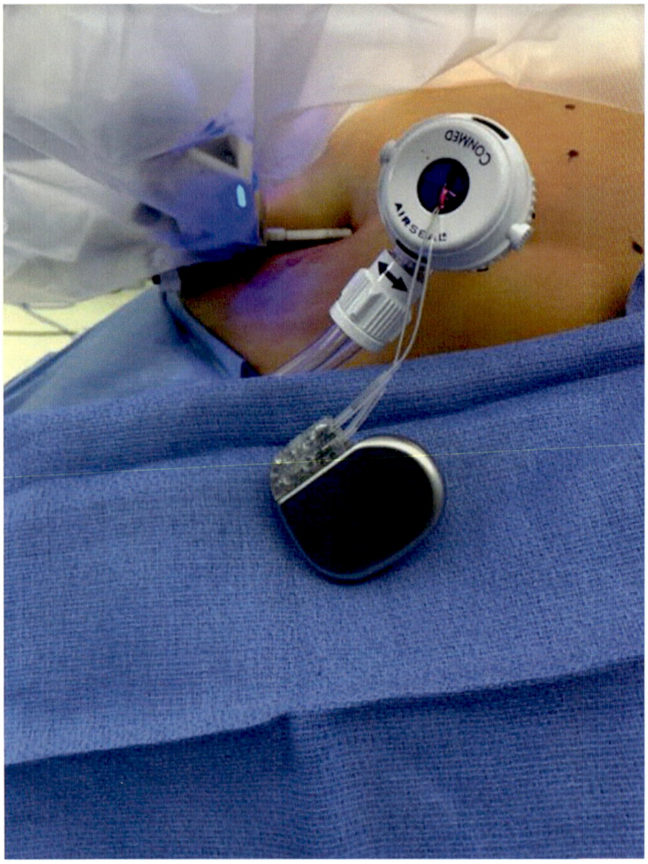

Fig. 5.18 The leads are gently tugged to confirm they are securely anchored to the generator

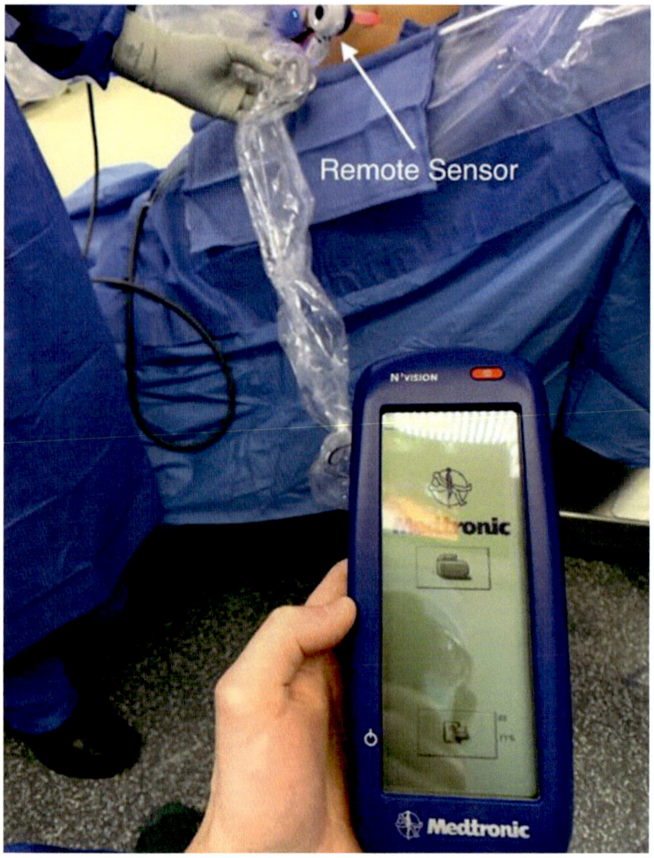

Fig. 5.19 The paddle of the programming device is then placed into a transparent, sterile cover and introduced into the surgical field. The paddle of the programmer is placed in contact with the neurostimulator generator. (The entire programmer can also be sterilely prepped into the field and controlled by the bedside assistant)

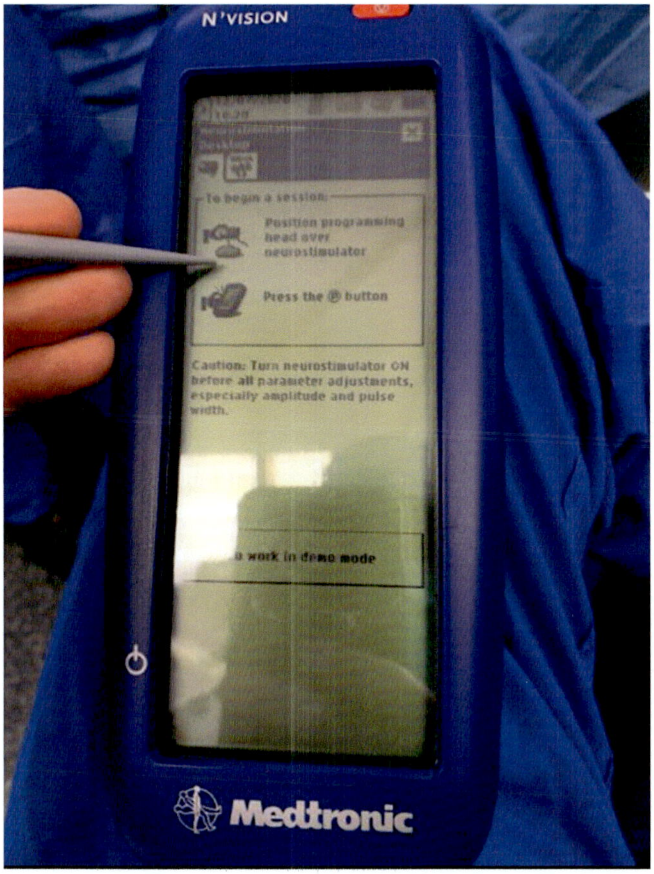

Fig. 5.20 Slide the "P" button on the side of the programmer to turn it on

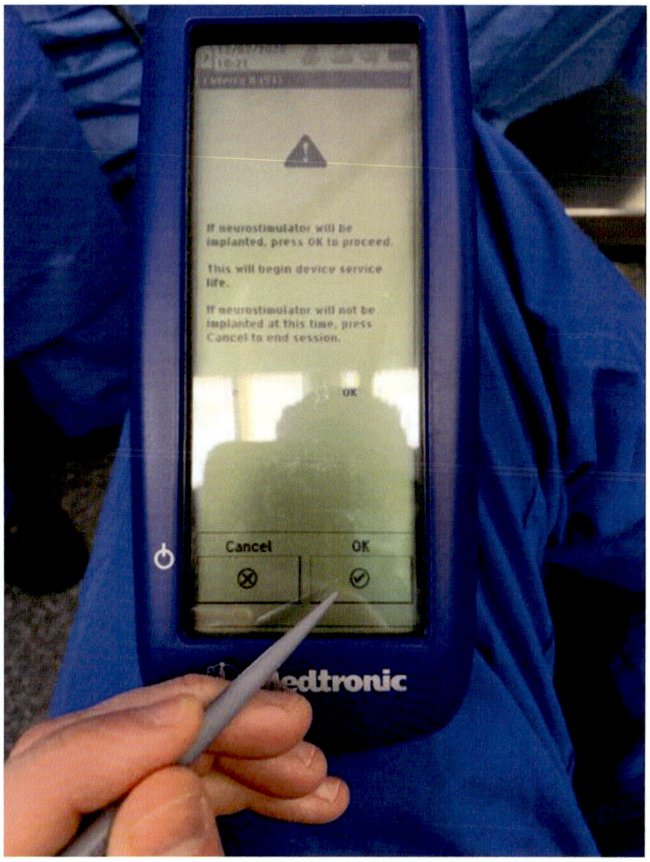

Fig. 5.21 Tap the "OK" icon to begin the diagnostic check

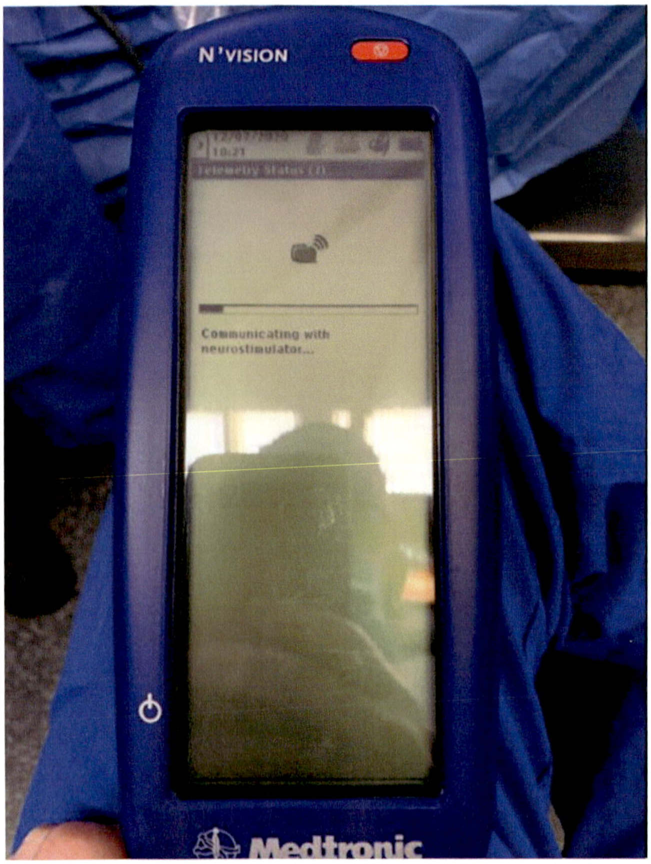

Fig. 5.22 The programmer will take a few moments to communicate with the neurostimulator generator

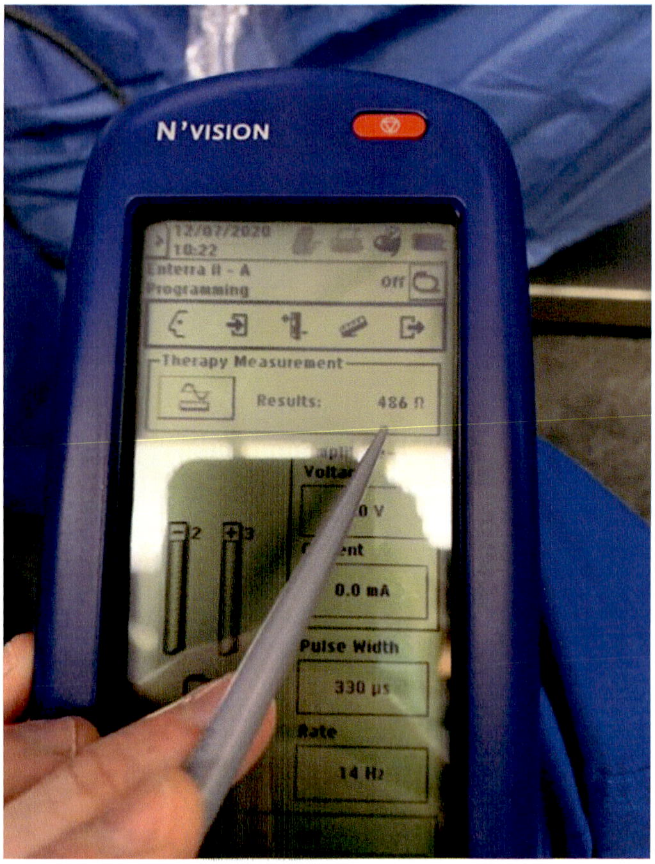

Fig. 5.23 Impedance through the circuit is checked. Leads are properly placed when the impedance is between 200 and 800 ohms

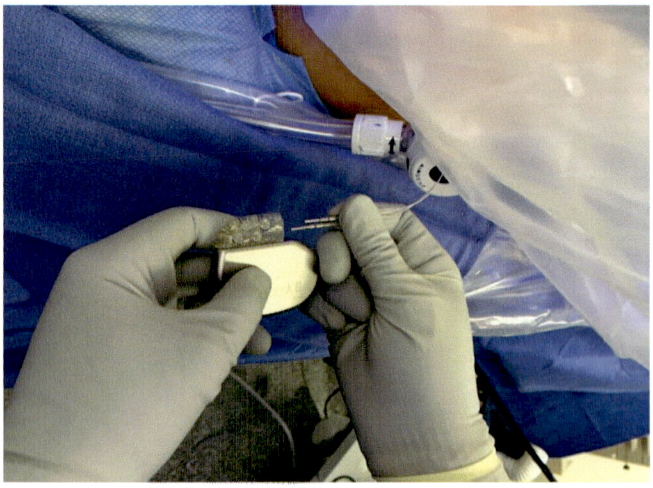

Fig. 5.24 Once these checks are successful, the neurostimulator leads can be secured to the gastric wall. The leads are then unscrewed from the stimulator using the torque wrench

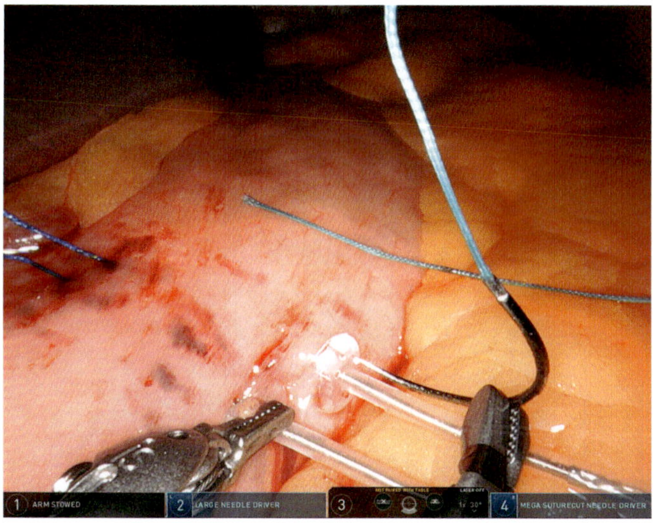

Fig. 5.25 Next, the silicone flanges of the two leads are secured to the gastric wall. This is performed by placing interrupted 2-0 Ethibond™ sutures between a serosal bite of the stomach wall and through the provided holes in the flanges. Care must be taken to avoid damage to the tunneled leads when placing these sutures

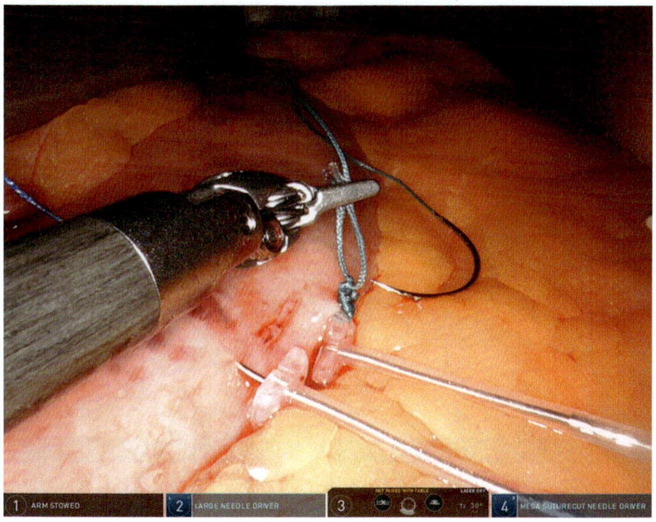

Fig. 5.26 Shown is the cranial stitch being placed for the proximal gastric lead

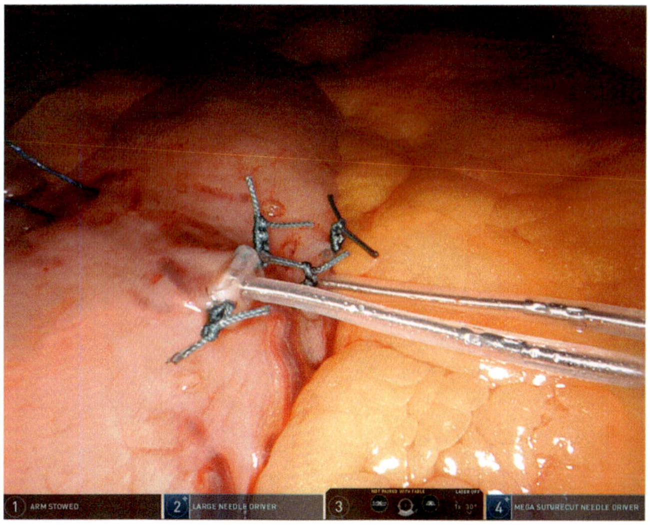

Fig. 5.27 Completed image showing all securing stitches placed through the flanges

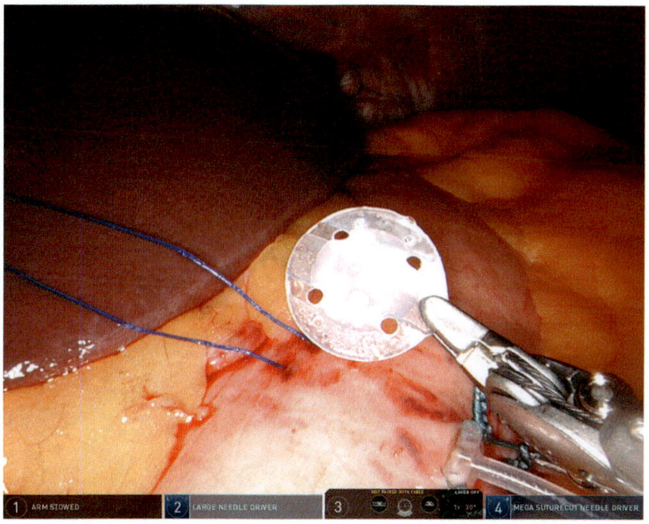

Fig. 5.28 The leads are further secured at their distal ends where they exit the stomach wall. The provided silicone discs are used for this purpose

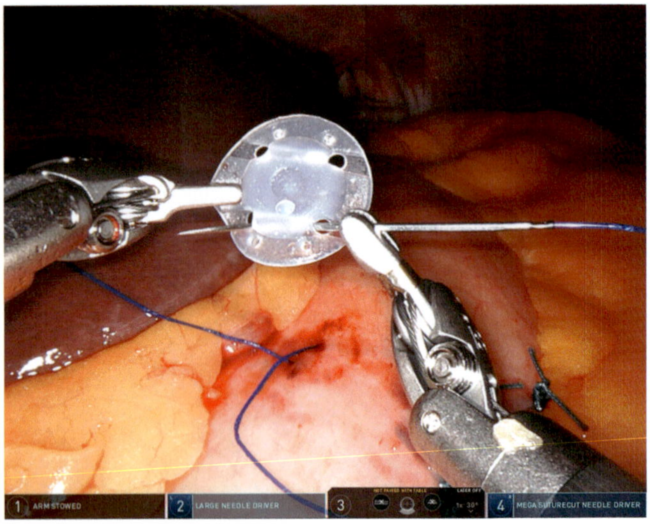

Fig. 5.29 The gastric neurostimulator ski needle is passed through the discs as shown, threading the Prolene suture portion of the lead through the appropriate holes

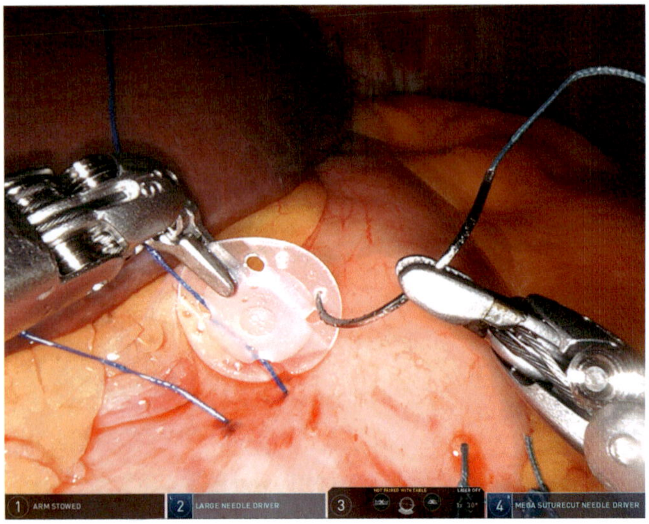

Fig. 5.30 The disc is then secured to the anterior stomach wall. Additional 2-0 Ethibond suture is placed through the provided side holes of the disc and then to the stomach wall using a serosal bite

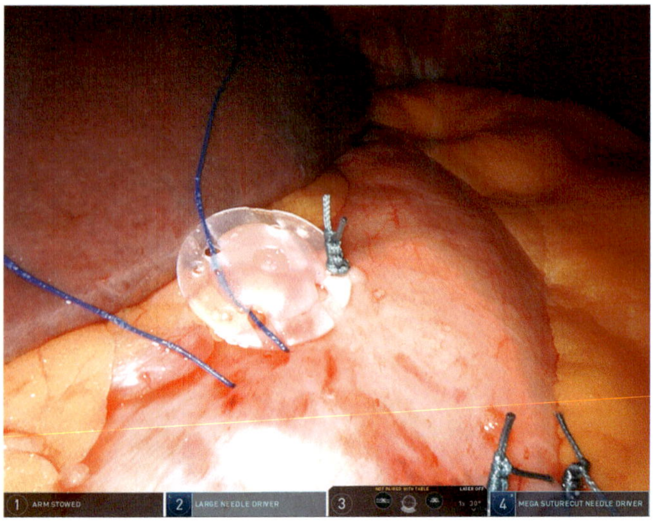

Fig. 5.31 Completed fixation of the disc to the anterior gastric wall is shown

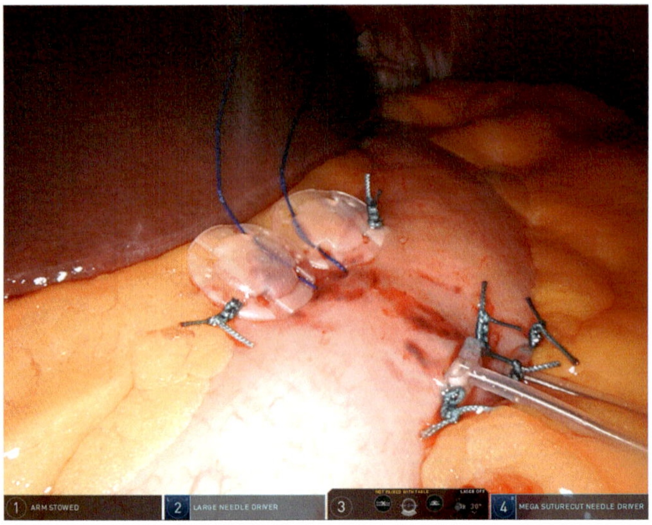

Fig. 5.32 The process is then repeated with the other neurostimulator lead using another silicone disc. The disc is secured away from the first one

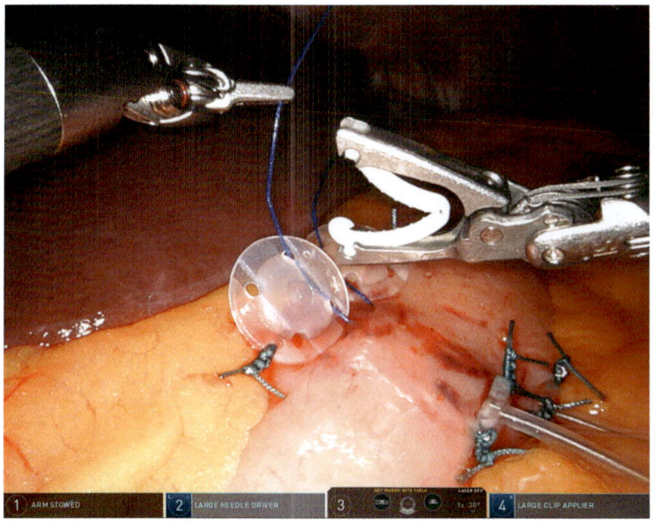

Fig. 5.33 A robotic clip applier is then used to further secure the leads where the Prolene suture portion exits the silicone discs

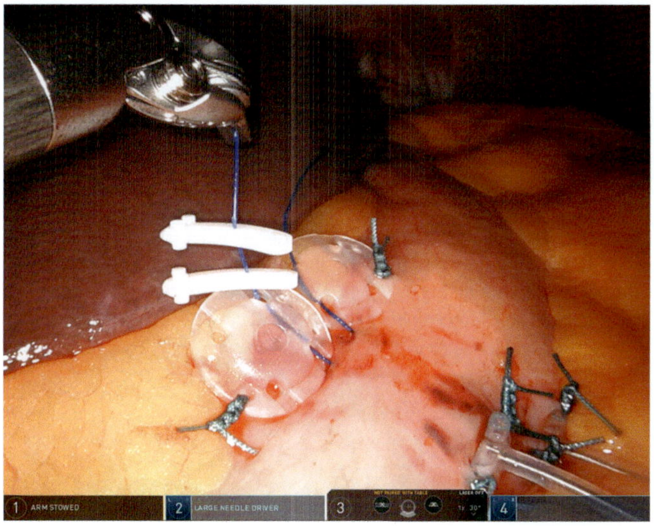

Fig. 5.34 Two clips are placed on each Prolene suture, close to where it exits the silicone disc

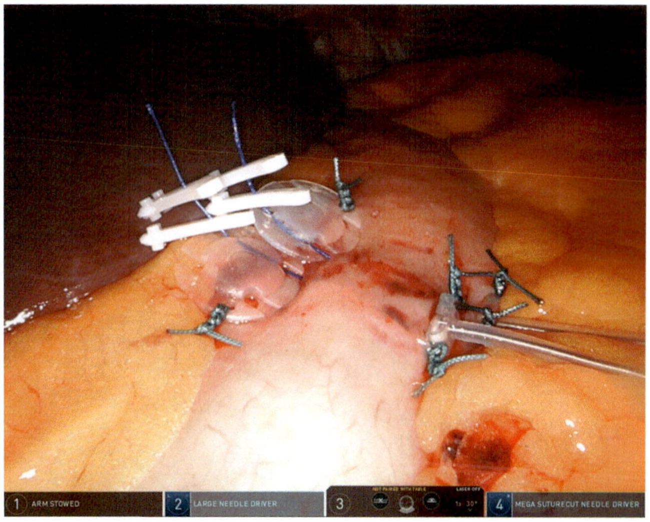

Fig. 5.35 The two ski needles are then cut off the suture and removed from the abdomen. Completed placement of the two gastric neurostimulator leads is shown. This concludes the robotic portion of the procedure

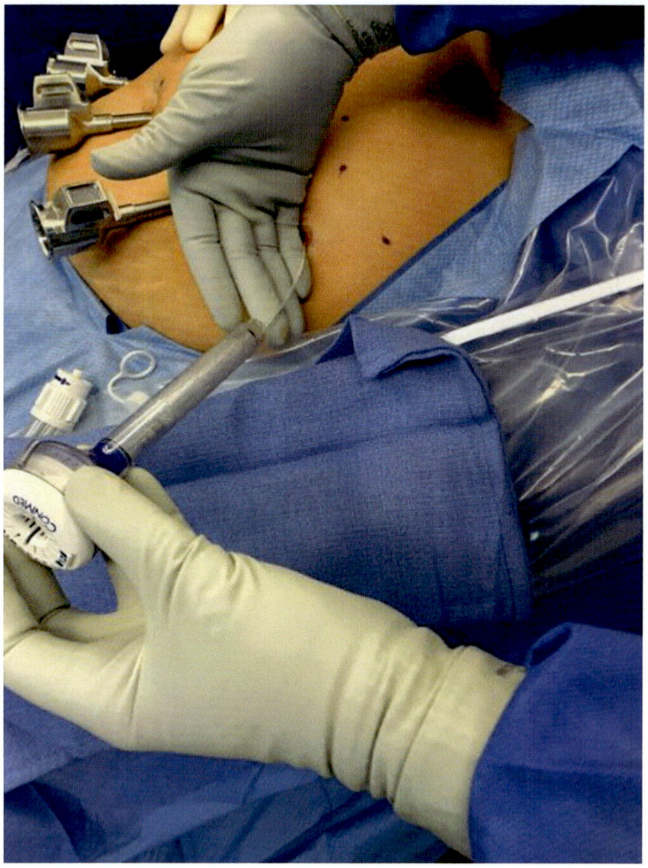

Fig. 5.36 The robot is undocked from the patient, pneumoperitoneum is released, and the 12 mm assistant trocar is carefully removed leaving the ends of the leads outside of the patient's body

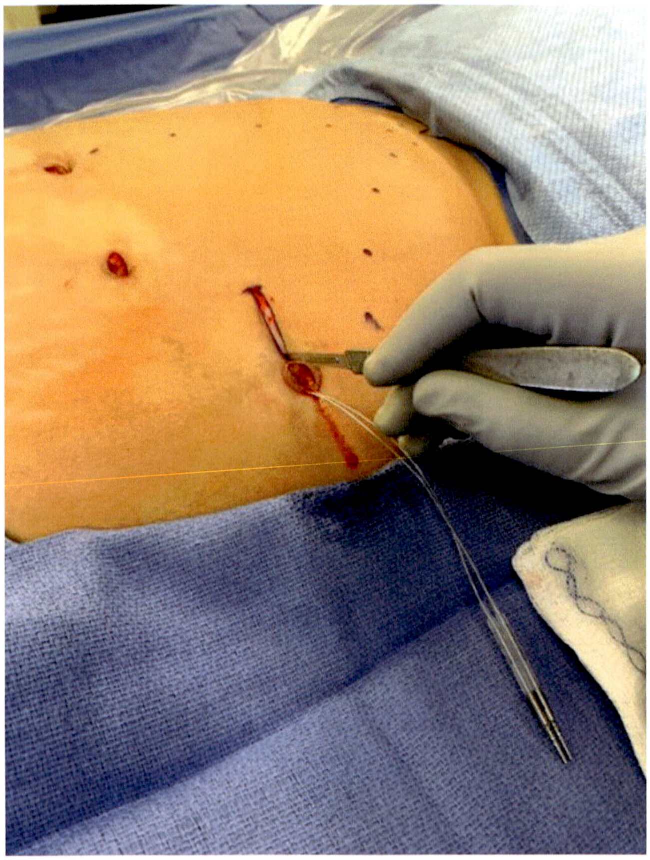

Fig. 5.37 The generator pocket is then prepared. The 12 mm trocar site incision is extended medially to 4 cm in length

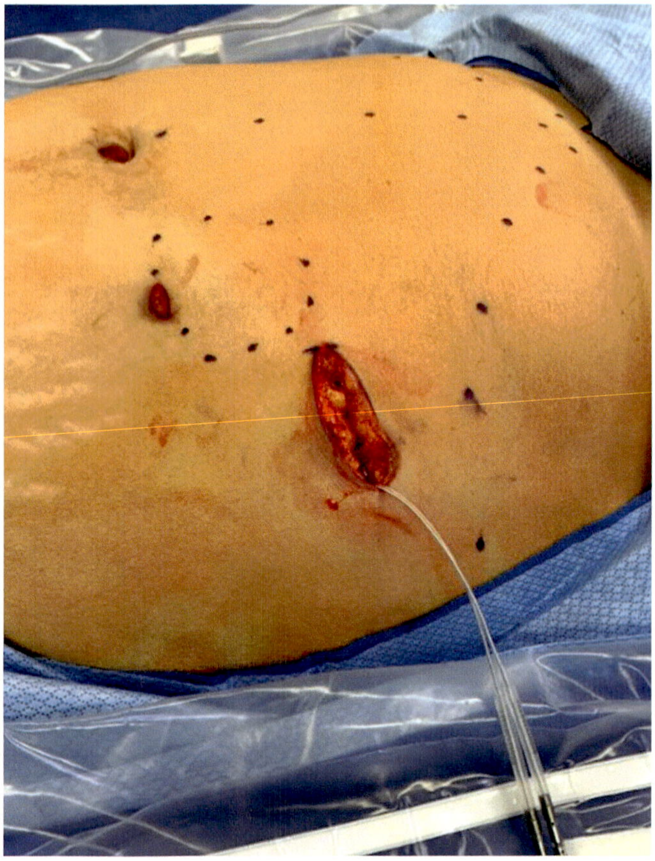

Fig. 5.38 Monopolar electrosurgical energy must *not* be used at any point in the remaining portion of the procedure. Current may travel through the leads causing stomach wall thermal injury or damaging the leads themselves. Hemostasis may be achieved with simple direct pressure or a bipolar forceps device

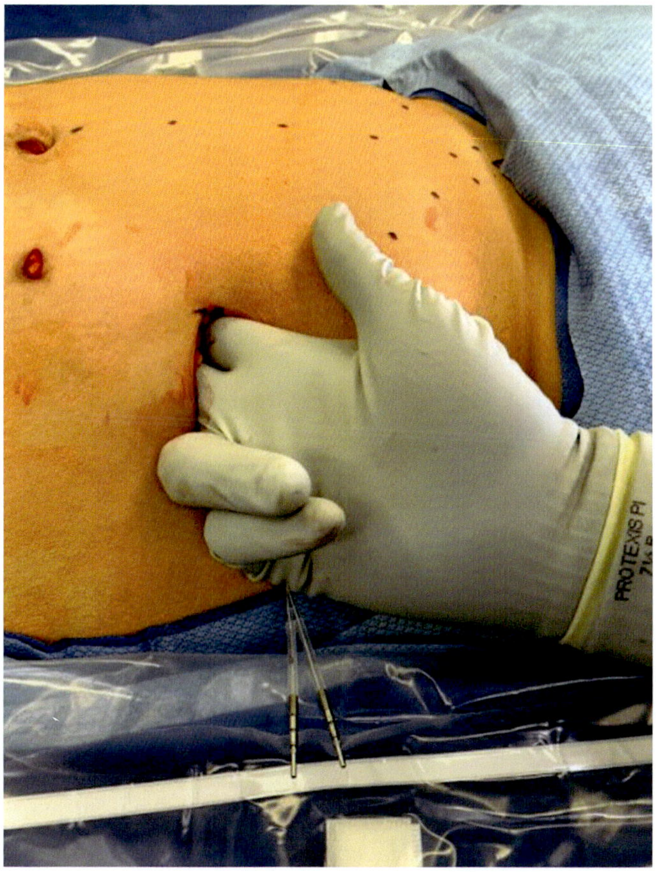

Fig. 5.39 Blunt dissection is performed on top of the anterior fascia to create a pocket for the neurostimulator generator. The pocket should not be made too large or else the generator will be free to rotate or flip

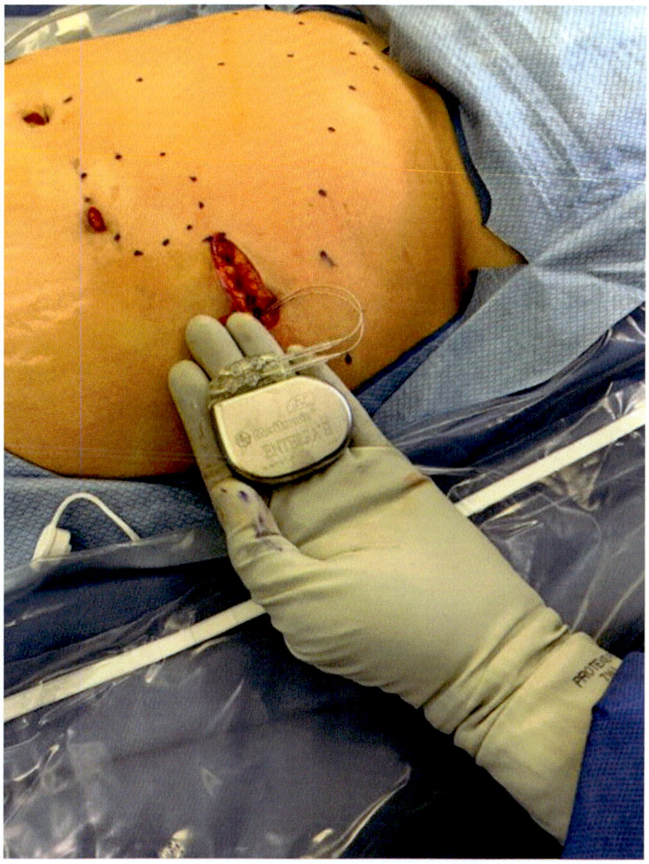

Fig. 5.40 Neurostimulator leads are then reattached to the generator and secured with the provided torque wrench

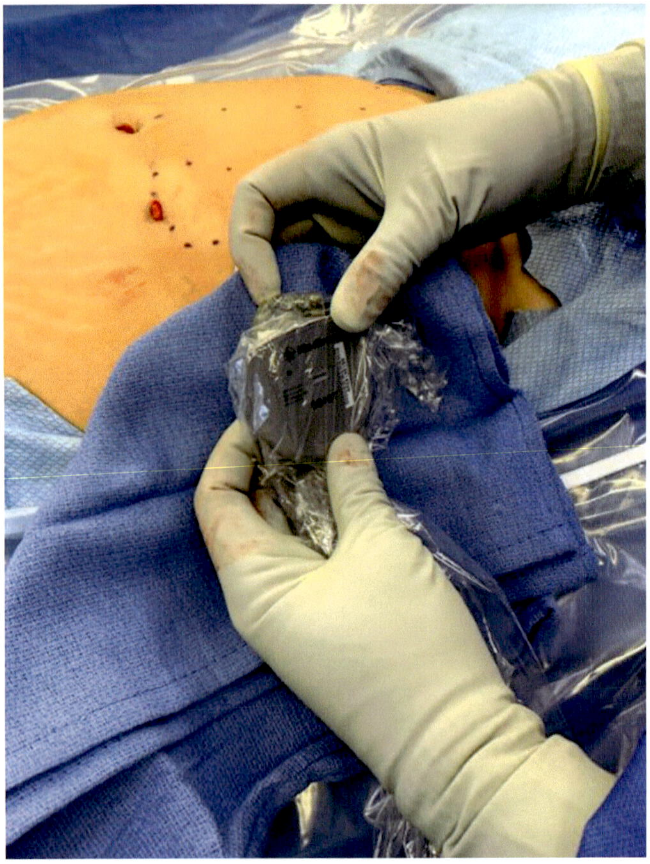

Fig. 5.41 The neurostimulator is once again checked for proper function by placing the programmer paddle over the generator

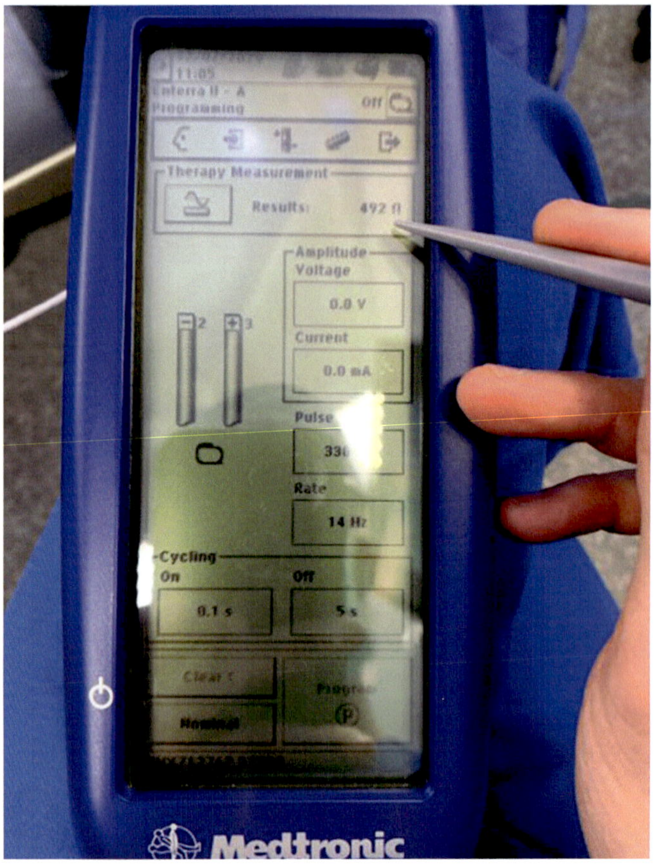

Fig. 5.42 The impedance is confirmed to be between 200 and 800 ohms

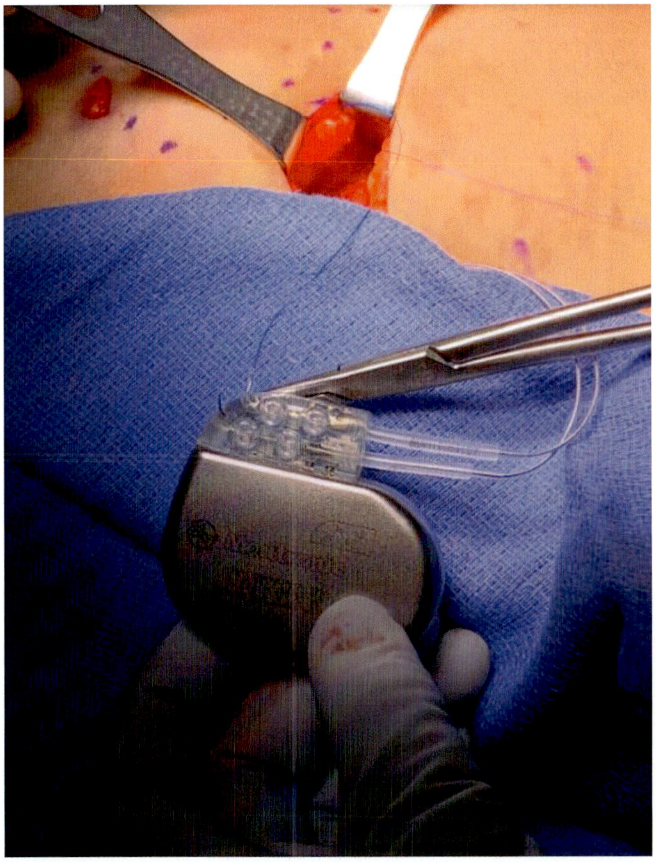

Fig. 5.43 The generator is next introduced into the pocket and secured. A 2-0 Prolene stitch is first placed through the provided holes in the plastic generator housing. Careful attention must be used at all times to avoid inadvertent damage to the leads

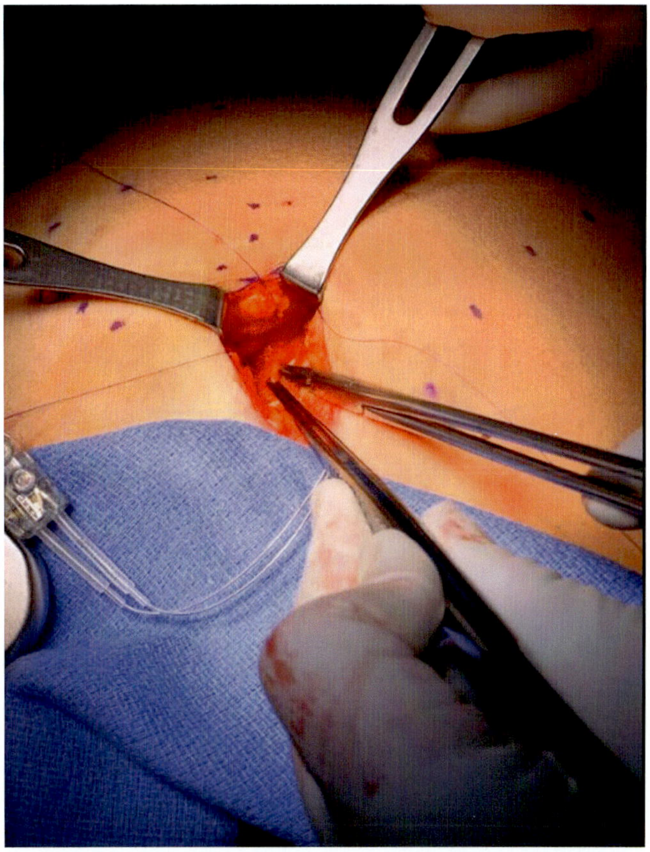

Fig. 5.44 The Prolene stitch is then placed through the anterior fascia inside the pocket where the generator is to be secured

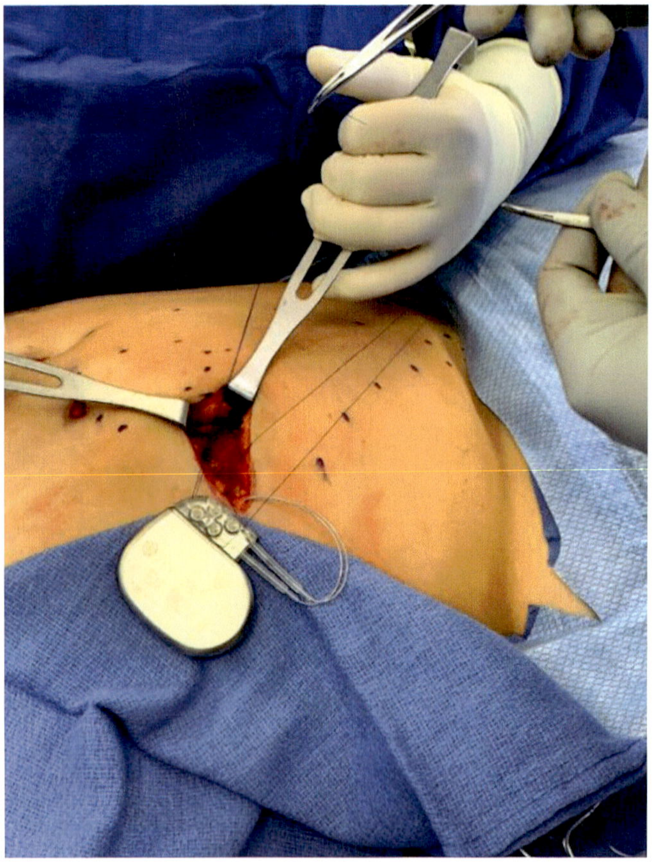

Fig. 5.45 A second 2-0 Prolene stitch is similarly placed through the other provided hole and to the fascia. These stitches secure the generator to the pocket and prevent it from flipping or rotating. The generator is then gently introduced into the pocket while the sutures are parachuted down along with it

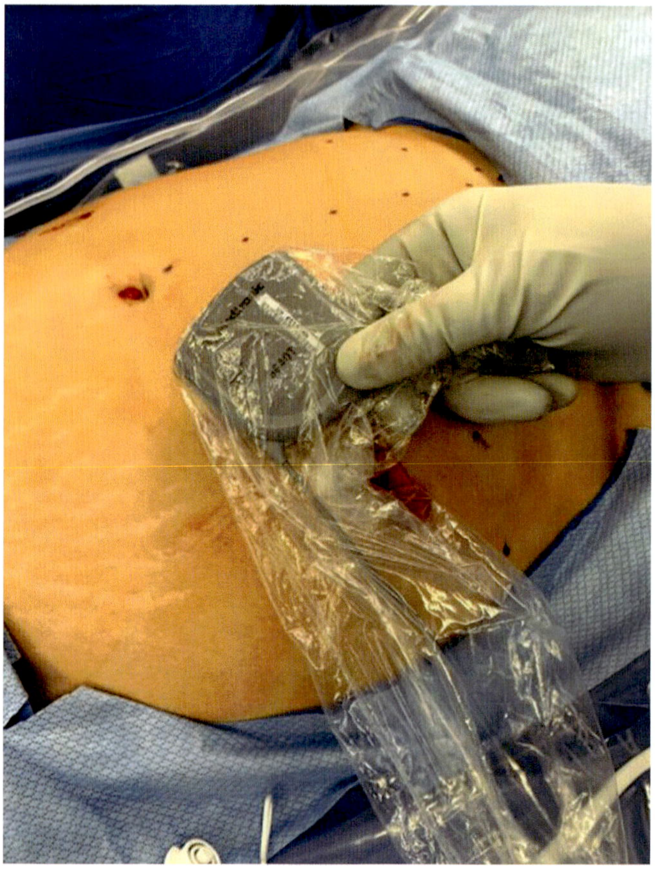

Fig. 5.46 The neurostimulator is then once again interrogated through the skin for proper function once it is in its final position in the subcutaneous pocket

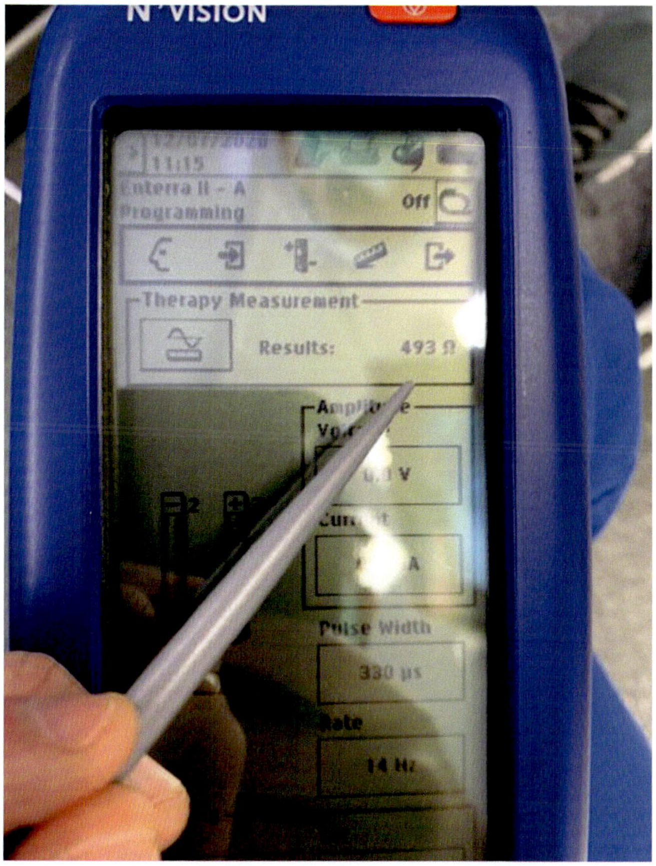

Fig. 5.47 During this third and final check, the impedance is once again confirmed to be within range and the neurostimulator is turned at its nominal settings

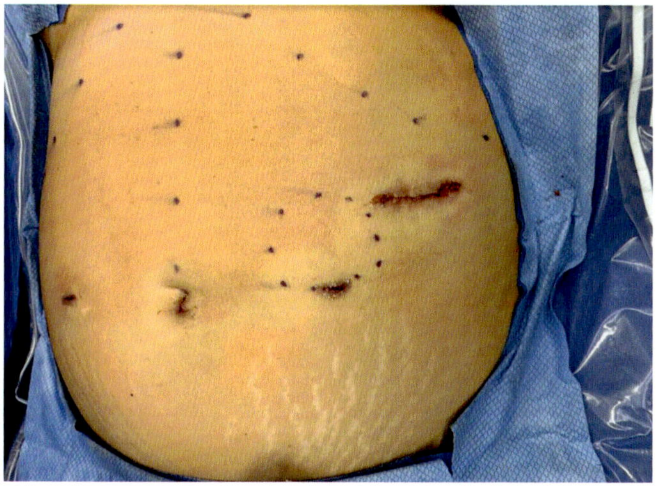

Fig. 5.48 Incisions are then closed using absorbable, running subcuticular suture and dressed

References

1. Mason RJ, Lipham J, Eckerling G, et al. Gastric electrical stimulation; an alternative surgical therapy for patients with gastroparesis. Arch Surg. 2005;140(9):841–8.
2. Fonseca Mora MC, Milla Matute CA, Aleman R, et al. Medical and surgical management of gastroparesis: a systematic review. Surg Obes Relat Dis. 2020:1–16. Online.
3. Revicki DA, Rentz AM, Dubois D, et al. Gastroparesis Cardinal Symptom Index (GCSI): development and validation of a patient reported assessment of severity of gastroparesis symptoms. Qual Life Res. 2004;13(4):833–44.

Robotic Paraconduit Hernia

6

Ashwini S. Poola, Torjborg Holtestaul, Laila Rashidi, and Prakash Gatta

Introduction

Diaphragmatic hernia following esophagectomy is a known yet rare complication. Hiatal enlargement during esophagectomy to allow for passage of gastric conduit can be a predisposing factor for the development of paraconduit hernias [1]. Paraconduit hernias following esophagectomy are increasingly common in the era of minimally invasive esophagectomy when compared to hybrid or open techniques. While the majority are asymptomatic and noted radiographically, symptoms warrant consideration of surgical repair. There are growing series advocating for a minimally invasive approach to repair [2].

As in standard hiatal hernia repair, the robotic approach to paraconduit repair offers advantages over laparoscopy [3, 4]. Visualization and identification of structures in the re-operative setting can be difficult; the robotic platform allows for careful identification of the gastric conduit and vascular supply. This is paramount when taking down adhesive bands between the conduit, the conduit's blood supply, and adjacent structures within the mediastinum. The utility of articulating instruments allows for an ergonomic approach to closing hiatal defects and precise placement of mesh and tension relieving measures on the crura.

When performing a paraconduit repair, the first step is identification of the gastric conduit, the gastro-epiploic artery or vascular pedicle, and the right and left crura. The firefly mode and injection of indocyanine green (ICG) can be used to identify the right gastro-epiploic artery and a safe dissection plane. Oftentimes, there is no discernible hernia sac in a paraconduit hernia. Both crura must be cleared of attachments to allow for a tension-free closure; this may include releasing the caudate lobe carefully from the right crura or creating relaxing incisions on the diaphragm. ICG can be again utilized to assess for hypoperfusion of the crura after suturing. Mesh is placed to reinforce the crural closure and sutured in place.

Procedures: Illustrated Steps

Figures 6.1, 6.2, 6.3, 6.4, 6.5, 6.6, 6.7, 6.8, 6.9, 6.10, 6.11, 6.12, 6.13, 6.14, 6.15, 6.16, 6.17, 6.18, 6.19, 6.20, 6.21, and 6.22 illustrate the technical aspects of robotic paraconduit hernia repair with mesh placement.

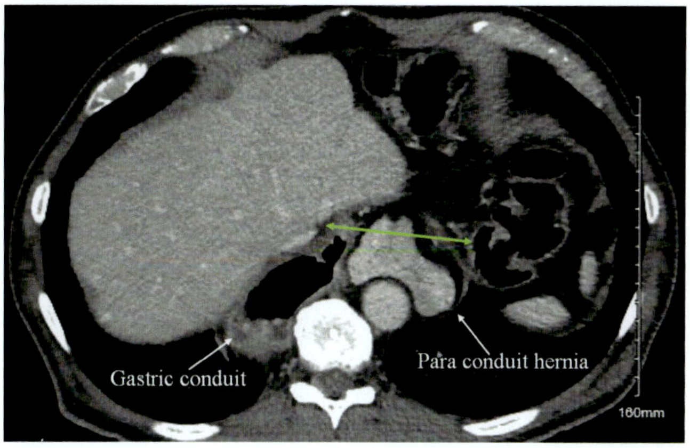

Fig. 6.1 Computed tomography (CT) chest transverse image. Level of the diaphragmatic hiatus. Paraconduit hiatal hernia of small intestine. Hiatal opening noted by green arrow

A. S. Poola · T. Holtestaul · P. Gatta (✉)
Department of Surgery, Multicare Health System, Tacoma, WA, USA
e-mail: prakash.gatta@wsu.edu

L. Rashidi
MultiCare Colon and Rectal Surgery – Tacoma Clinic, Tacoma, WA, USA

O. Y. Kudsi, P. P. Grimminger (eds.), *Atlas of Robotic Upper Gastrointestinal Surgery*,
https://doi.org/10.1007/978-3-030-86578-8_6

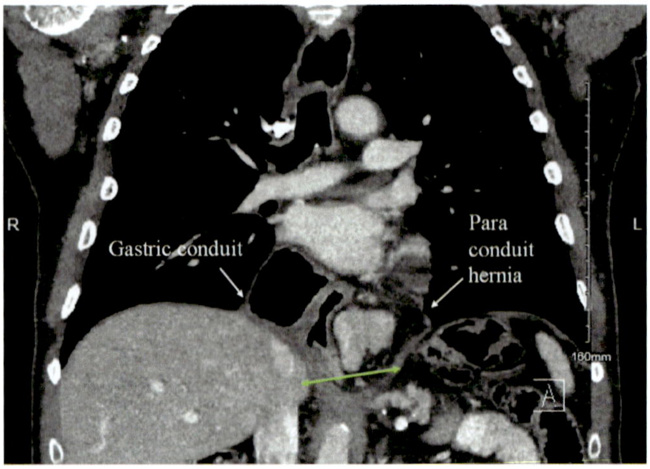

Fig. 6.2 Computed tomography (CT) chest coronal image. Level of the diaphragmatic hiatus. Paraconduit hiatal hernia of small intestine. Hiatal opening noted by green arrow

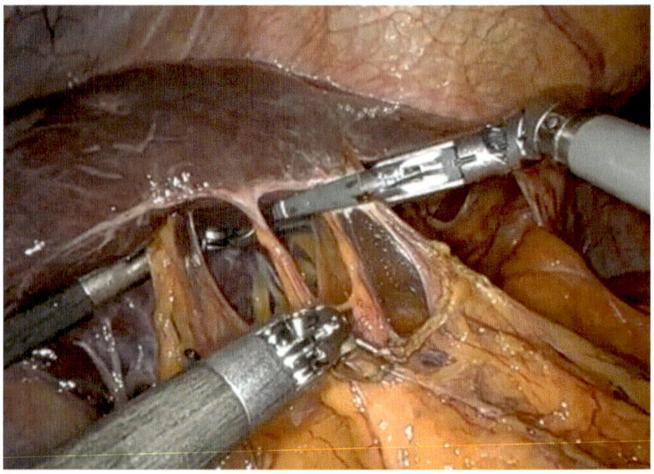

Fig. 6.5 Exposure. The short grasper is used as liver retractor. The vessel sealer is used to lyse adhesions between the liver and the previously mobilized duodenum and gastric conduit

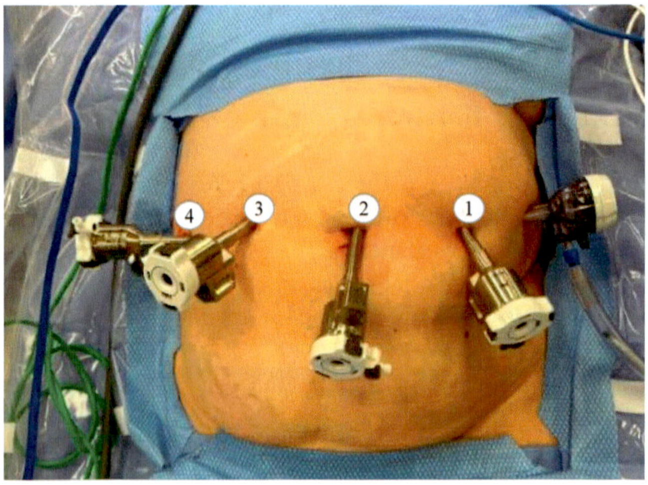

Fig. 6.3 Port placement. Arm 1: Vessel sealer. Arm 2: Camera. Arm 3: Fenestrated bipolar grasper. Arm 4: Short grasper used as liver retractor. 11 mm assist port

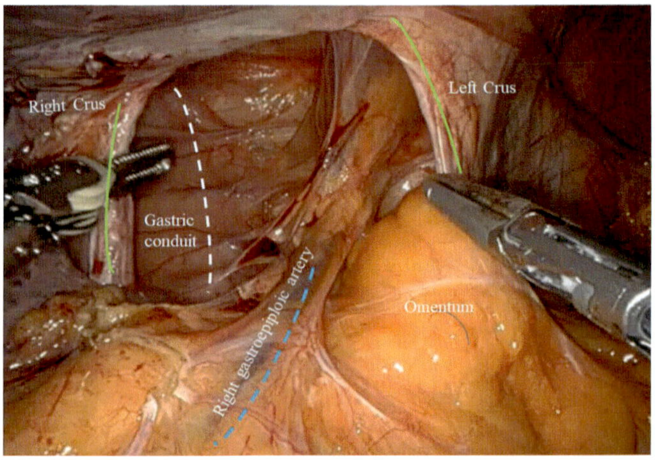

Fig. 6.6 Structure identification. Gastric conduit, right gastroepiploic artery and hernia contents are identified. Omentum is seen adjacent to the gastric conduit

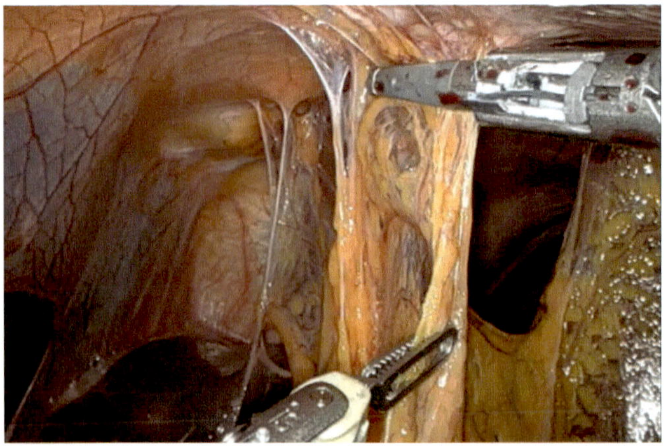

Fig. 6.4 Adhesiolysis. With revisional surgery, careful abdominal entry along with precise lysis of adhesions. The vessel sealer can be used for both sharp and thermal lyses

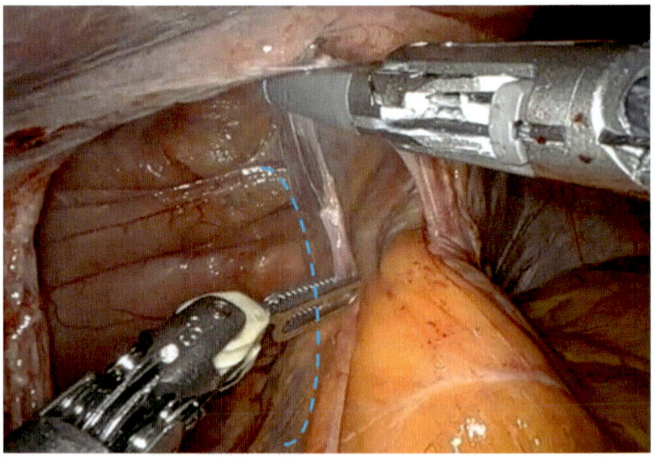

Fig. 6.7 Mediastinal dissection: Careful lysis of adhesions between conduit and mediastinum. Be mindful of the R. gastroepiploic artery/ conduit blood supply (blue dotted line)

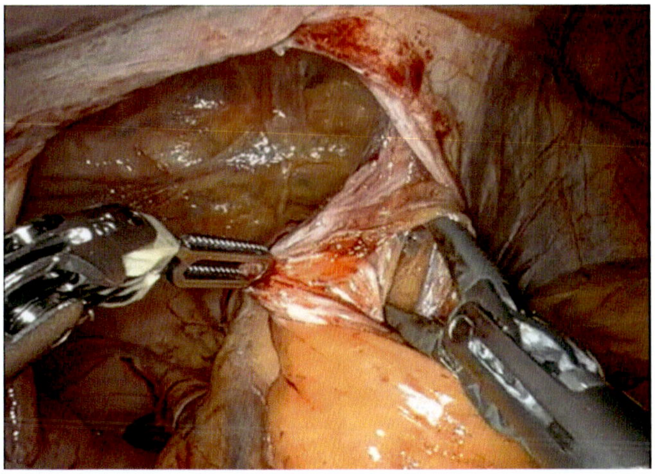

Fig. 6.8 Mediastinal dissection: Of note, paraconduit hernias do not have a defined hernia sac

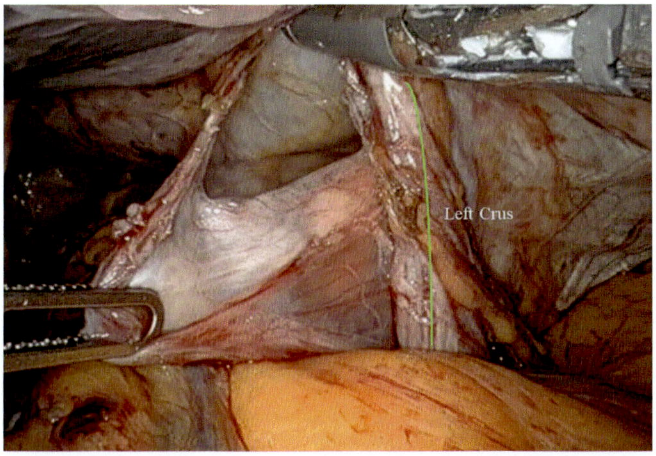

Fig. 6.9 Mediastinal dissection: Clear crura of attachments that may limit closure

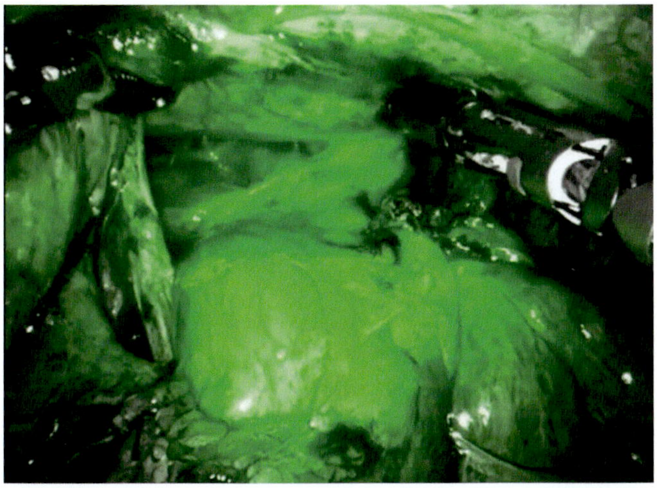

Fig. 6.10 Injection of intraoperative indocyanine green (ICG) is used to identify the conduit vascular supply and conduit perfusion

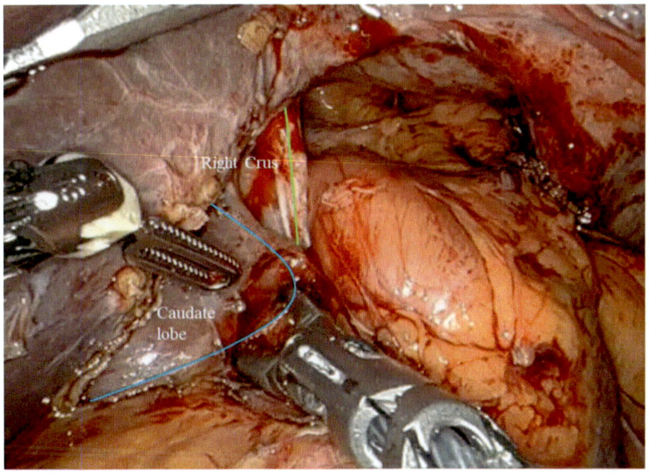

Fig. 6.11 Right crural dissection: Clearing the caudate lobe can be crucial to allow for less tension on the right crura during closure

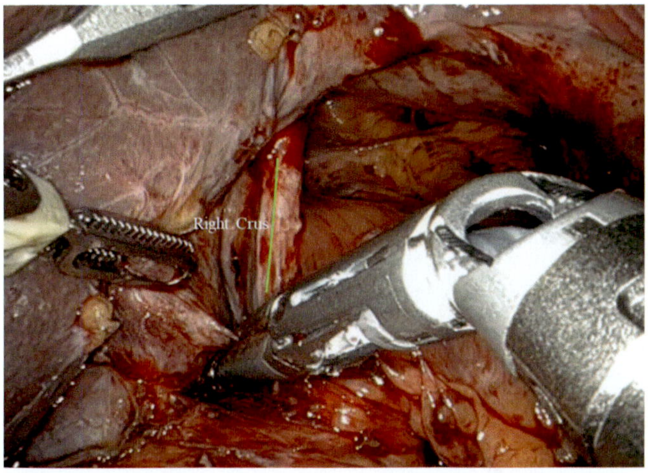

Fig. 6.12 Right crural dissection: Clearing the right crura of attachments

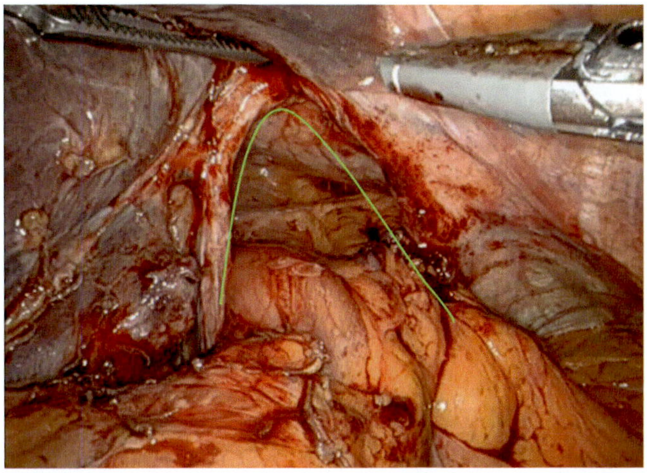

Fig. 6.13 Crural closure. The liver retractor is repositioned to grasp the apex of the hiatus and create a V-shaped opening for an anterior repair

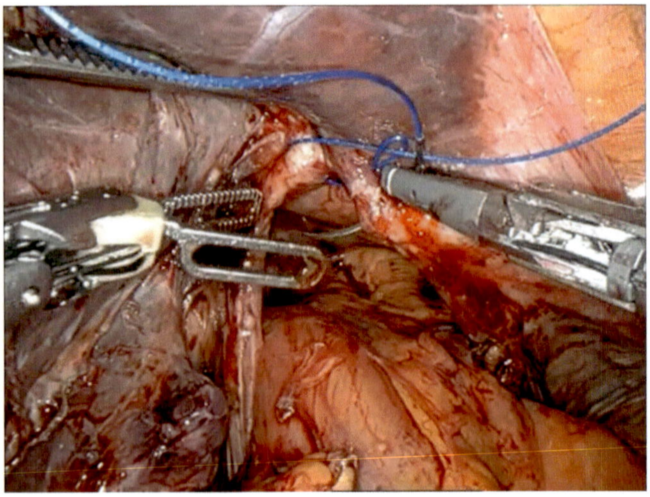

Fig. 6.14 Crural closure. Anterior closure is performed to decrease injury to the gastric conduit

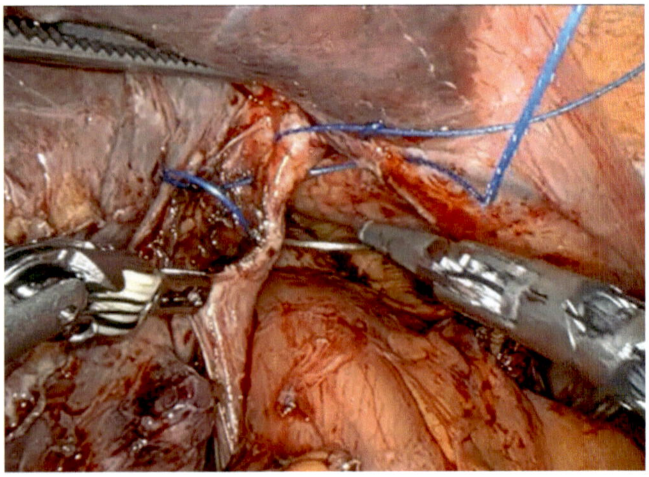

Fig. 6.15 Crural closure. Anterior closure is performed with a non-absorbable 0 V-Loc suture in a running horizontal mattress fashion

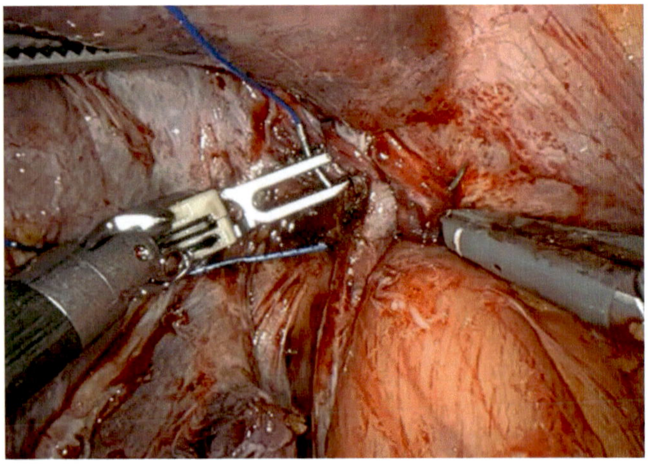

Fig. 6.16 Crural closure. The same V-lok suture is used to run back over the closure

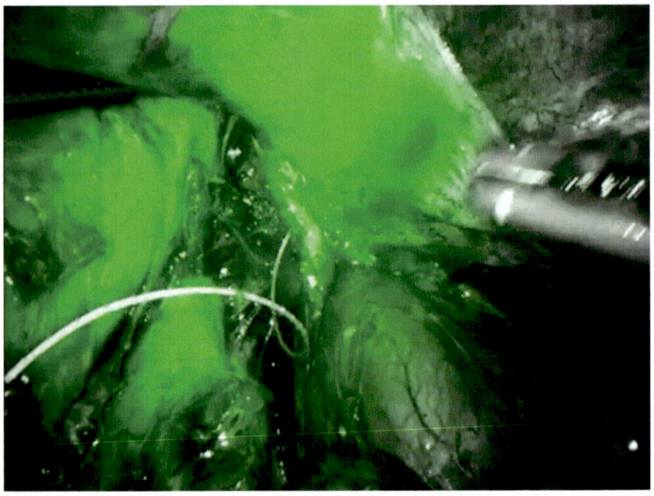

Fig. 6.17 Crural closure. ICG is utilized to assess for muscular ischemia post-closure. Crura are noted to be well-perfused bilaterally

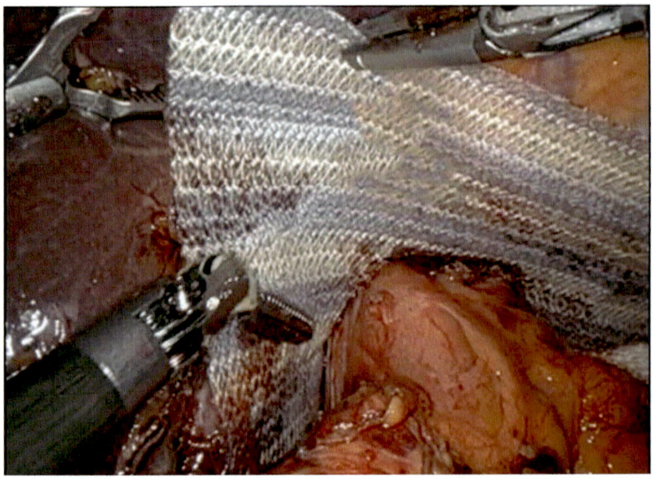

Fig. 6.18 Mesh Placement. Phasix ST Mesh is pre-cut with keyhole defect and tucked under the caudate lobe

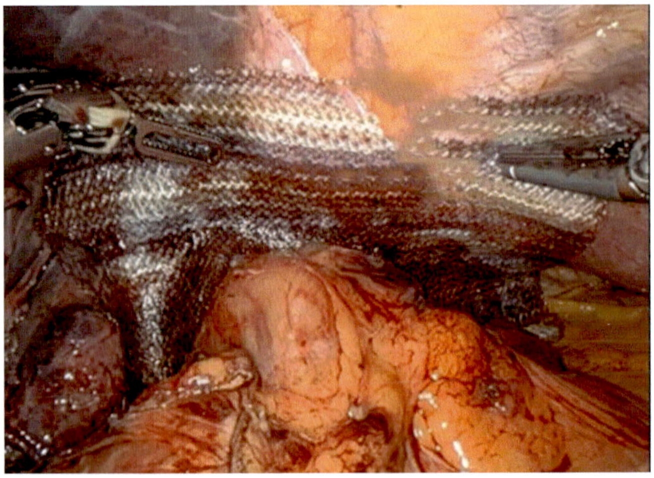

Fig. 6.19 Mesh Placement. Phasix ST Mesh is placed anteriorly in upside-down U to buttress crural closure

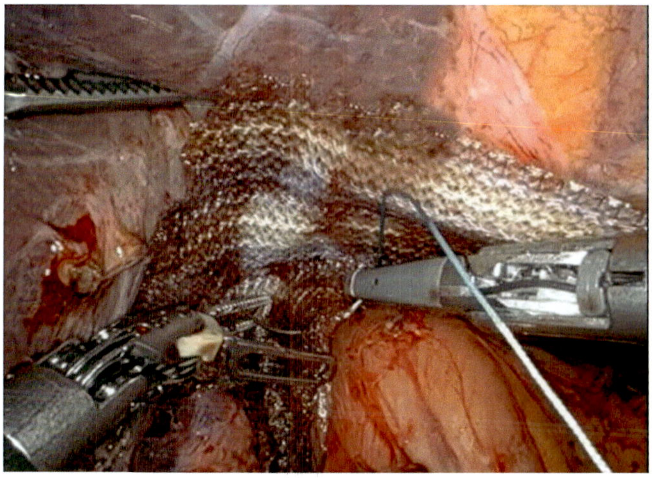

Fig. 6.20 Mesh Placement. Mesh is fixed in place with a 2-0 Ethibond stitch at three points. One simple stitch at the crural closure and medially

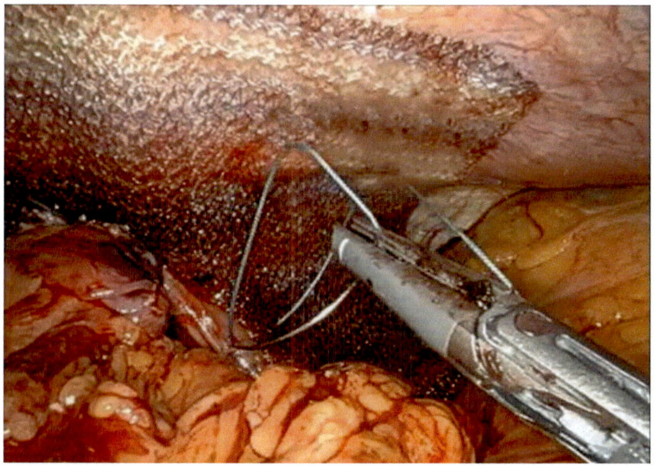

Fig. 6.21 Mesh Placement. Mesh is fixed in place with a 2-0 Ethibond stitch at three points. One simple stitch is placed laterally, taking care to not to injure the pericardium

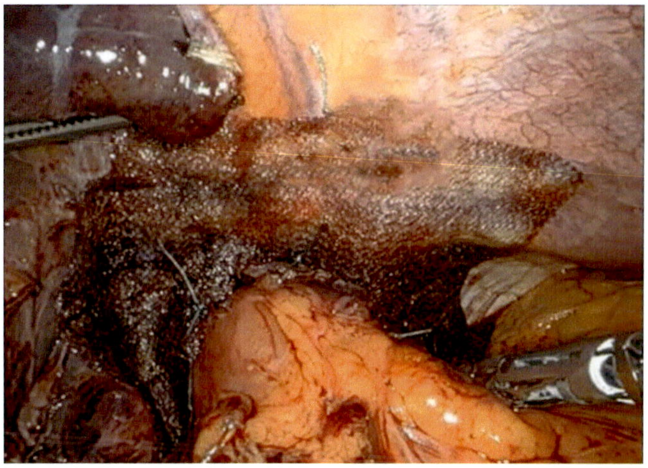

Fig. 6.22 Post repair. Gastric conduit in position with reduced herniated contents

References

1. Ganeshan DM, Correa AM, Bhosale P, Vaporciyan AA, Rice D, Mehran RJ, Walsh GL, Iyer R, Roth JA, Swisher SG, Hofstetter WL. Diaphragmatic hernia after esophagectomy in 440 patients with long-term follow-up. Ann Thorac Surg. 2013;96:1138–45. https://doi.org/10.1016/j.athoracsur.2013.04.076.
2. Lung K, Carroll PA, Rogalla P, Yeung J, Darling G. Paraconduit hernia in the era of minimally invasive esophagectomy: underdiagnosed? Ann Thorac Surg. 2020; https://doi.org/10.1016/j.athoracsur.2020.07.047.
3. O'Connor SC, Mallard M, Desai SS, Couto F, Gottlieb M, Ewing A, Cobb WS, Carbonell AM, Warren JA. Robotic versus laparoscopic approach to hiatal hernia repair: results after 7 years of robotic experience. Am Surg. 2020;86(9):1083–7. https://doi.org/10.1177/0003134820943547. Epub 2020 Aug 18. PMID: 32809844.
4. Gerull WD, Cho D, Kuo I, Arefanian S, Kushner BS, Awad MM. Robotic approach to paraesophageal hernia repair results in low long-term recurrence rate and beneficial patient-centered outcomes. J Am Coll Surg. 2020;231(5):520–6. https://doi.org/10.1016/j.jamcollsurg.2020.07.754. Epub 2020 Aug 3. PMID: 32758533.

Robotic Partial Fundoplication and Hiatal Hernia Repair

7

Frank J. Voskens, Jelle P. Ruurda, and Ivo A. M. J. Broeders

Introduction

The da Vinci surgical robot is increasingly applied as a clinically safe technique in the surgical treatment of large paraesophageal hernias [1, 2]. Robotic-assisted repair of large and recurrent hiatal hernias remains a technically demanding procedure and consists of some challenging key steps [3]. A successful robotic-assisted (para)esophageal hernia repair should be performed according to the following three principles: (1) complete reduction of the stomach and hernia sac with extensive mediastinal dissection to optimize esophageal length, (2) primary closure of the crus using nonabsorbable sutures, and (3) the addition of a fundoplication. The emphasis of this chapter lies on these specific key steps. Furthermore we would like to emphasize the importance of a dedicated surgical team. Understanding the robotic system and necessary steps during this procedure provides proper positioning, optimal surgical exposure, and workflow and increases efficiency.

In this chapter we present a case of an elderly patient with a large paraesophageal hernia. Preoperative symptoms included early satiety, nausea, vomiting, and atrial arrhythmias. The patient was planned for robotic hiatal hernia repair with an anterior 180° partial fundoplication. Various modifications have been described in the literature on hiatal hernia repair, including the need for prosthetic reinforcement of the crural repair and the location (anterior or posterior) and/or degree (90–360°) of the fundoplication wrap [3]. An anterior 180° partial fundoplication is currently considered standard treatment in our hospital for patients with large paraesophageal hernias. Reflux is usually not a predominant symptom, and focus is on restoration of anatomy, with an adequate but not exaggerated valve function [3].

Procedure: Illustrated Steps

Figures 7.1, 7.2, 7.3, 7.4, 7.5, 7.6, 7.7, 7.8, 7.9, 7.10, 7.11, 7.12, 7.13, 7.14, 7.15, 7.16, 7.17, 7.18, 7.19, 7.20, 7.21, 7.22, 7.23, 7.24, 7.25, 7.26, 7.27, 7.28, 7.29, 7.30, 7.31, 7.32, 7.33, and 7.34 illustrate the procedure.

F. J. Voskens · Ivo A. M. J. Broeders
Department of Surgery, Meander Medical Center, Amersfoort, The Netherlands

University of Twente, Robotics and Mechatronics, Enschede, The Netherlands

J. P. Ruurda (✉)
Department of Gastro-intestinal and Oncologic Surgery, University Medical Center, Utrecht, The Netherlands
e-mail: J.P.Ruurda@umcutrecht.nl

O. Y. Kudsi, P. P. Grimminger (eds.), *Atlas of Robotic Upper Gastrointestinal Surgery*,
https://doi.org/10.1007/978-3-030-86578-8_7

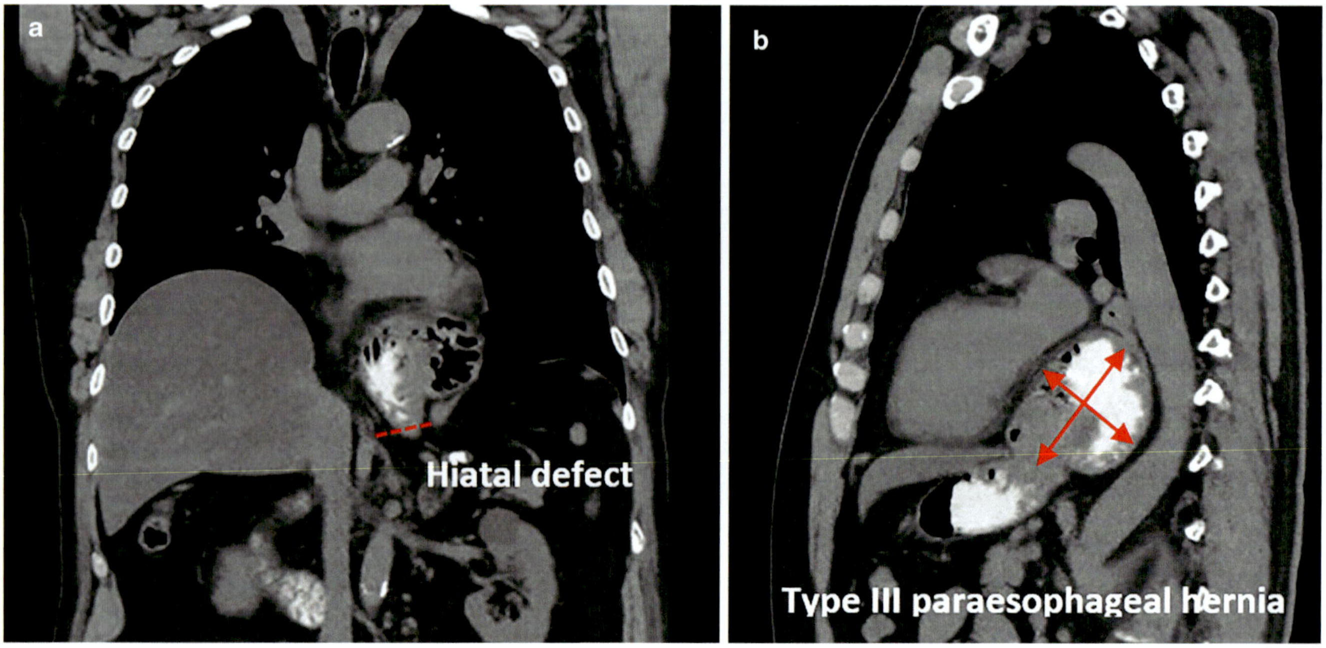

Fig. 7.1 Preoperative view of the computerized tomography (CT) with oral contrast, showing a large type III paraesophageal hiatal hernia

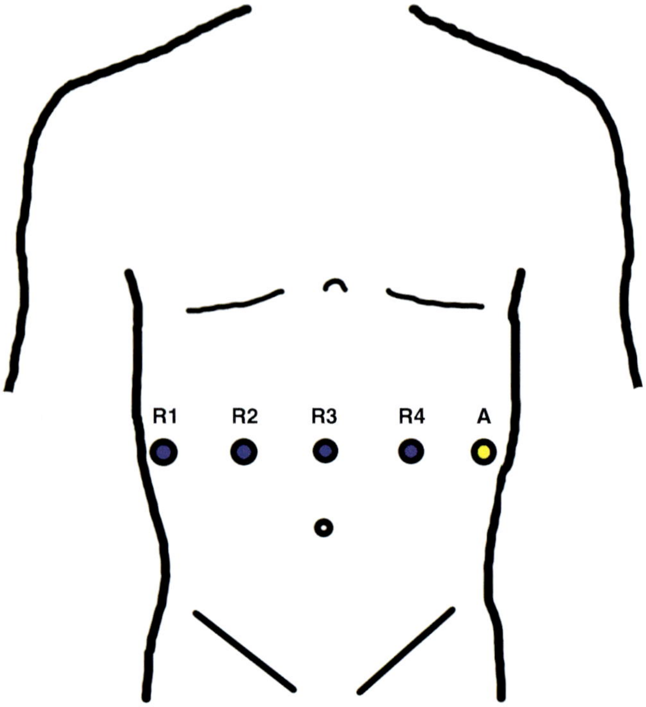

Fig. 7.2 Trocar placement for robotic-assisted transabdominal hiatal hernia repair with the da Vinci Xi. The camera (R3) is placed in a supra-umbilical position, approximately 2/3 the distance from the xiphoid to umbilicus. Subsequently three robotic trocars and one assistant trocar are placed at the same level as the camera port: R1, small grasping retractor (liver retractor); R2, cadiere forceps; R4, cautery hook/suture cut needle driver; A, assistant port. Alternatively, a liver retractor with a low arm out of the way of the robotic arm can be used in a subxiphoid position. Arm port R1 can be left out in that approach or used for exposition in complex cases

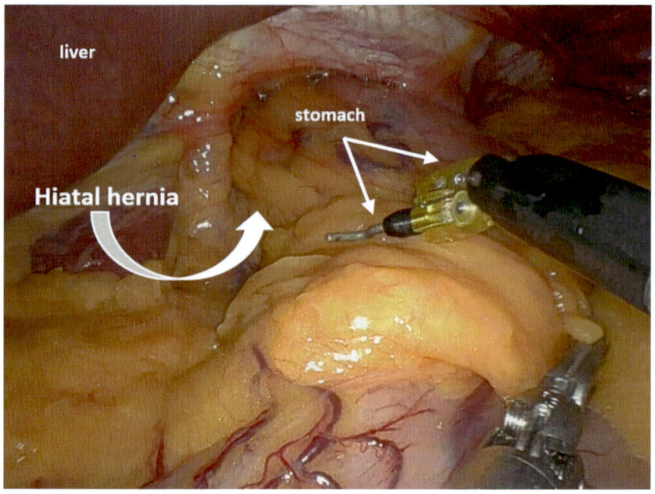

Fig. 7.3 After trocar insertion the patient is placed in steep reverse Trendelenburg, the robot is docked, and instruments are introduced. The small grasping retractor is placed to retract the left lateral segment of the liver superiorly. A type III hiatal hernia is revealed

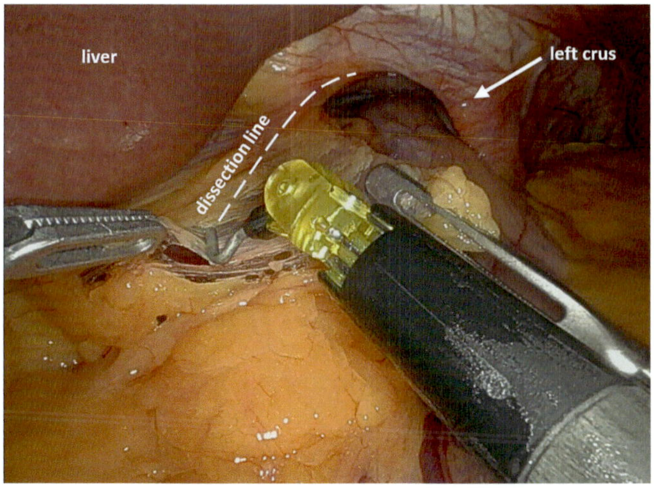

Fig. 7.4 The procedure starts with the incision of the pars flaccida of the gastrohepatic ligament. Surgeons should take care to avoid transection of a large aberrant left hepatic artery in this area (not present in this case). Vagal branches can be saved only when this does not hinder adequate sac resection and hiatal repair

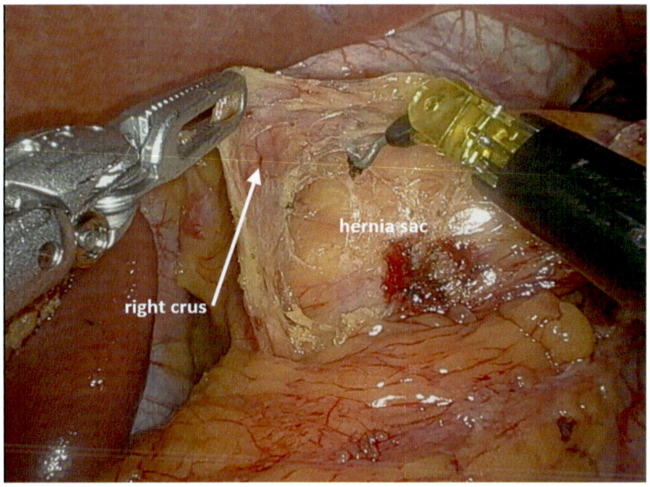

Fig. 7.6 Careful dissection to enter the plane on the outside of the hernia sac. The medial side of the right crus is grasped with the left instrument and retracted laterally

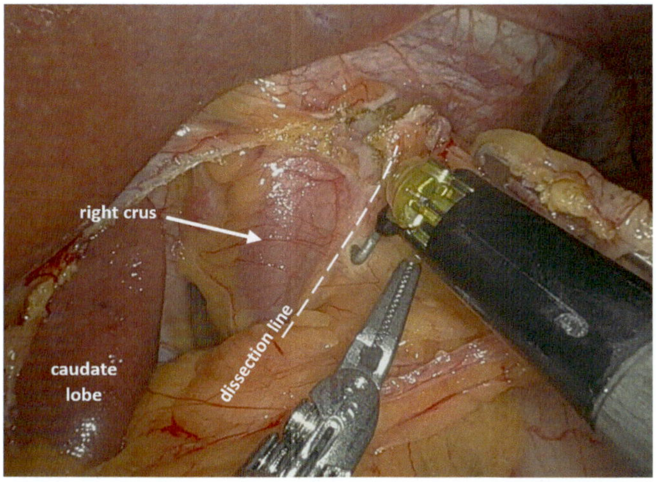

Fig. 7.5 Incision of the phrenoesophageal membrane with preservation of the peritoneum of the right crus. The bedside assistant retracts the gastrohepatic ligament in lateral and caudal direction

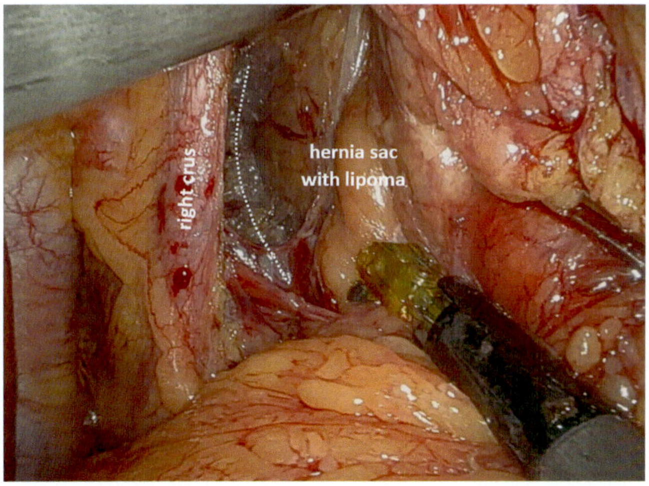

Fig. 7.7 Further dissection at the medial aspect of the right crus, separating the hernia sac from the mediastinum. Recognizing the right tissue plane allows blunt mobilization of the tissue with minimal bleeding. The pleura is to be preserved, and great care is required to avoid damage to the vagal nerves who may present at substantial distance from the esophagus

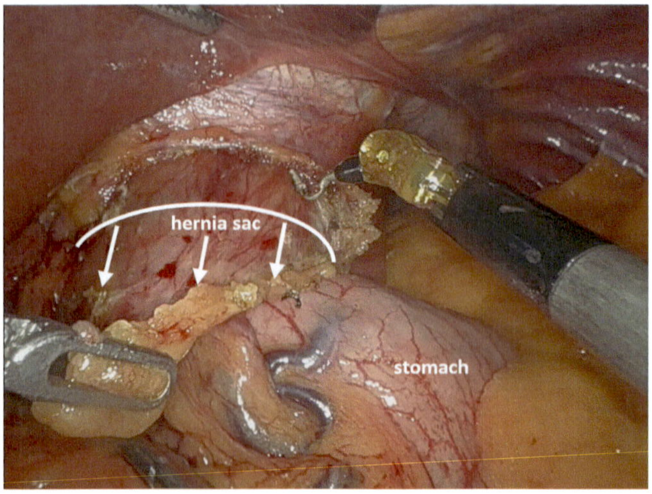

Fig. 7.8 The hernia sac is retracted and dissected in a clockwise direction around the arch of the crus to the left crus. Blunt maneuvers are alternated with diathermic coagulation. Great care is taken to avoid transection of the anterior vagal nerve

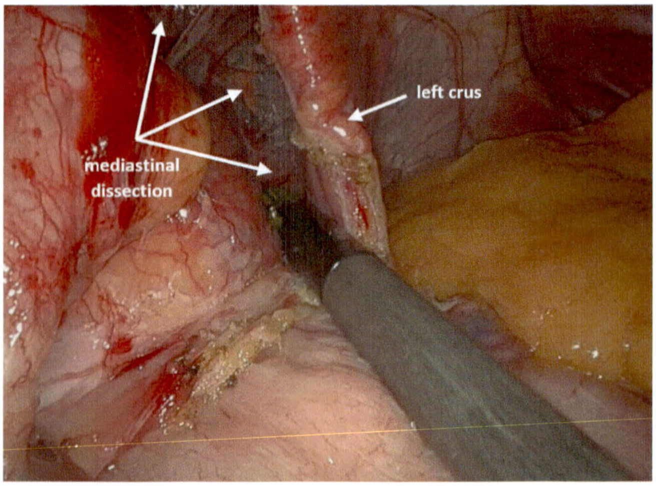

Fig. 7.10 The surgeon's left instrument elevates the left crus away from the esophagus, allowing dissection between the peritoneal sac and mediastinum. The bedside assistant provides countertraction of the stomach inferiorly

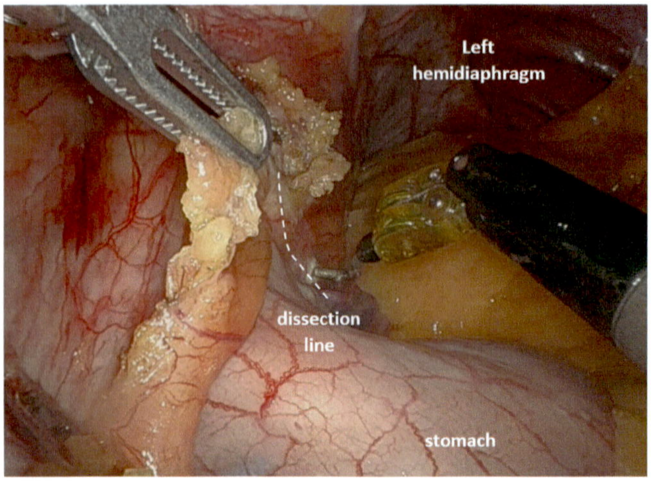

Fig. 7.9 Incision of the phrenogastric attachments to the medial border of the left crus

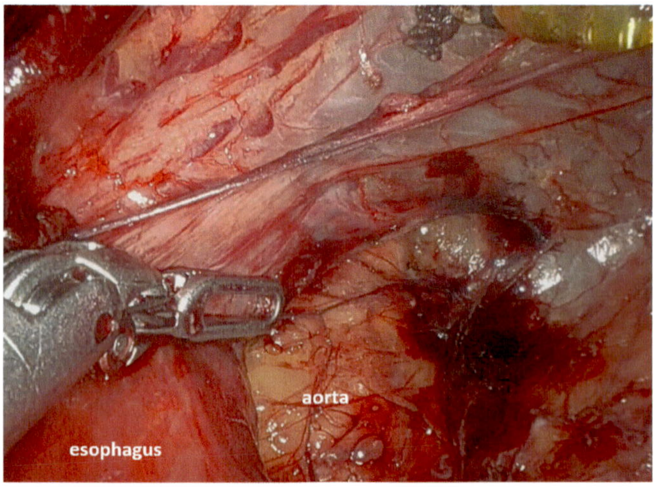

Fig. 7.11 Circumferential esophageal dissection is performed, and the esophagus is mobilized high in the mediastinum. The anterior and posterior vagal nerves should be identified

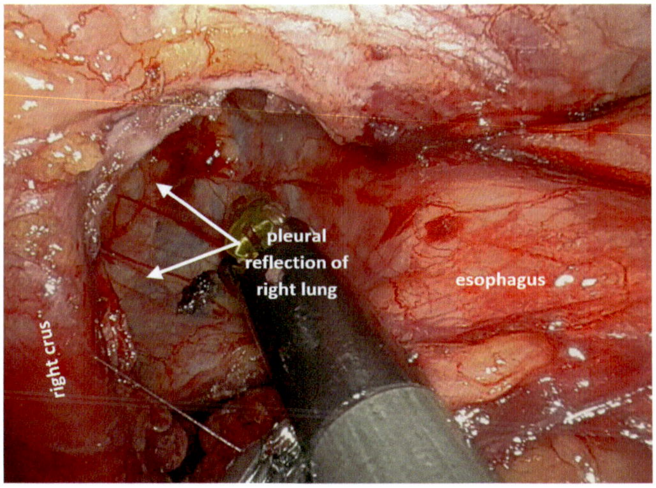

Fig. 7.12 Mediastinal dissection on the right side of the esophagus. Care is taken not to breach the pleura, since an iatrogenic pleural defect can result in a capnothorax. In the event of a capnothorax, conservative care with the addition of positive end-expiratory pressure equivalent to the abdominal insufflation pressure is generally sufficient. Drains are not required as resulting pneumothorax is rare. A direct postoperative chest X-ray should confirm absence of pneumothorax in case of pleural tears

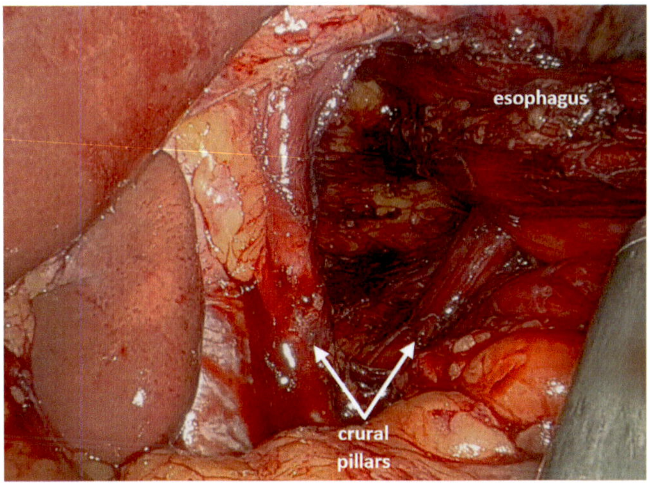

Fig. 7.14 Situation after mediastinal retroesophageal mobilization, with a proper intra-abdominal length of the distal part of the esophagus to achieve a tension-free repair. The bedside assistant lifts the esophagus to the left

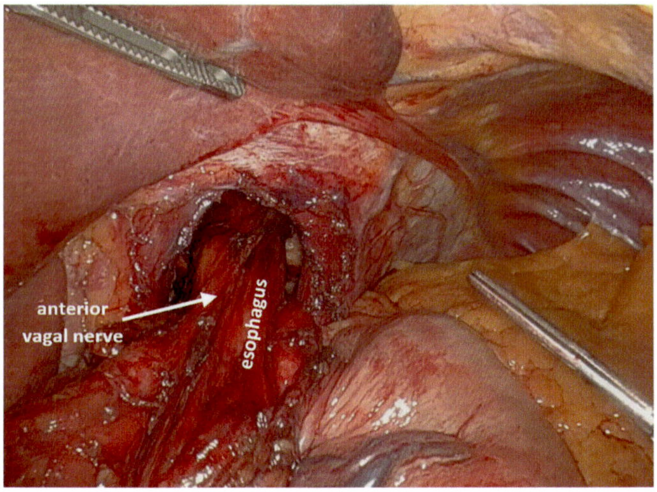

Fig. 7.13 The hernia sac is mobilized down to the gastroesophageal junction, and the anterior and posterior vagal nerve are identified and spared. We do not routinely excise the hernia sac to avoid injury of adherent vagus nerves

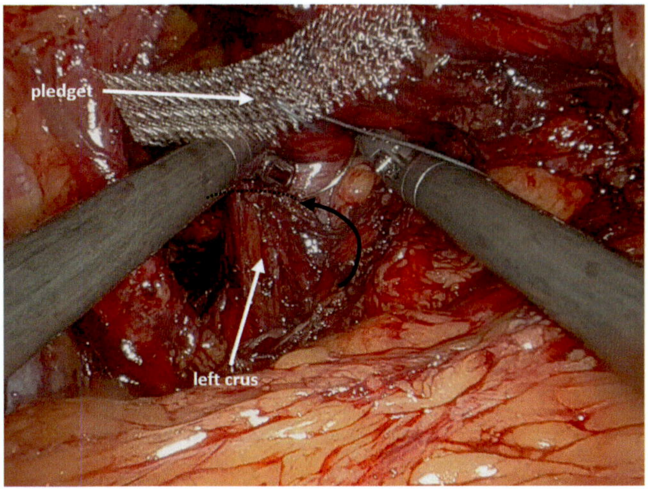

Fig. 7.15 Posterior crural repair. A suture cut needle driver is positioned on the right arm (robotic arm 4). We prefer the use of interrupted nonabsorbable braided sutures and Prolene strips measuring 40 mm × 8 mm to reinforce the crural repair and support the sutures. The strip is first loaded onto the needle

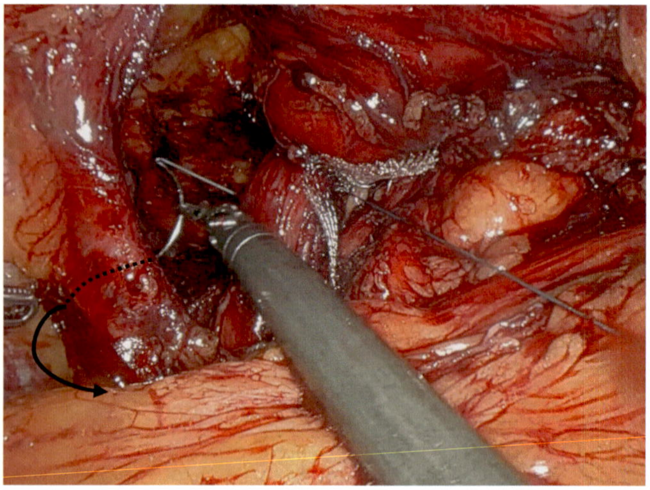

Fig. 7.16 Starting posterior, substantial bites of the left and right crural pillars are taken, including the crural fascia. The left hiatal pillar can be lifted with the cadiere forceps to tilt the pillar away from the aorta and allow a sufficient bite

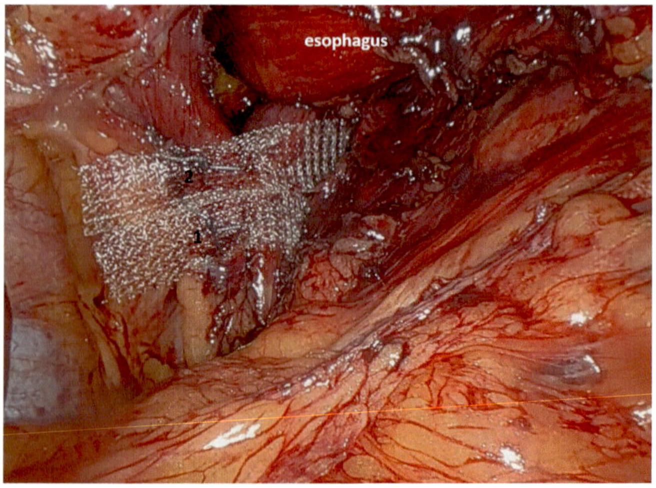

Fig. 7.18 A second interrupted suture with a strip is placed as an onlay over the crura. Artificial material only to bridge the gap should be avoided at all times to avoid erosion into the esophagus

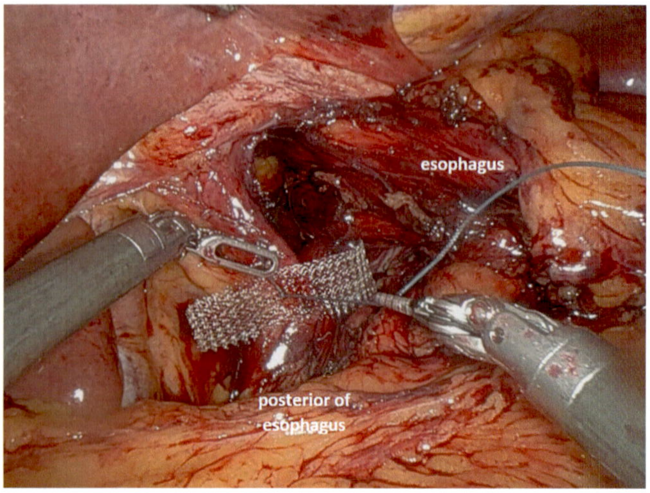

Fig. 7.17 The needle is passed back through the strip and tied using an intracorporeal suturing technique, ensuring adequate overlap of the strip ends on the left and right crural pillars

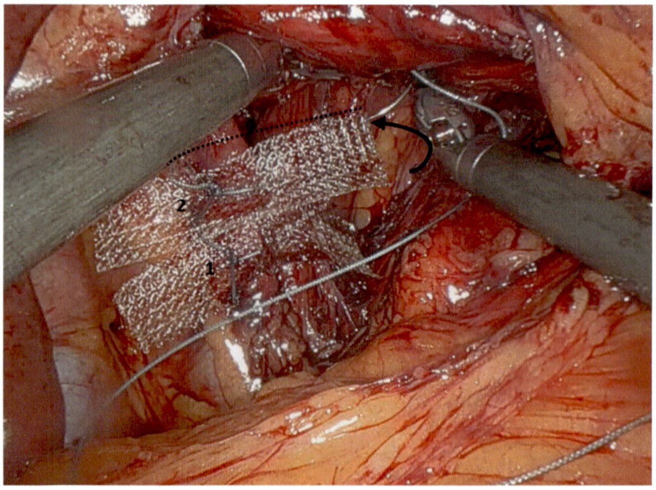

Fig. 7.19 An additional suture, without strip, is placed posterior to the esophagus. This suture helps to avoid direct contact with the upper border of the closest strip

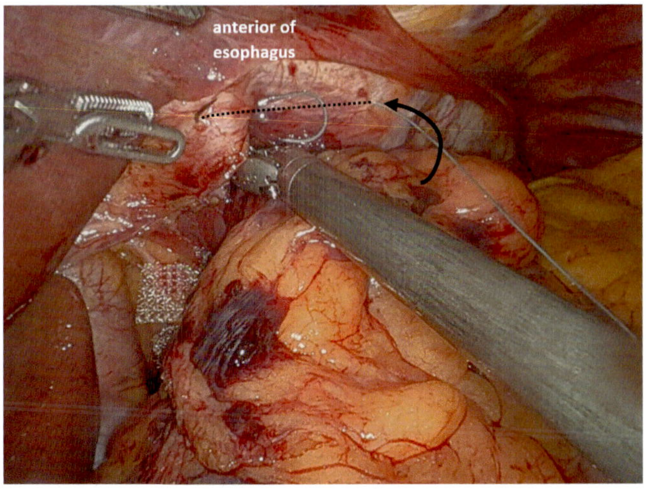

Fig. 7.20 A third suture is placed high on the anterior portion of the hiatus and is enforced with a strip

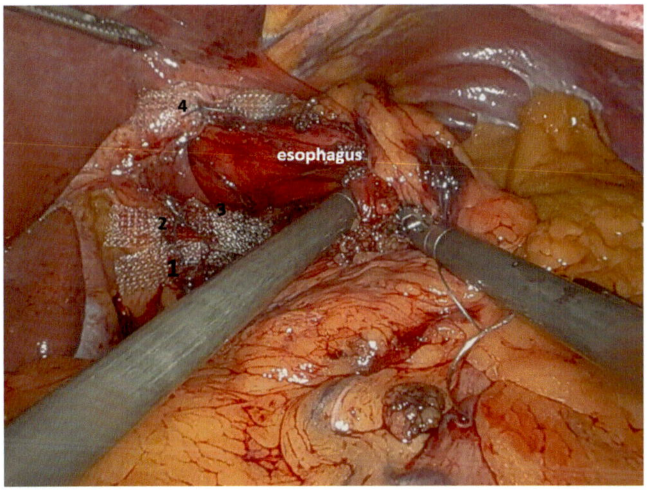

Fig. 7.22 Situation after four interrupted sutures, including three with reinforcing polypropylene strips. No intraesophageal bougie is placed; this is open for personal preference

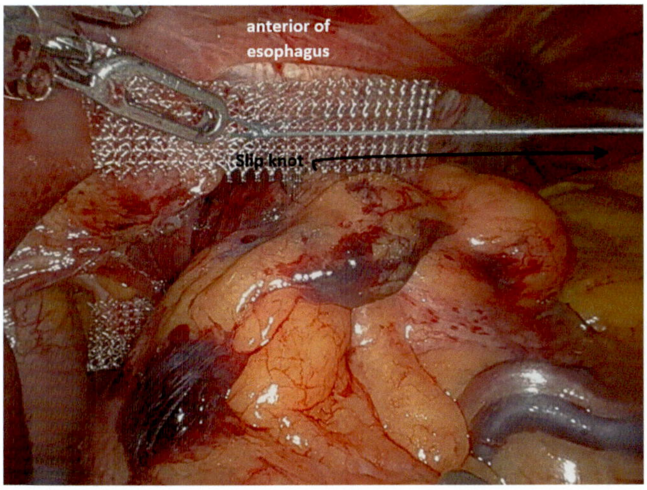

Fig. 7.21 The anterior cruroplasty reinforces the anterior crural junction and allows the formation of a more elliptical shaped hiatus. Intracorporeal slip knots are used throughout the operation, assisting in approximating the pillars under slight tension

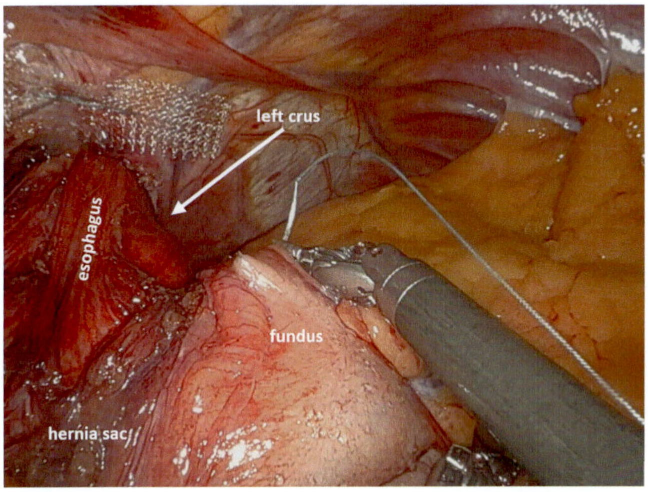

Fig. 7.23 The construction of the anterior 180° partial fundoplication. The first suture is placed in the most superior area of the fundus edge. The fundoplication is set up in an anticlockwise manner (left side first), facilitating better exposure of the left crural pillar

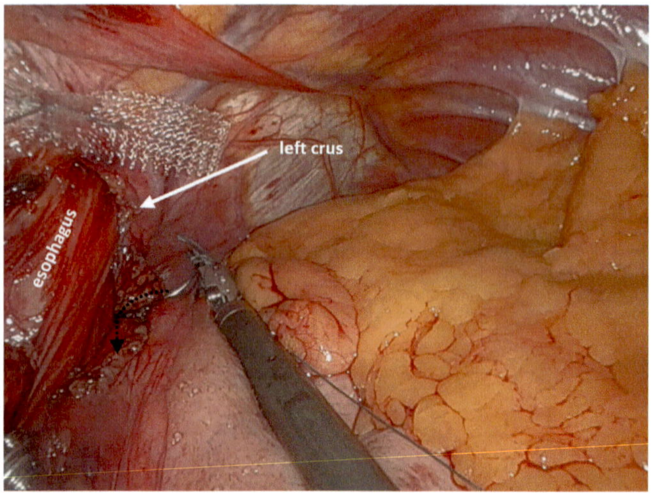

Fig. 7.24 The first suture is fixed dorsally on the left hiatal pillar, in an effort to avoid recurrence

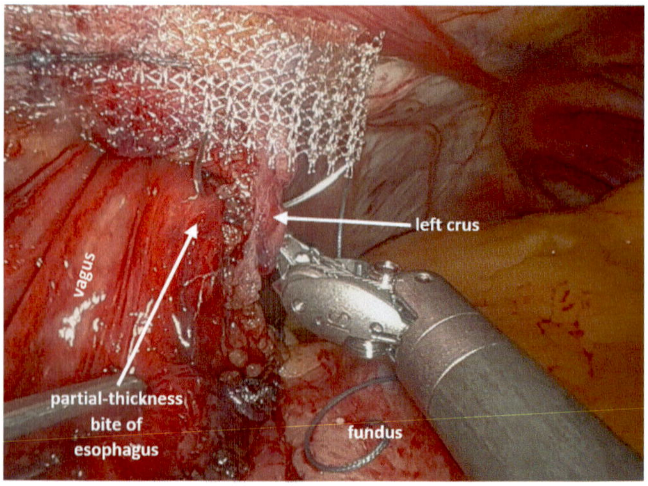

Fig. 7.26 This second suture incorporates the left crus and a muscular bite in the left side of the intra-abdominal esophagus, lateral of the anterior vagal nerve

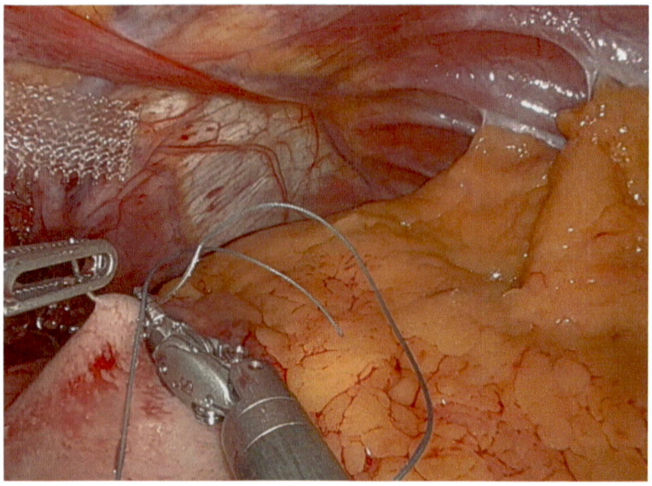

Fig. 7.25 The second suture is placed on the medial wall of the fundus, inferior from the first suture when retracting the stomach downward. It is important to ensure deep seromuscular bites of the fundus

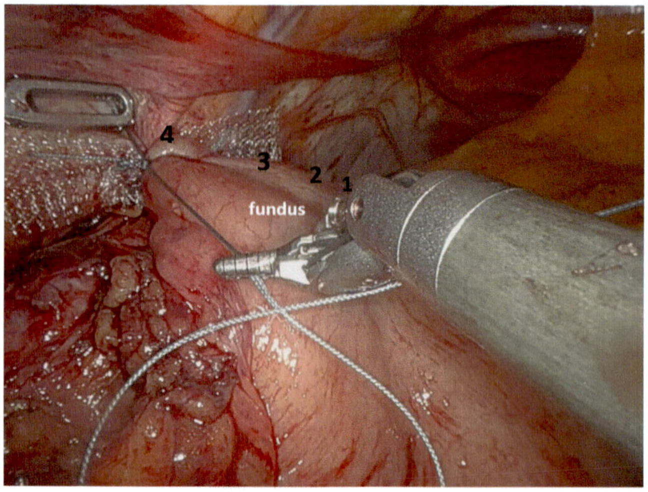

Fig. 7.27 A third and fourth suture is placed through the ridge of the anterior fundus and attached to the diaphragm adjacent to the hiatal rim

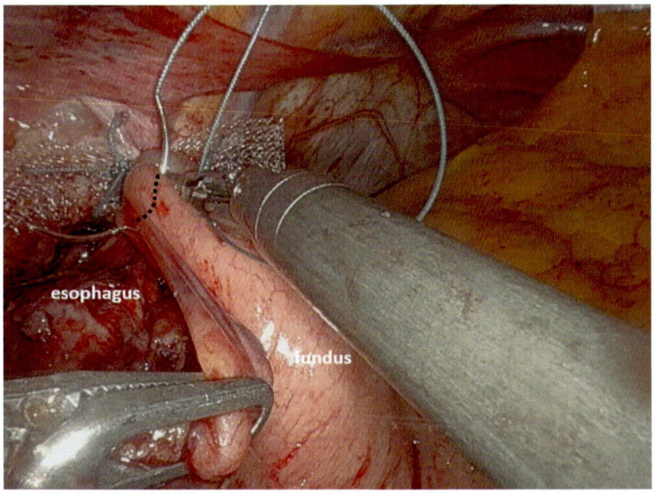

Fig. 7.28 A fifth suture is placed further medial on the fundus

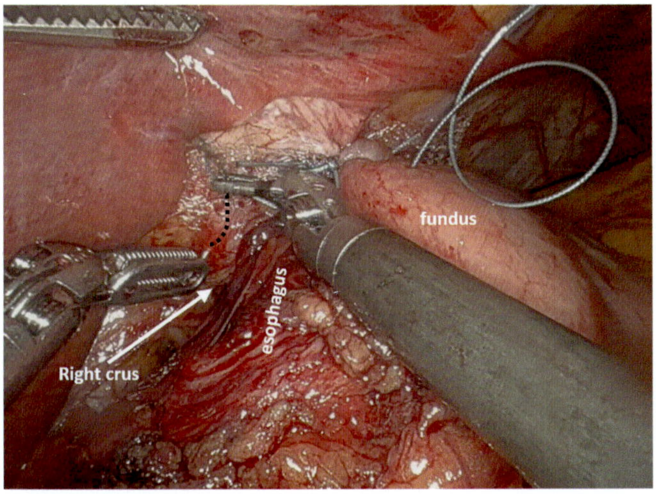

Fig. 7.29 This suture is fixed on the peritoneum of the right crus, fixing the fundus to the diaphragm

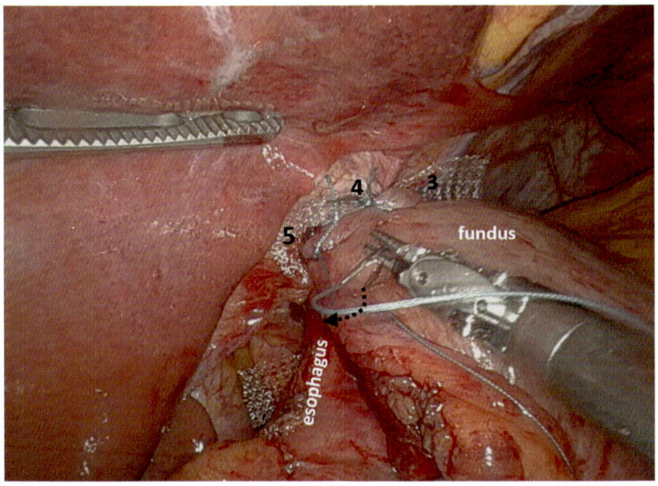

Fig. 7.30 Finally, the last suture is placed through the fundus

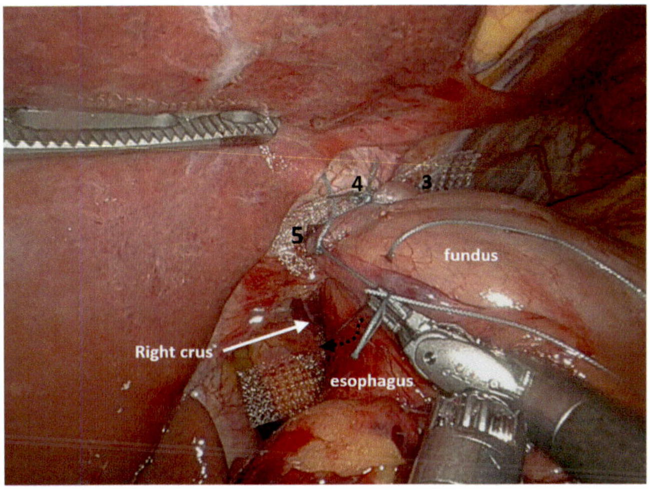

Fig. 7.31 In this suture the right anterolateral side of the esophagus is taken. This is the second and last suture to incorporate the esophageal muscular wall

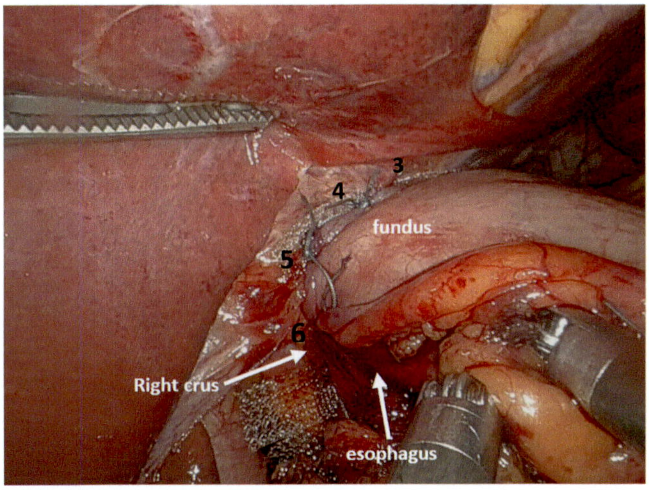

Fig. 7.32 This last suture anchors the fundus and the right side of the esophagus to the right limb of the crus and closes the port to avoid migration of hernia sac remnants or lipomas into the mediastinum

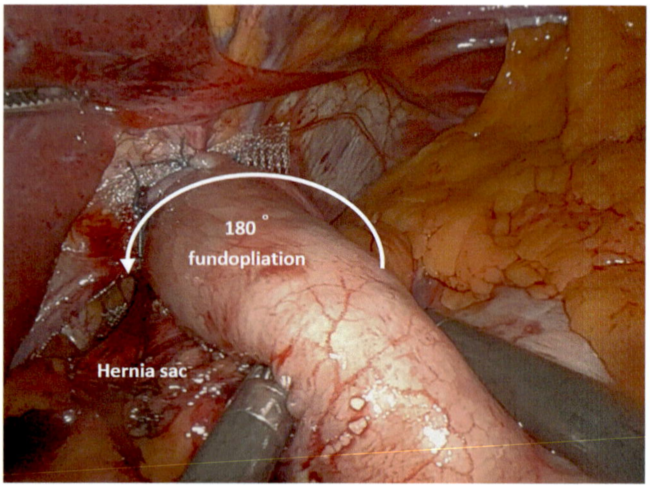

Fig. 7.33 Final situation after a completed anterior 180° partial fundoplication

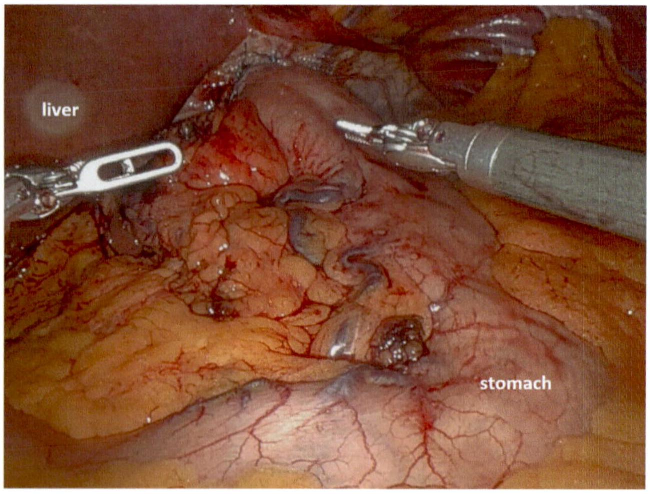

Fig. 7.34 Final aspect of a floppy anterior fundoplication valve

References

1. Mertens AC, Tolboom RC, Zavrtanik H, Draaisma WA, Broeders I. Morbidity and mortality in complex robot-assisted hiatal hernia surgery: 7-year experience in a high-volume center. Surg Endosc. 2019;33:2152–61. https://doi.org/10.1007/s00464-018-6494-4.
2. Brenkman HJ, Parry K, van Hillegersberg R, Ruurda JP. Robot-assisted laparoscopic hiatal hernia repair: promising anatomical and functional results. J Laparoendosc Adv Surg Tech A. 2016;26:465–9. https://doi.org/10.1089/lap.2016.0065.
3. Tolboom RC, Broeders IA, Draaisma WA. Robot-assisted laparoscopic hiatal hernia and antireflux surgery. J Surg Oncol. 2015;112:266–70. https://doi.org/10.1002/jso.23912.

Robotic Toupet Fundoplication

8

Mickael Chevallay, Marco Augusto Bonino, Minoa Karin Jung, and Stefan Paul Mönig

Gastroesophageal reflux disease (GERD) is a widespread benign disorder of the distal oesophagus and gastroesophageal junction that severely affects a patient's quality of life. GERD pathophysiology presents several causes, among them hiatal hernia with abnormal transdiaphragmatic pressure gradient and with an obtuse angle [1]. Despite the extensive adoption of medical therapy with proton pump inhibitors, this treatment fails to resolve the GERD symptoms completely in almost 40% of all patients [2]. Surgery was formerly considered only for severe cases. However, with the evolution of the minimally invasive approach, indications for anti-reflux surgery have broadened. Patients with failed medical management, with preference over life-long medication, Barrett's oesophagus or extra-oesophageal manifestations, should be offered surgical management. A score calculated during a 24-hour oesophageal pH monitoring, the DeMeester score, higher than 14.7 is another indication for surgical treatment. The measure of impedance during the pH monitoring can detect also reflux with low acidity, which could also benefit from surgical correction. Oesophageal manometry completes the GERD work-up and allows diagnosis oesophageal motility abnormalities. Studies show that anti-reflux surgery in Barrett's oesophagus patients effectively achieves relief of GERD symptoms, induction of histologic regression and prevention of progression of intestinal metaplasia to dysplasia or invasive carcinoma [3].

Minimally invasive fundoplication has proven to be the gold standard surgical treatment for GERD over the open approach, with comparable efficacy and lower mortality [4]. The goal of the surgery is to restore the anti-reflux mechanism of the gastro-oesophageal junction by correcting the crural diaphragm, as well as the geometry and pressures of the gastro-oesophageal junction. The surgery starts with the dissection of the hiatal region to expose both diaphragmatic crus and a reduction of a potential hiatal hernia with resection of the sac. A transhiatal mobilisation allows obtaining approximately 3 centimetres of intra-abdominal oesophagus. Short gastric vessels are divided to free the gastric fundus, and a crural closure with non-absorbable sutures is completed. The surgery is concluded with the creation of a gastric wrap around the oesophagus. A previous debate was about the magnitude with which the gastric wrap should surround the oesophagus. A total (360°) wrap (Nissen fundoplication) was commonly performed with a good improvement of reflux symptoms, but with the risk of post-operative dysphagia and gas bloating [5].

A partial (270°) wrap (Toupet fundoplication) is now preferred in many centres, with less post-operative dysphagia and similar reduction in reflux symptoms [6].

Robotic surgery has been a revolution in minimally invasive surgery, with several advantages over the laparoscopic approach: three-dimensional visualisation, seven degrees of freedom with endowristed instruments and tremor filtration. In anti-reflux surgery, the robotic approach is accepted as an alternative for a minimally invasive procedure, with the ability to overcome some technical limitations associated with conventional laparoscopy and similar post-operative outcomes in high-volume centres [7].

Procedure: Illustrated Steps

We present the case of a 25-year-old patient with a long history of GERD with heartburn sensation and with no symptom relief after PPI medication. Pre-operative workup consisted of oeso-gastro-duodenal transit and gastroscopy, which confirmed a sliding hiatal hernia type 1 and oesophagitis. We planned for a robotic Toupet fundoplication for the patient. Figures 8.1, 8.2, 8.3, 8.4, 8.5, 8.6, 8.7, 8.8, 8.9, 8.10, 8.11, 8.12, 8.13, 8.14, 8.15, 8.16, 8.17, 8.18, 8.19, 8.20, 8.21, 8.22, 8.23, 8.24, 8.25, 8.26, and 8.27 illustrate the technical aspects of the procedure.

M. Chevallay · M. A. Bonino · M. K. Jung · S. P. Mönig (✉)
Division of Digestive Surgery, Department of Surgery, Geneva University Hospital and Faculty of Medicine, Geneva, Switzerland
e-mail: stefan.moenig@hcuge.ch

O. Y. Kudsi, P. P. Grimminger (eds.), *Atlas of Robotic Upper Gastrointestinal Surgery*,
https://doi.org/10.1007/978-3-030-86578-8_8

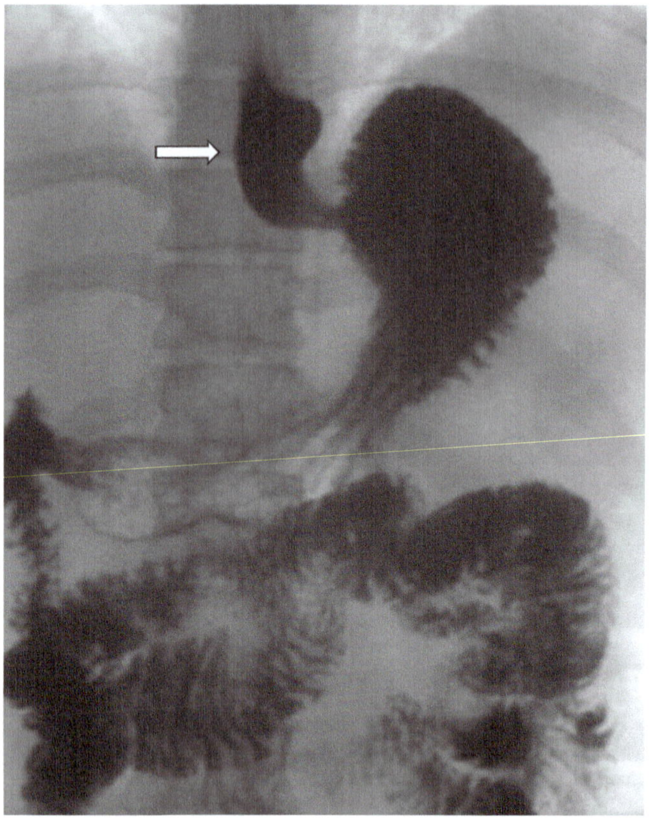

Fig. 8.1 Pre-operative oeso-gastro-duodenal transit showing a 3-centimetre sliding hiatal hernia (white arrow)

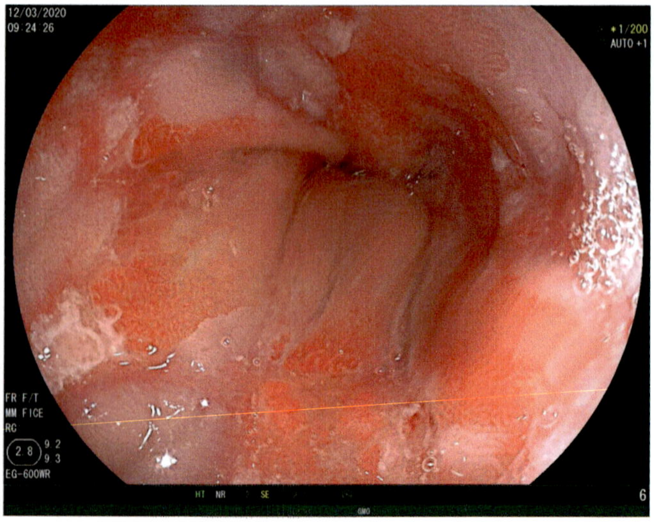

Fig. 8.2 Pre-operative gastroscopy with hiatal hernia and oesophagitis

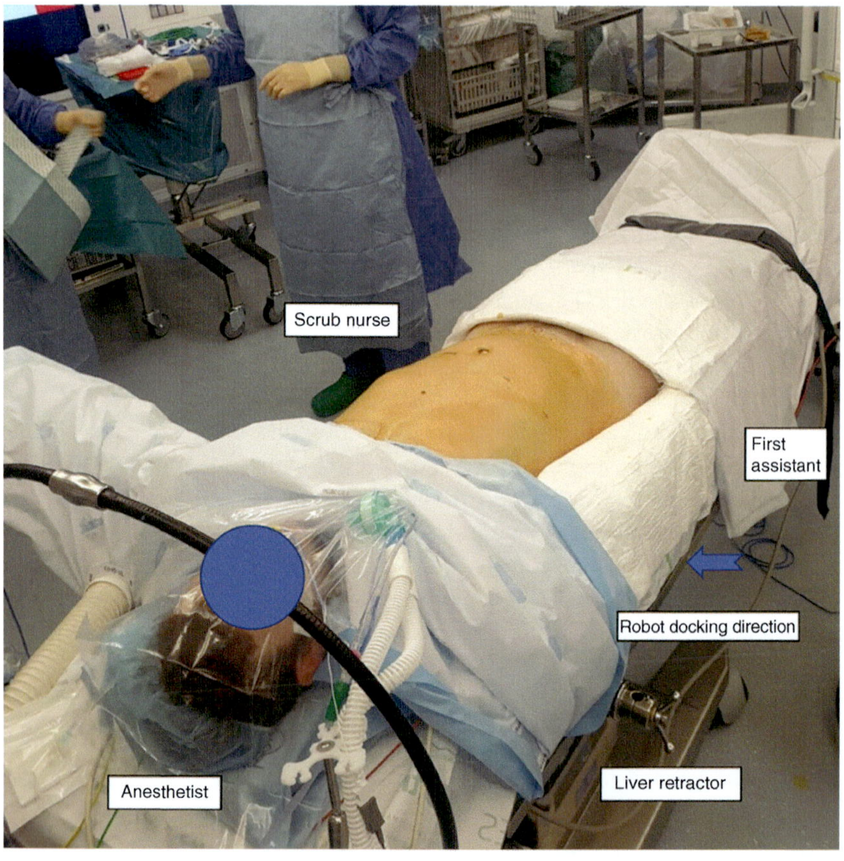

Fig. 8.3 Operating room set-up and patient positioning: supine position with leg straps, right arm adducted, left arm abducted, reverse Trendelenburg at 15° position

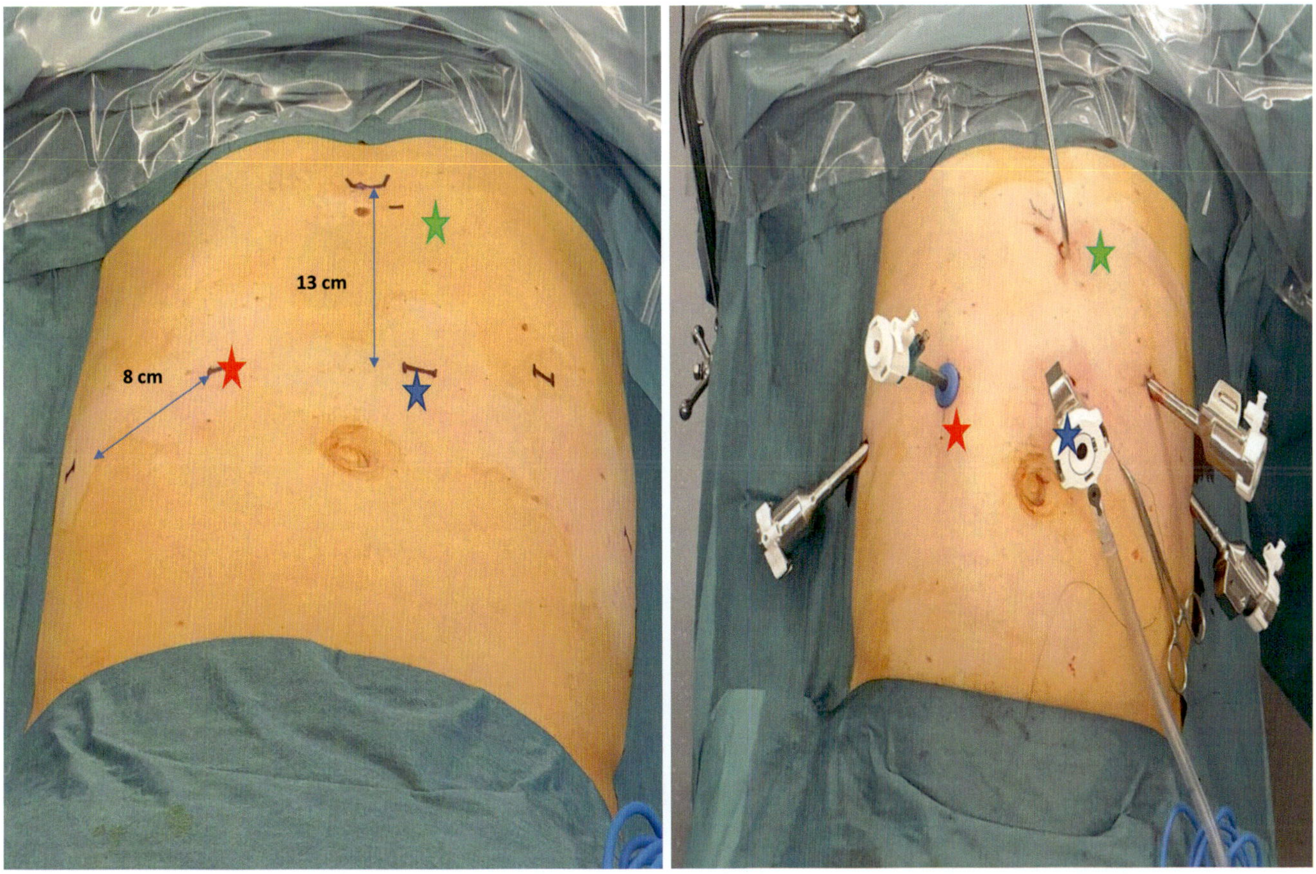

Fig. 8.4 Trocar positioning: The first trocar (for the camera) should be placed at 13 centimetres from the xiphoid process, left para-umbilical (blue star). Two robotic trocars should be placed on a horizontal line on the patient's left side. Two trocars, one laparoscopic for the assistant (red star) and one robotic, should be placed on the patient's right side. All trocars should have a space of 8 centimetres between them. The liver retractor should be placed in the epigastric region (green star)

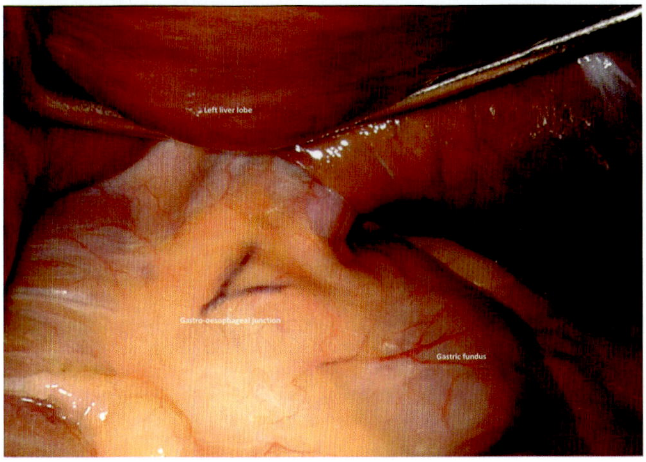

Fig. 8.5 After the trocars are introduced into the abdominal space, a liver retractor passed through the sub-xiphoid incision is positioned to lift the left hepatic lobe. This allows access to the gastro-oesophageal junction region

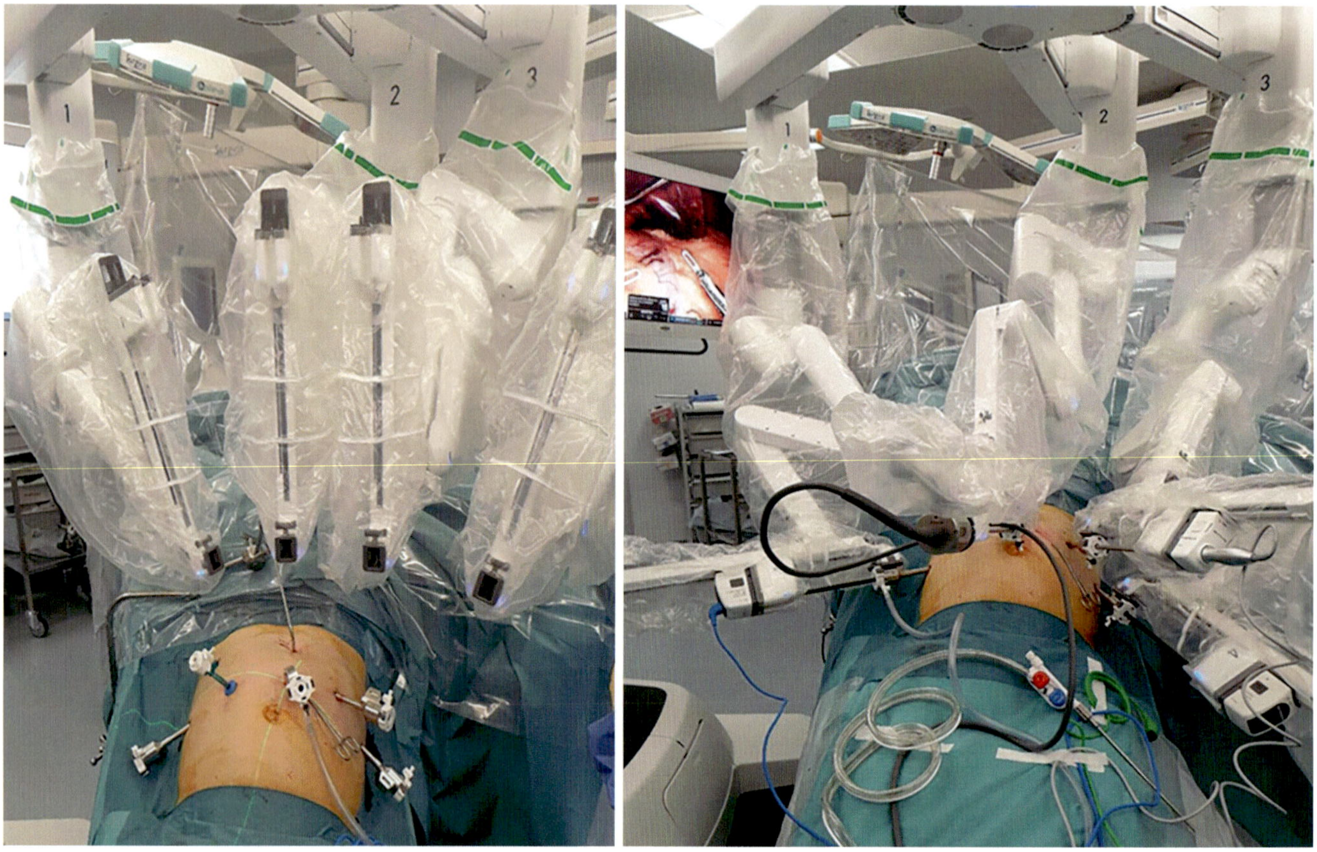

Fig. 8.6 Docking manoeuvre from the right of the patient to position the robot over the head

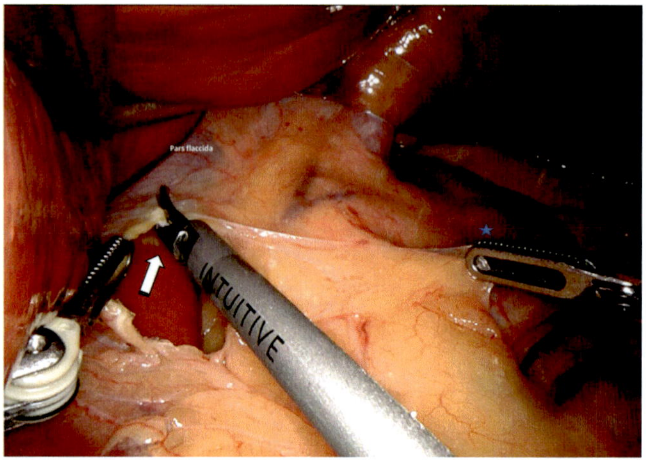

Fig. 8.7 An atraumatic grasper retracts the gastro-oesophageal junction to the left (blue star) Opening of the pars flaccida of the hepatogastric ligament to access the right diaphragmatic crus with the Ultracision™ (the white arrow indicates the direction of dissection)

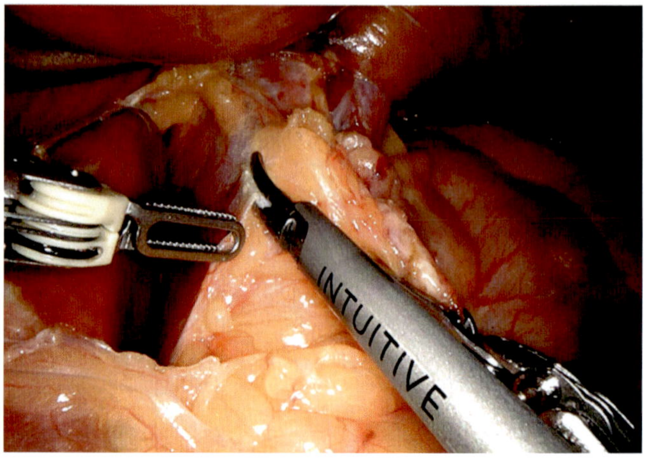

Fig. 8.8 Incision of the peritoneum on the right diaphragmatic crus

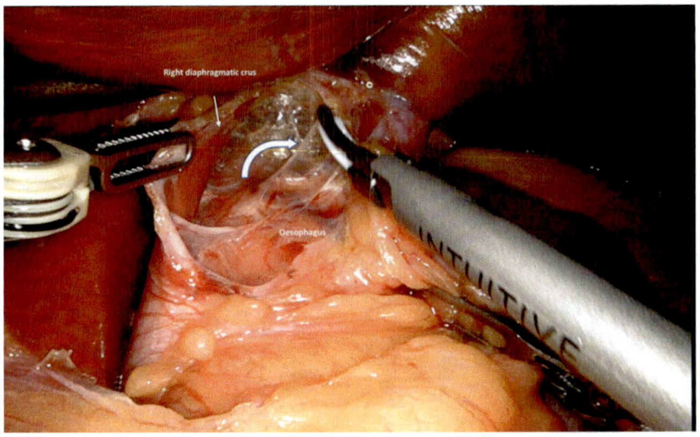

Fig. 8.9 Dissection follows the right crus superiorly with opening of the phreno-oesophageal membrane anteriorly. The white arrow indicates the direction of the dissection around the arch

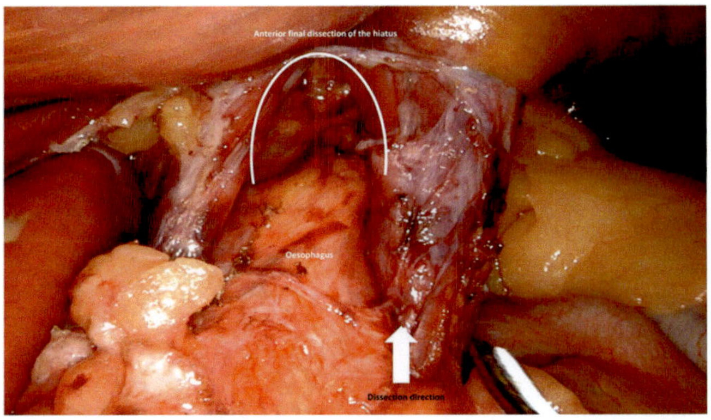

Fig. 8.10 After the arch has been dissected (white half-circle) and the anterior aspect of the oesophagus is clearly seen, the left aspect of the crus is dissected with the Ultracision™ from bottom to top. The hiatus is clearly identified at the end of the dissection

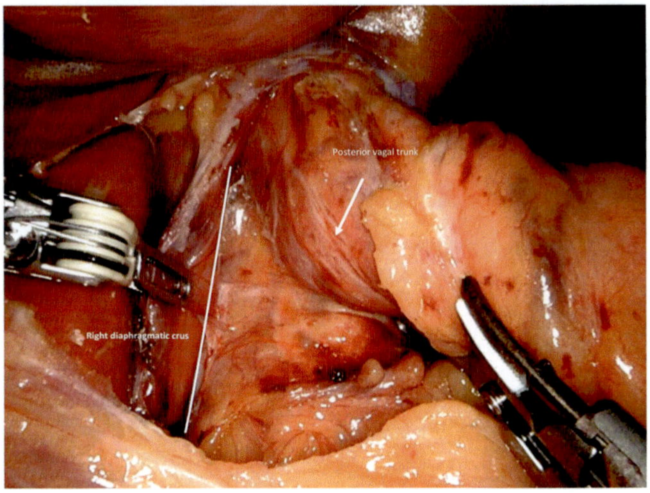

Fig. 8.11 After the anterior hiatus has been dissected, posterior dissection of the right crus is continued until the junction with the left crus is identified. The posterior vagal nerve is identified and preserved during the dissection

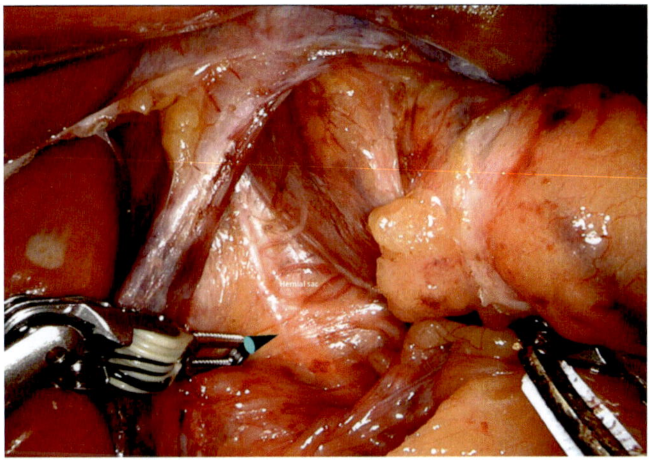

Fig. 8.12 A hernial sac can be identified (green cone). It should be dissected and completely resected. The vagal nerve is still visualised when separating the hernia sac from the oesophagus

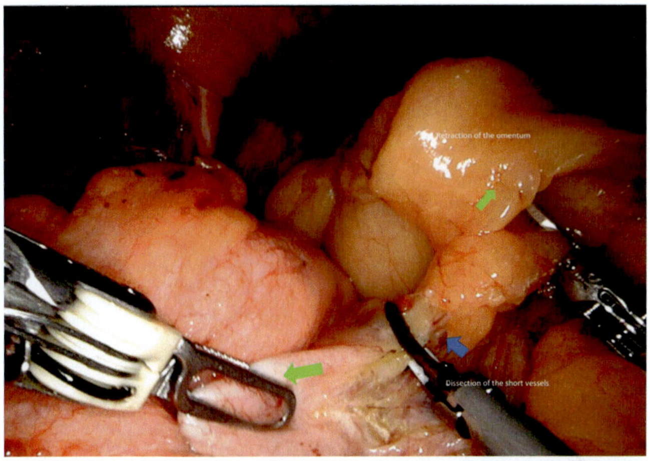

Fig. 8.13 Short gastric vessels are then divided in preparation for the fundoplication. This dissection allows for the freeing of the gastric fundus and ensures a tension-free wrap (green arrow, direction of retraction by two atraumatic robotic graspers; blue arrow, direction of dissection with the Ultracision™)

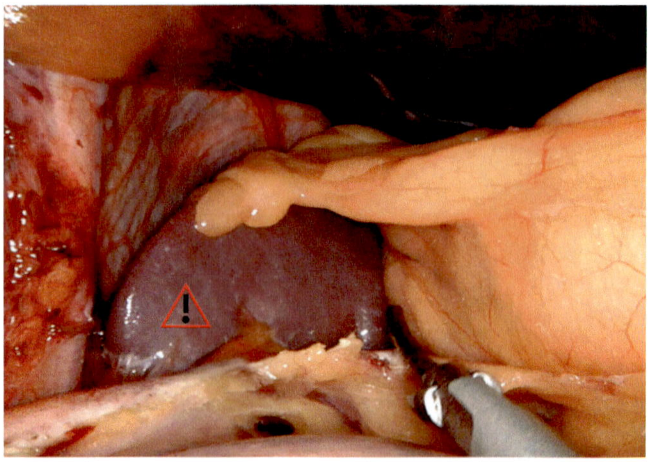

Fig. 8.14 Special care should be taken when approaching the proximal part of the fundus, as the spleen can be very close, with a high risk of bleeding by traction. At the end of the dissection, the stomach is completely freed from the spleen

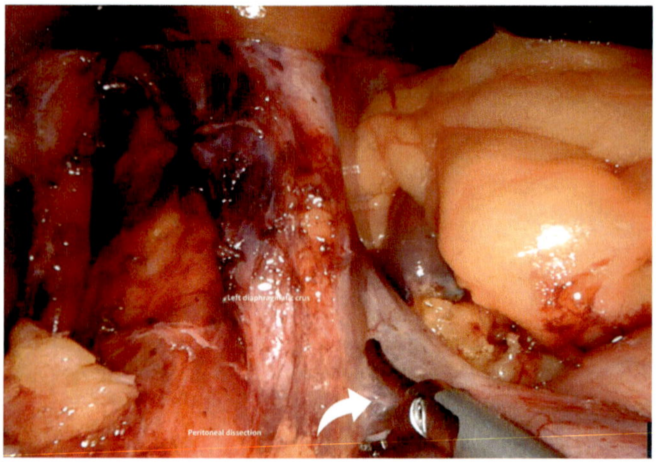

Fig. 8.15 Short vessel dissection is concluded by joining the dissection with the left diaphragmatic crus

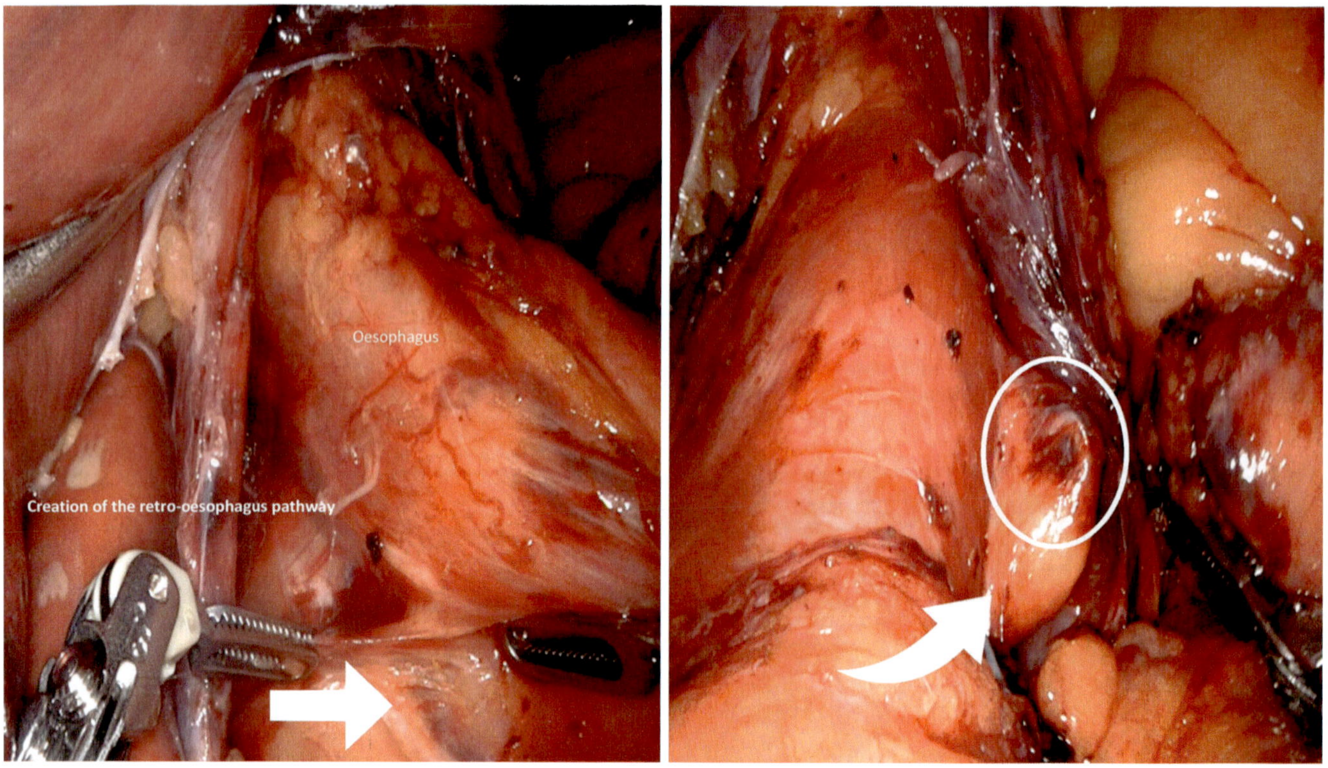

Fig. 8.16 A pathway is created in the posterior part of the oesophagus by inserting an atraumatic grasper until it appears on the other side of the oesophagus

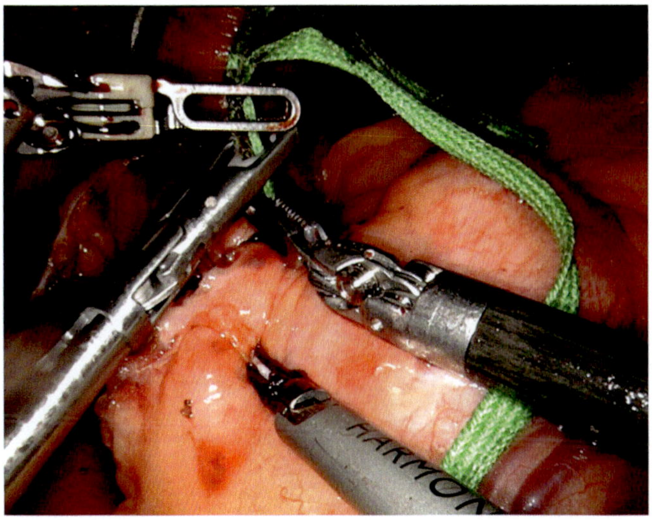

Fig. 8.17 A mesh or rubber band is then passed to the grasper behind the oesophagus to be placed around it. The surgeon fixes the two threads with two Hem-o-Lok. The assistant grasps the band to retract the oesophagus and the gastro-oesophageal junction

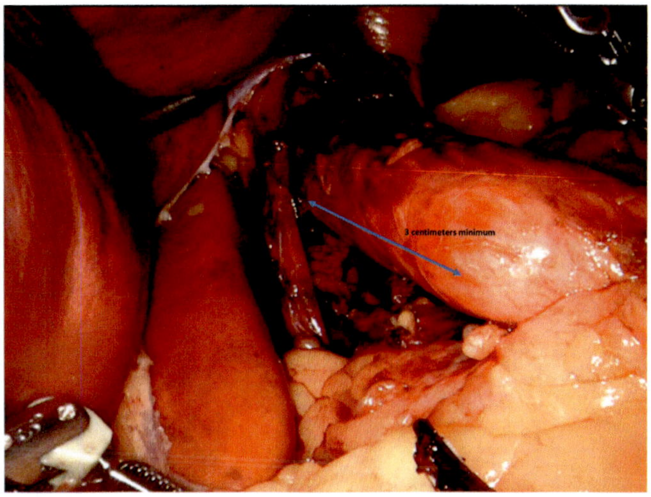

Fig. 8.19 At the end of the dissection, the oesophagus and GE junction are clearly visible and fully mobilised, with an intra-abdominal position. The transhiatal mobilisation should allow a minimum intra-abdominal oesophageal length of 3 centimetres

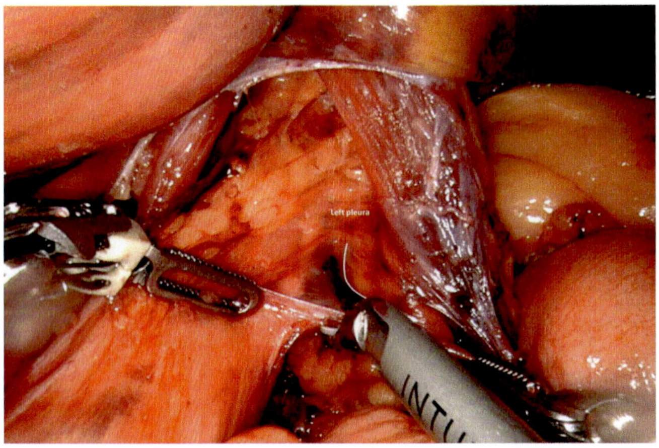

Fig. 8.18 The oesophagus is then dissected from any peritoneal and mediastinal attachments. Damage to pleura can happen during this step and should be recognised

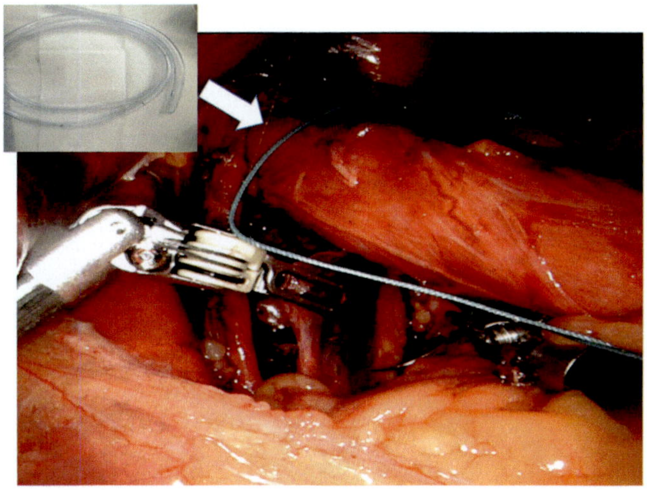

Fig. 8.20 After a 36 French bougie is inserted into the oesophagus for calibration, the crural defect is closed using non-absorbable (Ethibond 0) interrupted sutures

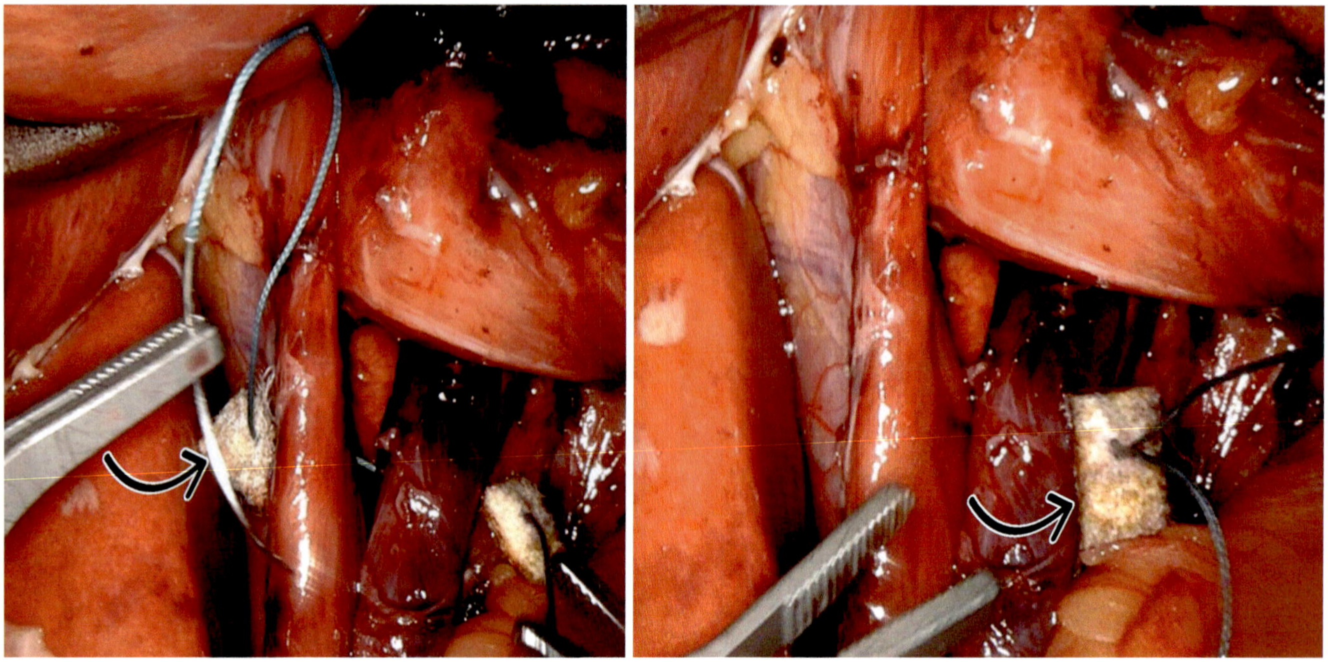

Fig. 8.21 0.5 × 0.5 cm pledgets reinforce the sutures. The first pledget is placed on the wire before the suture. After one passage through both crus, the wire is passed through a second pledget. The suture is then carried back through both crus and the first pledget

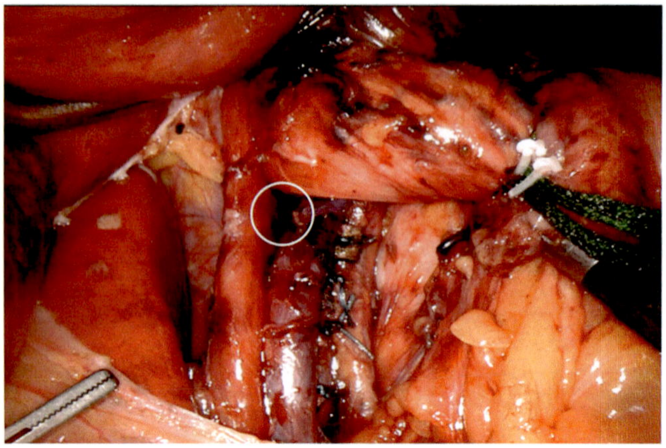

Fig. 8.22 The reapproximated crura should leave enough space for the oesophagus to expand during swallowing and avoid post-operative dysphagia

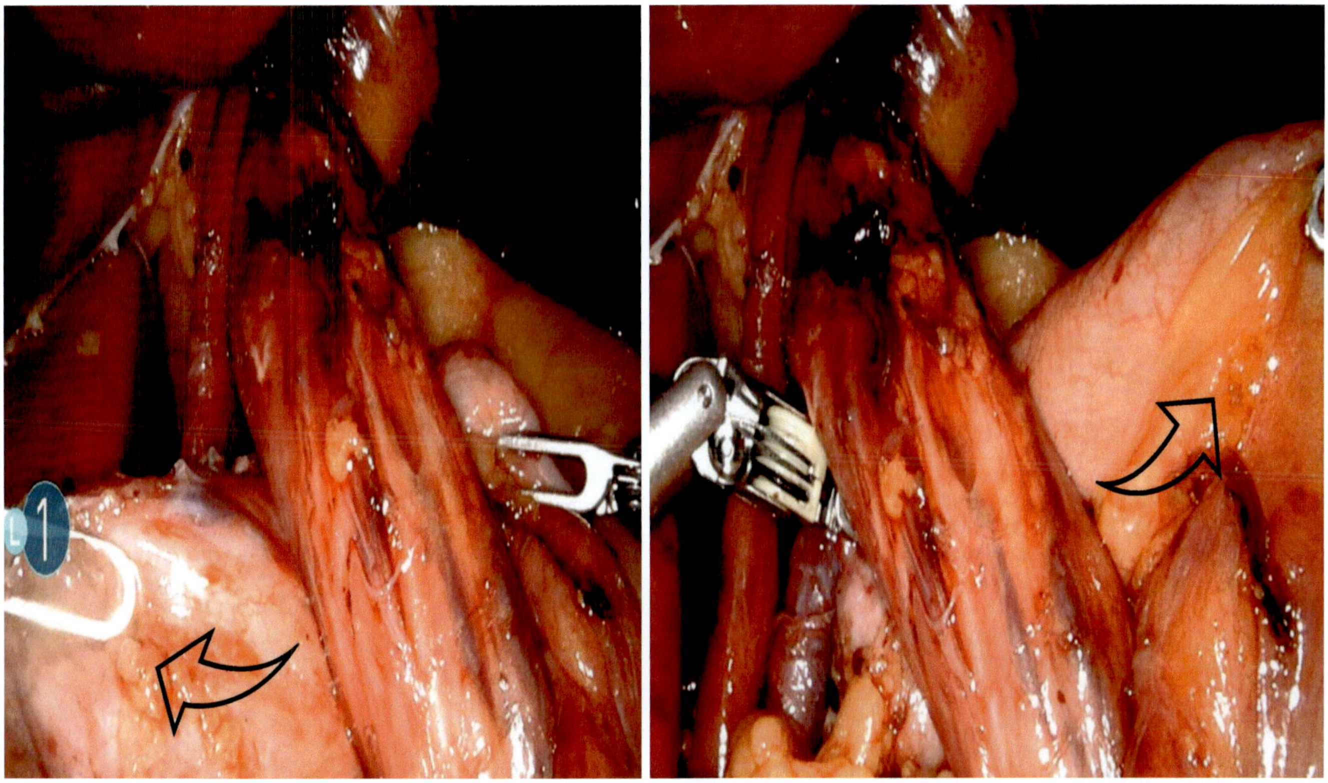

Fig. 8.23 An atraumatic robotic grasper is passed behind the oesophagus under direct vision. The fundus curvature is placed inside the grasper, and the fundus is pulled around behind the oesophagus. The 'shoeshine' manoeuvre is used so that the fundus has enough mobility to ensure a tension-free wrap

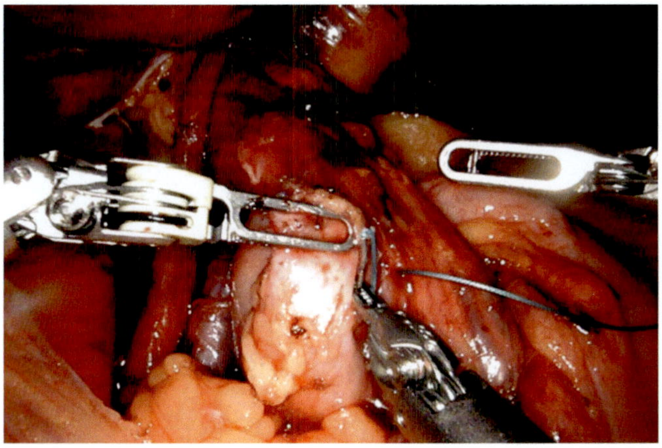

Fig. 8.24 A gastric wrap is created around 270° of the oesophagus (Toupet fundoplication). Interrupted non-absorbable sutures are used to fix the fundus with the anterior muscular part of the oesophagus. The 36 French bougie is left in the oesophagus lumen during the construction of the wrap for calibration

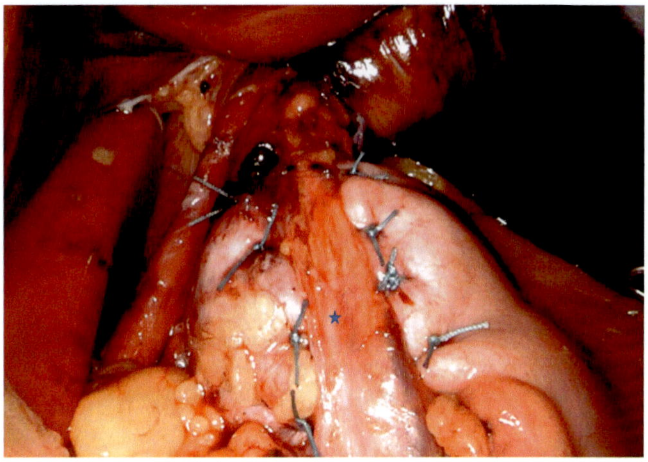

Fig. 8.25 Both left and right parts of the fundus are fixed to obtain a 3–4 cm wrap (3–4 stitches). Care should be taken to avoid suture over the anterior vagal nerve (blue star)

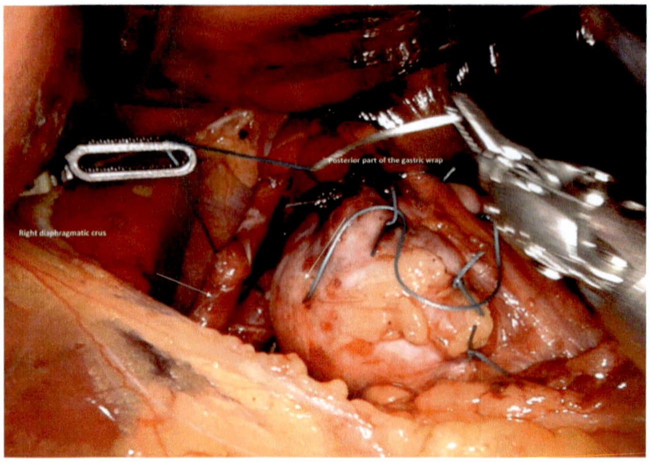

Fig. 8.26 The wrap is then fixed on both diaphragmatic crus with a single non-absorbable suture. In this picture, the posterior part of the gastric wrap is fixed on the right diaphragmatic crus

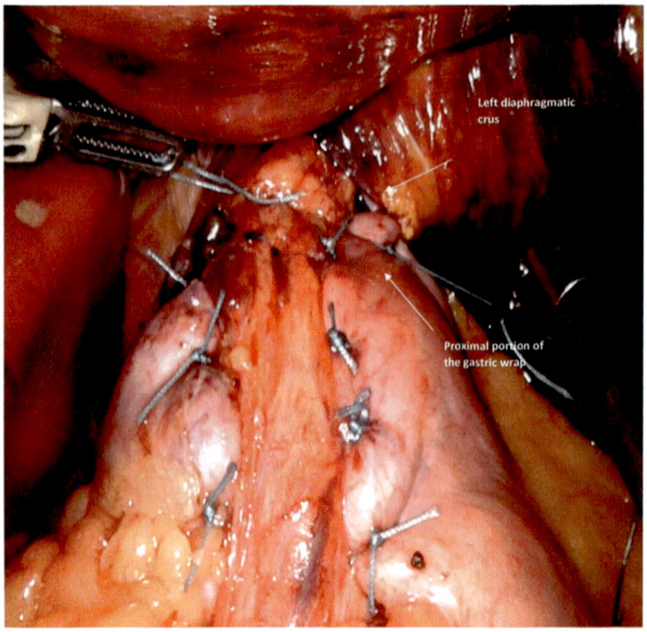

Fig. 8.27 Additionally, the left part of the wrap is fixed to the left diaphragmatic crux with a single non-absorbable suture to obtain a fundopexy. This secures the montage in an intra-abdominal position

References

1. Menezes MA, Herbella FAM. Pathophysiology of gastroesophageal reflux disease. World J Surg. 2017;41:1666–71.
2. Sifrim D, Zerbib F. Diagnosis and management of patients with reflux symptoms refractory to proton pump inhibitors. Gut. 2012;61:1340–54.
3. Peyre CG, Watson TJ. Surgical management of Barrett's esophagus. Gastroenterol Clin N Am. 2015;44:459–71.
4. Dallemagne B, Perretta S. Twenty years of laparoscopic fundoplication for GERD. World J Surg. 2011;35:1428–35.
5. Broeders JA, Mauritz FA, Ahmed Ali U, et al. Systematic review and meta-analysis of laparoscopic Nissen (posterior total) versus Toupet (posterior partial) fundoplication for gastro-oesophageal reflux disease. Br J Surg. 2010;97:1318–30.
6. Stefanidis D, Hope WW, Kohn GP, et al. Guidelines for surgical treatment of gastroesophageal reflux disease. Surg Endosc. 2010;24:2647–69.
7. Mertens AC, Tolboom RC, Zavrtanik H, et al. Morbidity and mortality in complex robot-assisted hiatal hernia surgery: 7-year experience in a high-volume center. Surg Endosc. 2019;33:2152–61.

Robotic Giant Paraesophageal Hernia Repair

9

Caitlin Houghton

Introduction

Foregut surgery is a relatively new indication for robotic surgery. Although surgeons have been utilizing the platform for these surgeries, FDA approval of the Xi da Vinci system just came in early 2021. Robotic foregut surgery is on an exponential rise largely due to the superior HD visualization; the ease in working in tight spaces, such as through the hiatus; and the precision of tissue dissection. The advancement in energy devices and instrumentation has also allowed the platform to be used in increasingly complex procedures such as cases of intra-thoracic stomach or giant paraesophageal hernias.

Procedure: Illustrated Steps

Figures 9.1, 9.2,9.3, 9.4, 9.5, 9.6, 9.7, 9.8, 9.9, 9.10, 9.11, 9.12, 9.13, 9.14, 9.15, 9.16, 9.17, 9.18, 9.19, 9.20, 9.21, 9.22, 9.23, 9.24, 9.25, 9.26, 9.27, 9.28, 9.29, 9.30, 9.31, and 9.32 show the procedure.

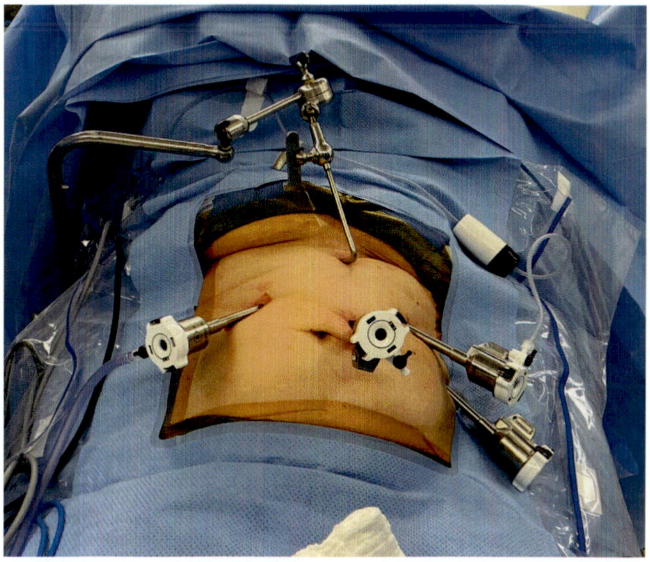

Fig. 9.1 Trocar placement includes four robotic trocars and a Nathanson retractor. The camera port is in the left paramedian space. Two trocars in the left upper quadrant: one in the midclavicular line and one in the anterior axillary line. One trocar in the RUQ placed to avoid the liver edge

C. Houghton (✉)
Department of Surgery, Keck School of Medicine, University of Southern California, Los Angeles, CA, USA
e-mail: caitlin.houghton@med.usc.edu

O. Y. Kudsi, P. P. Grimminger (eds.), *Atlas of Robotic Upper Gastrointestinal Surgery*,
https://doi.org/10.1007/978-3-030-86578-8_9

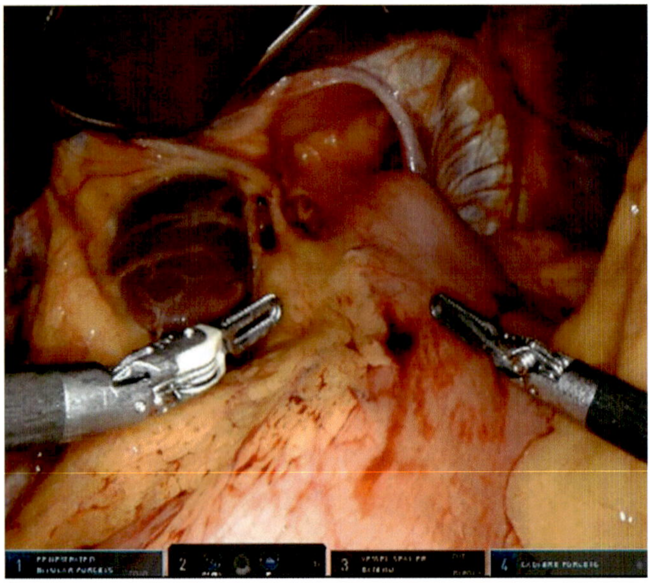

Fig. 9.2 Giant paraesophageal hernia noted on initial inspection

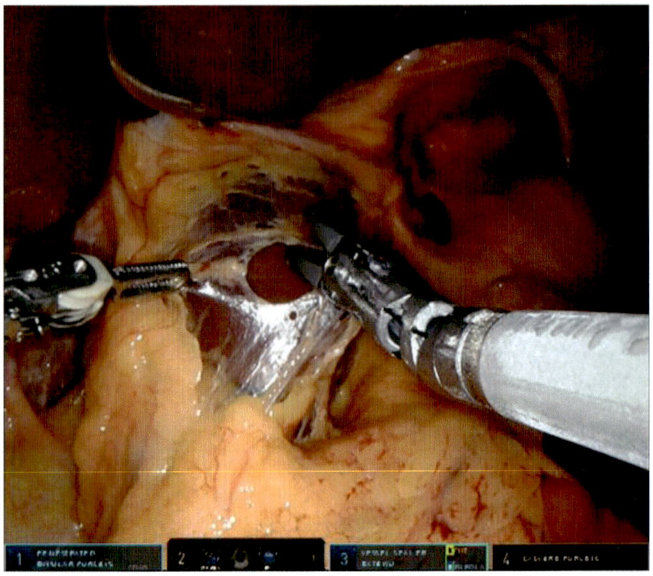

Fig. 9.4 Divide the pars flaccida and march up to the right crus

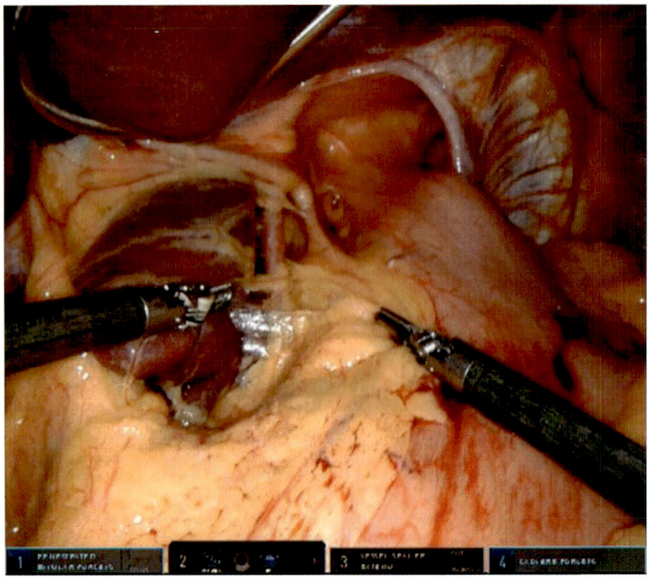

Fig. 9.3 Identify and expose the pars flaccida of the gastrohepatic ligament

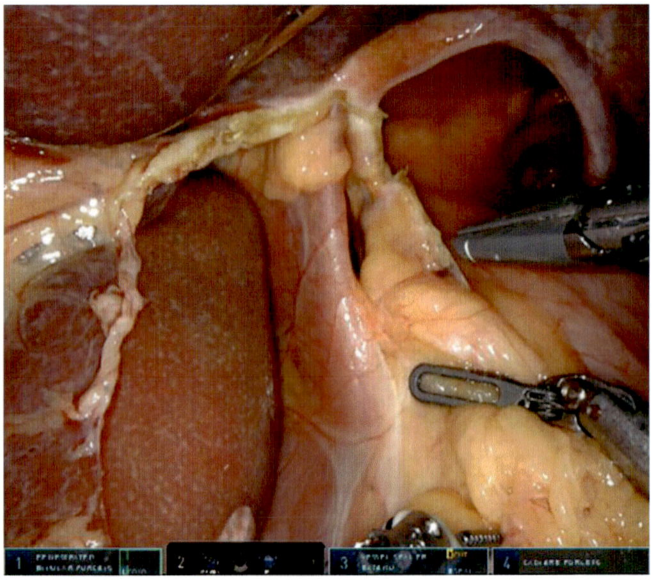

Fig. 9.5 Splay out the peritoneal covering of the right crus by retracting the adjacent fat

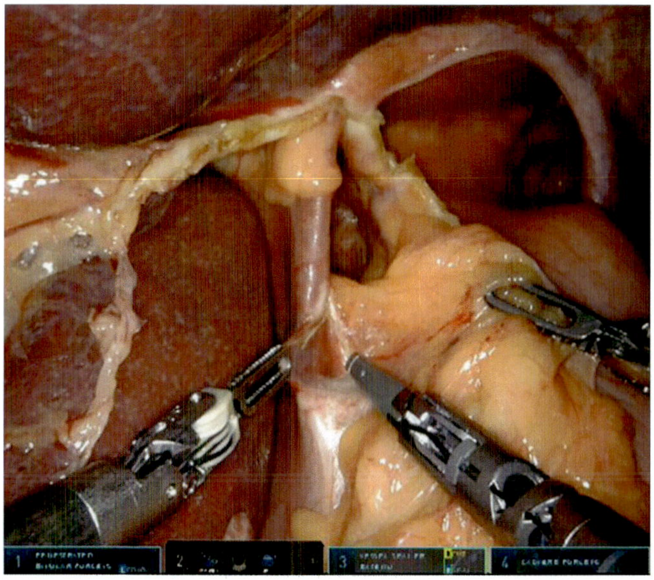

Fig. 9.6 Open the peritoneal covering using the vessel sealer extend down to muscle fibers

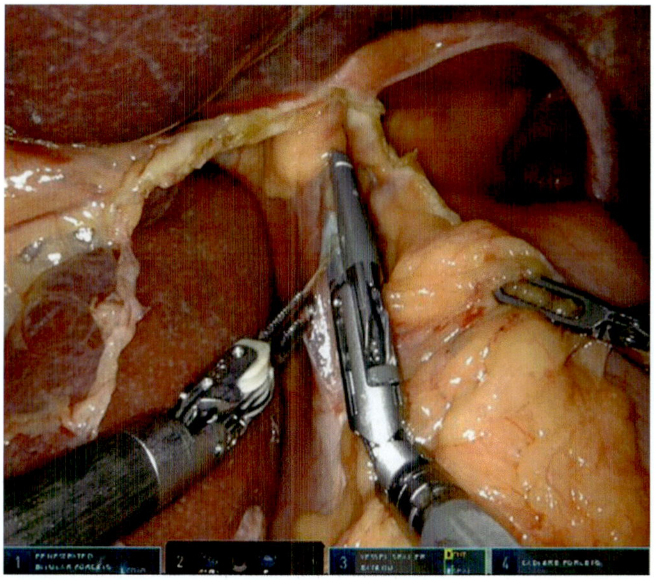

Fig. 9.7 Open along the entire length of the right crus

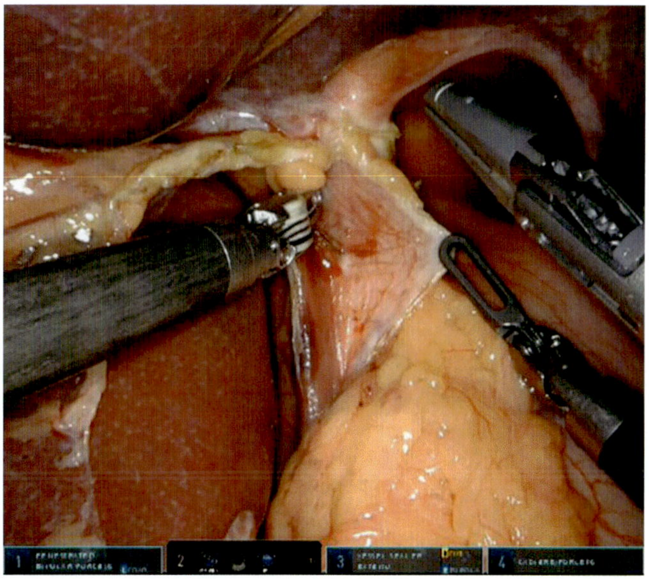

Fig. 9.8 Retract the hernia sac to see the muscle fibers which will be gently spread off the sac

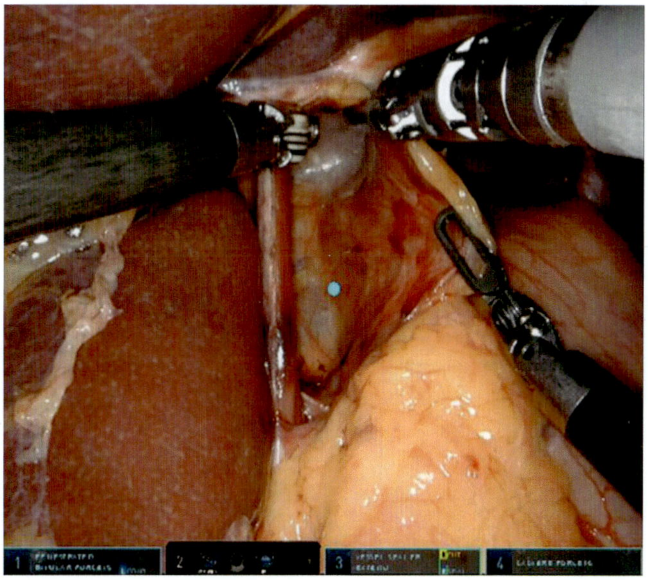

Fig. 9.9 Bluntly spreading the muscle fibers off the hernia sac lead to the areolar planes in the mediastinum

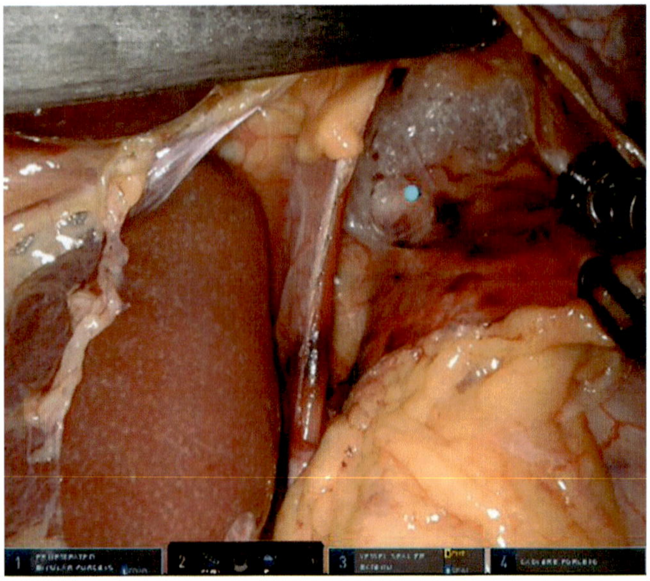

Fig. 9.10 Follow the areolar plane to mobilize the hernia sac away from the anterior mediastinum

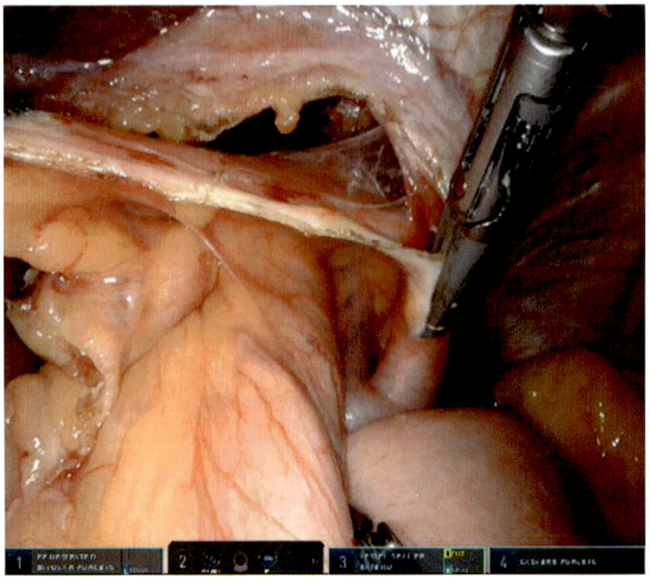

Fig. 9.11 Score the peritoneum down to muscle fibers along the left crus to separate the hernia sac from the crural muscle

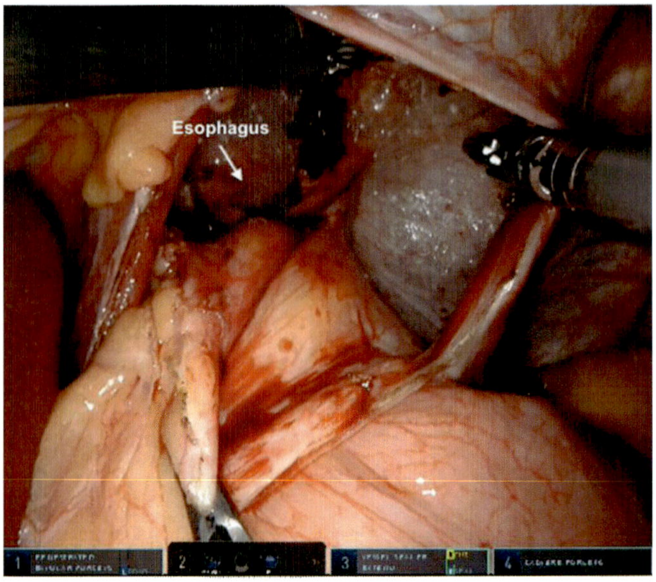

Fig. 9.12 Using blunt dissection and the areolar tissue planes as a guide continue to reduce the hernia sac from the mediastinal attachments. Once the hernia sac is reduced, the esophagus will come into view

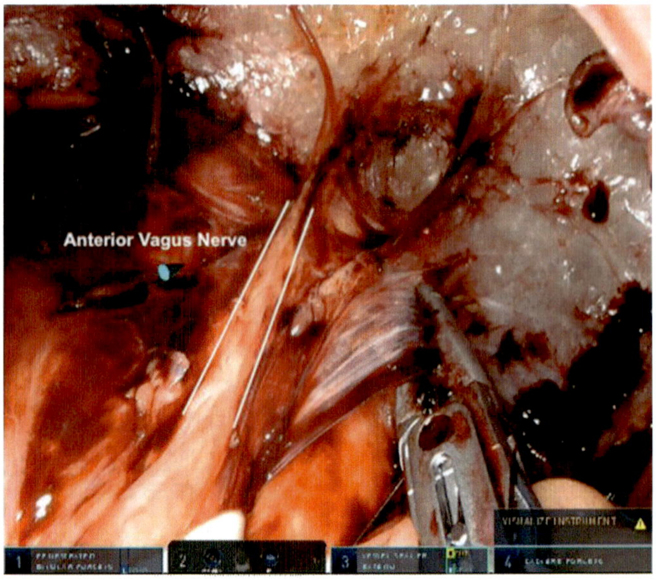

Fig. 9.13 Continue mobilizing the esophagus, identifying and preserving the anterior vagus nerve

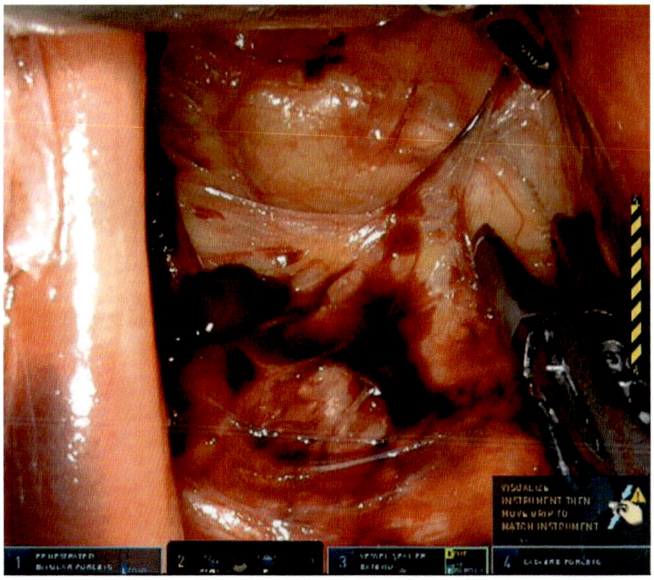

Fig. 9.14 Create the posterior window in the mediastinum by lifting the esophagus up and gently spreading the connective tissue until a window is made

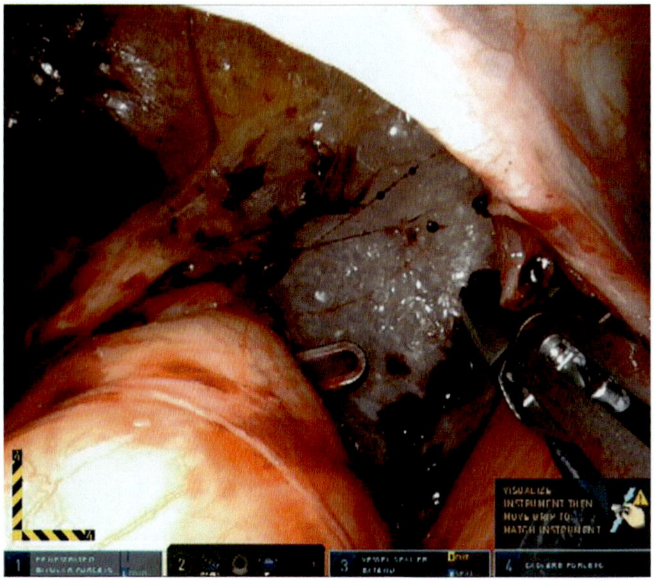

Fig. 9.15 Place a grasper through the window

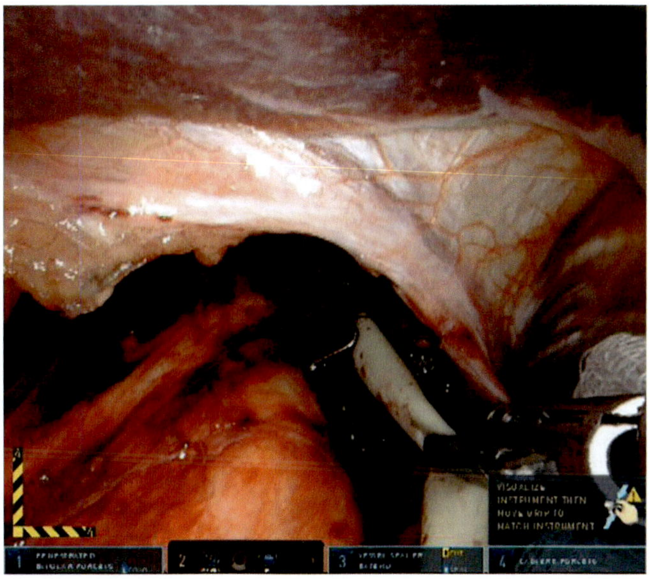

Fig. 9.16 Hand yourself a penrose to pull through the posterior window

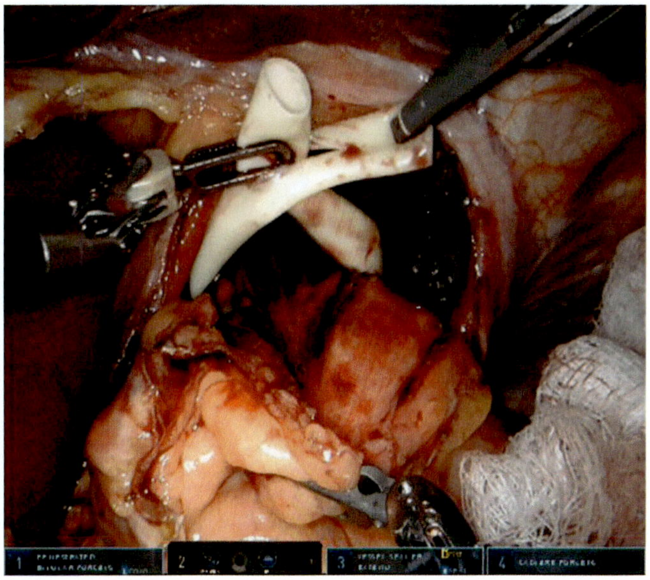

Fig. 9.17 Secure the penrose around the distal esophagus to aid in retraction for the rest of the case

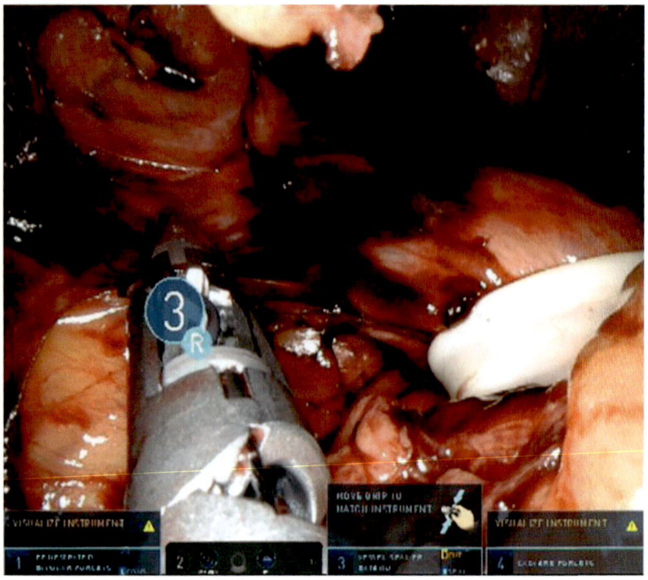

Fig. 9.18 Divide lateral attachments to continue esophageal mobilization

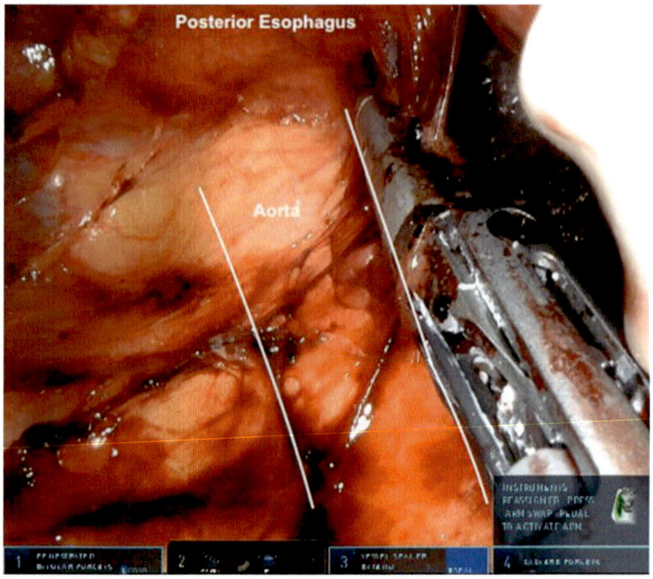

Fig. 9.20 March up along the aorta ligating tributary vessels along the way

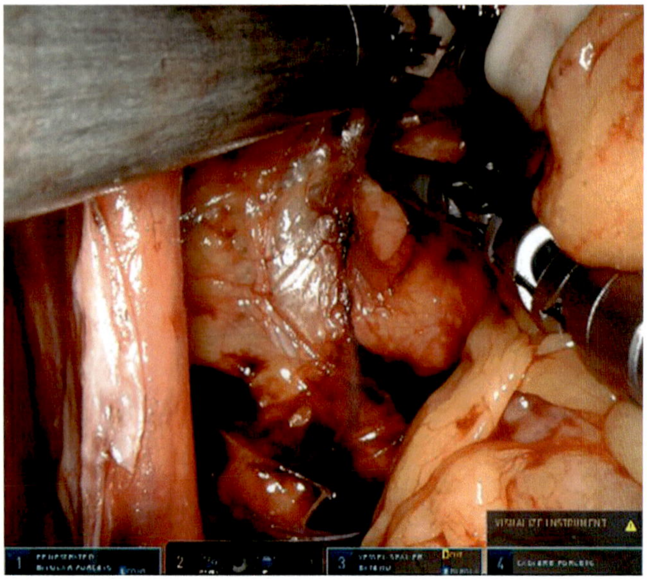

Fig. 9.19 Continue posterior dissection by dissection in the plane between the posterior esophagus and the aortic fat

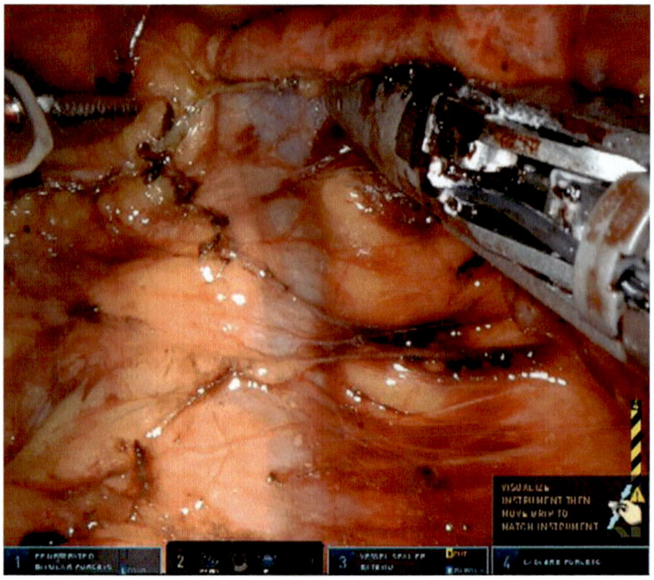

Fig. 9.21 Posterior dissection continues high into the mediastinum to relieve tension and tp gain intra-abdominal length on the esophagus

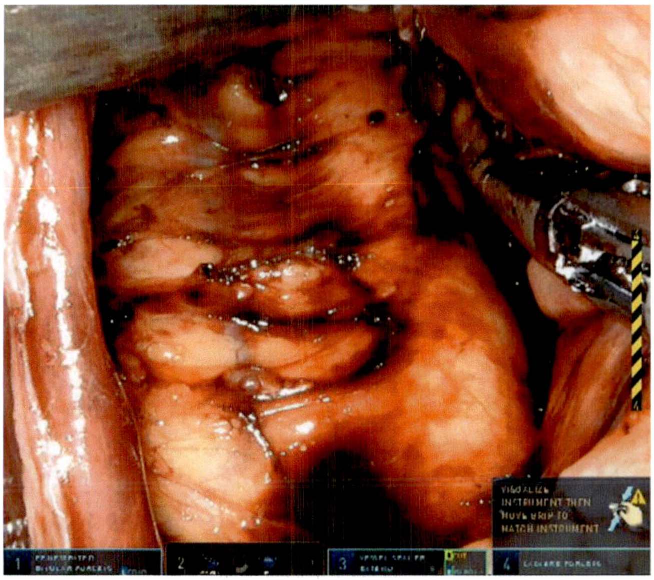

Fig. 9.22 Completed posterior esophageal dissection

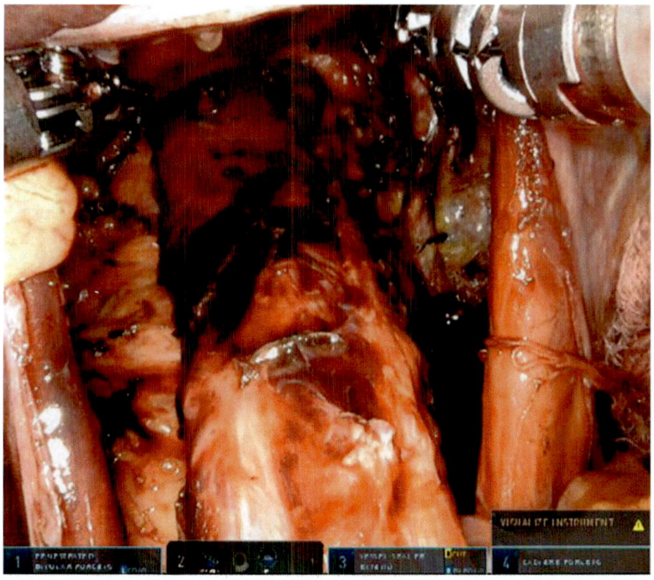

Fig. 9.23 Completed anterior esophageal dissection

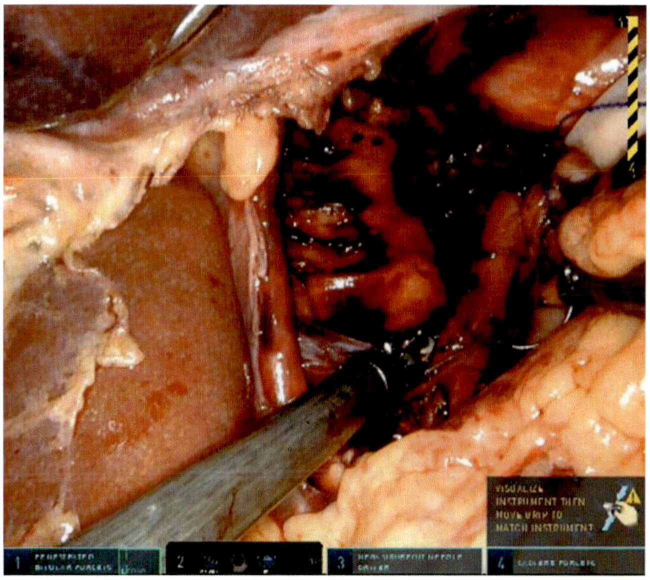

Fig. 9.24 Crural closure starts at the confluence of the crura. Protect the aorta with a grasper while taking a robust bite of the left crus. Non-absorbable barbed suture

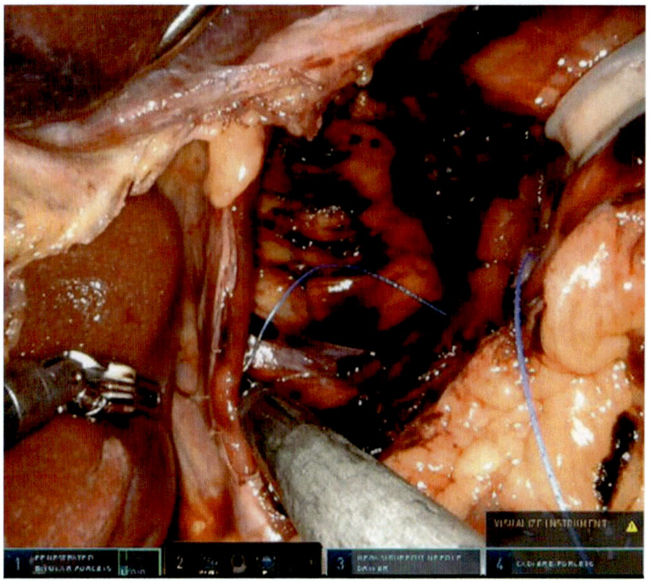

Fig. 9.25 Take a robust bite of the right crus catching the anterior peritoneal covering

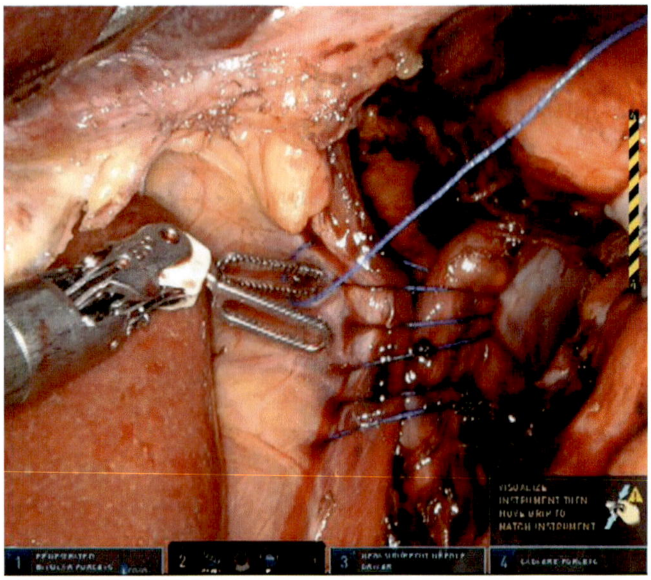

Fig. 9.26 Continue running the barbed suture to bring the crural muscles together posteriorly

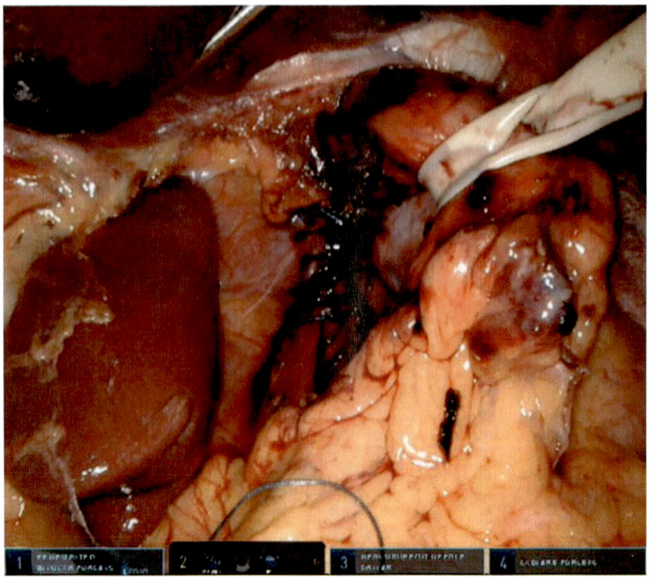

Fig. 9.27 Close the hiatus until it circumferentially approximates the esophagus without impinging on it

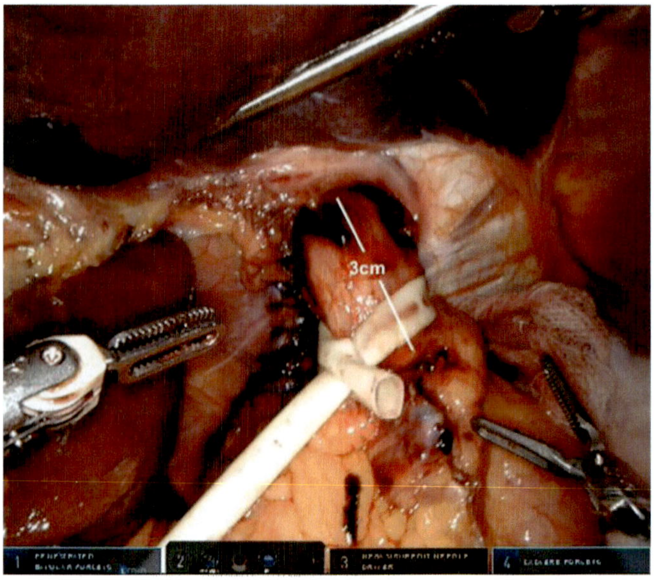

Fig. 9.28 Hernia is now repaired with 3 cm of intra-abdominal esophageal length

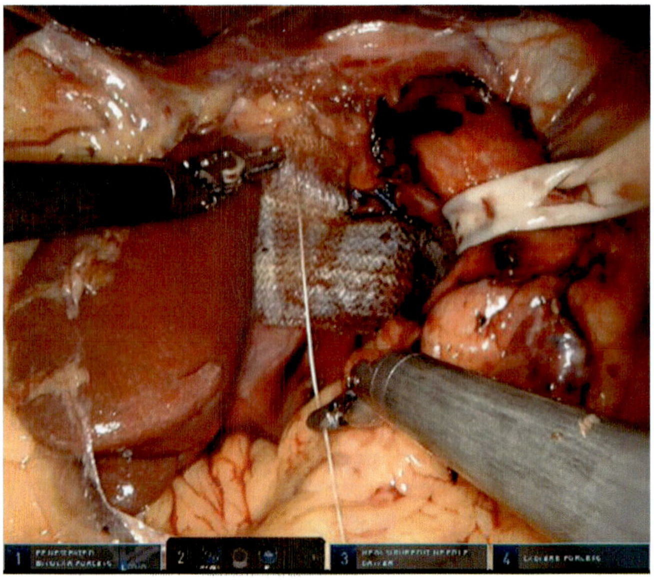

Fig. 9.29 Phasix ST mesh is cut and placed posteriorly to reinforce the hiatal closure

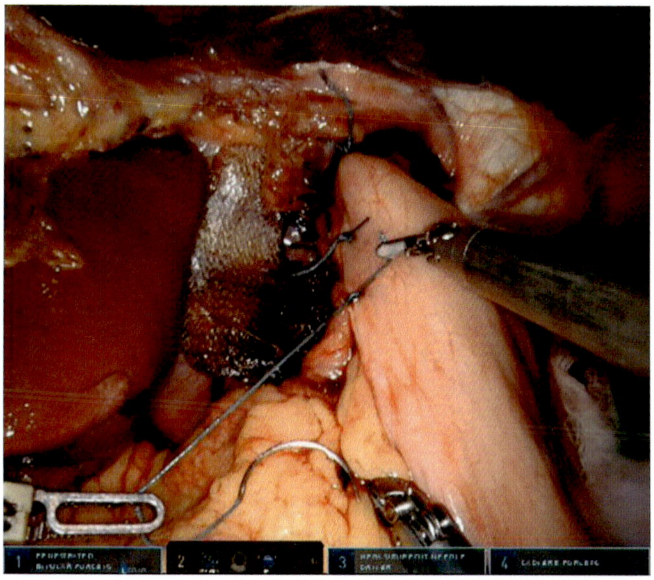

Fig. 9.30 Once the hernia is repaired, LES augmentation required. Anterior partial fundoplication (modified Watson fundoplication) is used in this case

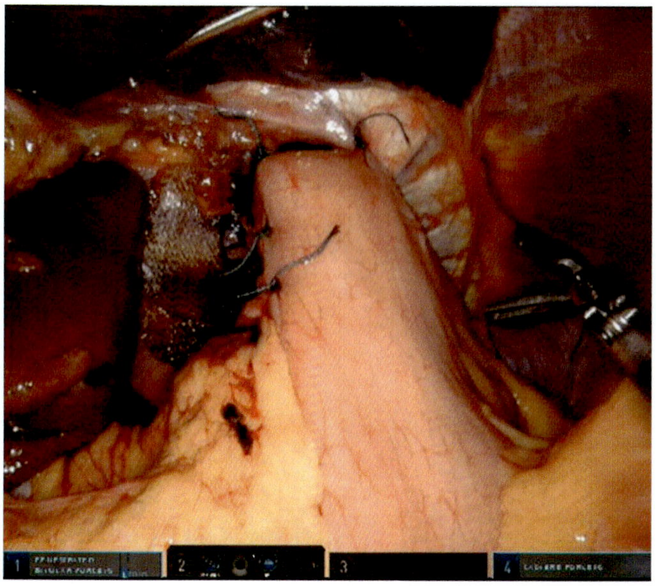

Fig. 9.31 Fundoplication completed

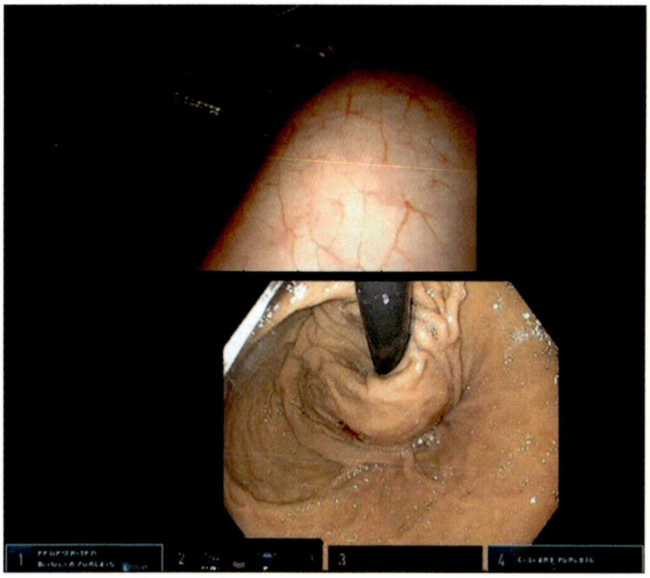

Fig. 9.32 Endoscopic evaluation of the valve shows a Hill grade 1 valve

References

1. Geoffrey P Kohn MBBS(Hons) MSurg FRACS, Raymond R Price MD FACS, Steven R Demeester MD FACS, Joerg Zehetner MD, Oliver J Muensterer MD, Ziad T Awad MD FACS, Sumeet K Mittal MD FACS, William S Richardson MD FACS, Dimitrios Stefanidis MD PhD FACS, Robert D Fanelli MD FACS and the SAGES Guidelines Committee. Guidelines for the management of hiatal hernia. 2013.
2. Kohn GP, Price RR, Demeester SR, et al. Guidelines for the management of hiatal hernia. Surg Endosc. 2013;27(12):4409–28. https://doi.org/10.1007/s00464-013-3173-3 [published Online First: Epub Date].
3. Hill LD, Kozarek RA, Kraemer SJM, et al. The gastroesophageal flap valve: in vitro and in vivo observations. Gastrointest Endosc. 1996;44(5):541–7.

10 Robotic Truncal Vagotomy and Antrectomy

Fazaldin Moghul and Abubaker A. Ali

Introduction

Peptic ulcer disease can cause complications requiring surgical intervention; acute complications include perforation and bleeding, while chronic complications include refractory ulcers, gastric outlet obstruction, and malignancy. The Johnson classification of peptic ulcers based on location can help tailor therapy. Type I ulcers occur on the body of the stomach along the lesser curve and are associated with normal acid secretion. Type II gastric ulcers occur in association with an active or previous duodenal ulcer. Type III ulcers are located in the prepyloric region. Type IV ulcers occur in the proximal stomach. Type V ulcers can occur anywhere in the stomach and are associated with chronic NSAID use. Type II and III ulcers are associated with hyperacid states and benefit from vagotomy and antrectomy or vagotomy and pyloroplasty. Performing antrectomy removes the portion of the stomach which contain the G cells that are responsible for secreting gastrin. Vagotomy removes the direct cholinergic stimulation for gastric acid secretion by the parietal cells and decreases the parietal cell response to histamine and gastrin [1]. Truncal vagotomy completely denervates the stomach, reduces acid secretion, and alters gastric motility. A gastric emptying procedure should be performed after truncal vagotomy.

The procedure can be performed open, laparoscopic, or robotic assisted. Robotic gastric surgery is associated with less blood loss and length of stay, though there are longer operative times [2]. The advantage of the robotic approach is the ability to perform meticulous dissection around a scarred stomach and duodenum with improved magnification and articulating movement of instruments.

A robotic antrectomy begins with dissection along the greater curve from the pylorus cephalad. The lesser curve is mobilized and the right gastric artery is ligated. The duodenal bulb is dissected off of the pancreas, which may have significant scarring. The proximal transection should extend from the incisura along the lesser curve to the terminal branch of the right gastroepiploic artery on the greater curve. The distal transection should be on to the duodenum to avoid retained antrum syndrome. An anastomosis to restore gastrointestinal continuity can be performed with a gastroduodenal or gastrojejunal anastomosis. The patient shown in this chapter underwent a gastrojejunal, or Billroth II, reconstruction. Truncal vagotomy involves resecting a 1–2 cm portion of the anterior and posterior vagal trunks as the nerves pass through the esophageal hiatus in the diaphragm. The nerve segments are sent to pathology to confirm the segment is nerve tissue [3].

Procedure: Illustrated Steps

Figures 10.1, 10.2, 10.3, 10.4, 10.5, 10.6, 10.7, 10.8, 10.9, 10.10, 10.11, 10.12, 10.13, 10.14, 10.15, 10.16, 10.17, 10.18, 10.19, 10.20, 10.21, 10.22, 10.23, 10.24, 10.25, 10.26, 10.27, 10.28, 10.29, 10.30, 10.31, 10.32, 10.33, 10.34, 10.35, 10.36, 10.37, and 10.38 illustrate the technical aspects of robotic vagotomy and antrectomy. The enteric reconstruction is performed with a stapled retrocolic retrogastric Billroth II gastrojejunostomy.

F. Moghul · A. A. Ali (✉)
Department of General Surgery, Wayne State University, Detroit, MI, USA
e-mail: aaali@med.wayne.edu

O. Y. Kudsi, P. P. Grimminger (eds.), *Atlas of Robotic Upper Gastrointestinal Surgery*,
https://doi.org/10.1007/978-3-030-86578-8_10

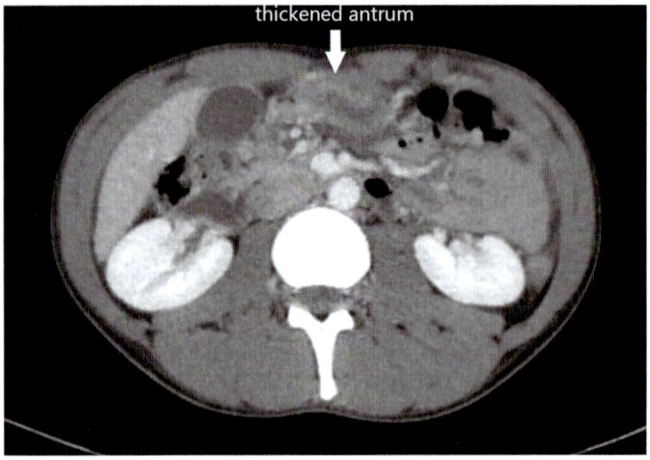

Fig. 10.1 Computerized tomography (CT), transverse image, thickened antrum

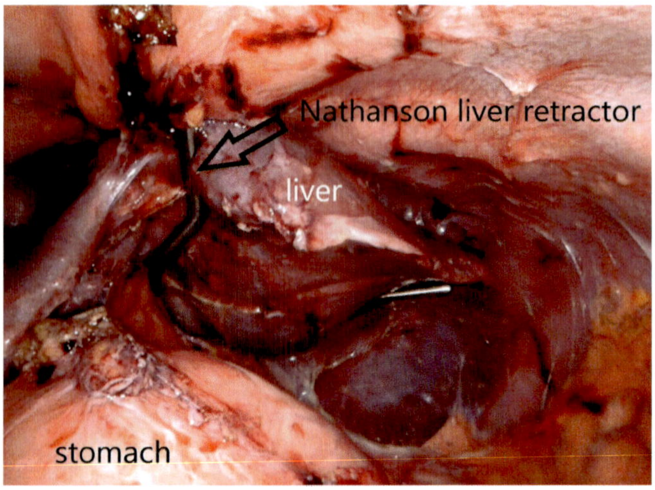

Fig. 10.2 After the trocars are inserted, a liver retractor is placed. A Nathanson retractor or snake liver retractor can be used. Alternatively, an 18 inch barbed suture can be used to suspend the left lateral segment of the liver anteriorly. The patient is placed in reverse Trendelenberg, and the patient side cart of the robot is docked

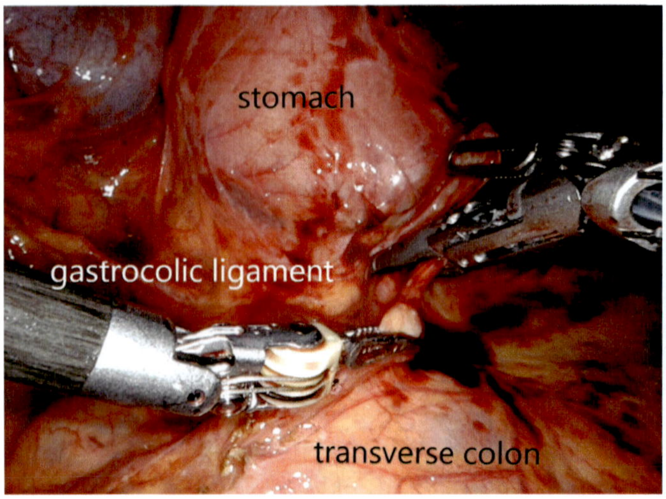

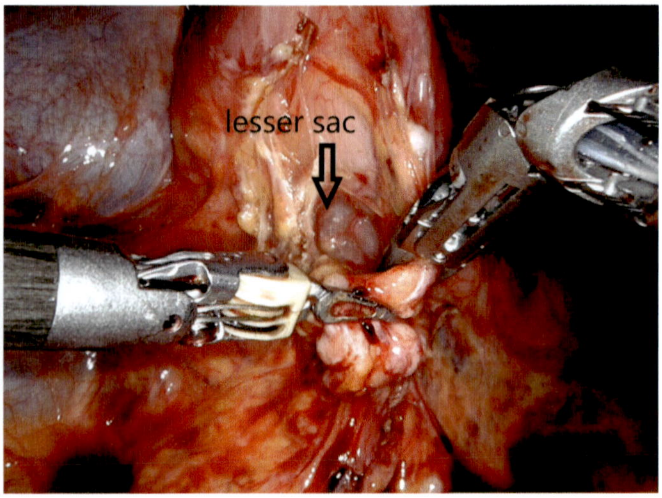

Figs. 10.3 and 10.4 The stomach is retracted cephalad, and the colon is retracted caudad. The vessel sealer is used to enter the lesser sac by incising the gastrocolic ligament in an avascular plane

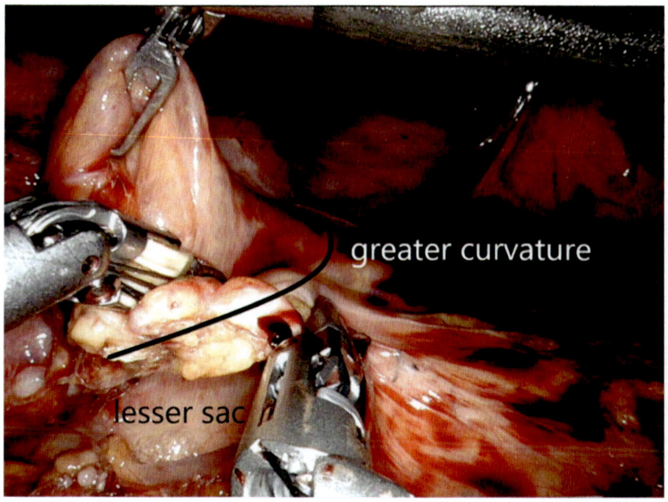

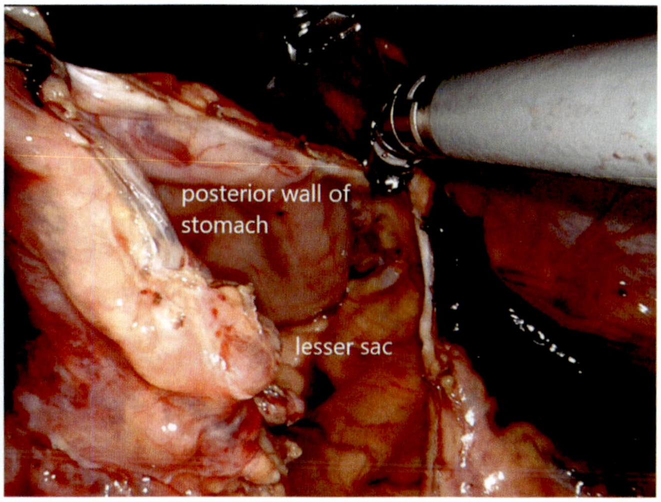

Figs. 10.5 and 10.6 The dissection is continued along the greater curvature cephalad until the junction of the right and left gastroepiploic arteries. The right gastroepiploic artery runs in closer proximity to the greater curvature of the stomach compared to the left gastroepiploic artery

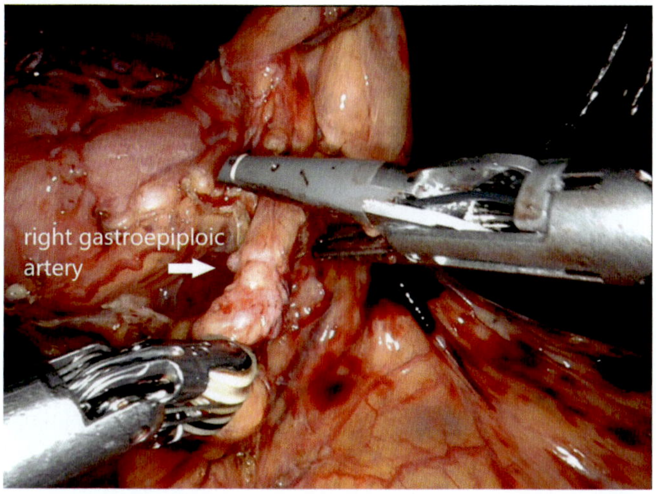

Fig. 10.7 The dissection continues distally along the greater curve past the pylorus with ligation of the right gastroepiploic artery

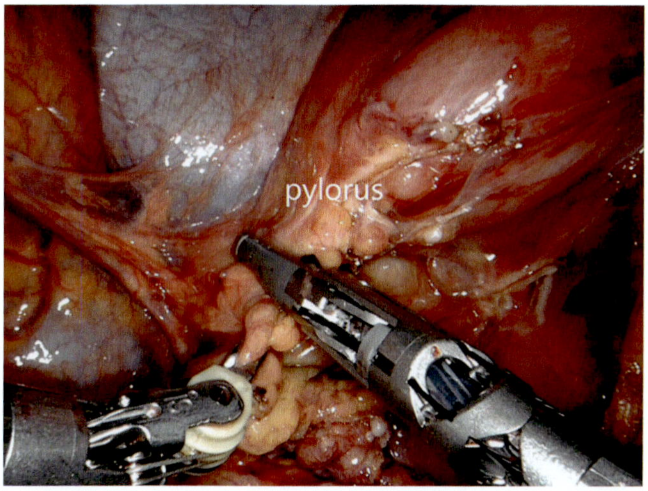

Fig. 10.9 The distal dissection should continue until the pylorus is mobilized enough to staple the duodenum approximately 1 cm past the pylorus

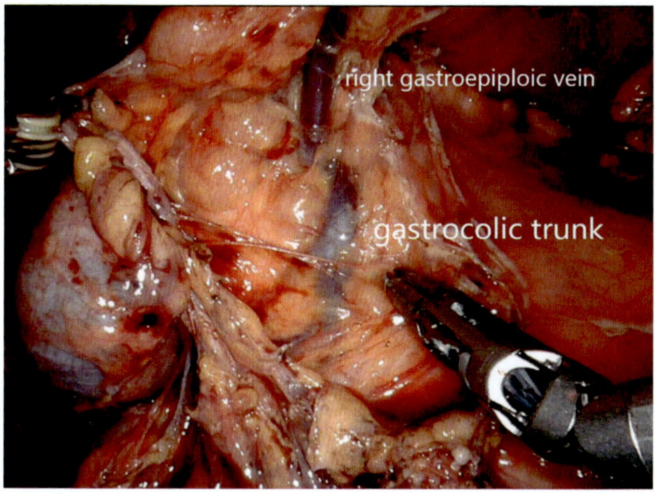

Fig. 10.8 The gastrocolic trunk is identified and the right gastroepiploic vein is ligated

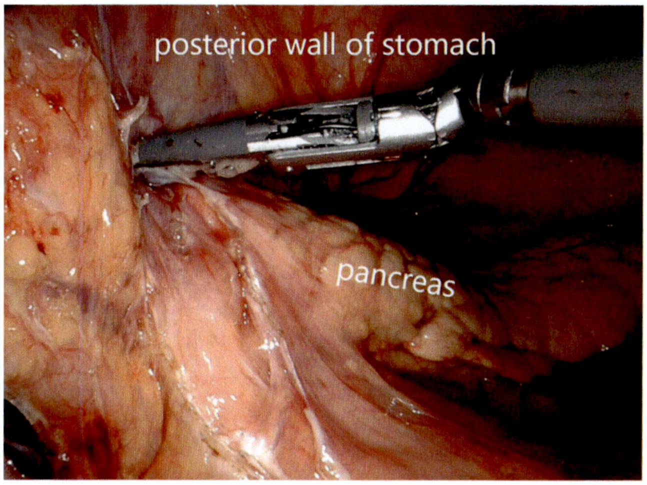

Fig. 10.10 Dissection is performed to free the posterior wall of the stomach from the anterior surface of the pancreas

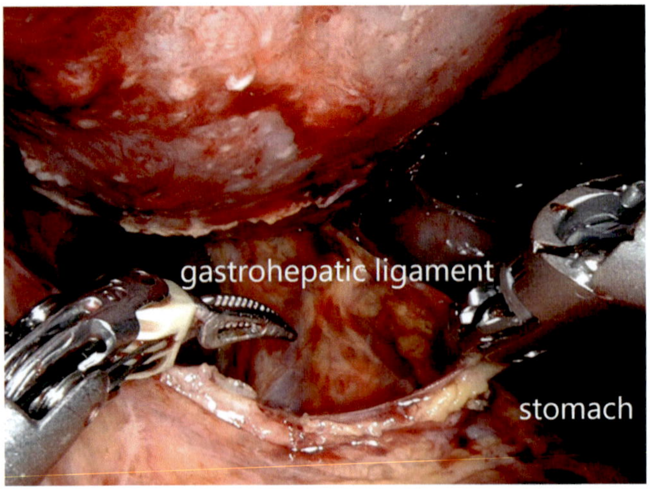

Fig. 10.11 The lesser curve is mobilized by incising the gastrohepatic ligament at the pars flaccida. The dissection should continue from the incisura toward the pylorus

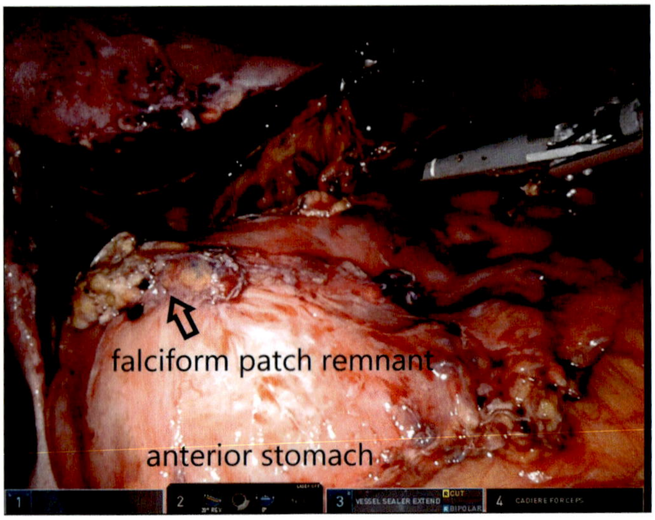

Fig. 10.13 The falciform patch from the previous prepyloric gastric perforation is seen on the anterior wall of the stomach

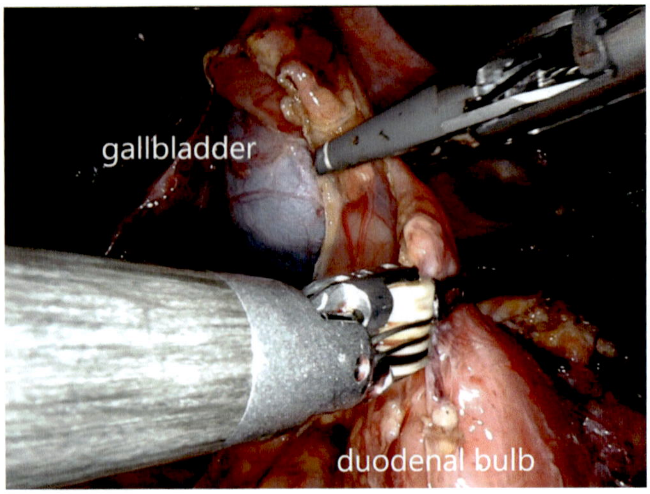

Fig. 10.12 The gallbladder is grasped and retracted cephalad. The adhesions between the gallbladder and duodenum are taken down to expose the duodenal bulb. The patient shown below had previous a previous gastric perforation that was repaired with a falciform ligament patch

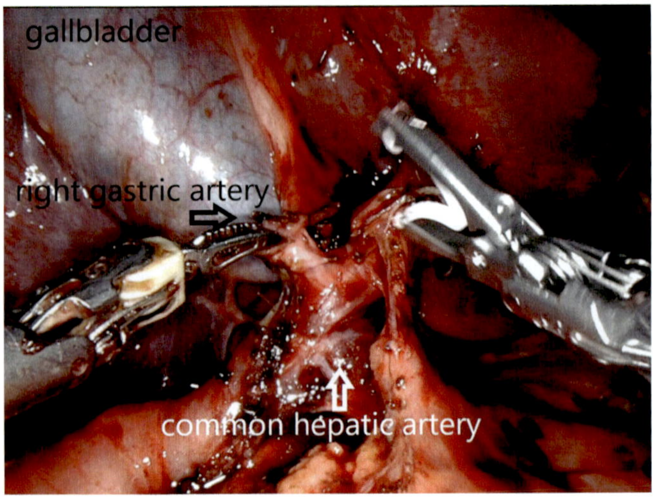

Fig. 10.14 The right gastric artery is ligated

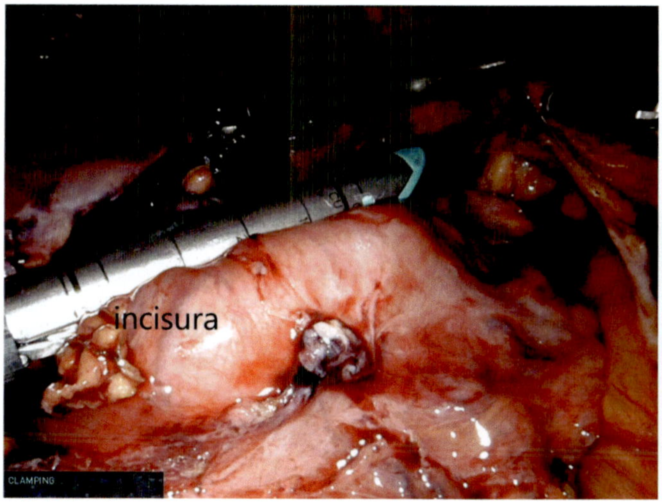

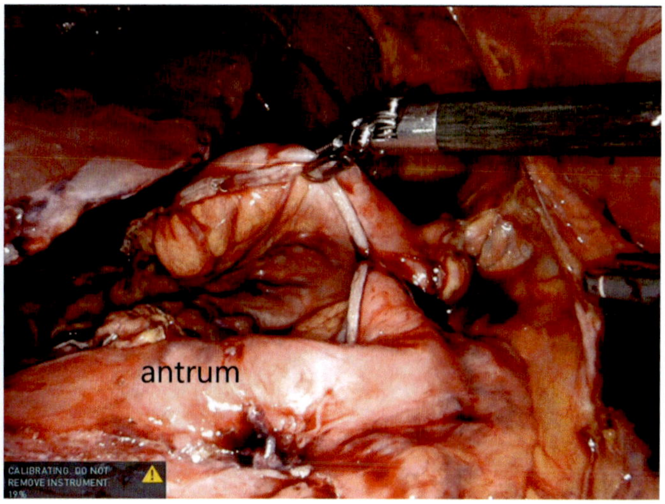

Figs. 10.15 and 10.16 The proximal transection is performed with the staple device in the left hand, from the middle of the lesser curve, or incisura, to the terminal branch of the right gastroepiploic artery

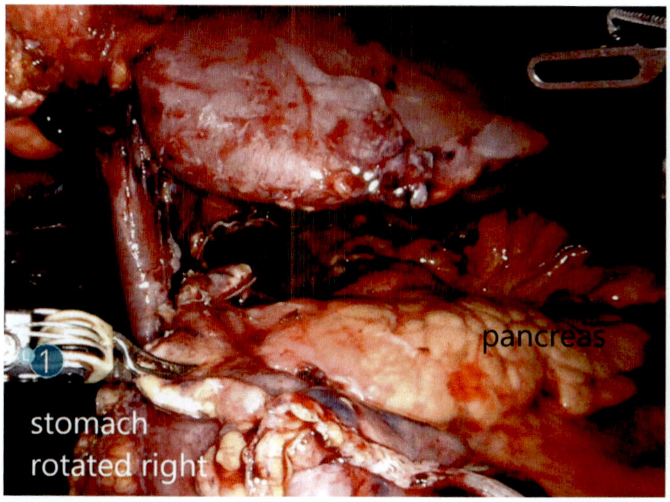

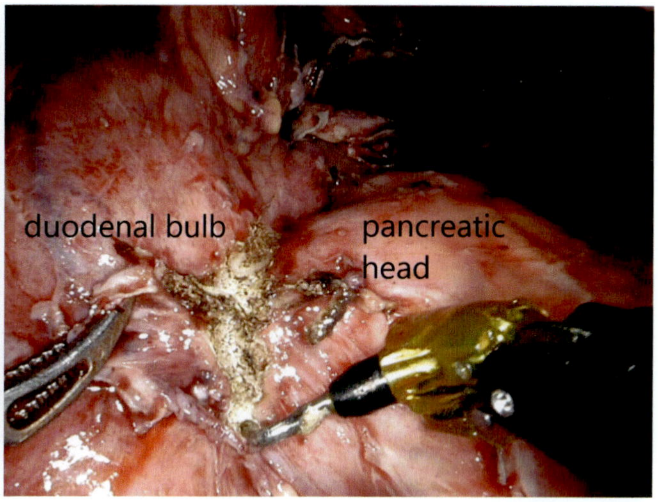

Figs. 10.17 and 10.18 Once the proximal transection is complete, the distal stomach is rotated to the patient's right side to expose the posterior wall of the duodenal bulb. Meticulous dissection should be performed to free the posterior duodenal bulb off of the pancreas, as there may be significant adhesions present. If encountered, bleeding typically arises from injuring the capsule of the pancreas, which can be controlled with suture ligature or bipolar device

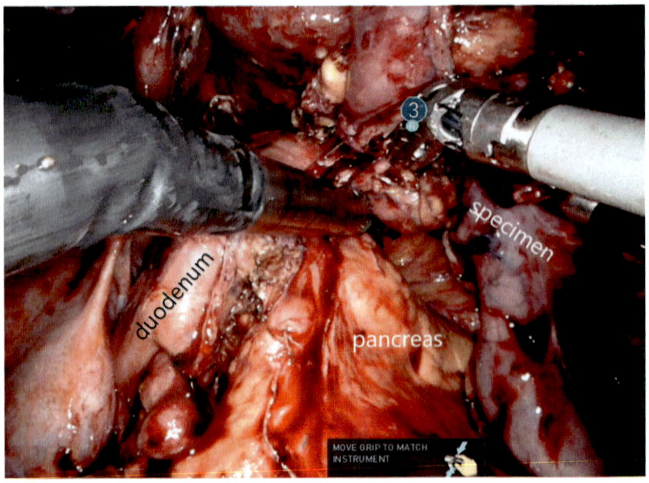

Fig. 10.19 Distally, the dissection should be carried onto the duodenum until the pylorus is mobilized. A helpful anatomic landmark is the prepyloric vein of Mayo, which is a tributary of the right gastric vein that passes anteriorly to the junction of the pylorus and duodenum. In patients with chronic peptic ulcer disease, there can be deformity of the stomach and duodenal bulb which can make distinction between the pylorus and duodenum difficult. In these cases, the distal transection margin should be sent to pathology for frozen section to identify the presence of duodenal cells (Brunner glands) and avoid retained antrum syndrome. The proximal duodenum is transected with care to avoid injury to the common bile duct by visualizing the tip of the stapler. The stomach should be rotated anteriorly while stapling

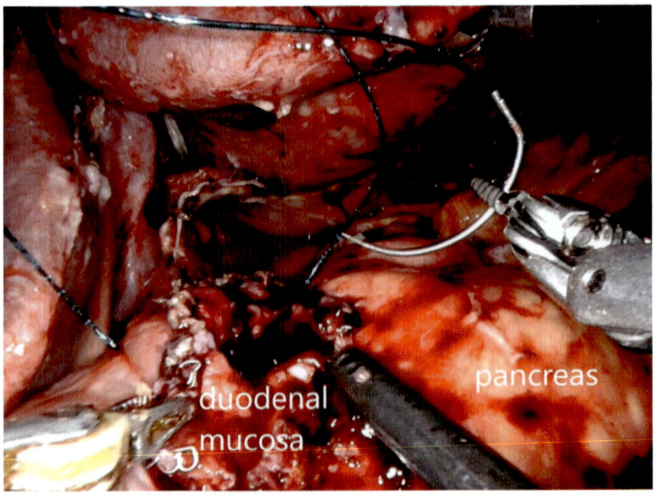

Fig. 10.20 The distal staple line should be examined. The patient below had staple line dehiscence due to wall edema and thickness. Options for repair include duodenal stump closure with suture or further mobilization of the duodenum to healthy, soft tissue for additional transection

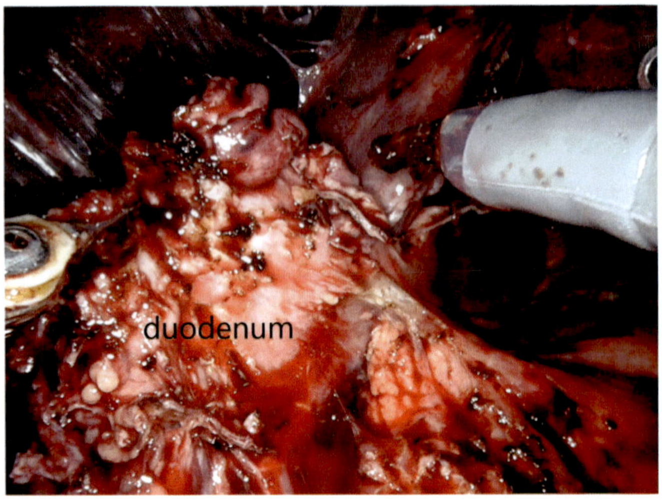

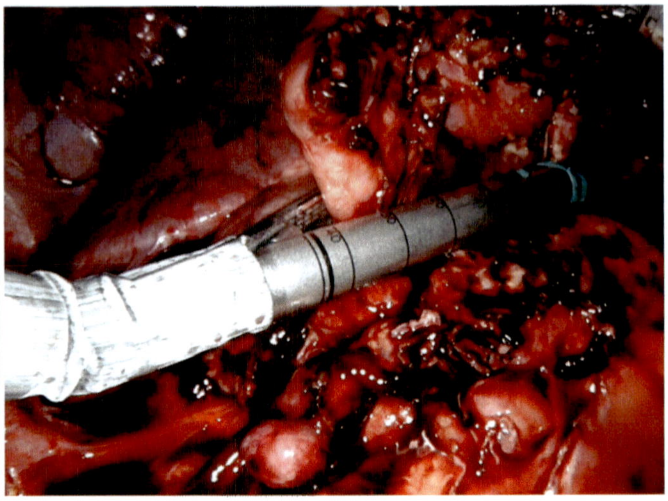

Figs. 10.21 and 10.22 The specimen can be removed through a Pfannenstiel incision and sent to pathology as a frozen section. If there is no duodenal mucosa identified, additional duodenal mobilization and transection must be performed

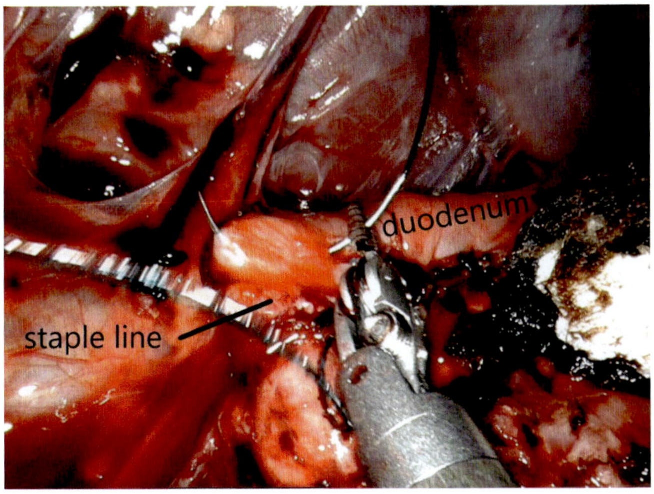

Fig. 10.23 The duodenal stump staple line can be reinforced by oversewing with a running suture in a full-thickness or imbricating fashion. A drain should be left at the duodenal stump to monitor for duodenal stump leak or blowout

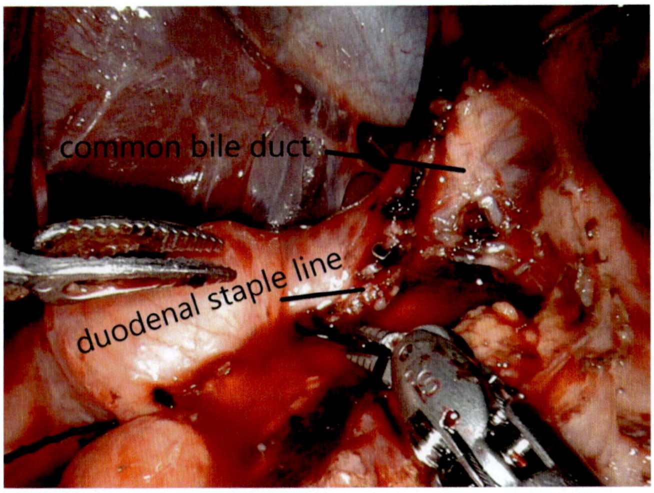

Fig. 10.24 The common bile duct is in close proximity to the staple line

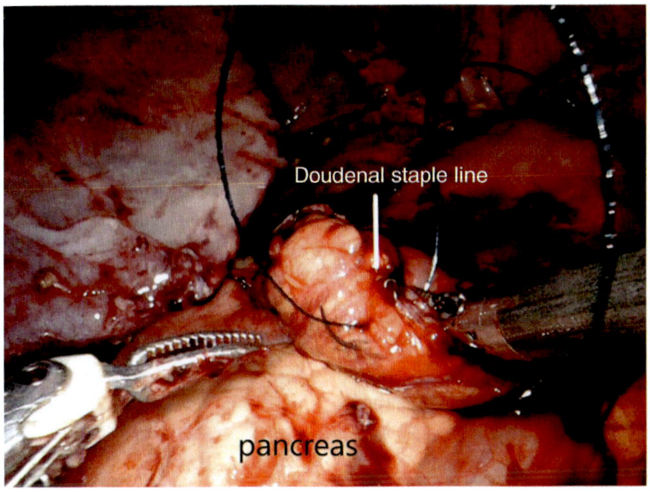

Fig. 10.25 The gastric transection can be reinforced with imbricating or full-thickness oversewing suture

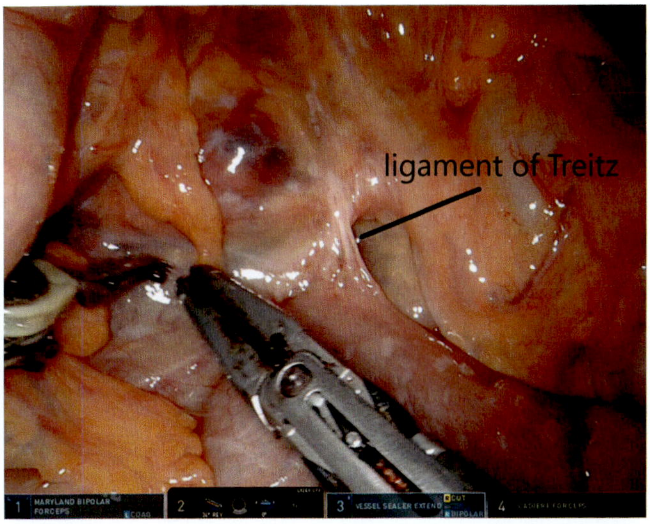

Fig. 10.26 The transverse colon should be retracted cephalad to identify the ligament of Treitz. An appropriate loop of jejunum approximately 20 cm distal to the ligament of Treitz is selected. A longer afferent limb can cause kinking and afferent loop obstruction

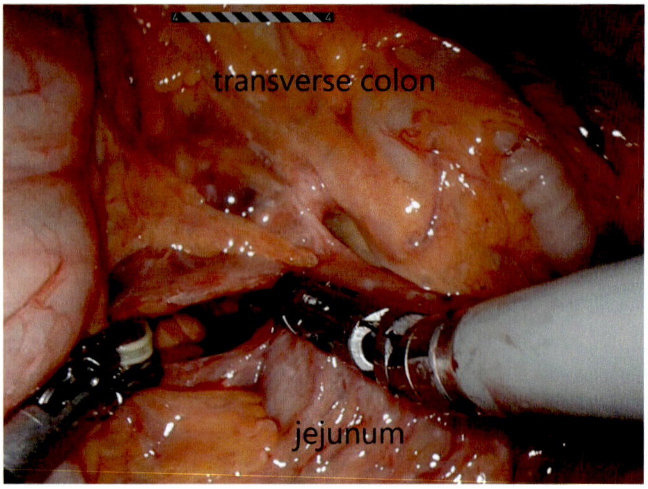

Fig. 10.27 A mesenteric window is created in the avascular plane at the base of the transverse mesocolon

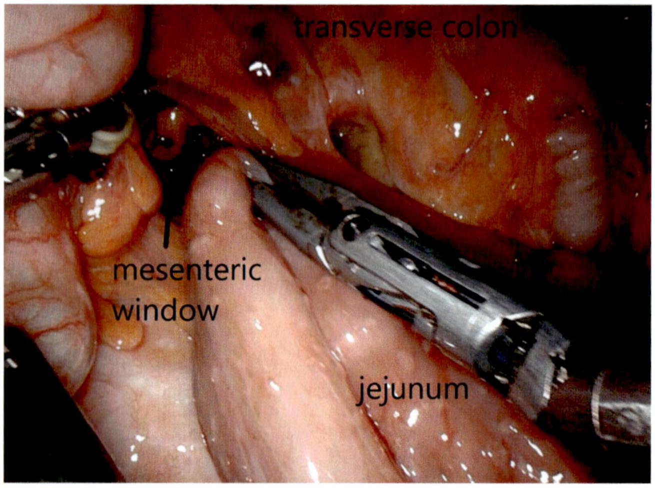

Fig. 10.28 The jejunal loop is delivered through the transverse mesocolon for our retrocolic anastomosis. Alternatively, the jejunum can be brought anterior to the transverse colon for an antecolic anastomosis. The anastomosis should not be under tension and the jejunal mesentery not twisted. A retrocolic approach allows for a shorter afferent limb

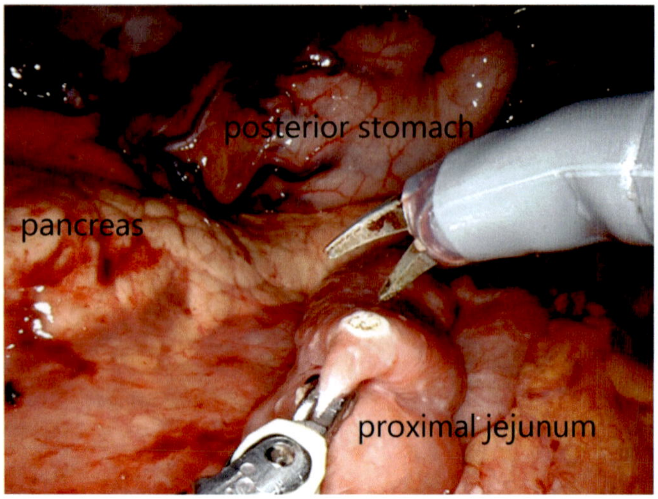

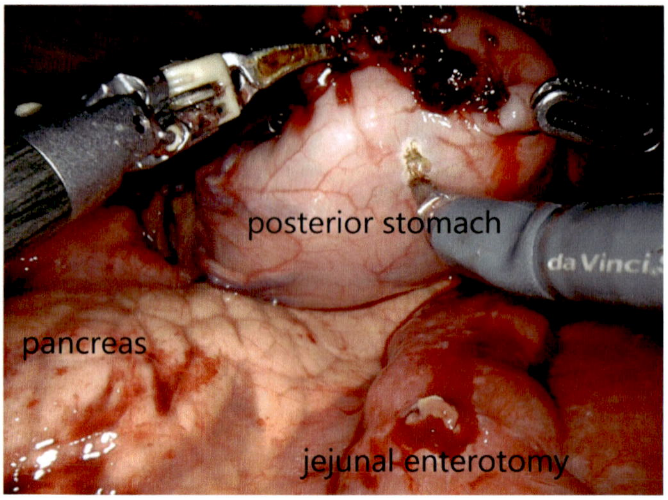

Figs. 10.29 and 10.30 Interrupted seromuscular traction sutures should be placed between the stomach and jejunum to line up the adjacent lumens. Matching incisions are created on the antimesenteric border of the jejunum and posterior wall of the stomach using electrocautery. This will allow for a retrogastric anastomosis. Alternativley, the anastomosis can be created in an antegatric fashion

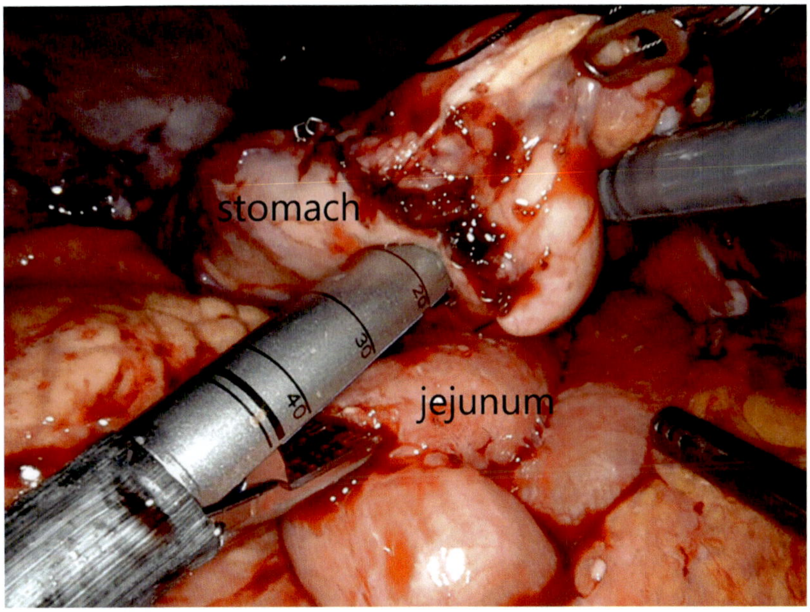

Fig. 10.31 The EndoGIA stapler is inserted into each lumen to create the anastomosis. Alternatively, a hand-sewn anastomosis can be performed

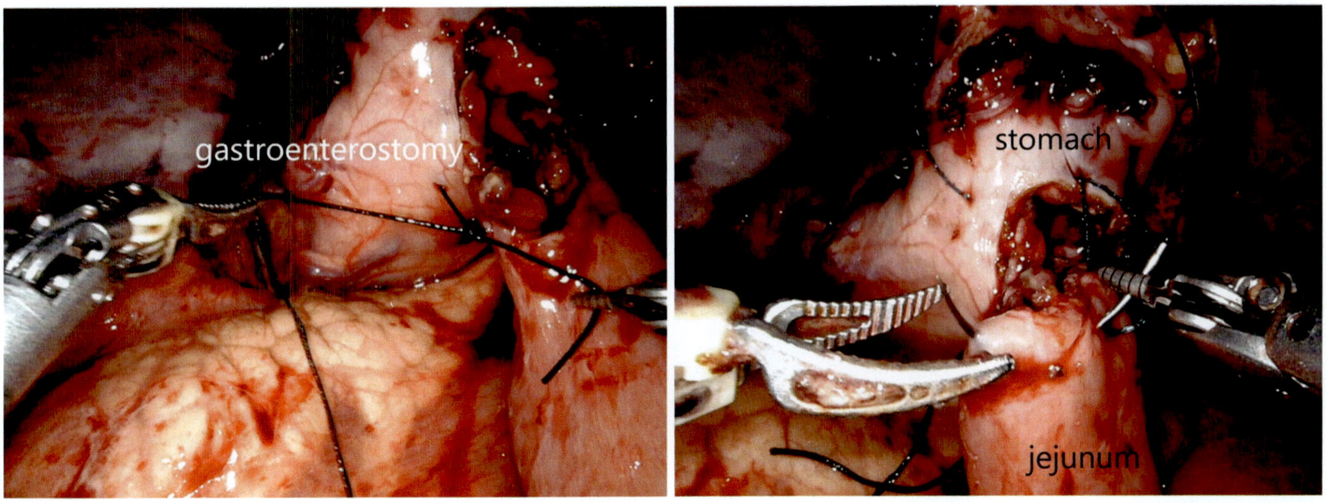

Figs. 10.32 and 10.33 The enterotomy is closed using a barbed suture in a continuous fashion. A silk suture is placed to facilitate retraction and identify the corner of the gastroenterotomy

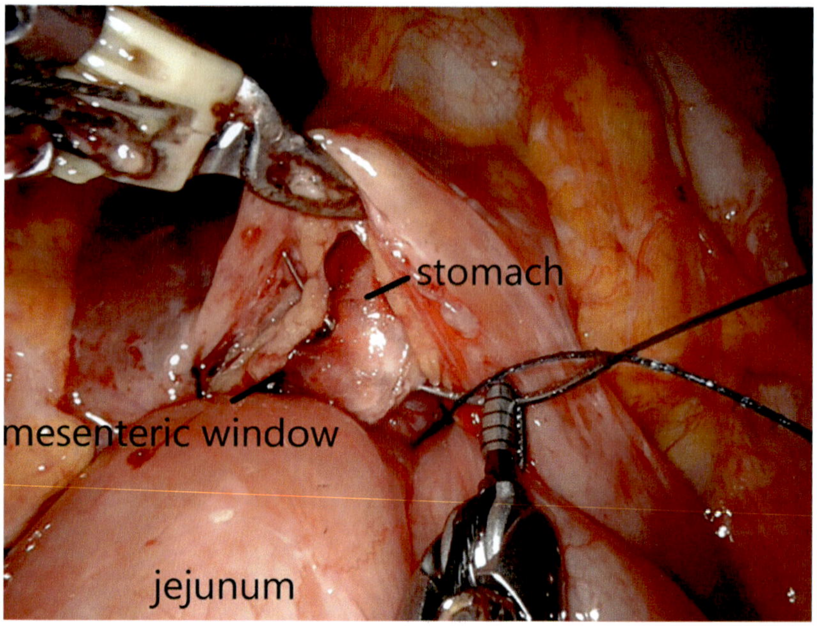

Fig. 10.34 The anastomosis is brought below the defect in the transverse mesocolon. Suturing the stomach to the mesentery prevents jejunal herniation through the defect and kinking of the afferent and efferent limbs

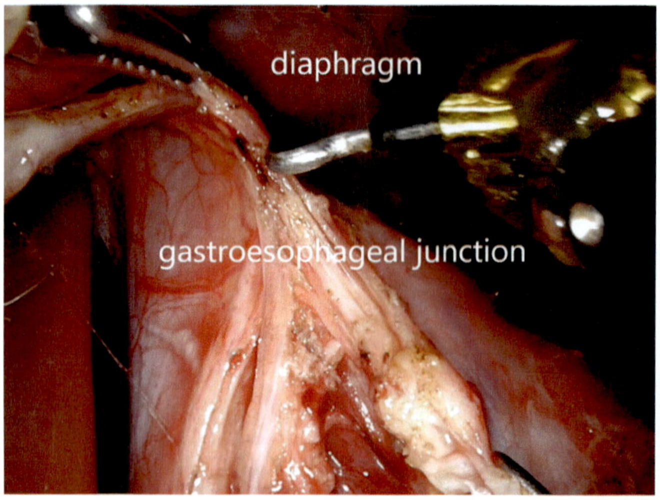

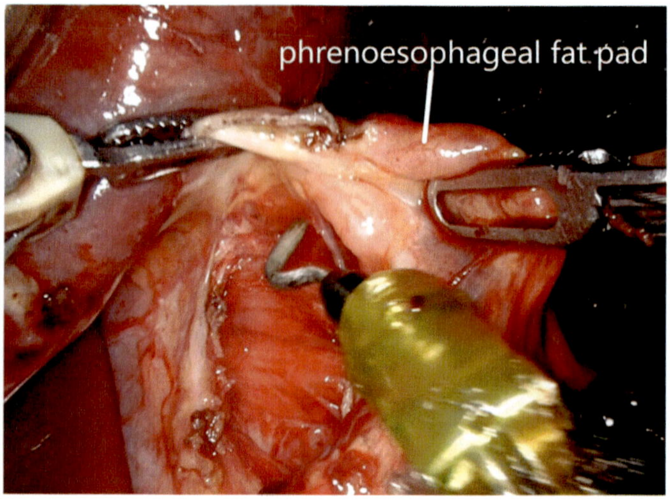

Figs. 10.35 and 10.36 To perform truncal vagotomy, the peritoneum is incised at the gastroesophageal junction horizontally from the lesser curvature to the cardiac notch on the greater curvature. The phrenoesophageal fat pad is mobilized. Blunt dissection is performed to encircle the esophagus with a Penrose drain to facilitate effective retraction

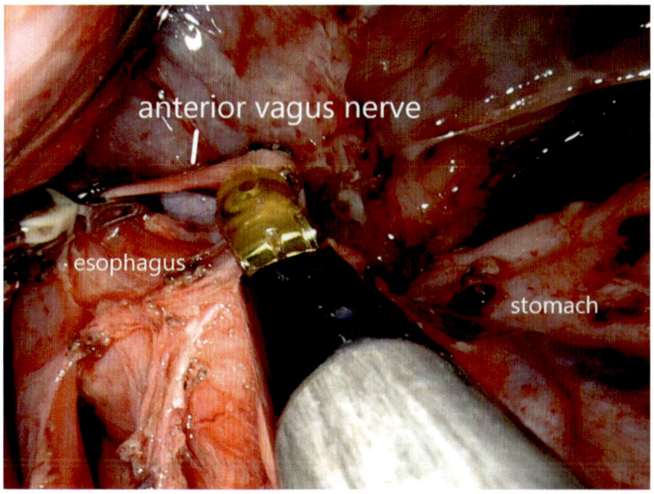

Fig. 10.37 The anterior vagal trunk can be identified in the anterior mid portion of the esophagus, 2 to 4 cm above the gastroesophageal junction. The anterior vagus can branch into two or three smaller cords. 2 to 4 cm of the vagal trunk should be freed off the surrounding tissues, and 1 to 2 cm of the nerve should be clipped and cut

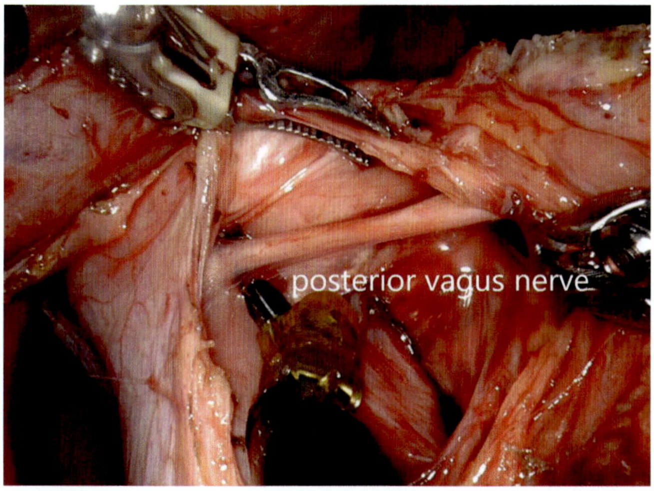

Fig. 10.38 The posterior vagal trunk appears as a taut cord anterior to the aorta above the gastroesophageal junction on the right side of the esophagus. If the anterior vagus has already been divided, downward traction on the gastroesophageal junction will cause the posterior vagus to "bowstring" and make it easier to identify. The "criminal nerve" of Grassi can be identified wrapping around the cardiac notch, originating from the posterior trunk. The resected portions of the vagal trunks should be sent to pathology for frozen section if there is question that the specimen is in fact nerve

References

1. Matthews JB, Silen W. Operations for peptic ulcer disease and early operative complications. In: Sleisenger MH, Fordtran JS, editors. Gastrointestinal disease. Philadelphia: Saunders; 1993.
2. Caruso S, Patriti A, Roviello F, et al. Robot-assisted laparoscopic vs open gastrectomy for gastric cancer: systematic review and meta-analysis. World J Clin Oncol. 2017;8(3):273–84. https://doi.org/10.5306/wjco.v8.i3.273.
3. Ali AA. Surgery for peptic ulcer disease. In: Yeo CJ, editor. Shackelford's surgery of the alimentary tract. 8th ed. Philadelphia, PA: Elsevier; 2019. https://doi.org/10.1016/C2015-1-00854-7.

Robotic Pyloroplasty

11

Katherine Fay and Ankit D. Patel

Introduction

Pyloroplasty is usually performed as a gastric drainage procedure in conjunction with truncal and selective vagotomies for peptic ulcer disease, in the setting of prior bleeding or perforated peptic ulcers causing strictures, or for patients with delayed gastric emptying. It is traditionally performed during esophagectomies to improve gastric emptying. Surgical intervention has also been shown to benefit patients with medically refractory gastroparesis [1].

There are three types of pyloroplasties—Heineke-Mikulicz, Finney, and Jaboulay. The Heineke-Mikulicz consists of transecting the pyloric sphincter longitudinally with a transverse closure and is generally the most preferred technique. A Finney pyloroplasty is a side-to-side gastroduodenostomy with incision of the pylorus muscle fibers. Similarly, a Jaboulay pyloroplasty is a side-to-side gastroduodenostomy; however, it is performed without incision of the pylorus sphincter. Finney pyloroplasty is preferred when ulcers occur in the second portion of duodenum; in cases of significant fibrosis of the pylorus, a Jaboulay technique is generally favored [2]. Pyloroplasty is performed over gastrojejunostomy due to the maintenance of true anatomic drainage and increased risk of bile reflux with duodenal diversion; gastrojejunostomy is generally reserved for when the duodenum and duodenal bulb are significantly scarred in setting of chronic ulcer disease.

Pyloroplasties can be performed open, laparoscopically, robotically, or endoscopically [3]. Regardless of technique, it is important to make the incision an adequate length on each side of the pylorus (3 cm on stomach and 2 cm on duodenum) and to be mindful that the gastric wall tissue is significantly thicker than the duodenal wall. The closure can be performed in a single or double interrupted or continuous suture layer; our preference is interrupted inner layer followed by continuous outer layer. An intraoperative upper endoscopy leak test and/or postoperative fluoroscopic radiographic study is performed to ensure patency. Most patients are discharged the following day on a liquid diet.

Procedure: Illustrated Steps

Figures 11.1, 11.2, 11.3, 11.4, 11.5, 11.6, 11.7, 11.8, 11.9, 11.10, 11.11, 11.12, 11.13, 11.14, 11.15, 11.16, 11.17, 11.18, 11.19, 11.20, 11.21, 11.22, 11.23, 11.24, 11.25, 11.26, 11.27, 11.28, 11.29, and 11.30 illustrate the technical aspects of a robotic Heineke-Mikulicz pyloroplasty.

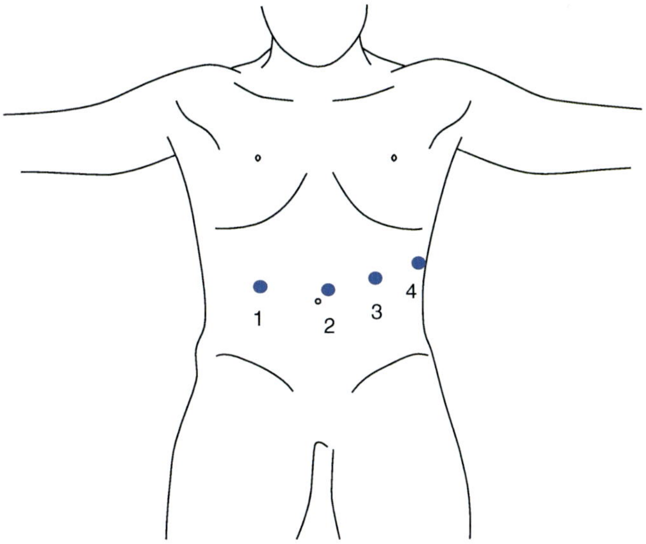

Fig. 11.1 Optimal robotic port placement. Instruments needed for this operation include a cadiere, a prograsp (which we find better to assist with suturing), a hook or monopolar scissors for dissecting, and a needle driver (with or without suture cut per surgeon preference)

K. Fay · A. D. Patel (✉)
Department of Surgery, Emory University School of Medicine, Atlanta, GA, USA
e-mail: apatel7@emory.edu

O. Y. Kudsi, P. P. Grimminger (eds.), *Atlas of Robotic Upper Gastrointestinal Surgery*,
https://doi.org/10.1007/978-3-030-86578-8_11

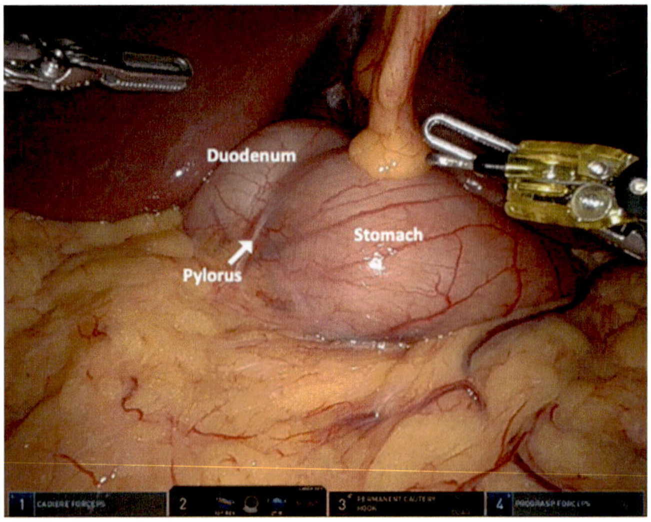

Fig. 11.2 Identification of the pyloric sphincter

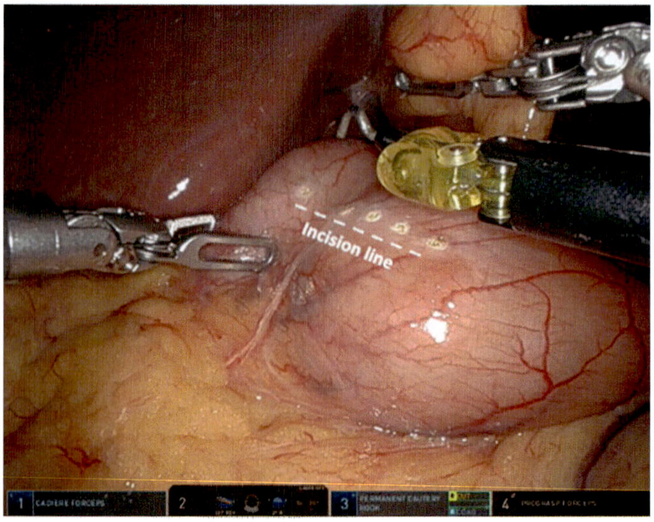

Fig. 11.4 Electrocautery is used to mark the longitudinal incision overlying the pylorus, at least 3 cm in length on the stomach and 2 cm on the duodenum

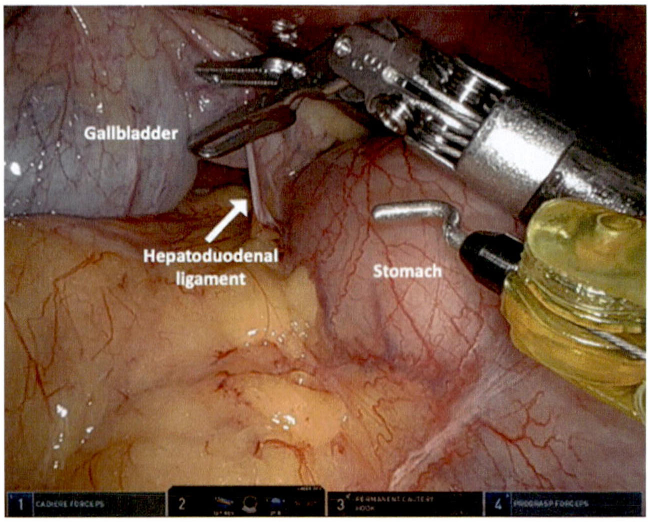

Fig. 11.3 Identification of the hepatoduodenal ligament. This is divided to allow for mobilization of the duodenum. Sometimes a formal Kocher maneuver is necessary for full visualization

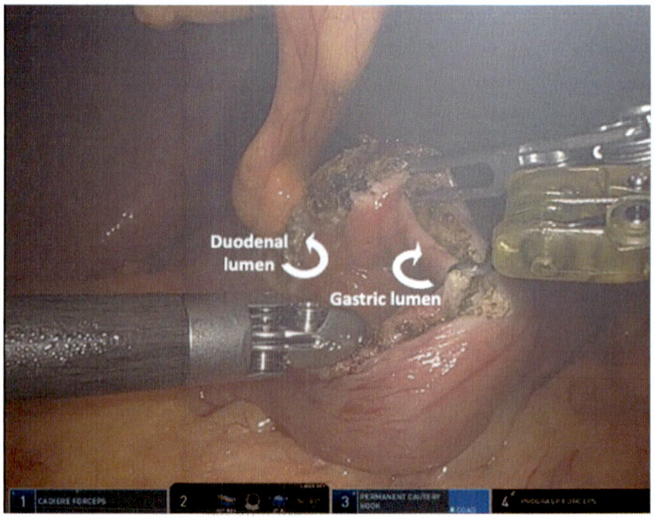

Fig. 11.5 A monopolar hook (or scissor) is used to incise the pylorus along with the perigastric and duodenal tissues

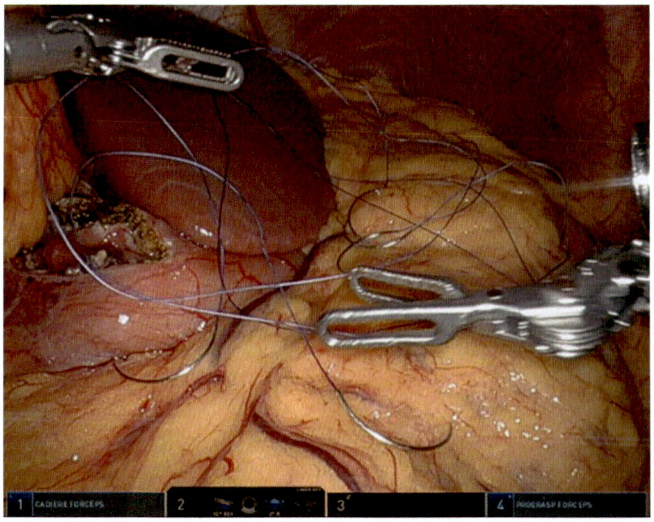

Fig. 11.6 Several 9-inch absorbable polyfilament sutures are introduced into the abdominal cavity. We prefer 2-0 Vicryl® on SH needle. A barbed absorbable suture could also be used in a running fashion

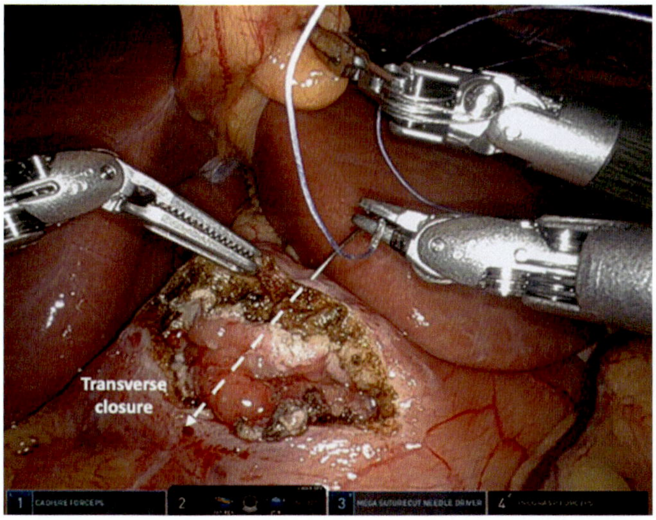

Fig. 11.7 A transverse closure is used to prevent luminal narrowing and potential gastric outlet obstruction

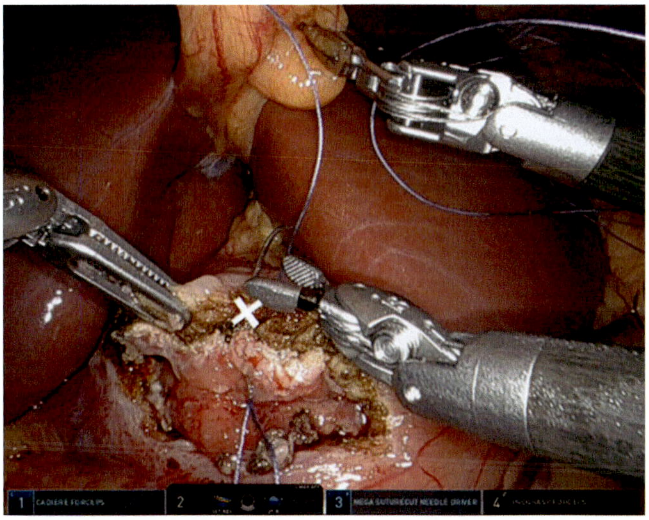

Fig. 11.8 A stay stitch is placed in the apex of the planned transverse closure

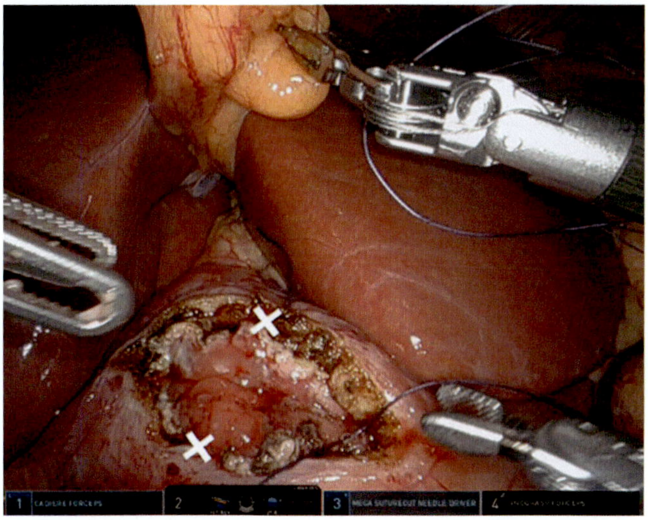

Fig. 11.9 Another stitch is placed in the opposite corner to help align the closure

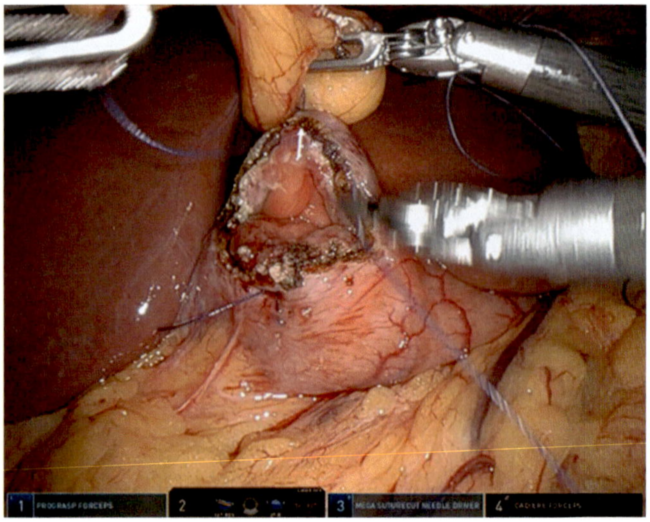

Fig. 11.10 The third robotic arm is used to suspend the apex of the closure and allow for ease of suturing

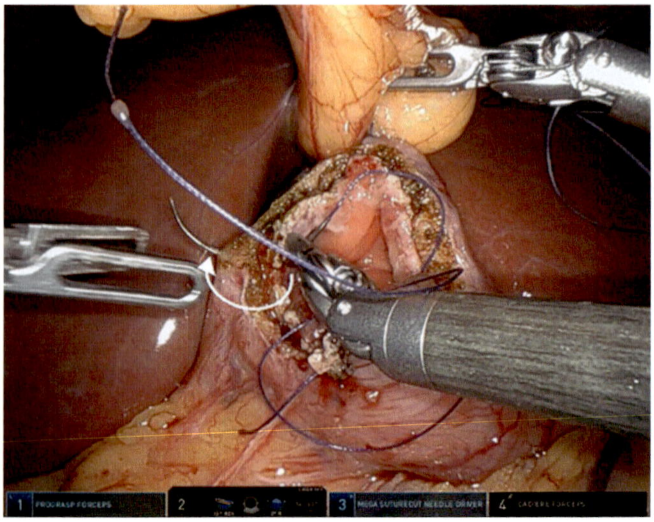

Fig. 11.12 This stitch is then placed in the center of the defect in the duodenum

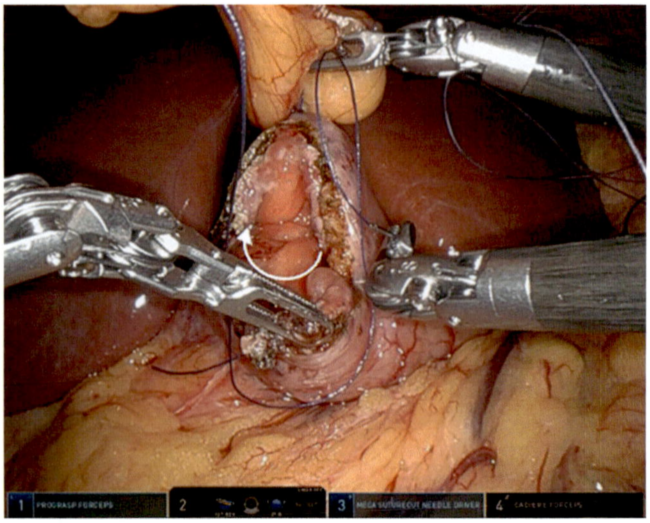

Fig. 11.11 A single interrupted stitch is placed in the center of the defect

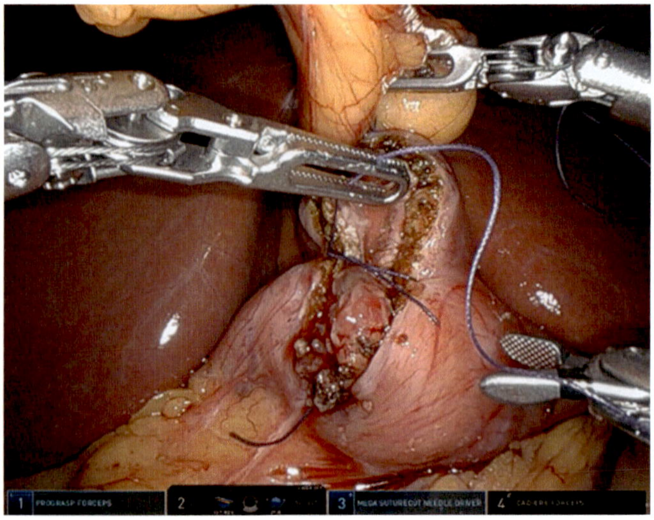

Fig. 11.13 This stitch is loosely tied as a slipknot to approximate the edges of the closure leaving room to visualize the lumen

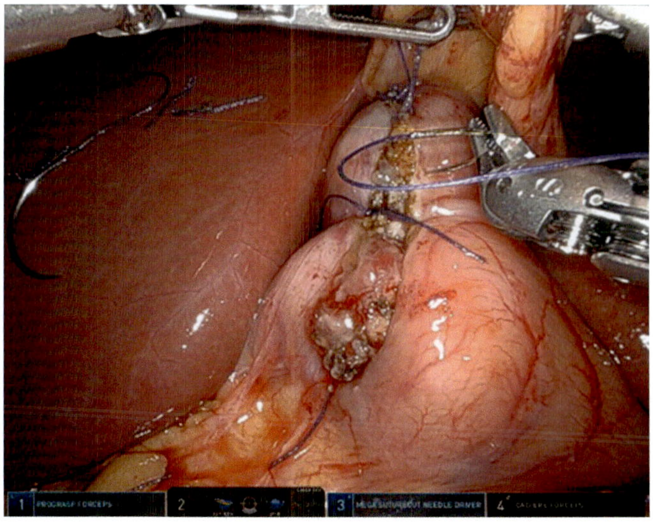

Fig. 11.14 A new interrupted suture is placed between the apex and middle suture essentially dividing the length in half

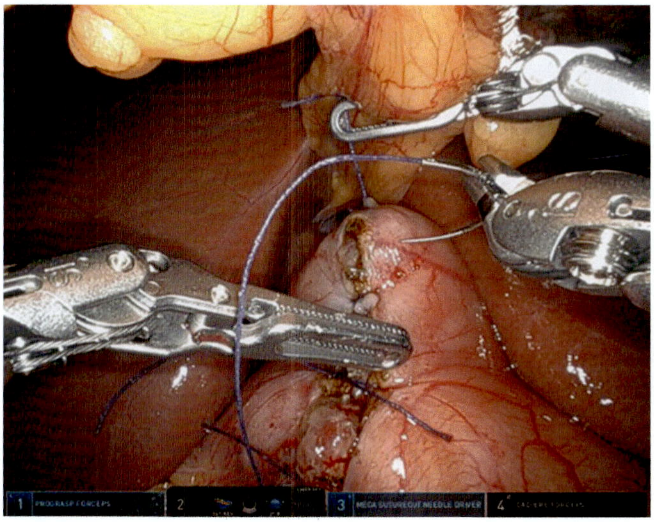

Fig. 11.15 Additional sutures are placed until the upper portion of the closure is complete

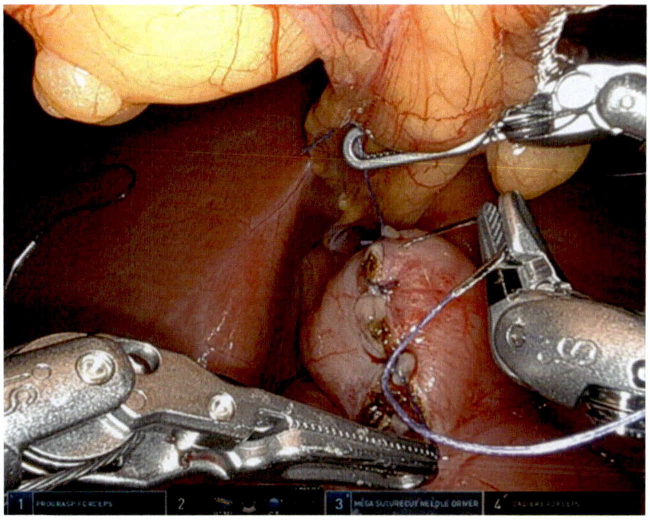

Fig. 11.16 Additional sutures are placed until the entire upper half of the closure is complete

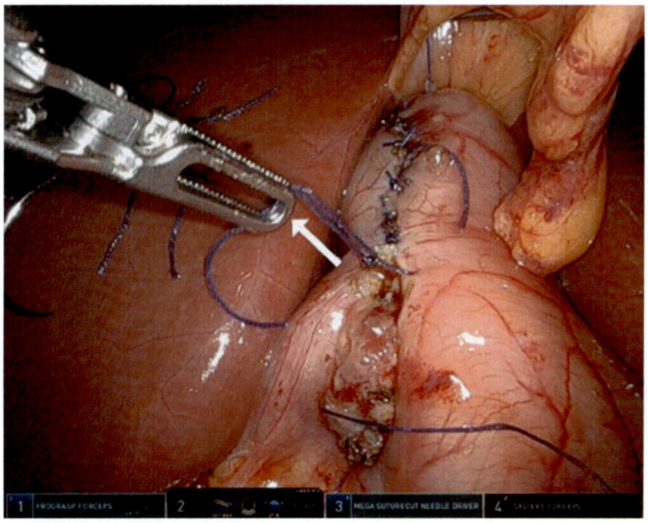

Fig. 11.17 Once the upper portion of the pyloroplasty is closed, the third robot arm moves to retract the initial central suture to expose and align the bottom portion of the closure

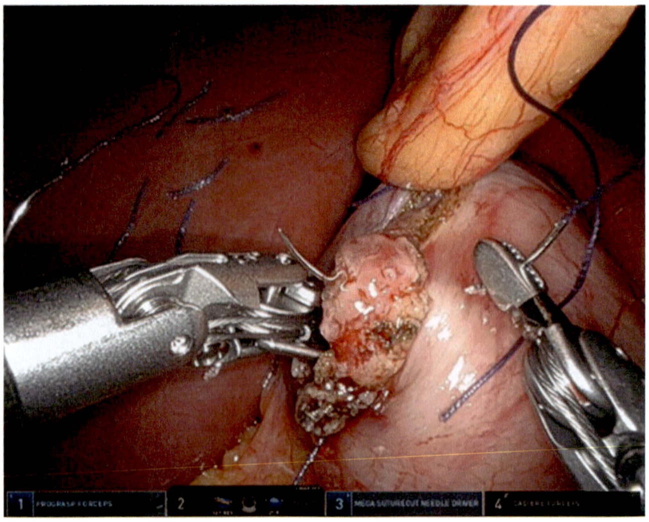

Fig. 11.18 Interrupted sutures are similarly placed to close the lower portion of the incision

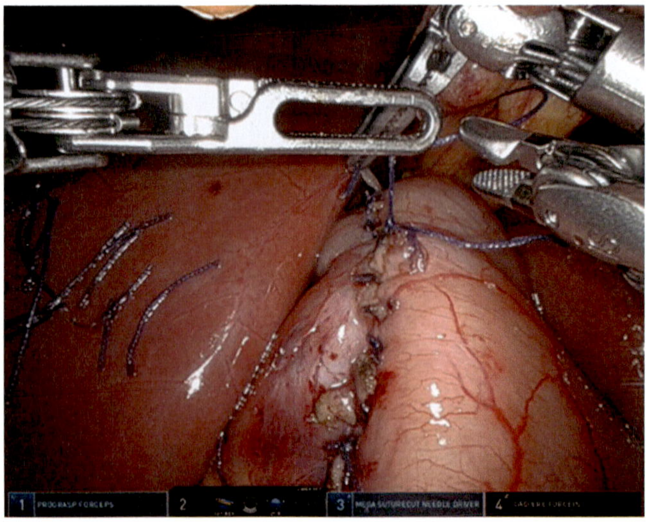

Fig. 11.19 Once the closure is complete, the central suture knot is secured down. Any weak areas are further reinforced. Suture fragments and needles are removed from the abdominal cavity

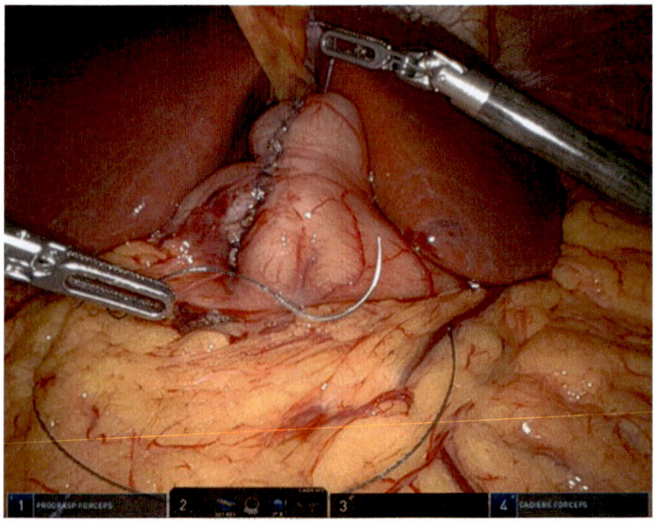

Fig. 11.20 The third robotic arm regrasps the apex suture to align the entire closure

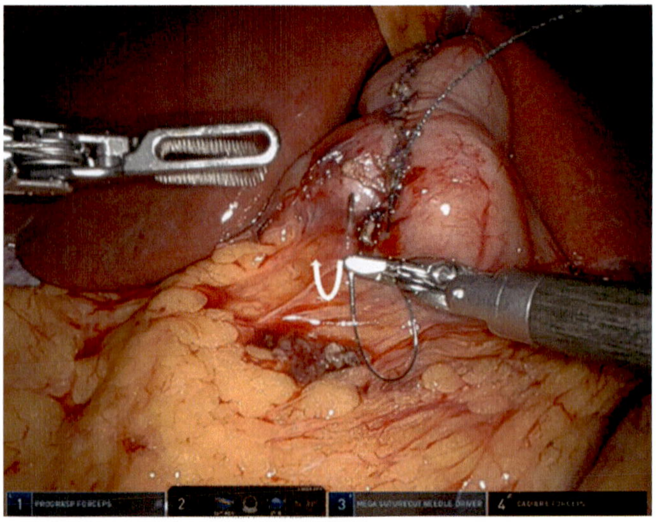

Fig. 11.21 Starting at the opposite end, an absorbable barbed monofilament suture is used to oversew the primary closure to imbricate the suture line. We prefer to use 2-0 suture

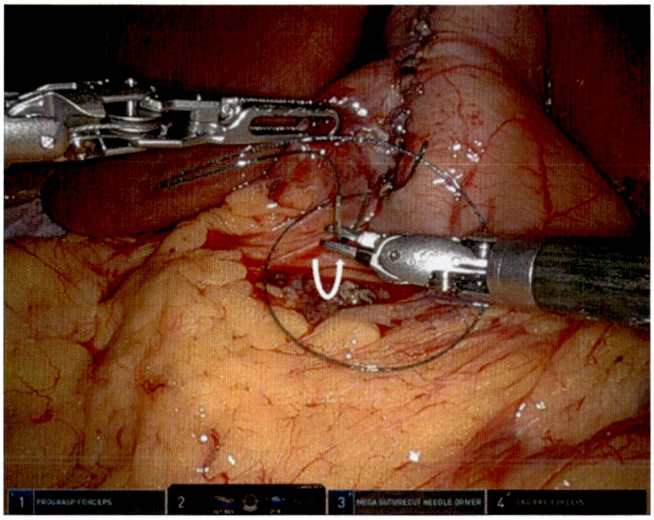

Fig. 11.22 The suture is continued in the cephalad direction after the corner is secured

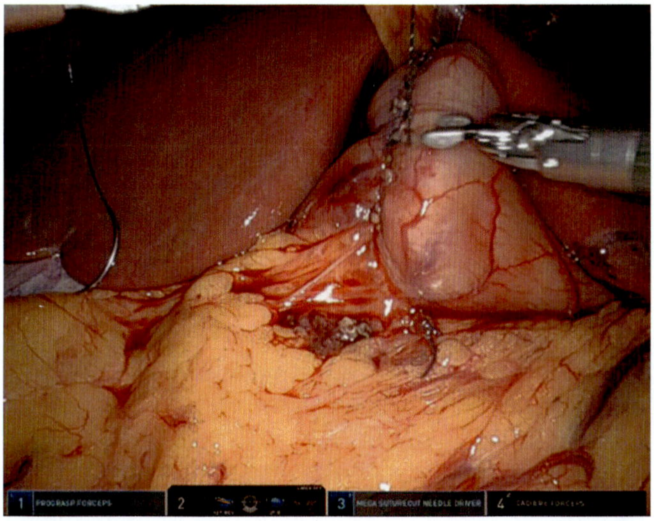

Fig. 11.23 As the suture line continues, the overlying serosa inverts to cover the interrupted sutures

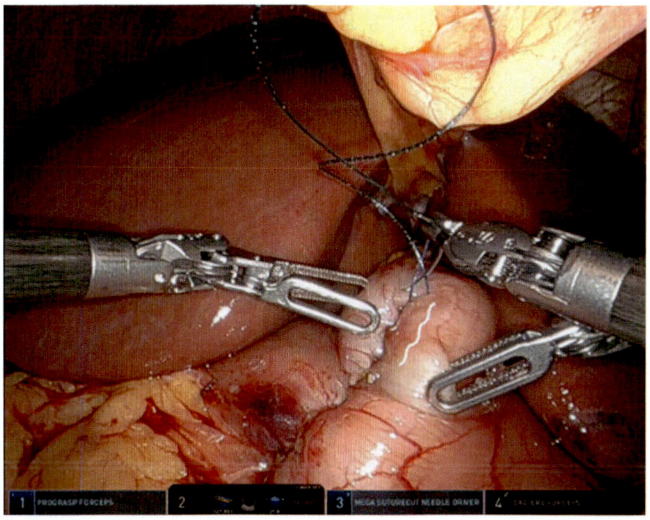

Fig. 11.24 At the superior aspect, a few bites are taken in the opposite direction to lock the suture

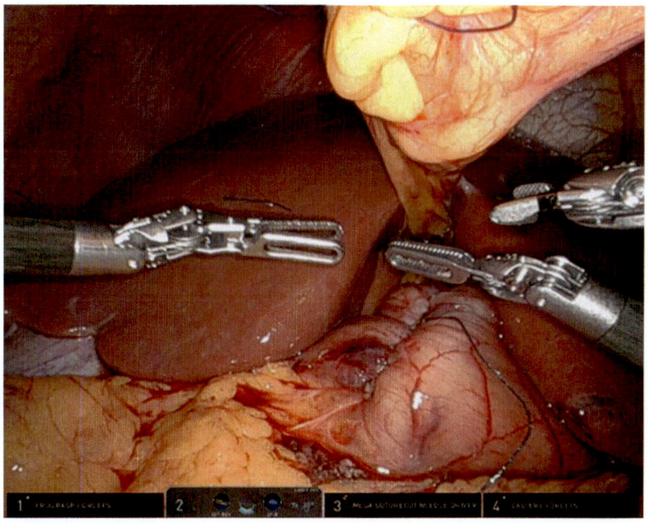

Fig. 11.25 Once completed, the tail of the interrupted apex suture is removed. We keep the second suture attached

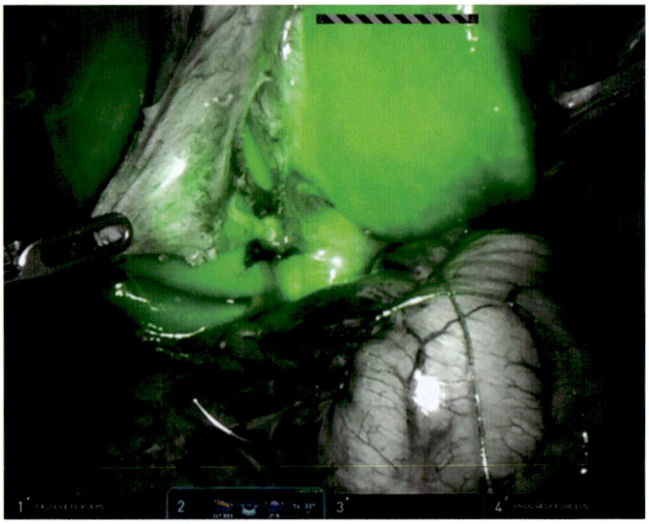

Fig. 11.26 If a gallbladder is present, it is removed prophylactically. Utilization of a robotic approach allows for use of indocyanine green-enhanced fluorescence to assess biliary drainage

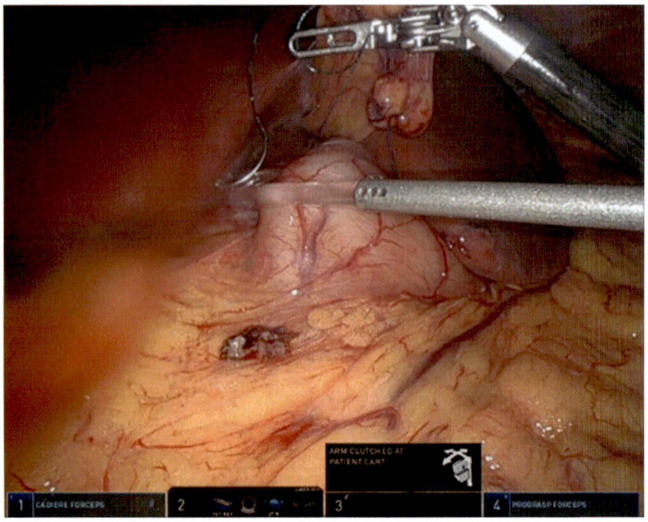

Fig. 11.27 Irrigation is placed in the abdomen in anticipation of an endoscopic leak test to assess the suture line

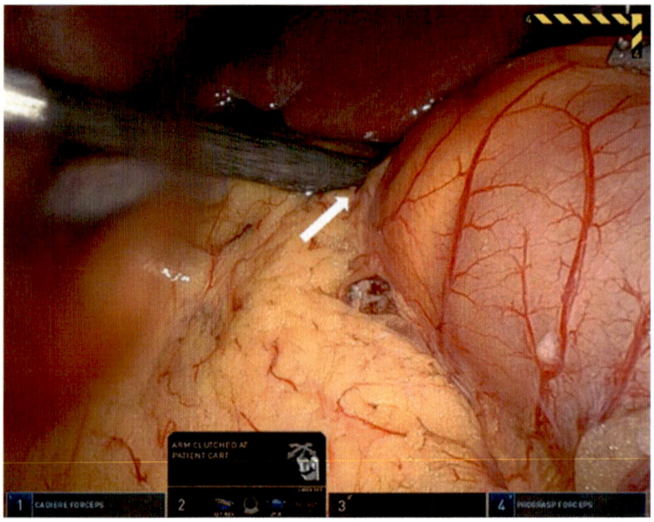

Fig. 11.28 An endoscope is used to evaluate for patency and leaks. An instrument is used to obstruct outflow of gas distal to the pyloroplasty to preferentially drive gas through a leak if it exists

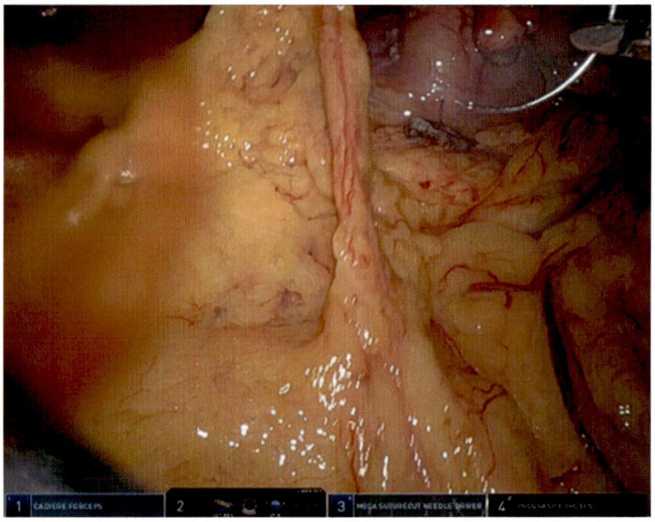

Fig. 11.29 A portion of mobile omentum is identified to be used to cover the suture line

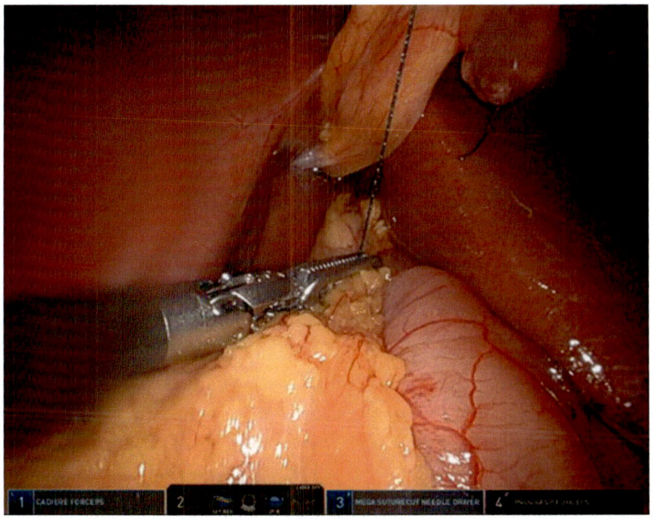

Fig. 11.30 The omental patch is fixated in place with our remaining suture. The suture is removed and counts are confirmed

References

1. Toro JP, Lytle NW, Patel AD, Davis SS Jr, Christie JA, Waring JP, Sweeney JF, Lin E. Efficacy of laparoscopic pyloroplasty for the treatment of gastroparesis. J Am Coll Surg. 2014;218(4):652–60.
2. Sawyers JL, Richards WO. Selective vagotomy and pyloroplasty. In: Baker RJ, Fisher JE, editors. Mastery of surgery. 4th ed. Philadelphia: Lippincott Williams & Wilkins; 2001. p. 933–41.
3. Gonzalez C, Kwak JM, Davrieux F, Watanabe R, Marescaux J, Swanstrom L. Hybrid endoluminal stapled pyloroplasty: an alternative treatment option for gastric outlet obstruction syndrome. Surg Endosc. 2019;33(1):303–8.

12 Robotic Duodenectomy

Torben Glatz and Dirk Bausch

Introduction

Pancreas-sparing duodenectomy is a challenging procedure. It is rarely used, and the required surgical extent varies from small segmental resections to complete duodenectomy with reinsertion of the major duodenal papilla.

Indications for pancreas-sparing duodenectomy are nonmalignant duodenal lesions without involvement of the pancreas itself [1], such as gastrointestinal stromal tumors (GIST), duodenal adenomas not feasible for endoscopic resection, and familial adenomatous polyposis (FAP). Due to its rare use, literature on minimally invasive duodenectomy techniques and their results are limited to case reports and small case series [1–3].

The available retrospective studies demonstrate the well-known advantages of minimally invasive surgery for this procedure too [2]. The use of the robotic platform with its enhanced vision, magnification, and improved dissection techniques allows for a safer and faster procedure. However, its major advantage is the ability to easily reconstruct the duodenal segment with a hand-sewn anastomosis after resection.

The surgical extent of the procedure depends on the location and size of the lesion within the duodenum. While lesions of the duodenal bulb and superior part as well as lesions of the horizontal and ascending part of the duodenum can usually be treated with a limited resection, lesions of the descending part and conditions that require a total duodenectomy (mainly FAP) require careful examination of a possible involvement of the major duodenal papilla and possibly its reinsertion into the proximal jejunum.

Minimally invasive resection of the duodenum requires subtle dissection of the pancreatic head from the duodenum and has a permanent risk for bleeding due to the ample blood supply to the duodenum originating in the pancreatic head. For lesions of the descending part of the duodenum with proximity to the major duodenal papilla, identification of the bile and pancreatic duct and their preservation are crucial. While utilization of Indocyanine Green (Firefly®) can be helpful, insertion of a catheter via the cystic duct into the major duodenal papilla remains the safest method to avoid its accidental dissection or injury. If reconstruction or reinsertion of the major duodenal papilla is not possible, or the lesion extends into the pancreas, a pancreaticoduodenectomy is usually required.

Procedure: Illustrated Steps

Figures 12.1, 12.2, 12.3, 12.4, 12.5, 12.6, 12.7, 12.8, 12.9, 12.10, 12.11, 12.12, 12.13, 12.14, 12.15, 12.16, 12.17, 12.18, 12.19, 12.20, 12.21, 12.22, 12.23, 12.24, 12.25, 12.26, 12.27, 12.28, 12.29, 12.30, 12.31, 12.32, 12.33, 12.34, 12.35, 12.36, 12.37, 12.38, 12.39, 12.40, and 12.41 illustrate the technical aspects of a robotic partial duodenectomy of a GIST of the descending duodenum.

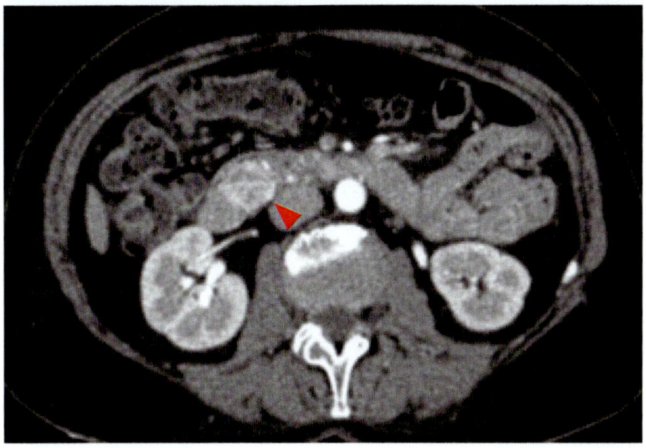

Fig. 12.1 Preoperative Computerized Tomography (CT, transverse image) demonstrating a lesion of the duodenum biopsied as a GIST

T. Glatz · D. Bausch (✉)
Department of Surgery, Marien Hospital Herne, Universitätsklinikum der Ruhr-Universität Bochum, Herne, Germany
e-mail: Dirk.Bausch@ruhr-uni-bochum.de

O. Y. Kudsi, P. P. Grimminger (eds.), *Atlas of Robotic Upper Gastrointestinal Surgery*,
https://doi.org/10.1007/978-3-030-86578-8_12

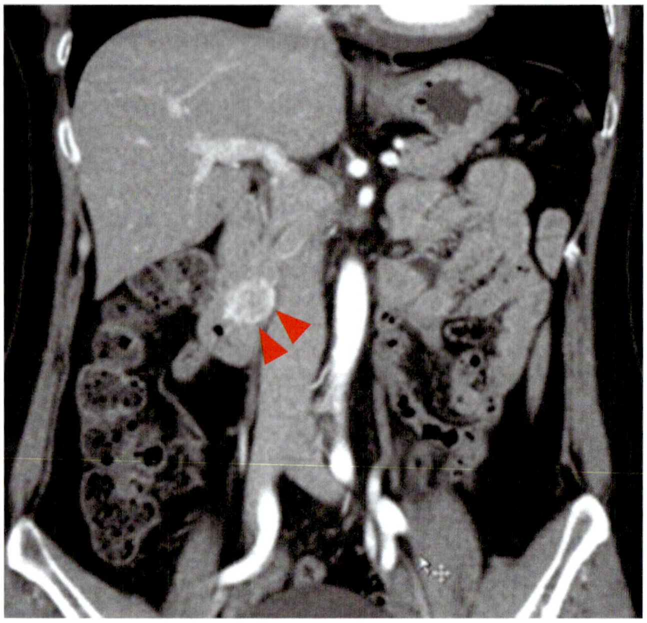

Fig. 12.2 Preoperative CT (coronary image) demonstrates the location of the GIST within the descending part of the duodenum

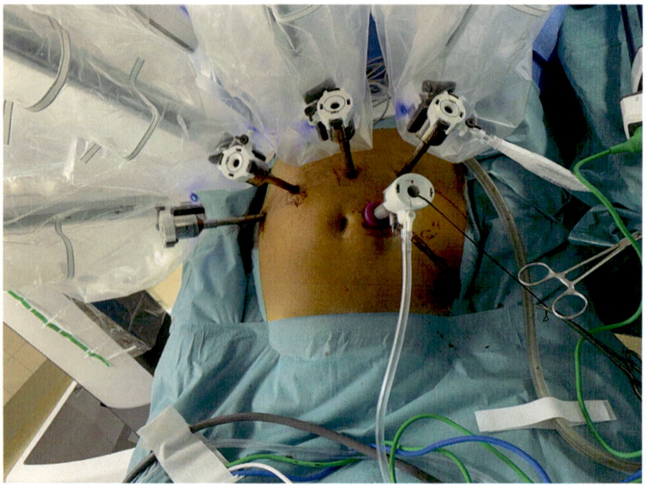

Fig. 12.3 Trocar positioning: right-sided supraumbilical position of the robotic trocars with angulated 12 mm assistant trocar between arms 3 and 4

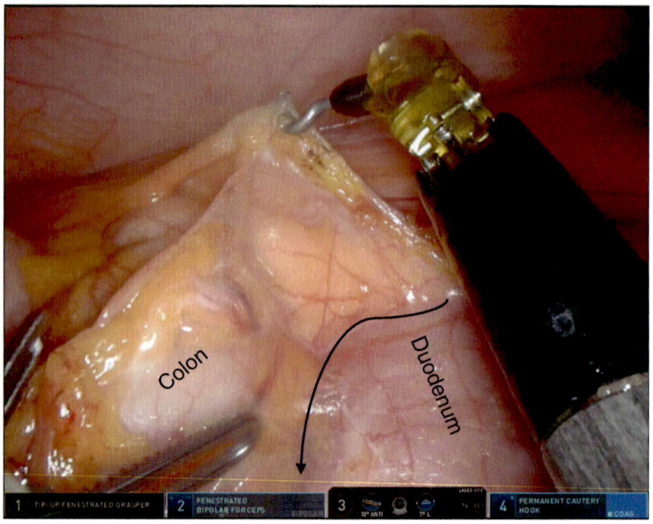

Fig. 12.4 Mobilization of the hepatic flexure and exposure of the duodenum with the monopolar hook

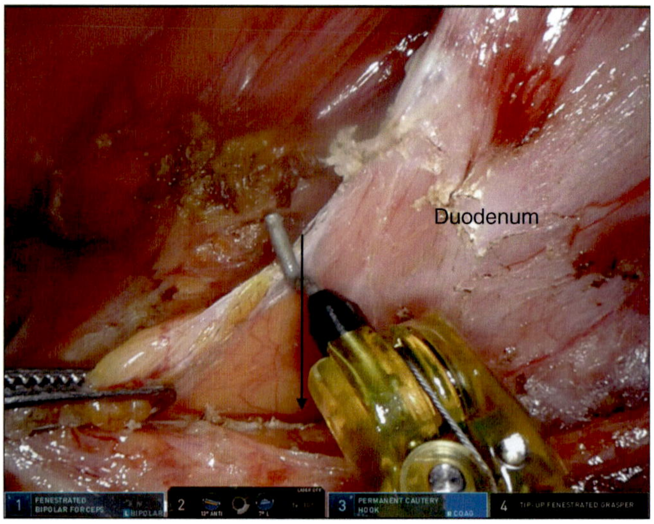

Fig. 12.5 Kocher maneuver: the duodenum is retracted upward with the third arm to create maximum tension

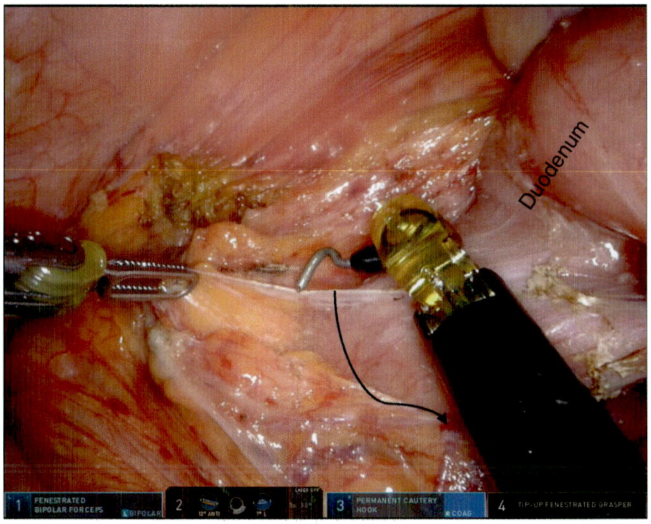

Fig. 12.6 Kocher maneuver: incision of the dorsal attachments

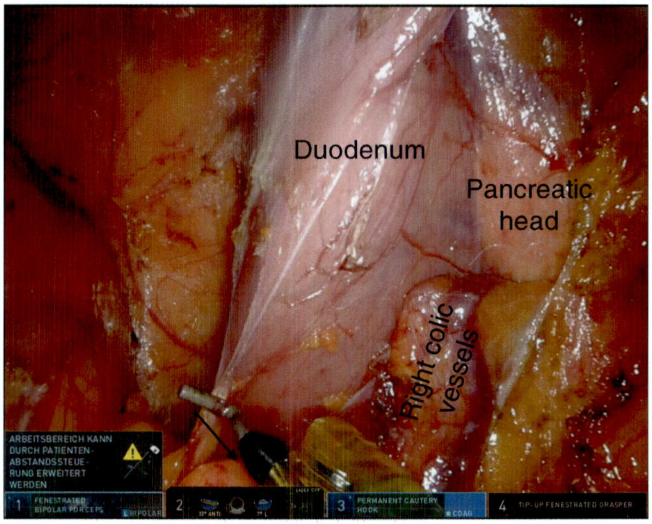

Fig. 12.7 Kocher maneuver: visualization of the pancreatic head and the right colonic vessels

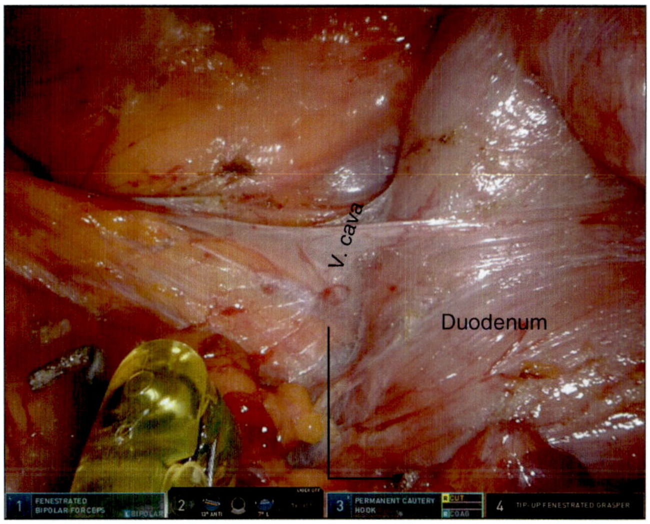

Fig. 12.8 Kocher maneuver: dissection of the duodenum from the vena cava

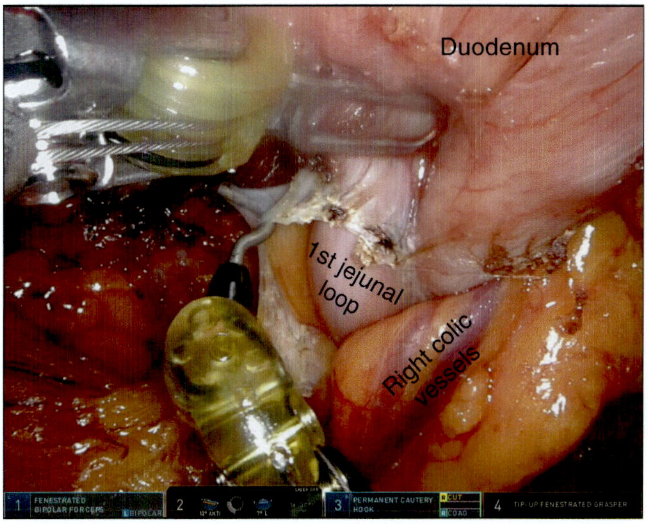

Fig. 12.9 Kocher maneuver: completion by incision of the ligament of Treitz and visualization of the first jejunal loop

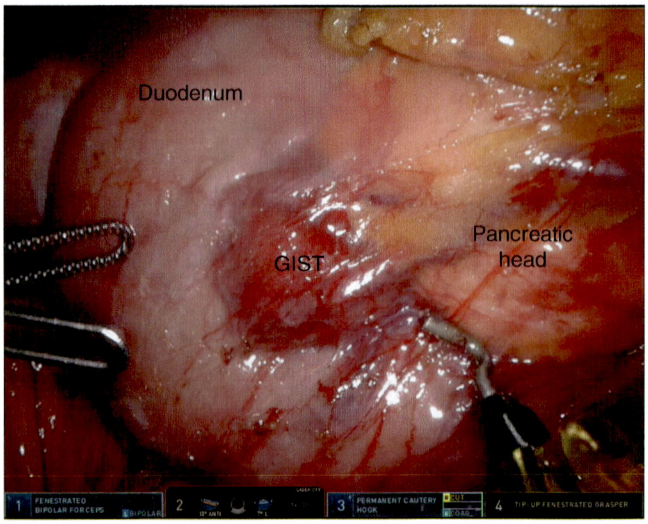

Fig. 12.10 Exposure of the GIST within the descending part of the duodenum

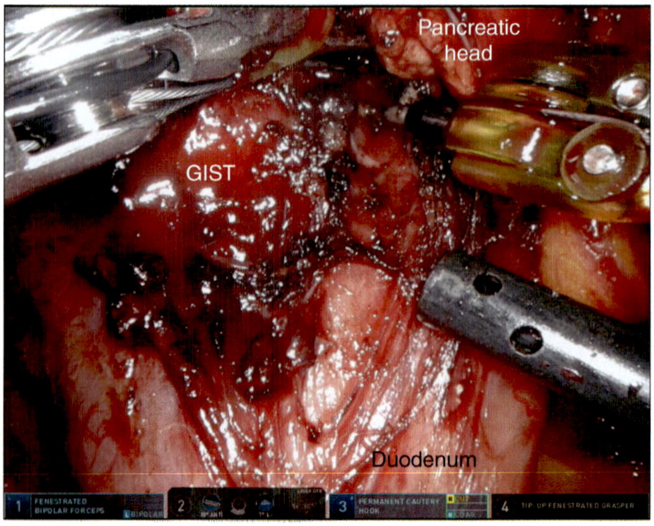

Fig. 12.12 Dissection of the tumor from the pancreatic head

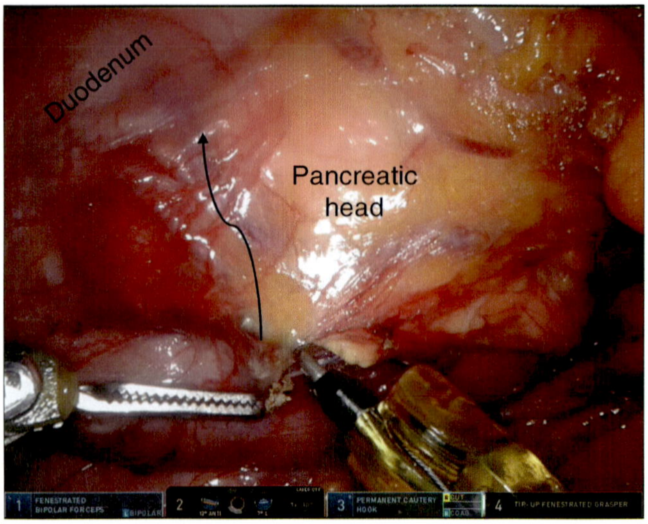

Fig. 12.11 Dissection of the duodenum from the pancreatic head

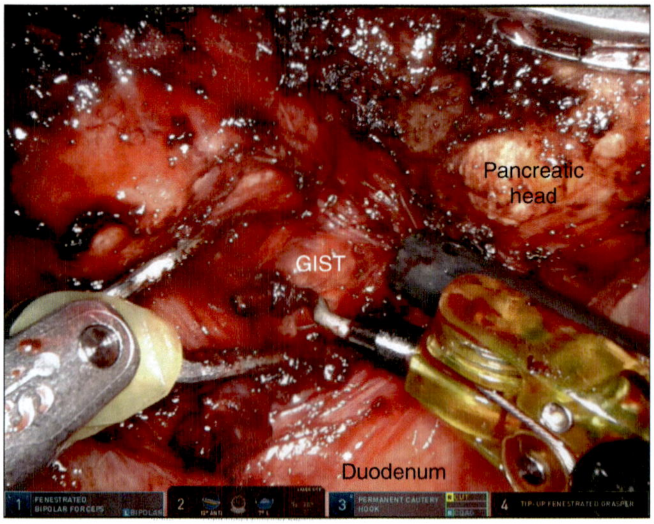

Fig. 12.13 Exposure of the proximal duodenum

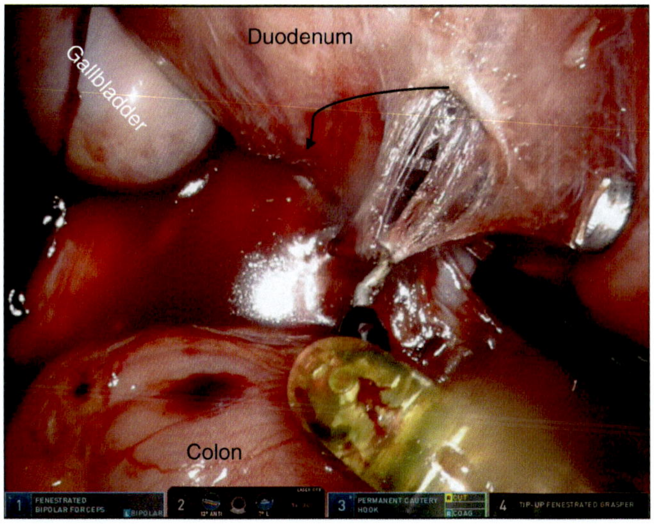

Fig. 12.14 Dorsal completion of the duodenal mobilization

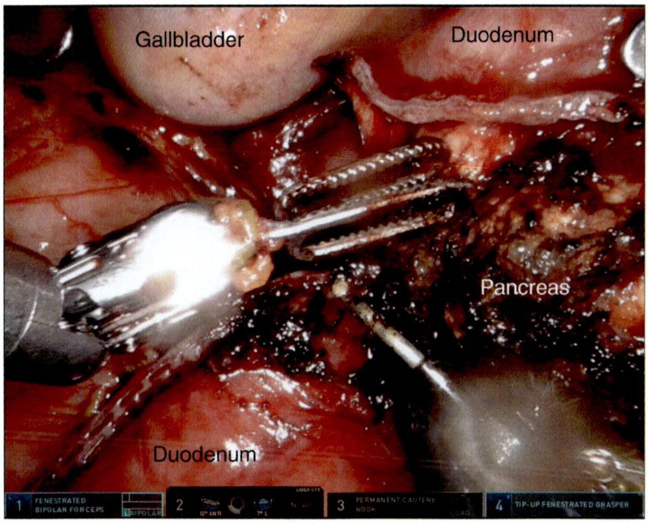

Fig. 12.16 Completion of the duodenal dissection from the pancreatic head

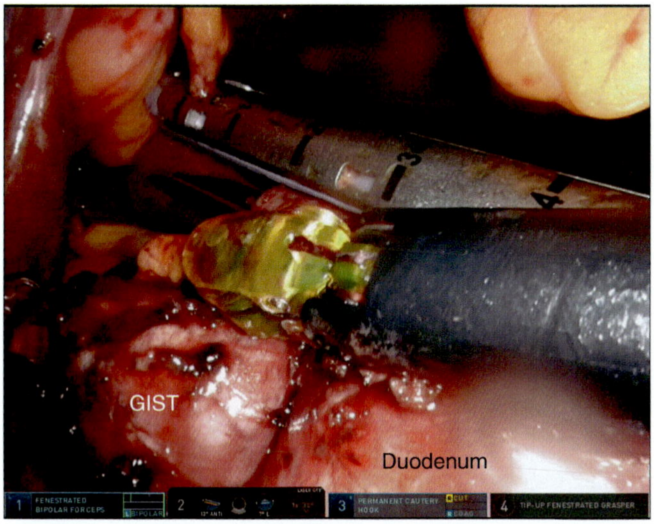

Fig. 12.15 Transection of the proximal duodenum the robotic stapler

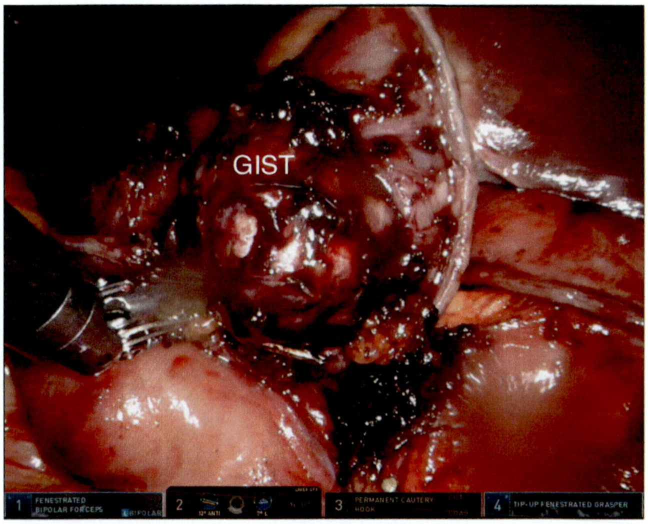

Fig. 12.17 Resected tumor with distal duodenum

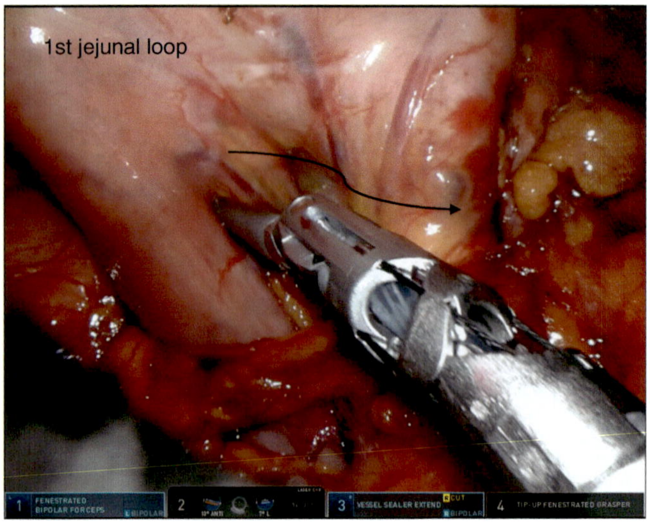

Fig. 12.18 Dissection of the jejunal mesentery with a bipolar sealing device

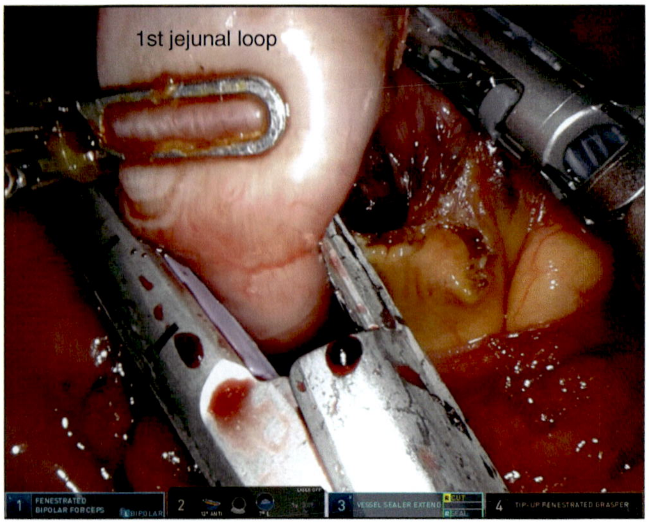

Fig. 12.19 Transection of the jejunum with the robotic stapler

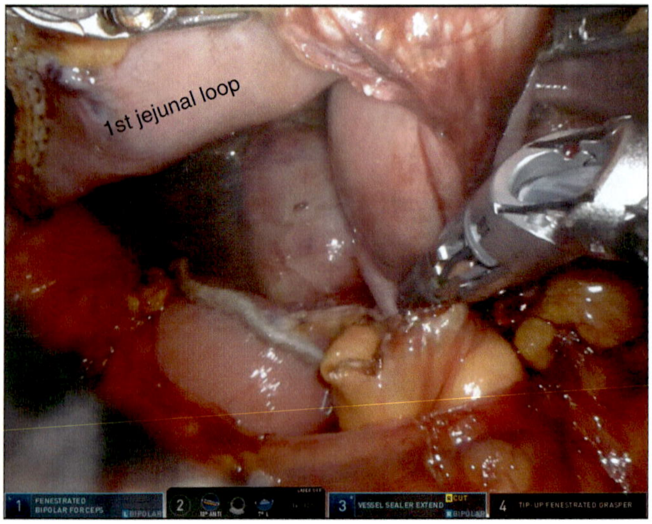

Fig. 12.20 Completion of the mobilization of the first jejunal loop

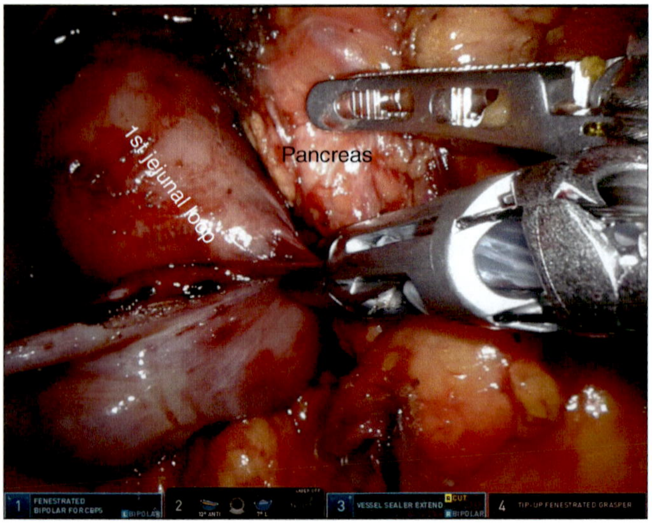

Fig. 12.21 Pull-through of the first jejunal loop under the mesenteric root

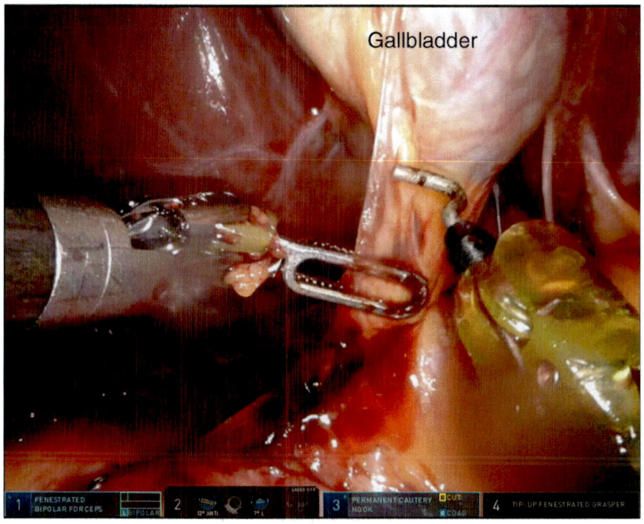

Fig. 12.22 Cholecystectomy: mobilization of the gallbladder

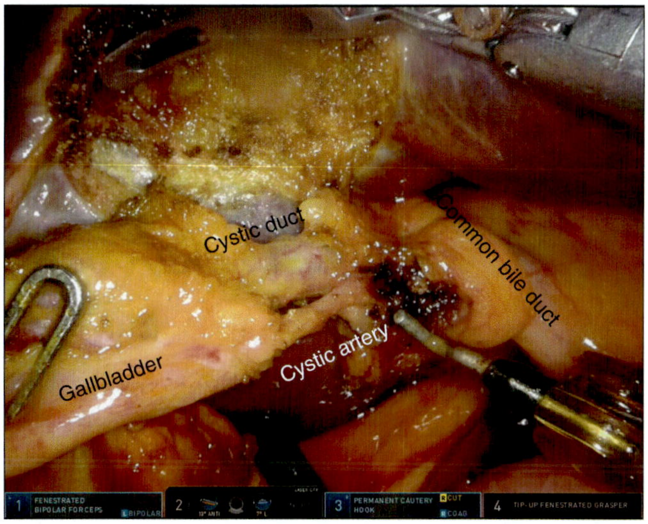

Fig. 12.24 Cholecystectomy: identification of the cystic artery and duct

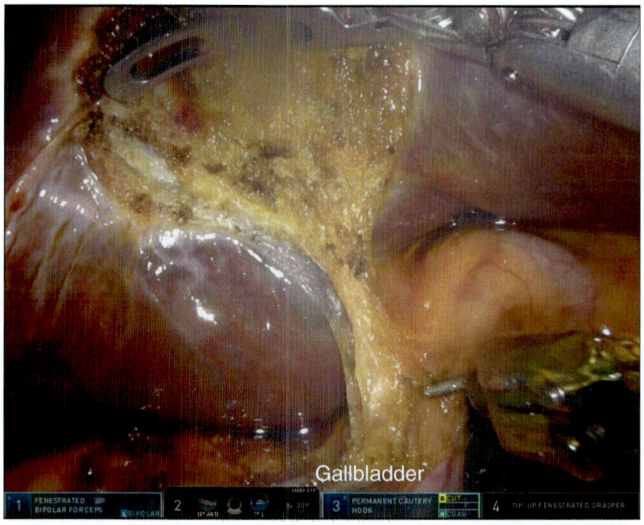

Fig. 12.23 Cholecystectomy: dissection of the gallbladder from the liver

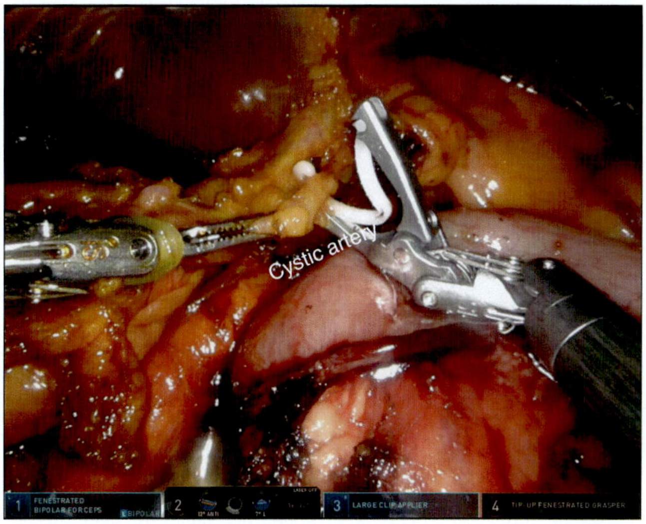

Fig. 12.25 Cholecystectomy: ligation of the cystic artery by clipping

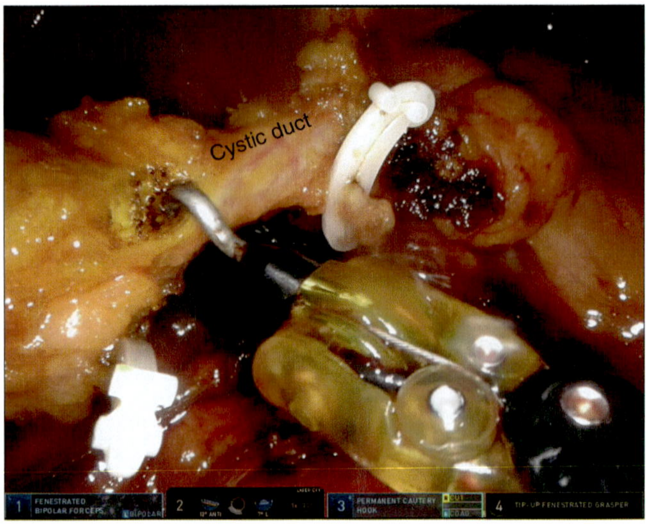

Fig. 12.26 Incision of the cystic duct

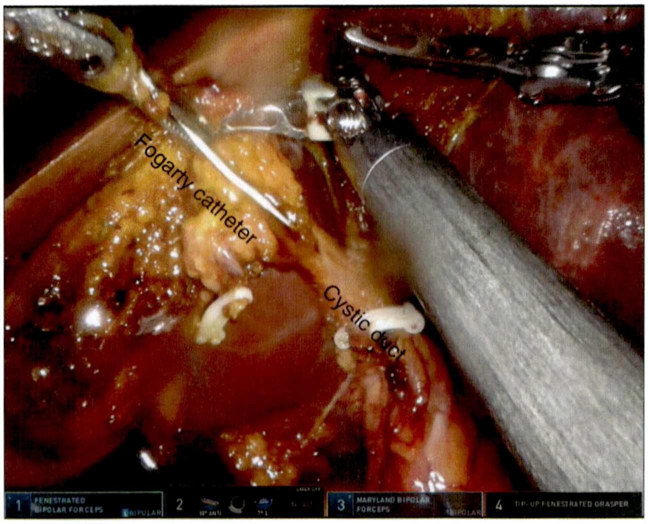

Fig. 12.27 Insertion of a Fogarty catheter into the cystic duct

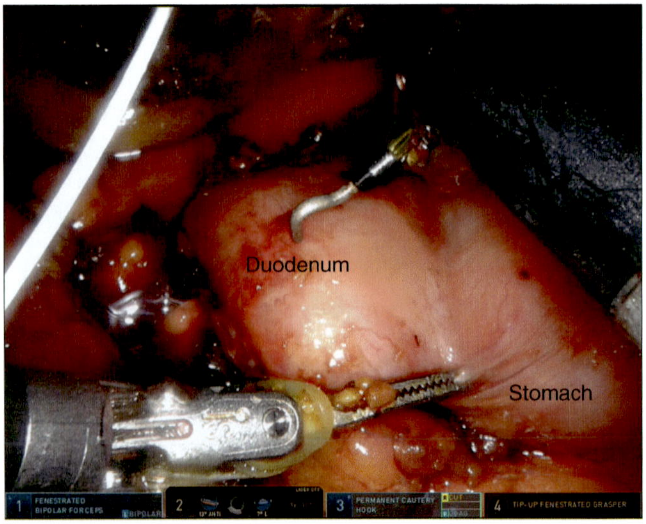

Fig. 12.28 Incision of the duodenum

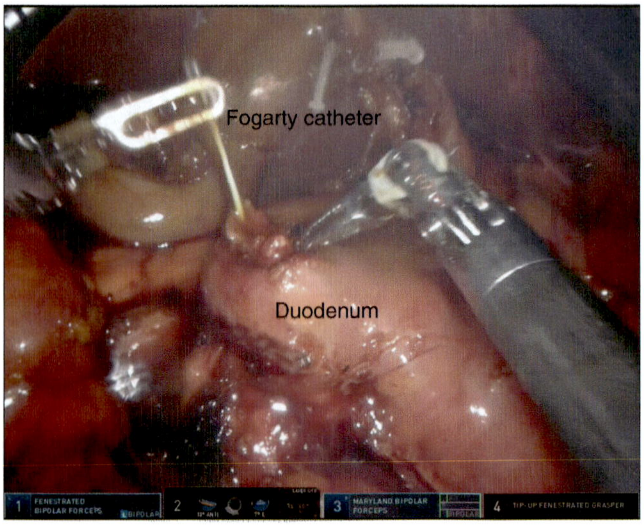

Fig. 12.29 Guaranteeing the preservation of the major duodenal papilla by visualizing the Fogarty catheter within the duodenum

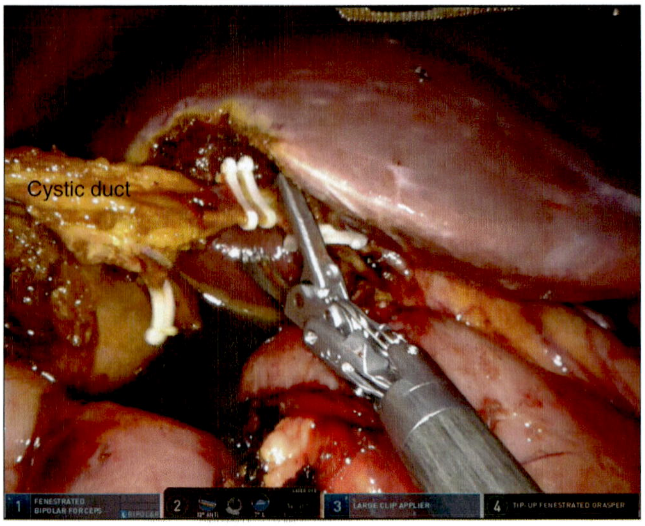

Fig. 12.30 Ligation of the cystic duct after removal of the catheter by double clipping

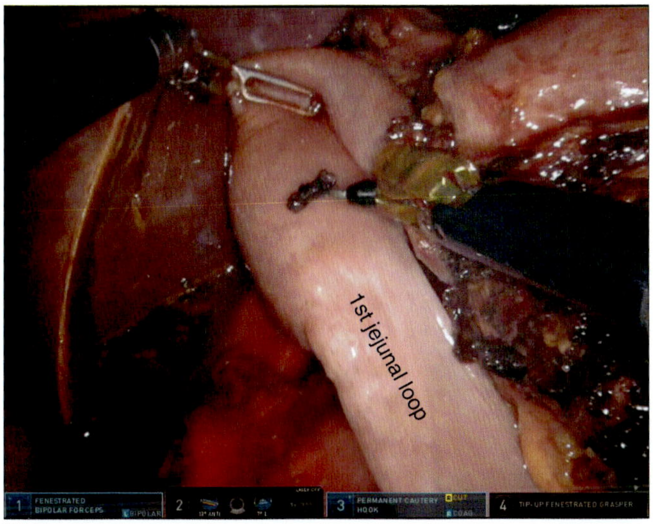

Fig. 12.31 Positioning of the jejunum for double-layered side-to-side anastomosis

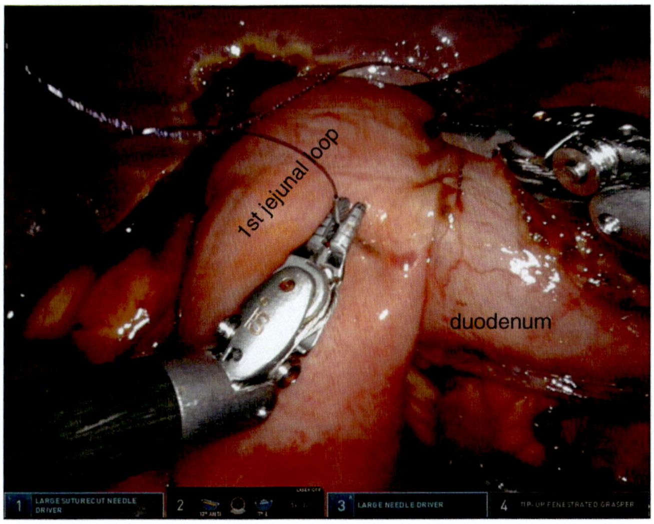

Fig. 12.32 Anastomotic technique: side-to-side alignment of the duodenum and jejunum by a running 4-0 barbed suture (PDS)

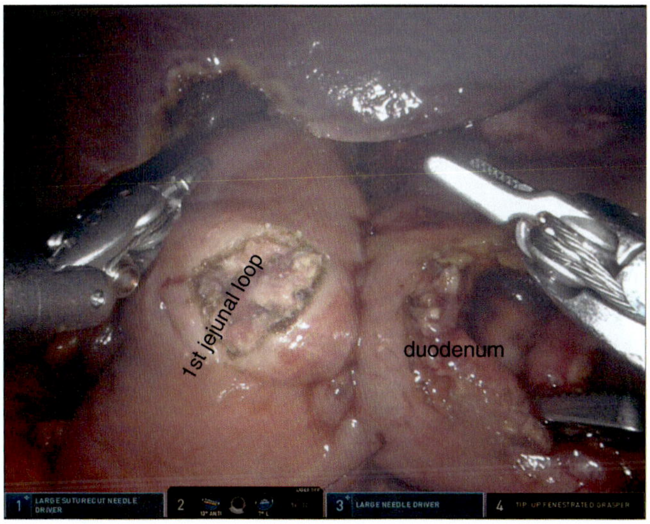

Fig. 12.33 Anastomotic technique: incision of the jejunum and enlargement of the duodenal incision

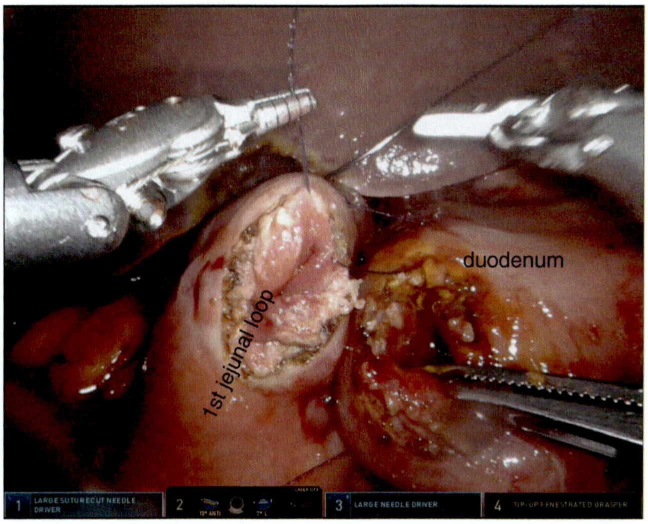

Fig. 12.34 Anastomotic technique: fashioning of the second dorsal layer by running 4-0 barbed suture (PDS)

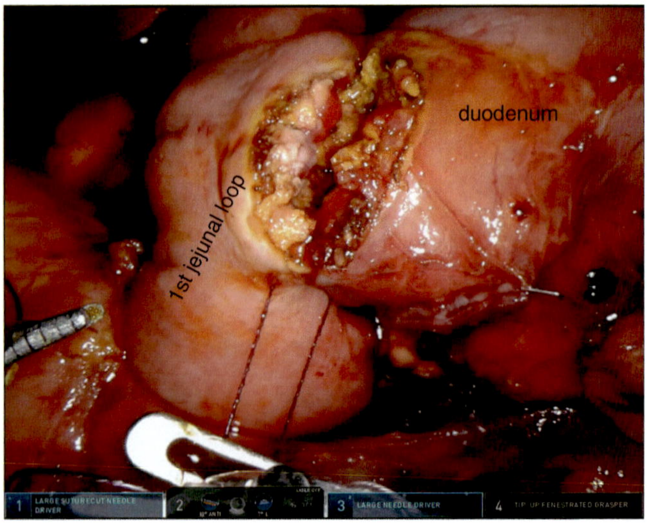

Fig. 12.35 Anastomotic technique: completion of the dorsal layers

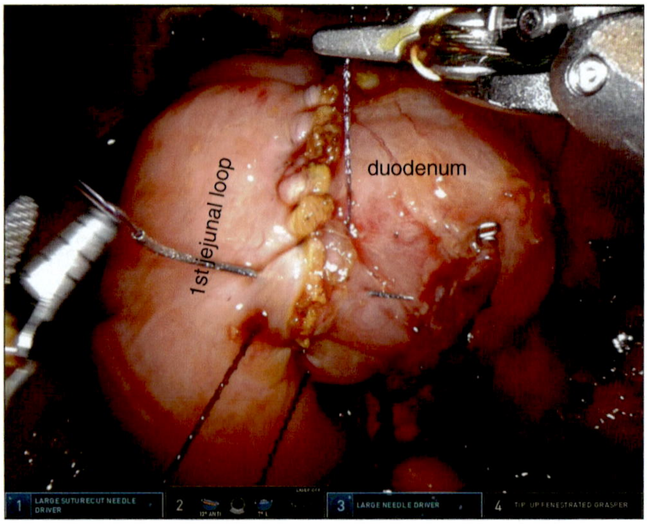

Fig. 12.36 Anastomotic technique: fashioning of the inner front layer by a separate running 4-0 barbed suture (PDS)

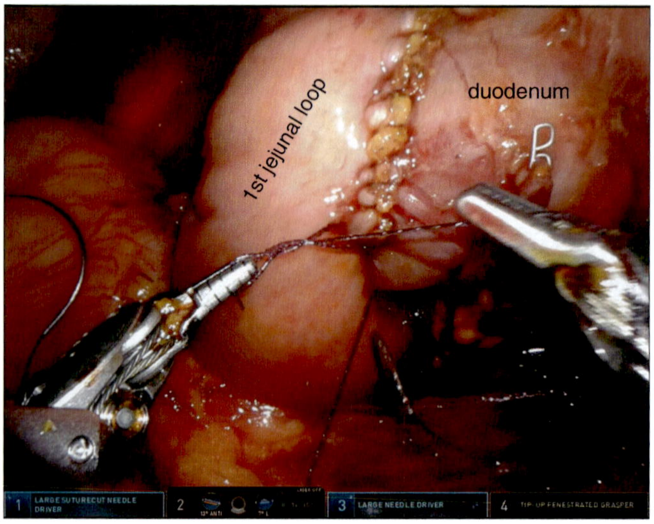

Fig. 12.37 Anastomotic technique: completion of the inner front layer and securing of the inner layer by knotting of the two sutures

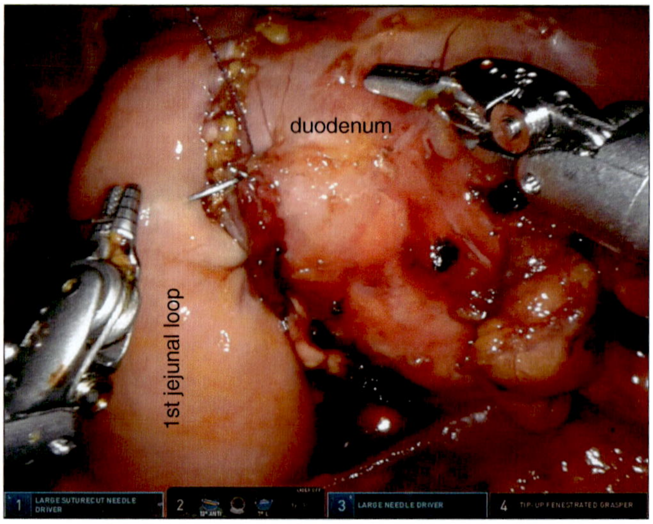

Fig. 12.38 Anastomotic technique: fashioning of the second front layer

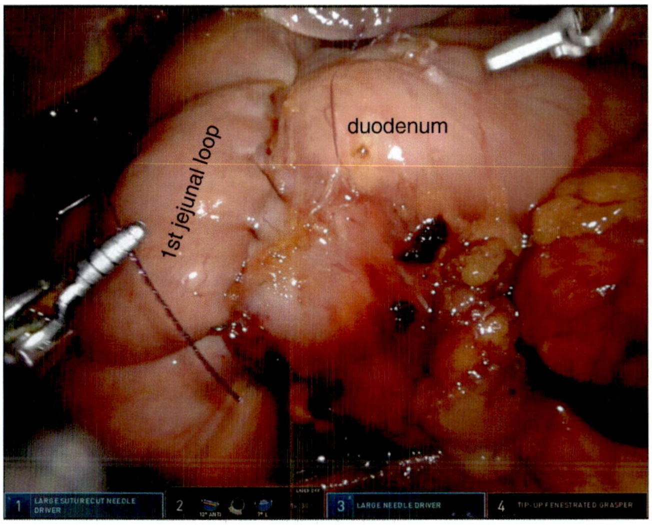

Fig. 12.39 Double layered side-to-side duodenojejunostomy after completion

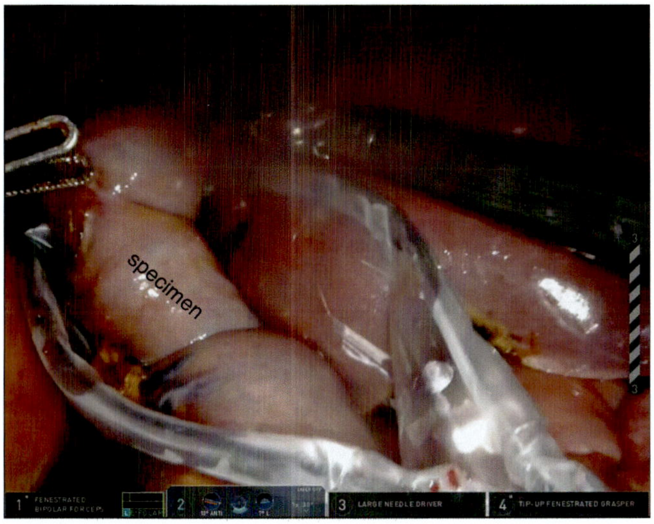

Fig. 12.40 Extraction of the specimen via assistant port

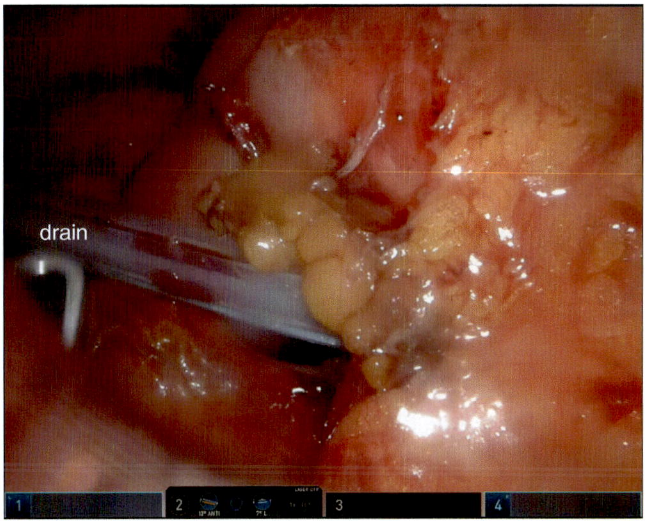

Fig. 12.41 Drain placement at the anastomosis

References

1. Chung RS, Church JM, van Stolk R. Pancreas-sparing duodenectomy:indications, surgical technique, and results. Surgery. 1995;117(3):254–9.
2. Kokosis G, Ceppa EP, Tyler DS, Pappas TN, Perez A. Laparoscopic duodenectomy for benign nonampullary duodenal neoplasms. Surg Laparosc Endosc Percutan Tech. 2015;25(2):158–62.
3. Ojima T, Nakamura M, Hayata K, Kitadani J, Katsuda M, Takeuchi A, Tominaga S, Yamaue H. J laparoscopic limited resection for duodenal gastrointestinal stromal tumors. Gastrointest Surg. 2020;24(10):2404–8.

Robotic Esophagectomy: Ivor Lewis

13

Peter P. Grimminger, Giovanni Capovilla, and Evangelos Tagkalos

Introduction

Transthoracic esophageal resection with gastric conduit reconstruction (Ivor Lewis esophagectomy) represents a widely adopted approach for the treatment of junctional and thoracic esophageal cancer. The Ivor Lewis procedure consists of an abdominal phase including a D2 level lymphadenectomy followed by the preparation of a gastric conduit and the thoracic phase involving the esophageal resection, the mediastinal lymphadenectomy, and the esophagogastric anastomosis. The procedure can nowadays be performed using a laparoscopic-thoracoscopic approach (fully *minimally invasive esophagectomy* – MIE), with superior short-term outcomes and equivalent oncologic results compared to the conventional open approach. The *robot-assisted minimally invasive thoraco-laparoscopic esophagectomy* (RAMIE) has recently been developed to overcome the technical complexity of MIE [1]. The robotic approach offers the advantages of the magnified three-dimensional vision and the use of intracorporeally articulated instruments, thus facilitating the technically demanding dissection phase required during esophagectomy [2]. A recent randomized trial demonstrated the superiority of RAMIE compared to the conventional open approach [3]. The results of a prospective randomized trial comparing RAMIE and conventional MIE are awaited.

We present here our technique for RAMIE using the da Vinci Xi® Surgical System (Intuitive Surgical, Sunnyvale, CA, USA) [4]. Briefly, a gastric conduit is prepared by stapling the stomach along the lesser curvature (Endo GIA™, Covidien, Mansfield, MA, USA) and preserving the right gastric vessels and the gastroepiploic arcade to guarantee an adequate vascularization of the gastric conduit. Ideally, a lymphadenectomy of the D2 level should be performed. The thoracic phase consists of freeing the esophagus along with the lower, middle, and upper mediastinal lymph nodes, resecting the specimen and performing an end-to-side esophagogastric gastric anastomosis using a circular stapler (CEEA™, Covidien, Mansfield, MA, USA) (Figs. 13.1, 13.2, 13.3, 13.4, 13.5, 13.6, 13.7, 13.8, 13.9, 13.10, 13.11, 13.12, 13.13, 13.14, 13.15, 13.16, 13.17, 13.18, 13.19, 13.20, 13.21, 13.22, 13.23, 13.24, 13.25, 13.26, 13.27, 13.28, 13.29, 13.30, 13.31, 13.32, 13.33, 13.34, 13.35, 13.36, 13.37, 13.38, 13.39, 13.40, 13.41, 13.42, 13.43, 13.44, 13.45, 13.46, 13.47, 13.48, 13.49, 13.50, 13.51, 13.52, 13.53, 13.54, 13.55, 13.56, and 13.57).

P. P. Grimminger (✉) · G. Capovilla · E. Tagkalos
Department of General-, Visceral- and Transplant Surgery, University Medical Center Mainz, Mainz, Germany
e-mail: peter.grimminger@unimedizin-mainz.de

O. Y. Kudsi, P. P. Grimminger (eds.), *Atlas of Robotic Upper Gastrointestinal Surgery*, https://doi.org/10.1007/978-3-030-86578-8_13

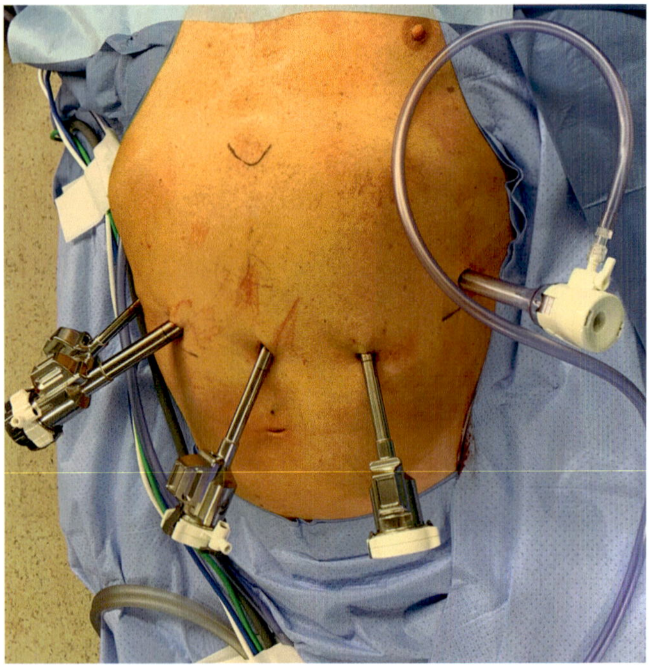

Fig. 13.1 Trocar position: the patient is placed in a normal supine position with a 15° reverse Trendelenburg. Pneumoperitoneum is applied with a Veress needle in the upper left abdominal quadrant, 2–3 cm above the umbilical line. Upon removal of the Veress needle, a 8 mm trocar is placed to be used for the energy dissection device (Vessel Sealer Extend or Monopolar-Hook). The 8 mm midline camera trocar is placed a certain distance above the umbilicus, depending on the location of the stomach in the CT scan. A 12 mm trocar used for the Fenestrated Bipolar Forceps and the Stapler is placed in the upper right quadrant. A fenestrated Tip-Up grasper is introduced with the third arm, through another 8 mm trocar placed in the right lateral subcostal area. Finally, a 12 mm assistant trocar is placed in the left lateral subcostal area and used for retraction, suction, and introduction/removal of any material during the dissection. The da Vinci® Xi robotic system is positioned on the right side of the patient. The position of the assistant is on the patient's left side

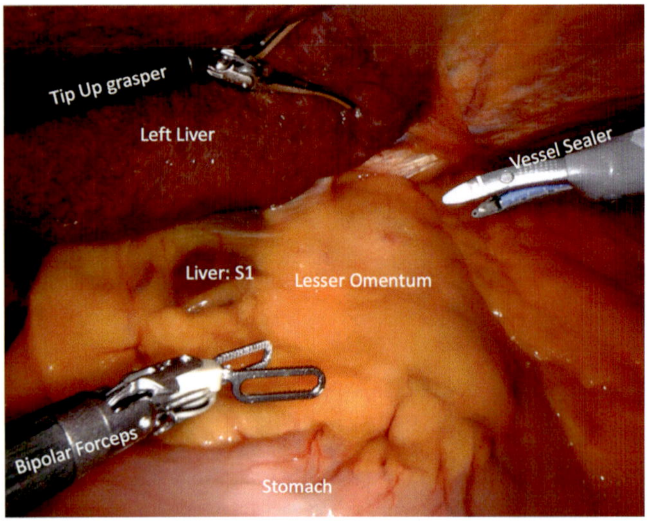

Fig. 13.2 The initial setting includes the use of the fenestrated bipolar forceps on the left arm and the Vessel Sealer on the right arm. The third robotic arm is equipped with a Tip-Up grasper and used to retract the left liver lobe

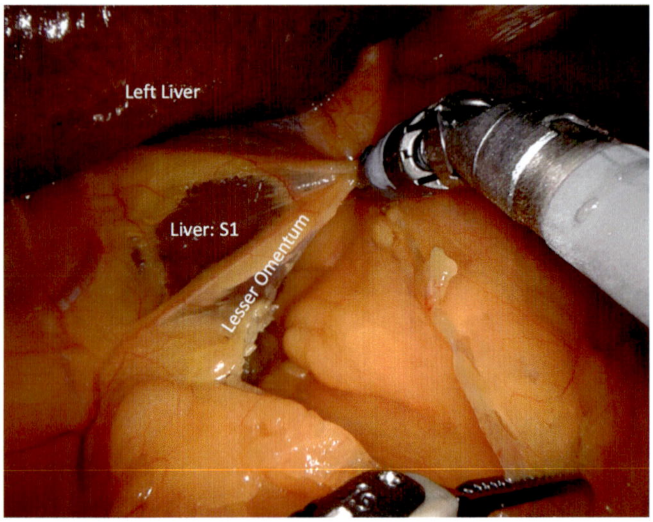

Fig. 13.3 The lesser omentum is opened, and the dissection is carried out toward the right diaphragmatic crus

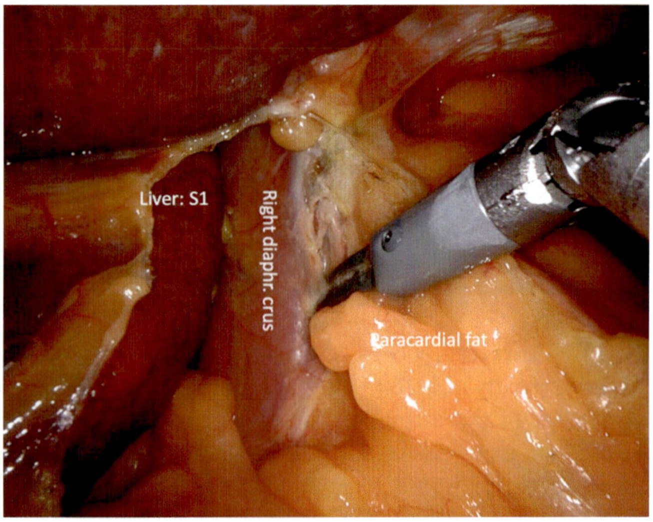

Fig. 13.4 The space between the right diaphragmatic crus and the pericardial fat is developed. The pericardial fat tissue is retracted to the left to provide tension and improve the field vision. The lower esophagus is completely freed on the right side. During this phase the lymph nodes of station 1 are collected and will be retrieved en bloc with the specimen

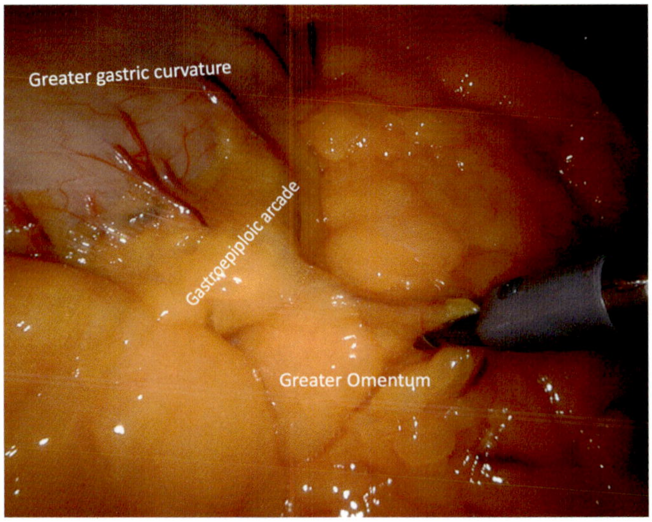

Fig. 13.5 In the next step, the greater omentum is retracted caudally, and the gastroepiploic arcade is identified along the greater curvature

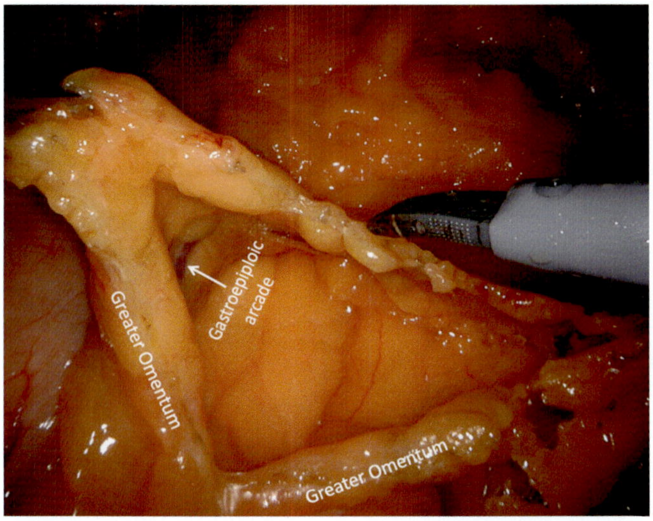

Fig. 13.6 The greater omentum is dissected, and a partial omentectomy is carried out along the greater curvature, toward the spleen. Direct vision of the gastroepiploic arcade can easily be acquired at the posterior aspect of the greater gastric curvature

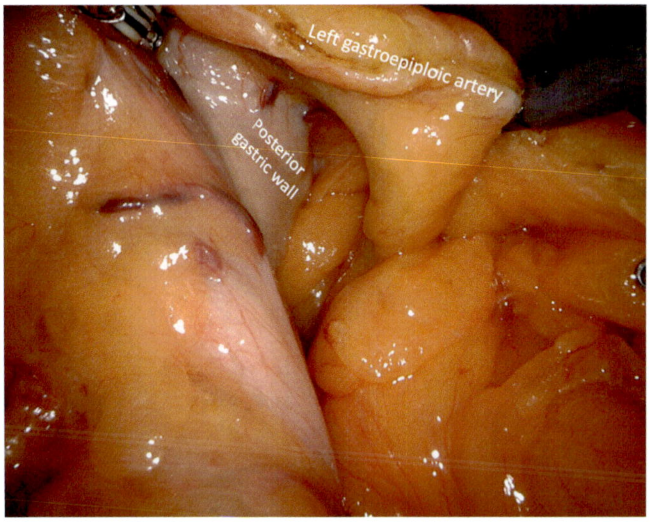

Fig. 13.7 The left gastroepiploic vessels are encountered and transected. The gastroepiploic arcade is preserved to provide an adequate vascularization of the gastric conduit. Lymph nodes of station 4sb and, above the left gastroepiploic artery, 4sa are retrieved during this phase and will be extracted en bloc with the specimen

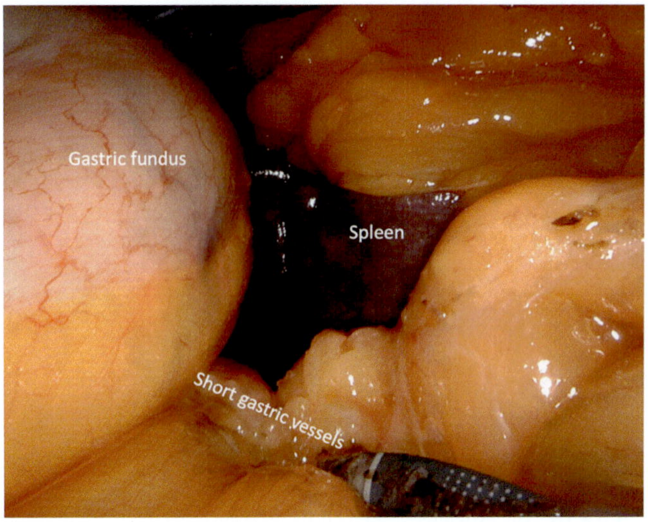

Fig. 13.8 The mobilization of the gastric fundus is completed by dividing the short gastric vessels. During this phase the stomach can be gently retracted toward the right using the third robotic arm (Tip Up grasper); the assistant can retract the fat pad toward the left side to provide tension

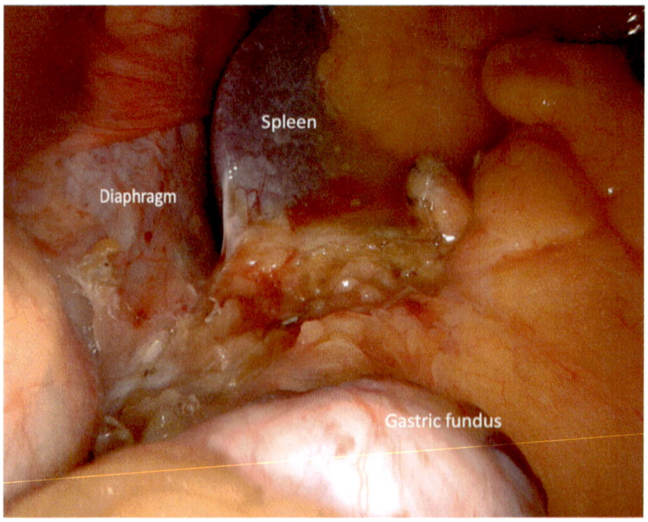

Fig. 13.9 Once fully mobilized from the spleen, the fundus can be retracted medially to access the left diaphragmatic crus. Lymph nodes of station 4sa are retrieved during this phase and will be extracted en bloc with the specimen

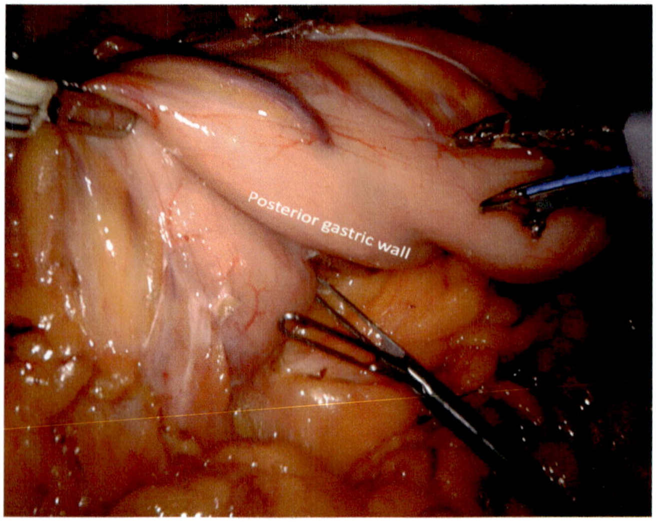

Fig. 13.11 The stomach is retracted cranially, and the partial omentectomy is continued toward the right gastroepiploic vessels

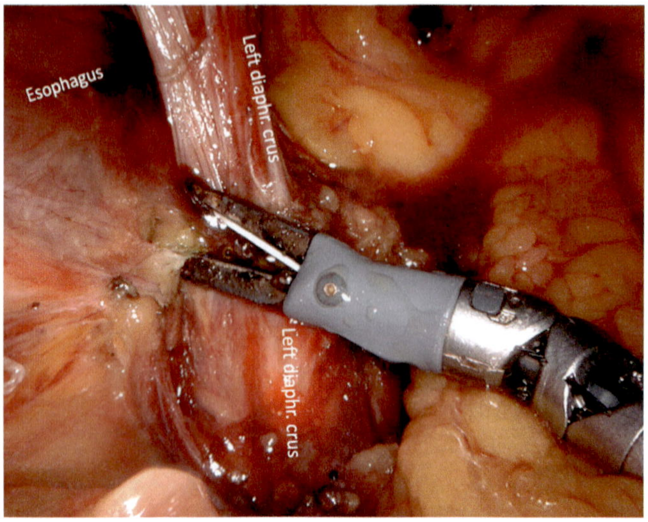

Fig. 13.10 The esophagus can be fully released from the left crus after complete dissection of lymph nodes station 2. The dissection plane is connected to the previously developed hiatal dissection plane on the right side

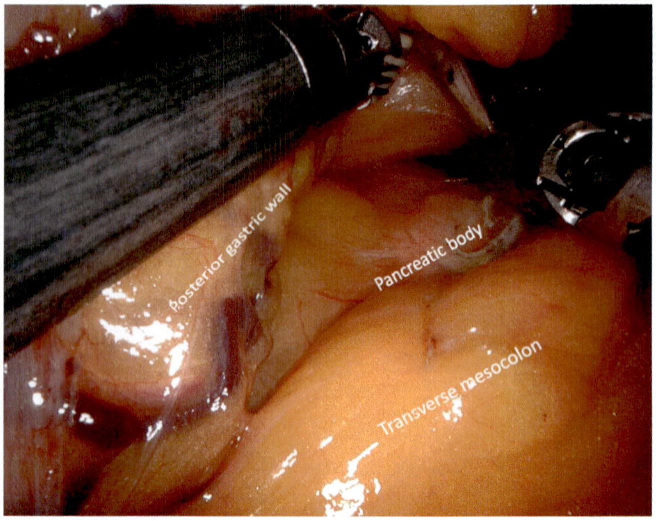

Fig. 13.12 During this phase any residual gastropancreatic ligament or adhesions with the transverse mesocolon are divided to achieve complete mobilization of the stomach

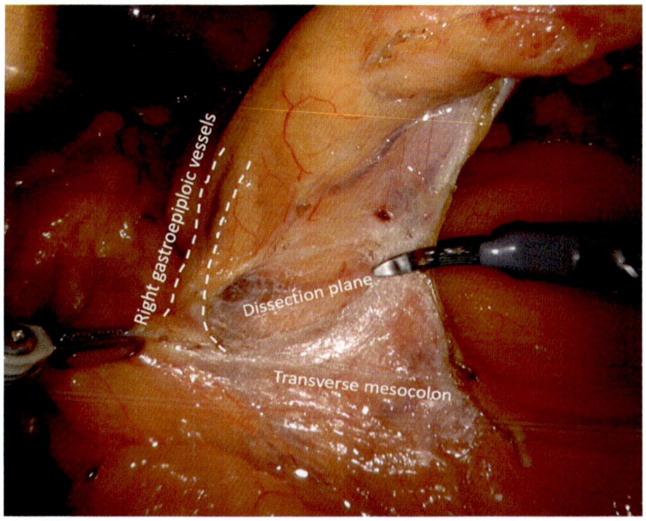

Fig. 13.13 The dissection is carried out toward the pylorus. The right gastroepiploic vessels are visualized and spared as they provide the vascularization to the gastric conduit. Care should be taken in separating the posterior gastric wall from the transverse mesocolon in this phase

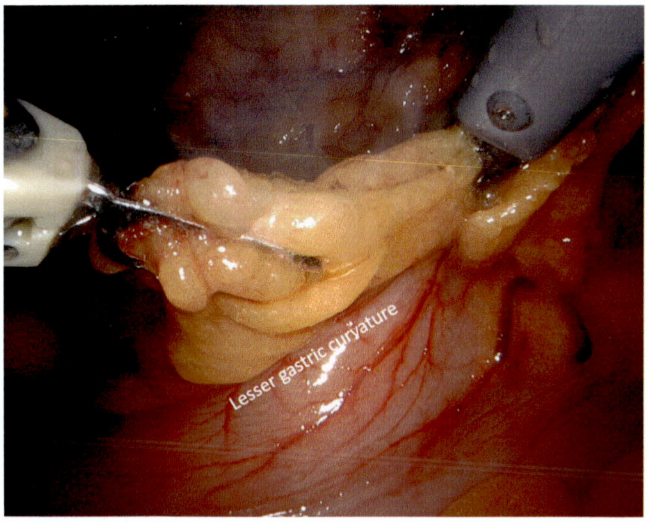

Fig. 13.15 The fat tissue is dissected from the lesser curvature to prepare the stomach for tubulization

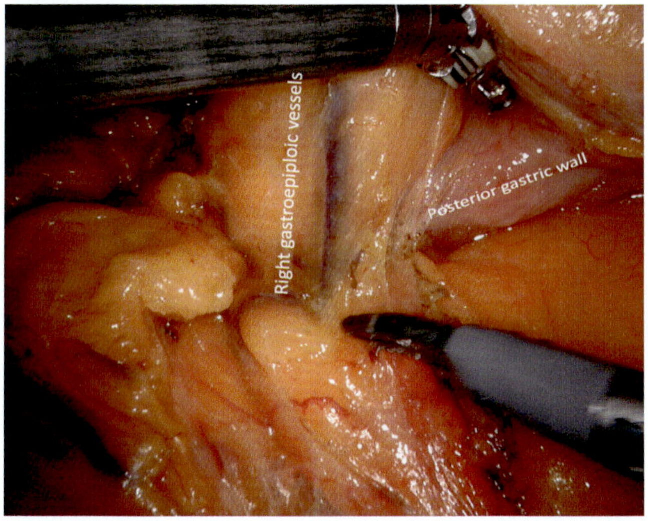

Fig. 13.14 During this step the antrum can be lifted up in order to bring the gastroepiploic vessels in orthogonal position and facilitate the dissection. The gastric mobilization should be extended toward the gallbladder until the postpyloric duodenum is visualized. The gastroduodenal artery is often visualized

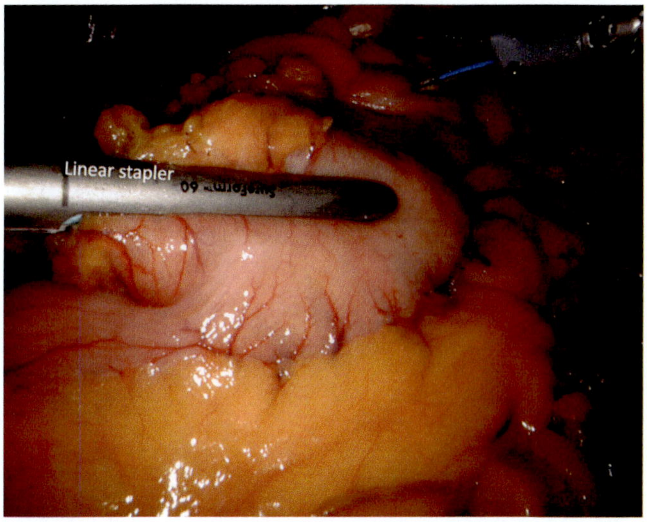

Fig. 13.16 The first stapler (*SureFormTM Stapler, Intuitive, Sunnyvale, California, USA*) is applied approximately between the distal third and the proximal two thirds of the lesser curvature

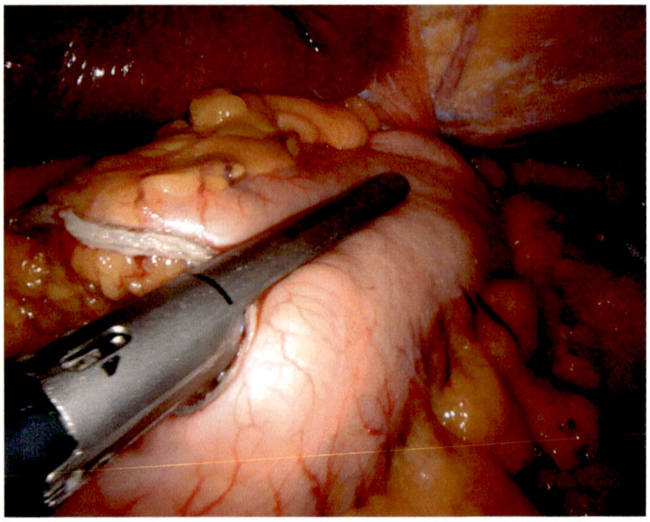

Fig. 13.17 Normally between three and four fires of the 60 mm stapler (blue or black magazines) are used

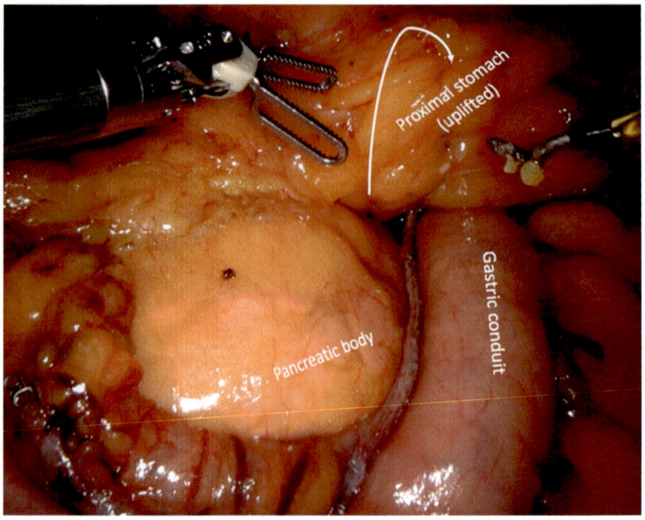

Fig. 13.19 After tubulization, the lesser curvature can be lifted cranially, thus improving the exposition for the subsequent lymphadenectomy

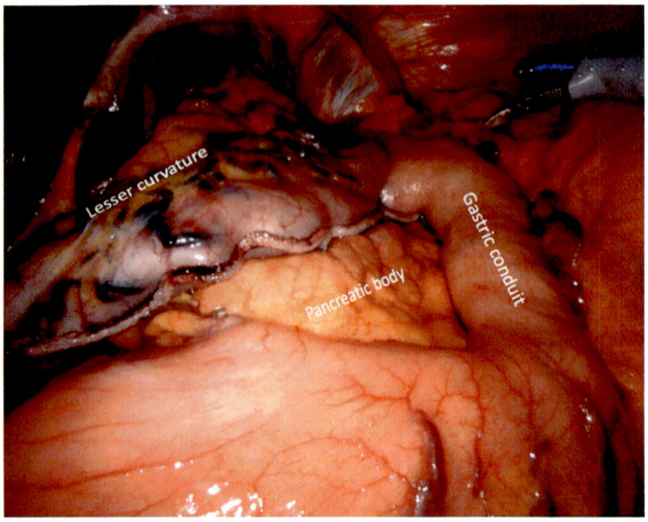

Fig. 13.18 A 4–5 cm tissue connection to the fundus is left, in order to later pull up the stomach by traction on the dissected esophagus

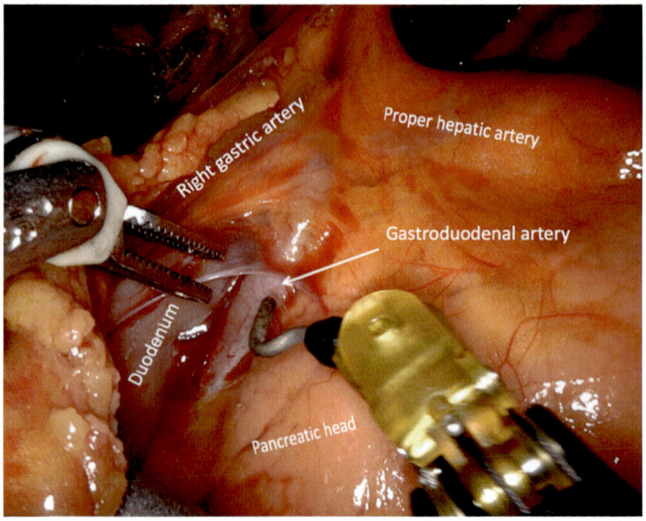

Fig. 13.20 The lymphadenectomy is started by dissecting the fat tissue medially from the right gastric artery

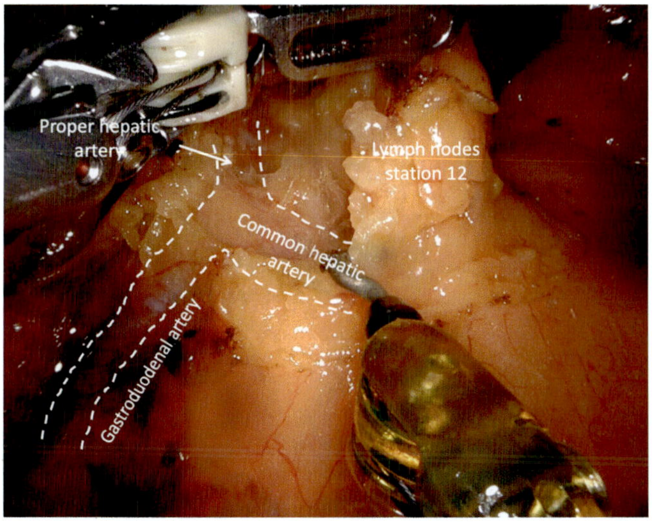

Fig. 13.21 Following the right gastric artery, the proper hepatic artery is identified. Dissection of the surrounding fat tissue is carried out toward the celiac trunk medially. The origin of the gastroduodenal artery from the common hepatic artery is identified. In this phase we prefer to use the Permanent Cautery Hook (monopolar). Station 12 lymph nodes are collected during this phase and will be extracted en bloc with the final specimen

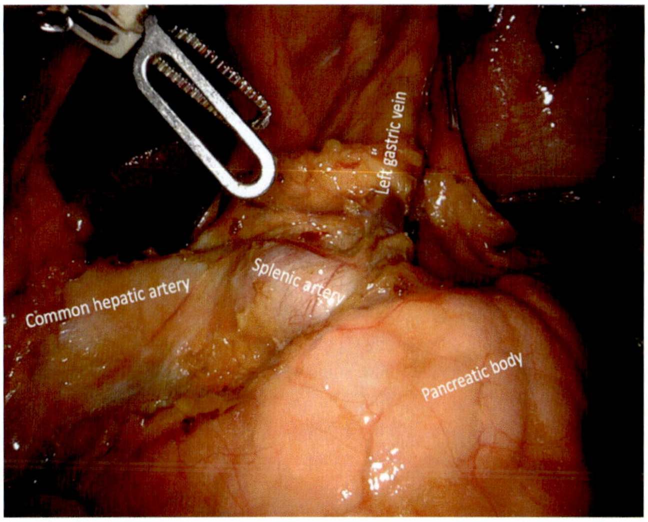

Fig. 13.23 The sovra-pancreatic fat is dissected medially along the superior border of the pancreatic body, and the celiac trunk and the proximal portion of the splenic artery are identified. Gentle cranial traction on the lesser gastric curvature facilitates the exposition of the left gastric vein. Station 9 and 11p lymph nodes are collected during this phase

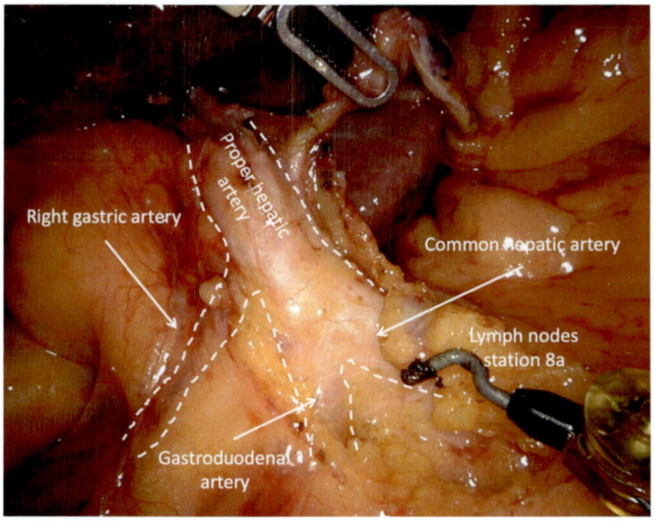

Fig. 13.22 Dissection of the anterior and posteromedial aspect of the common hepatic artery allows the retrieval of station 8 lymph nodes that will be resected en bloc with the final specimen

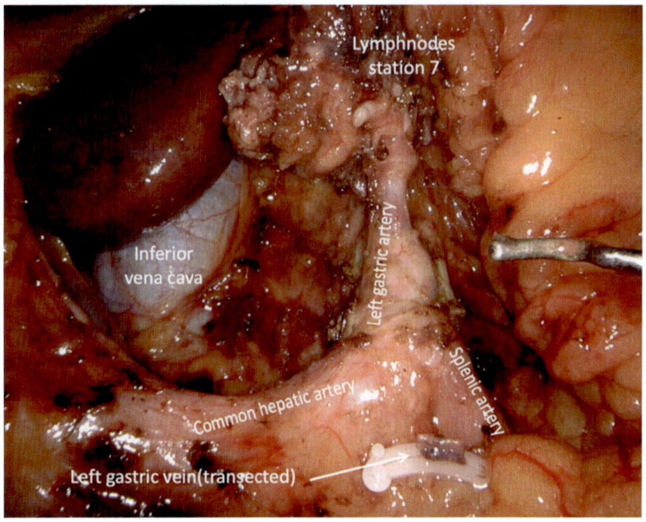

Fig. 13.24 After division of the gastric vein, the left gastric artery is identified and dissected posteriorly. During this phase the fat tissue surrounding the celiac trunk, the left gastric vessels, and the splenic artery is dissected and lifted cranially. This maneuver permits the retrieval of station 9, 7 and 11p lymph nodes that will be resected en bloc with the final specimen

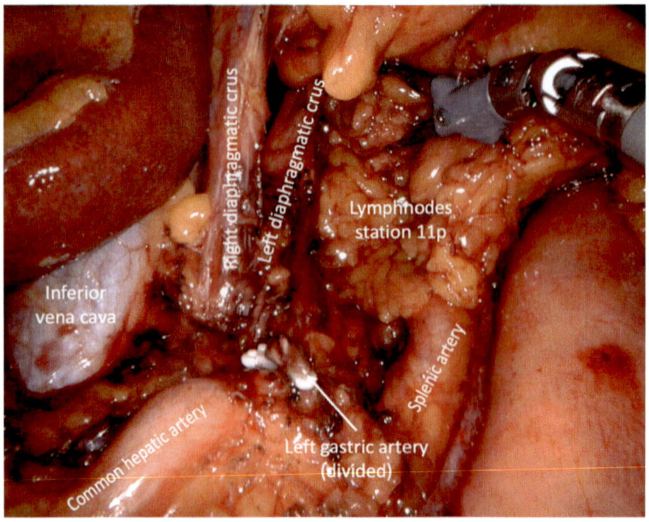

Fig. 13.25 After division of the left gastric artery, the dissection of the fat tissue is carried out posteriorly until the plane of the right and left diaphragmatic crura is reached

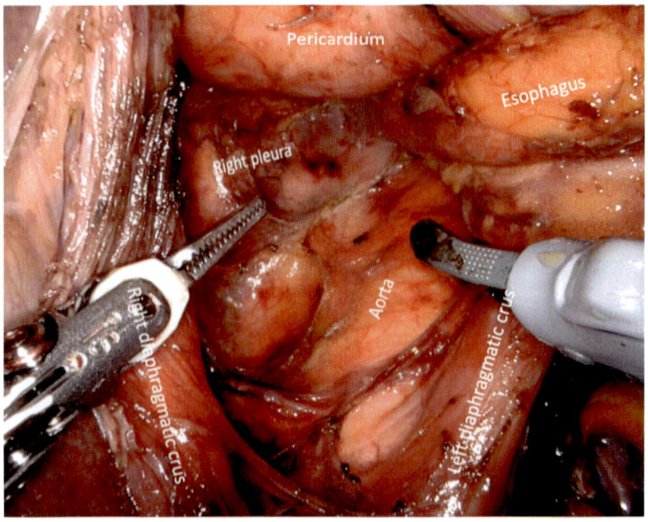

Fig. 13.26 After adequate mobilization of the lower esophagus and lymphadenectomy of pericardial lymph nodes, complete visualization of the left and right diaphragmatic crura and the aortal plane and the surrounding structures should be achieved

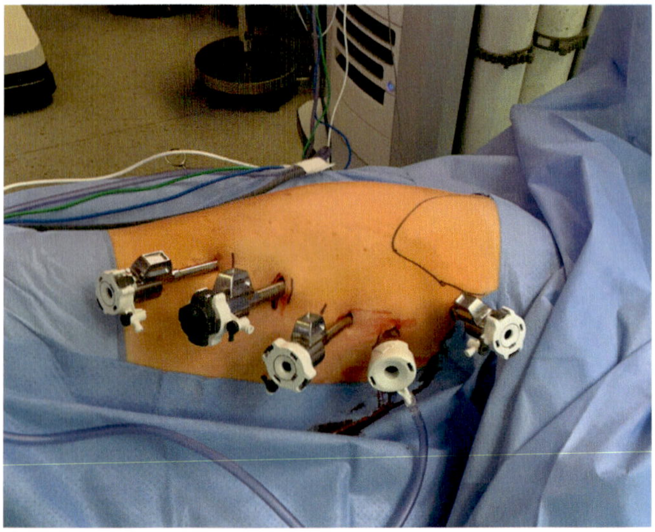

Fig. 13.27 For the thoracic phase of RAMIE, the patient is positioned in a semi-prone position. We normally prefer the patient to be tilted from the left-lateral position 45° toward the prone position. By using a dual-lumen endotracheal tube, the right lung is not ventilated. The first 12 mm assistant trocar is placed in the 5° intercostal space along the anterior axillary line and will be used for retraction, suction, and introduction/removal of any material during the dissection. The 8 mm camera trocar is placed in the 6° intercostal space between the middle and anterior axillary line. The Vessel Sealer Extend and the Monopolar Hook are introduced through an 8 mm trocar placed at the 4° intercostal space along the posterior axillary line. Another 12 mm trocar is placed in the 8° intercostal space, at the posterior axillary line, and is used for the Fenestrated Bipolar Forceps and the Linear Stapler. Finally, an 8 mm trocar is placed inferiorly, in the 10° intercostal space, at the posterior axillary line; this trocar will be used for the Synchro Seal and Tip-Up Grasper, for dissection and to achieve retraction of the lung. The da Vinci® Xi robotic system is positioned on the right side of the patient. The position of the assistant is on the patient's left side

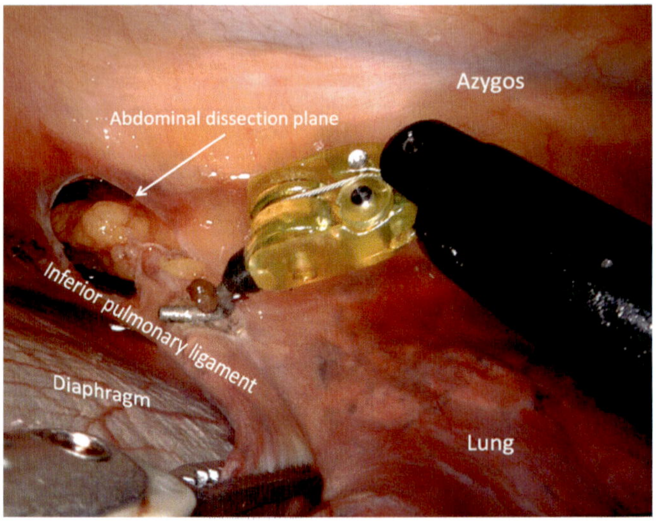

Fig. 13.28 The dissection is started from the inferior pulmonary ligament. The parietal pleura is incised along the anterior side of the esophagus on the pericardial layer

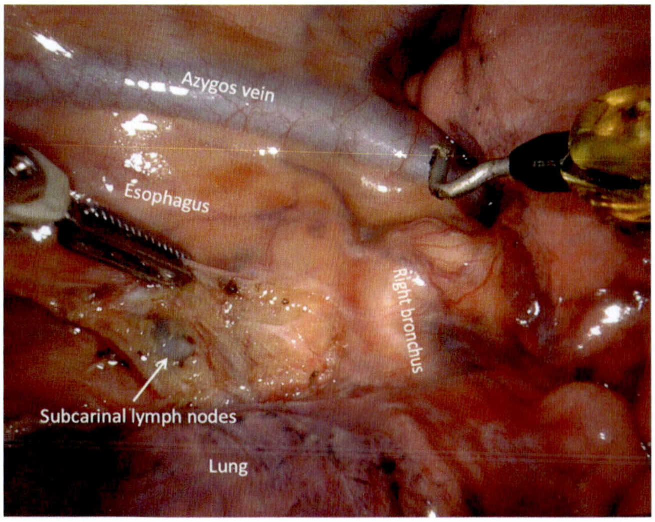

Fig. 13.29 The dissection is extended toward the azygos vein arch, which is clearly identifiable

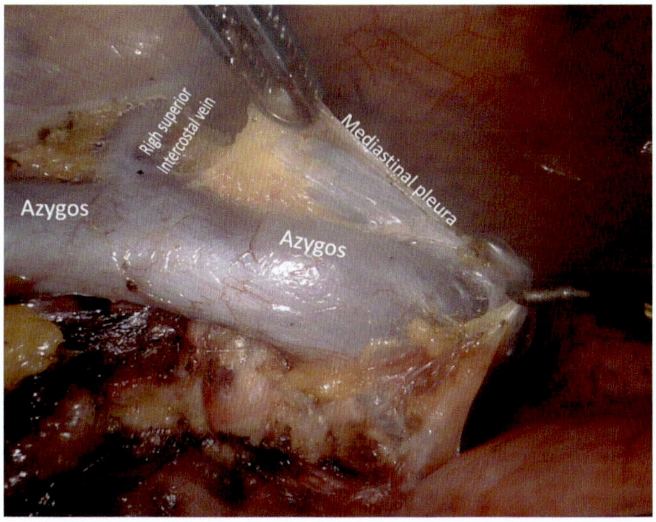

Fig. 13.30 The parietal pleura is further dissected above the azygos arch. This maneuver allows the retrieval of the right paratracheal lymph nodes

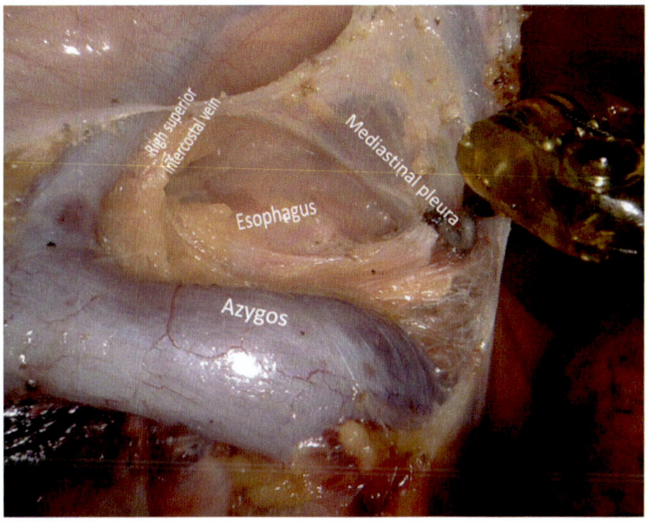

Fig. 13.31 The dissection is conducted above the azygos until visualization of the esophagus above is achieved

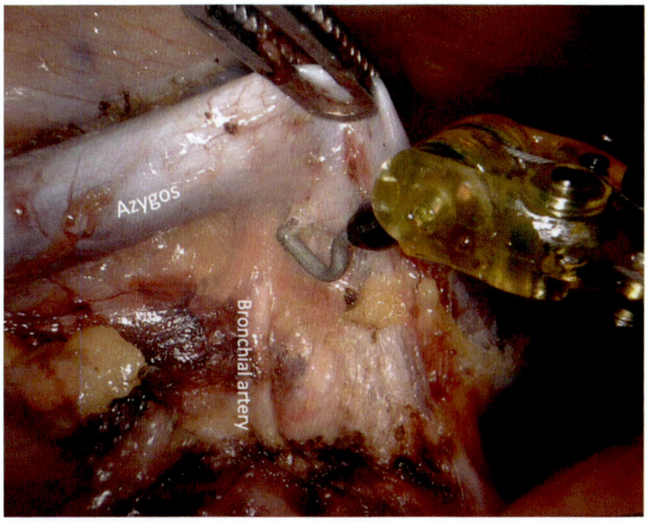

Fig. 13.32 Dissection at the posterior aspect of the azygos is conducted to develop a space for its transection. During this maneuver care should be taken to avoid bleeding from a bronchial artery that can be found underneath the azygos arch

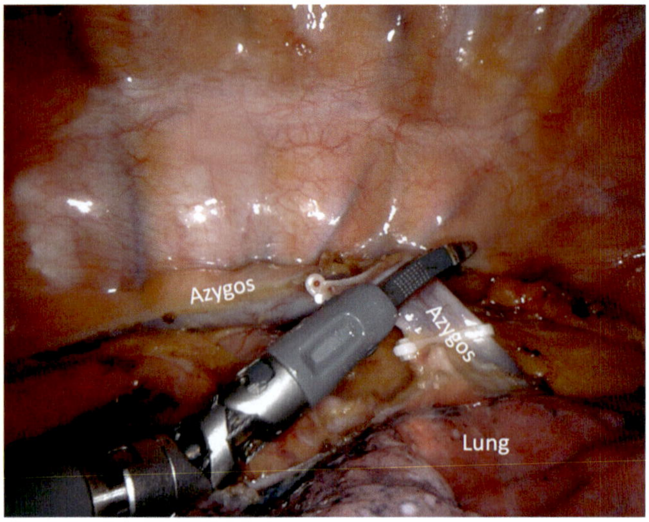

Fig. 13.33 The azygos is then clipped using Hem-o-lok (Teleflex Medical, Weck Drive, NC) and divided using a vessel sealer

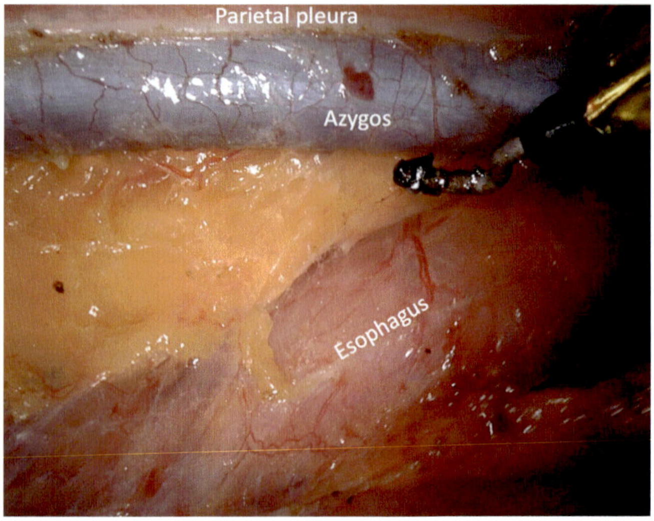

Fig. 13.35 The dissection is continued in a cranial-to-caudal direction at the posterior side of the esophagus along the azygos vein

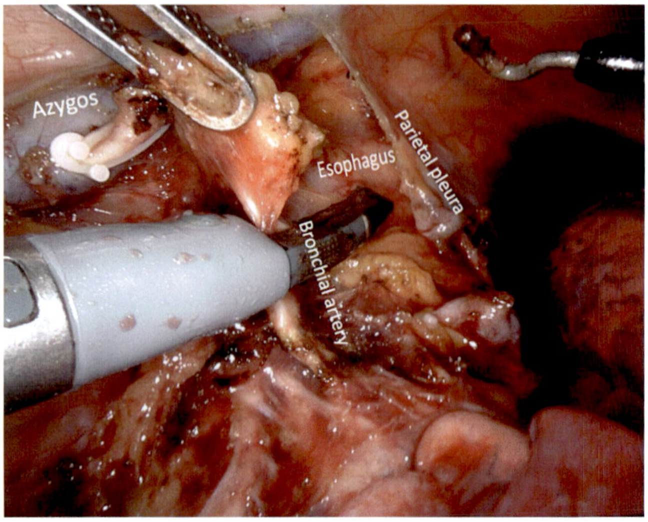

Fig. 13.34 To complete the dissection, the bronchial artery is selectively divided

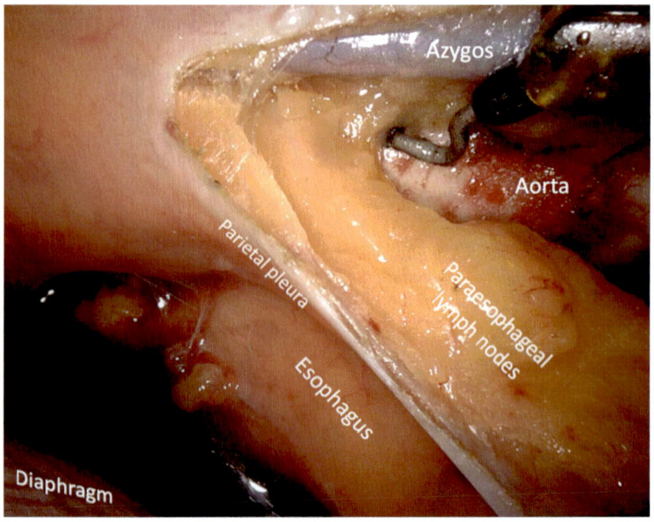

Fig. 13.36 The dissection is conducted until the aortal layer is reached. This dissection layer allows the retrieval of the paraesophageal lymph nodes

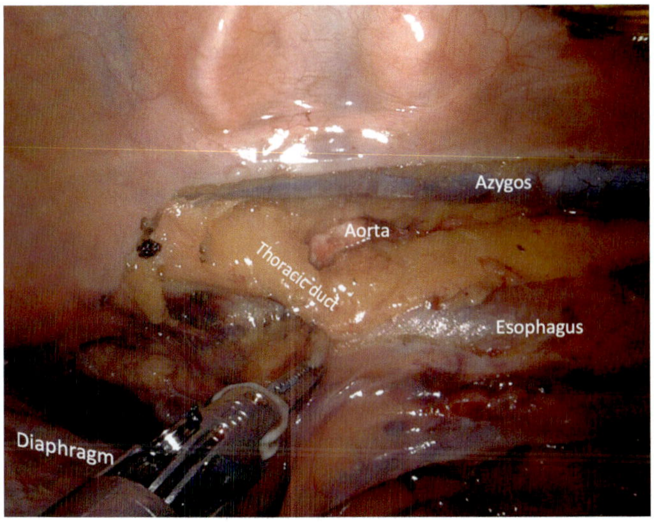

Fig. 13.37 The thoracic duct is dissected at the lower mediastinum

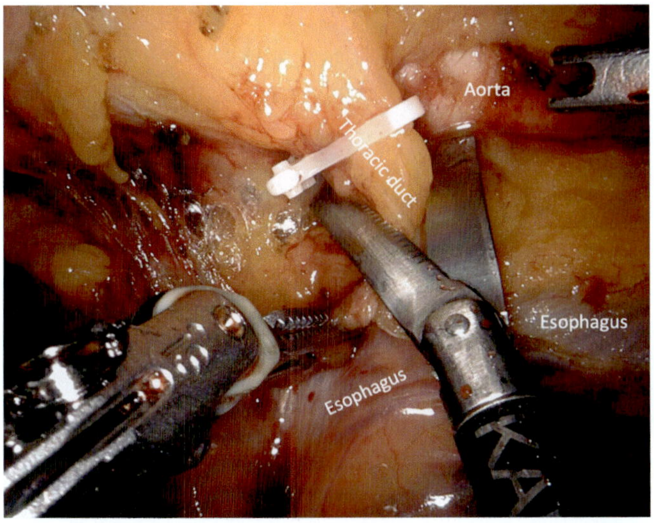

Fig. 13.38 The thoracic duct is then clipped and divided to prevent chylous leakage

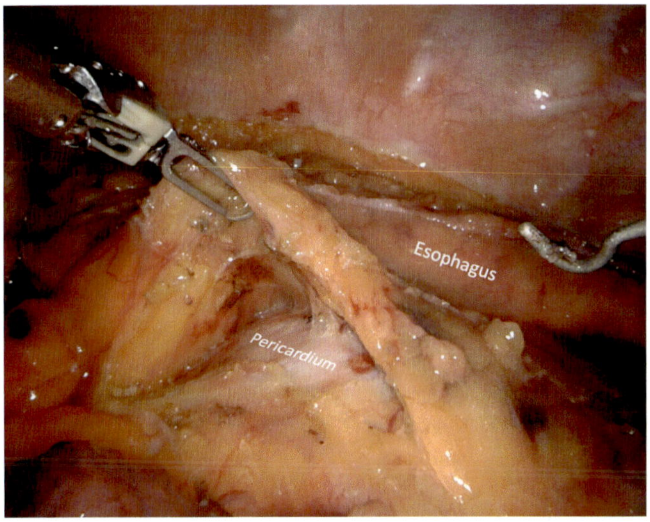

Fig. 13.39 The dissection plane at the anterior border of the esophagus is then further developed

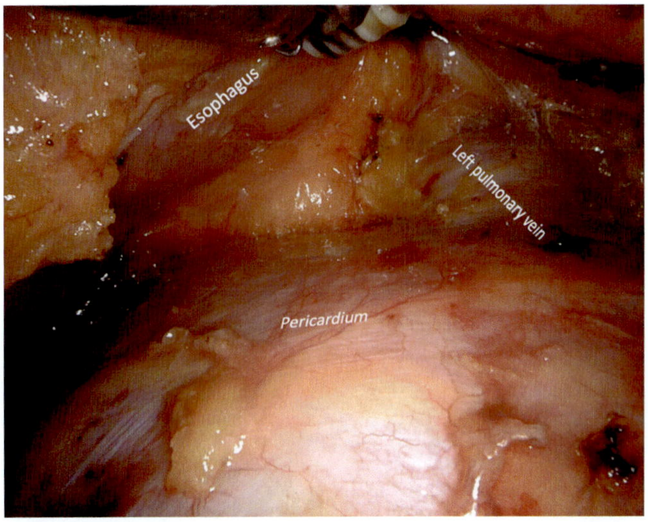

Fig. 13.40 The esophagus is completely dissected from the pericardial layer; during this phase the right and the left pulmonary veins can be identified

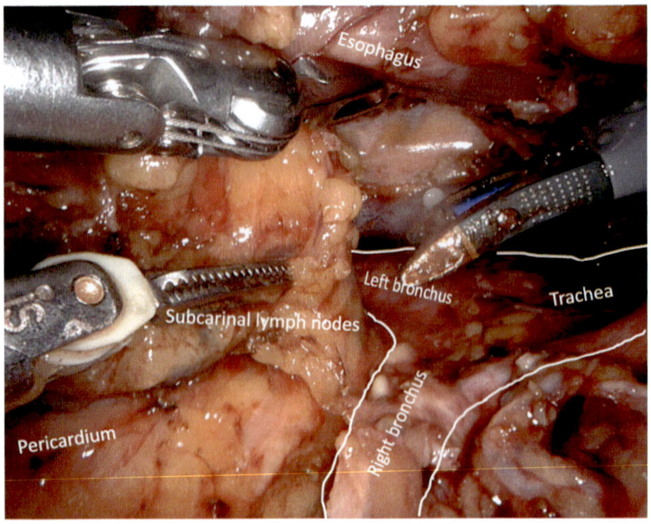

Fig. 13.41 The esophagus is then completely dissected from the trachea and the left and the right bronchi. During this phase care should be taken to avoid thermal injuries to the airways

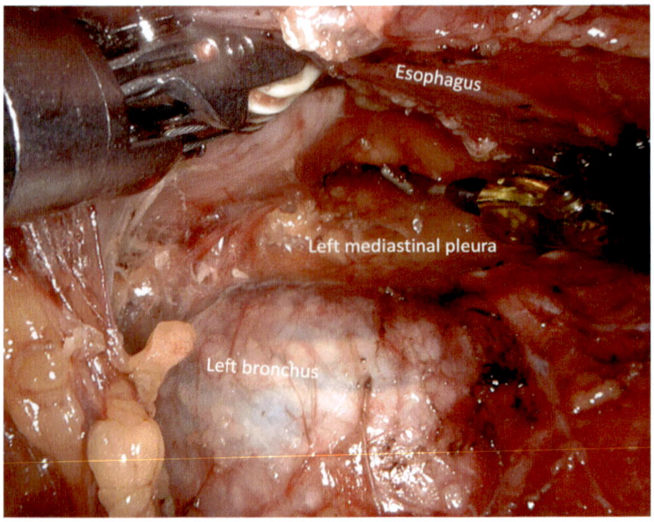

Fig. 13.43 The dissection plane with the left bronchus is usually more easily identifiable as the left bronchus is dilated by the dual lumen endotracheal tube balloon

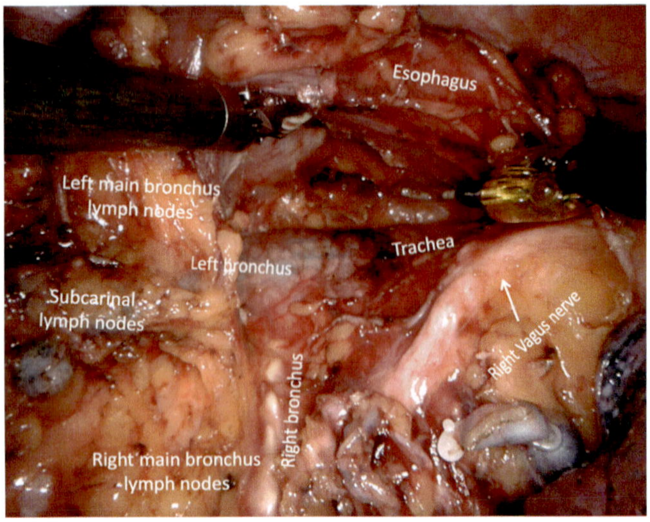

Fig. 13.42 During this phase the left and right main bronchus lymph nodes and the subcarinal lymph nodes can be collected and will be retrieved en bloc with the specimen

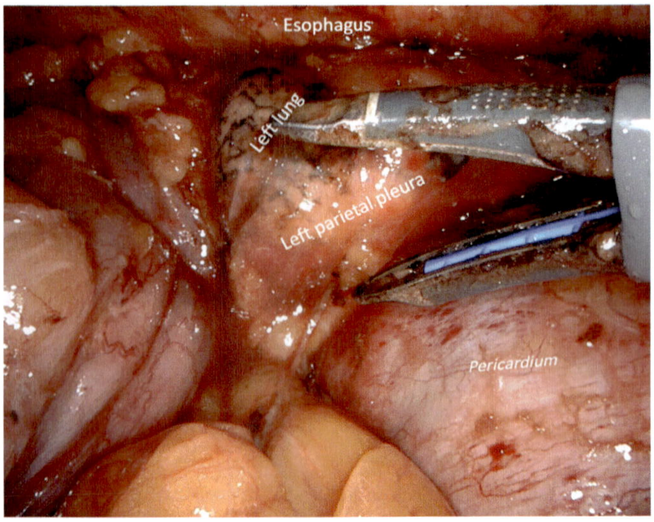

Fig. 13.44 The two dissection planes at the anterior and at the posterior esophageal border are connected at the level of the left parietal pleura

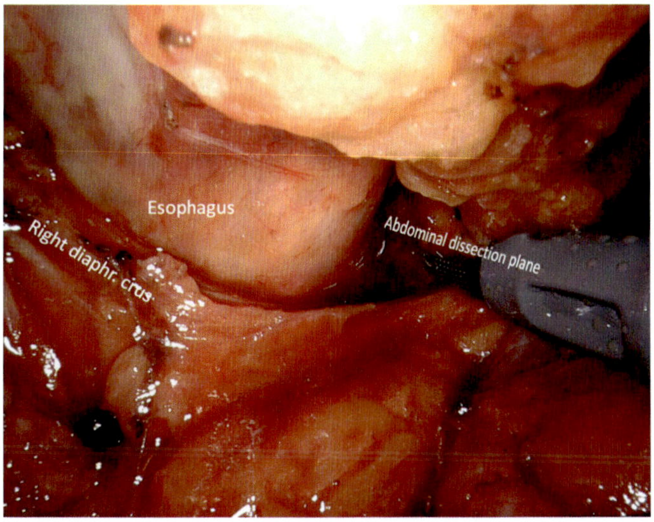

Fig. 13.45 The esophagus is dissected from the left and the right crura above the diaphragm. In this phase the posterior mediastinal and the supradiaphragmatic lymph nodes are collected and will be retrieved en bloc with the specimen

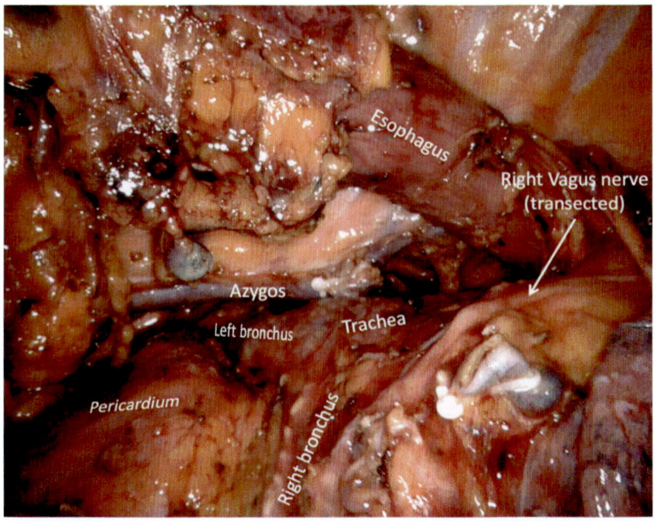

Fig. 13.46 The esophageal branches of the right vagus nerve are divided, while the bronchial branches are possibly preserved. Note that the paratracheal, bronchial, subcarinal, and periesophageal lymph nodes are included in the specimen

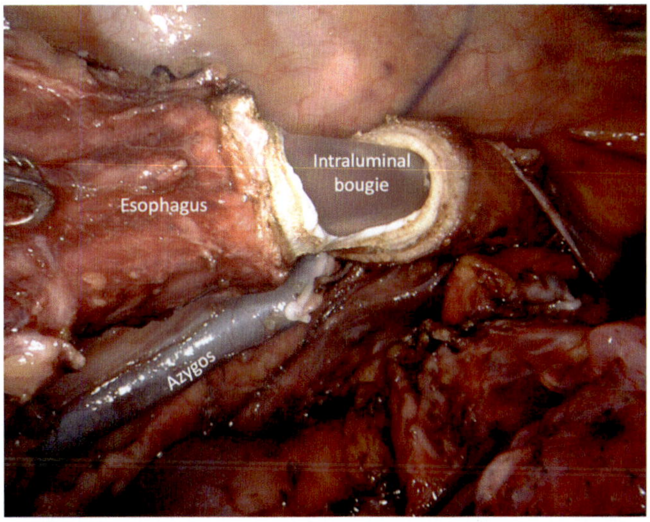

Fig. 13.47 The esophagus is divided using the Monopolar Hook. We normally place an intraluminal bougie at the beginning of the operation to facilitate the dissection; the bougie is then withdrawn to allow the esophageal transection

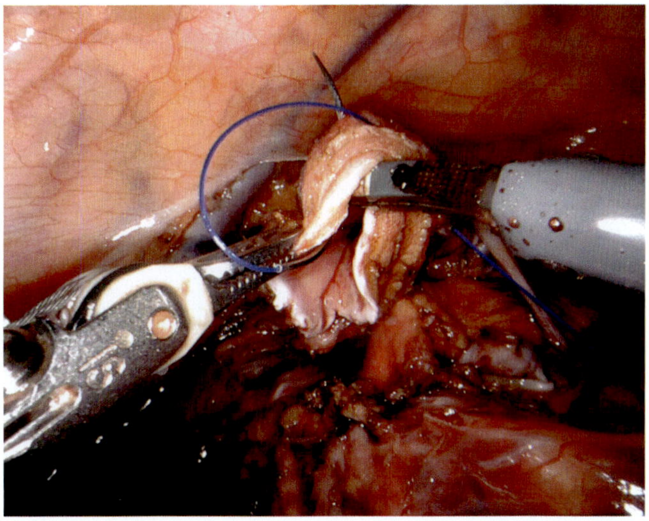

Fig. 13.48 We perform a monofilament purse string suture robotically, whose tails are exteriorized through the assistant trocar. The gastric conduit is brought into the right thorax by gentle traction of the omental fat at the greater curvature

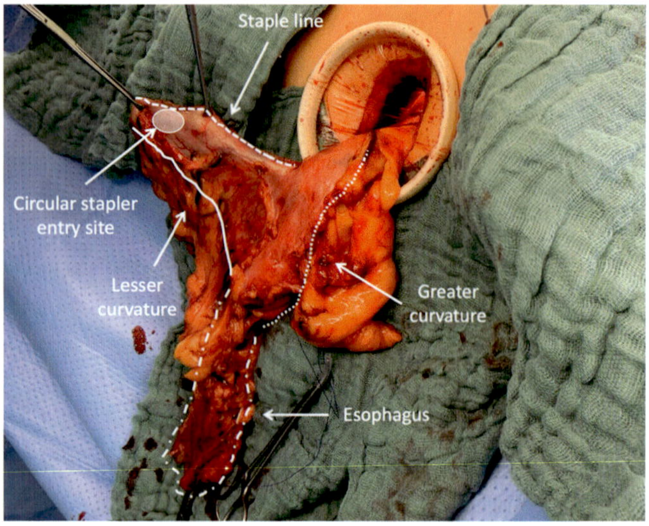

Fig. 13.49 The Robot is then undocked. The 12 mm assistant trocar incision is extended to a mini thoracotomy at the fifth intercostal space. An Alexis O Wound Protector/Retractor (Alexis™ Laparoscopic System, Applied Medical) is inserted. The specimen is exteriorized through the mini thoracotomy

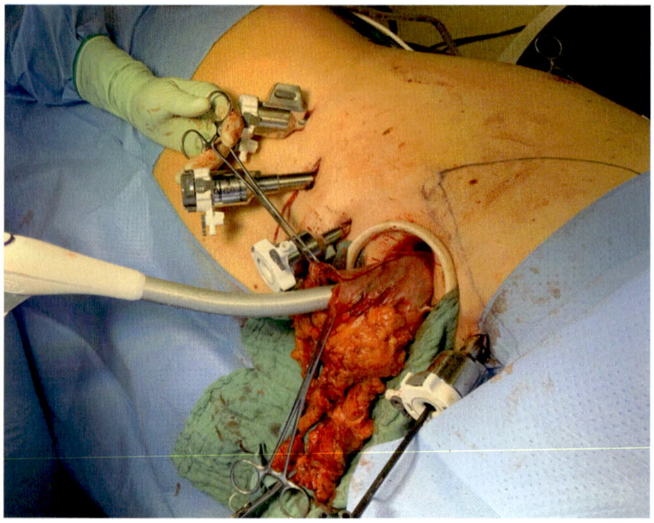

Fig. 13.51 The stapler is inserted through a small incision in the lesser curvature at the staple line

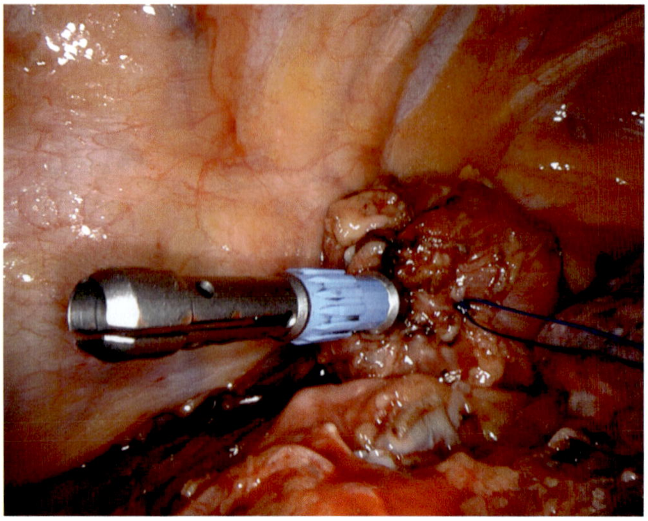

Fig. 13.50 The stapler head is brought through the mini thoracotomy and is secured into the esophageal stump using the prepared purse string suture. We normally use a 28 mm circular stapler (CEEA™, Covidien, Mansfield, MA, USA)

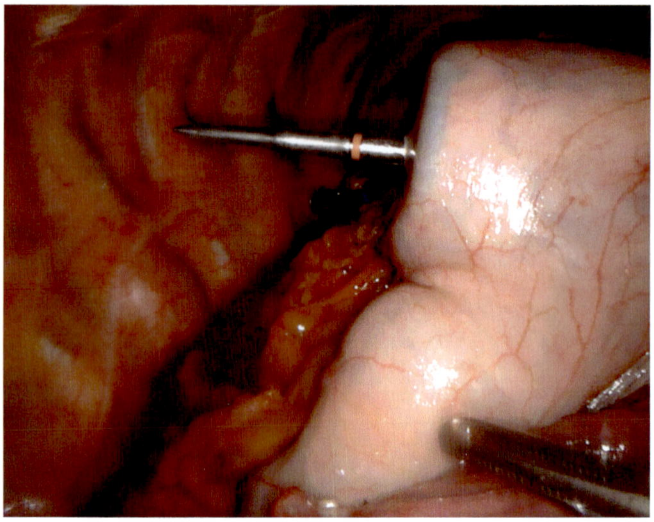

Fig. 13.52 The circular stapler shaft is exteriorized near the greater curvature region of the gastric conduit

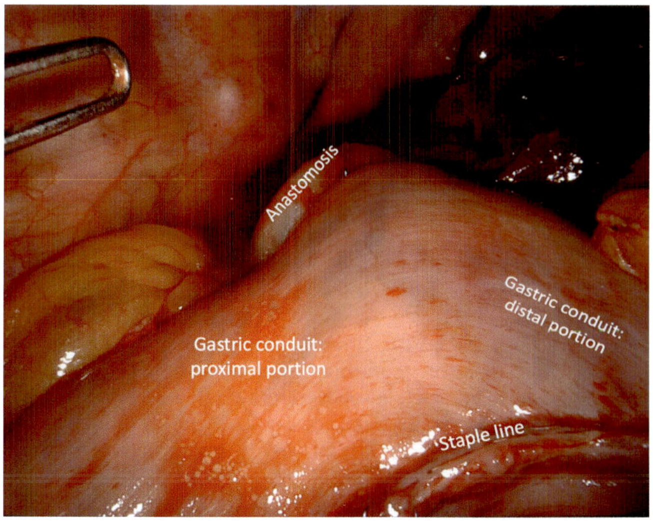

Fig. 13.53 The head and the shaft of the circular stapler are connected, and an end-to-side anastomosis is performed

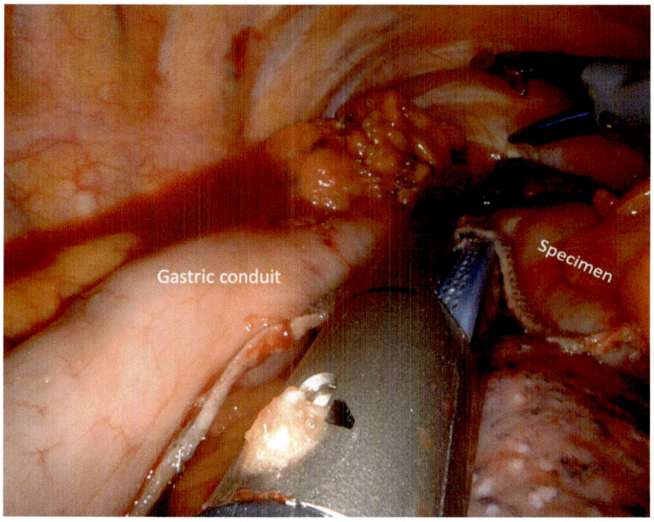

Fig. 13.54 The remaining gastric portion of the conduit is separated using a linear stapler (Endo-GIA™, Covidien, Mansfield, MA, USA). Before stapling, the bougie is reintroduced through the gastric conduit to prevent an accidental narrowing of the proximal conduit. The specimen is extracted through the mini thoracotomy

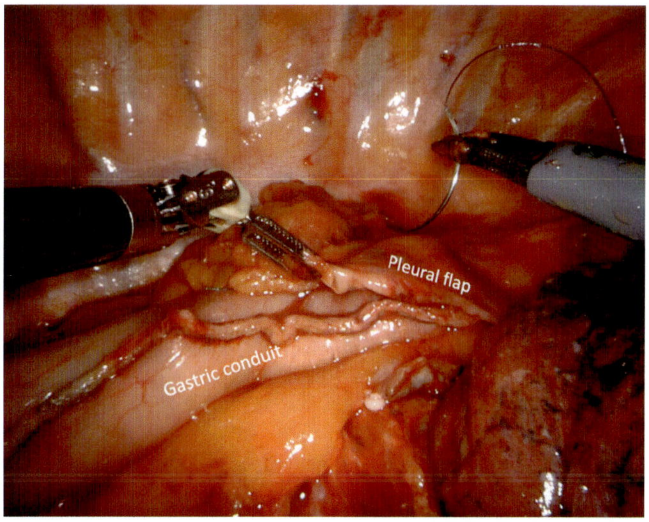

Fig. 13.55 The circular anastomosis is reinforced with single reabsorbable monofilament stitches or with a running suture using a barbed reabsorbable stich. An omental wrap and/or a parietal pleura flap is normally used to secure the anastomosis

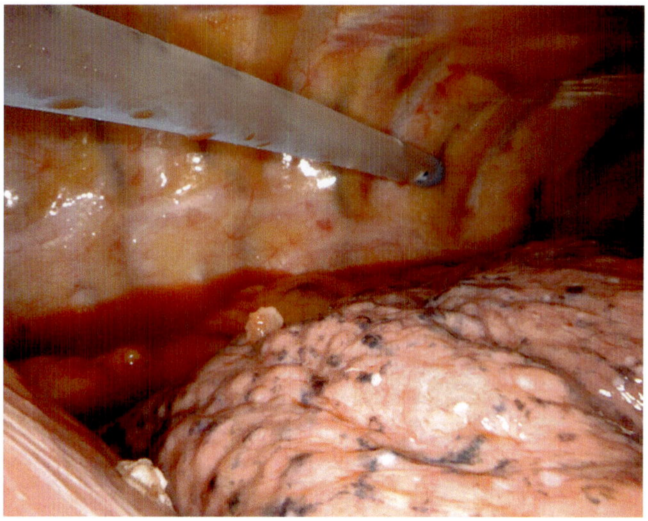

Fig. 13.56 A chest tube is routinely placed into the right chest via the trocar in the 10° intercostal space

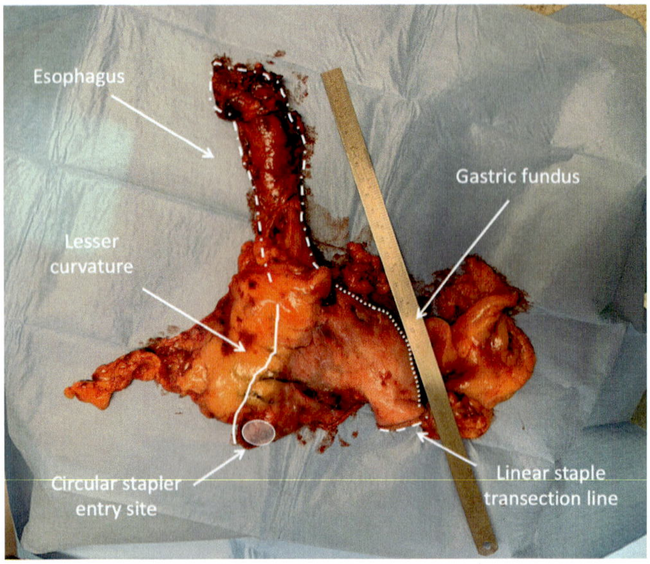

Fig. 13.57 The specimen is dissected at the back-table. The collected lymph node stations have been mentioned during the previous description

References

1. Tagkalos E, Goense L, Hoppe-Lotichius M, et al. Robot-assisted minimally invasive esophagectomy (RAMIE) compared to conventional minimally invasive esophagectomy (MIE) for esophageal cancer: a propensity-matched analysis. Dis Esophagus. 2020;33(4):doz060. https://doi.org/10.1093/dote/doz060.
2. van der Sluis PC, Tagkalos E, Hadzijusufovic E, et al. Robot-assisted minimally invasive esophagectomy with intrathoracic anastomosis (Ivor Lewis): promising results in 100 consecutive patients (the European experience). J Gastrointest Surg. 2021;25(1):1–8.
3. van der Sluis P, van der Horst S, May A, et al. Robot-assisted minimally invasive thoracolaparoscopic esophagectomy versus open transthoracic esophagectomy for resectable esophageal cancer: a randomized controlled trial (ROBOT trial). Ann Surg. 2019;269(4):621–30. https://doi.org/10.1097/SLA.0000000000003031.
4. Grimminger PP, Hadzijusufovic E, Babic B, van der Sluis PC, Lang H. Innovative fully robotic 4-arm Ivor Lewis esophagectomy for esophageal cancer (RAMIE4). Dis Esophagus. 2020;33(3):doz015. https://doi.org/10.1093/dote/doz015.

Robotic McKeown Esophagectomy

14

Richard van Hillegersberg, Eline de Groot, and Jelle P. Ruurda

Introduction

Curative treatment for locally advanced esophageal cancer is esophagectomy combined with neoadjuvant therapy. Various approaches for esophagectomy have been investigated including open, conventionally minimally invasive and robot-assisted minimally invasive esophagectomy (RAMIE). RAMIE was shown to be superior over open esophagectomy mainly in terms of overall postoperative complications, postoperative pain, and quality of life [1]. The merits of RAMIE over conventional minimally invasive surgery are mostly technical. RAMIE provides a superior three-dimensional view, increased dexterity due to articulating instruments, and tremor reduction technology. This is especially helpful in the areas that are hard to reach with conventional instruments, such as the upper mediastinum. Despite the technical benefits of robotic surgery, RAMIE remains a highly complex and invasive surgical procedure and is associated with a significant learning curve of 24–70 cases [2]. RAMIE is not yet a standardized procedure, and multiple different techniques exist including variations in anastomotic location and technique [3]. Factors such as tumor location and invasiveness, radiation field, and location of clinically positive lymph nodes determine the location of the anastomosis. The esophagogastric anastomosis may be located in either the thorax (Ivor Lewis) or the neck (McKeown). A typical reason to go to the neck are oncological purposes to reach a radical resection in mid-upper located esophageal tumors. In this chapter the robot-assisted McKeown procedure with a two-field lymphadenectomy is demonstrated. A McKeown procedure consists of three phases, the thoracic, abdominal, and cervical phase, respectively. The procedure is demonstrated step-by-step below.

Procedure: Illustrated Steps

Figures 14.1, 14.2, 14.3, 14.4, 14.5, 14.6, 14.7, 14.8, 14.9, 14.10, 14.11, 14.12, 14.13, 14.14, 14.15, 14.16, 14.17, 14.18, 14.19, 14.20, 14.21, 14.22, 14.23, 14.24, 14.25, 14.26, 14.27, 14.28, 14.29, 14.30, 14.31, 14.32, 14.33, 14.34, and 14.35 illustrate the technical aspects of robotic McKeown esophagectomy.

R. van Hillegersberg (✉) · E. de Groot
Department of Surgery, University Medical Center Utrecht, Utrecht, The Netherlands
e-mail: r.vanhillegersberg@umcutrecht.nl

J. P. Ruurda
Department of Gastro-intestinal and Oncologic Surgery, University Medical Center, Utrecht, The Netherlands

O. Y. Kudsi, P. P. Grimminger (eds.), *Atlas of Robotic Upper Gastrointestinal Surgery*,
https://doi.org/10.1007/978-3-030-86578-8_14

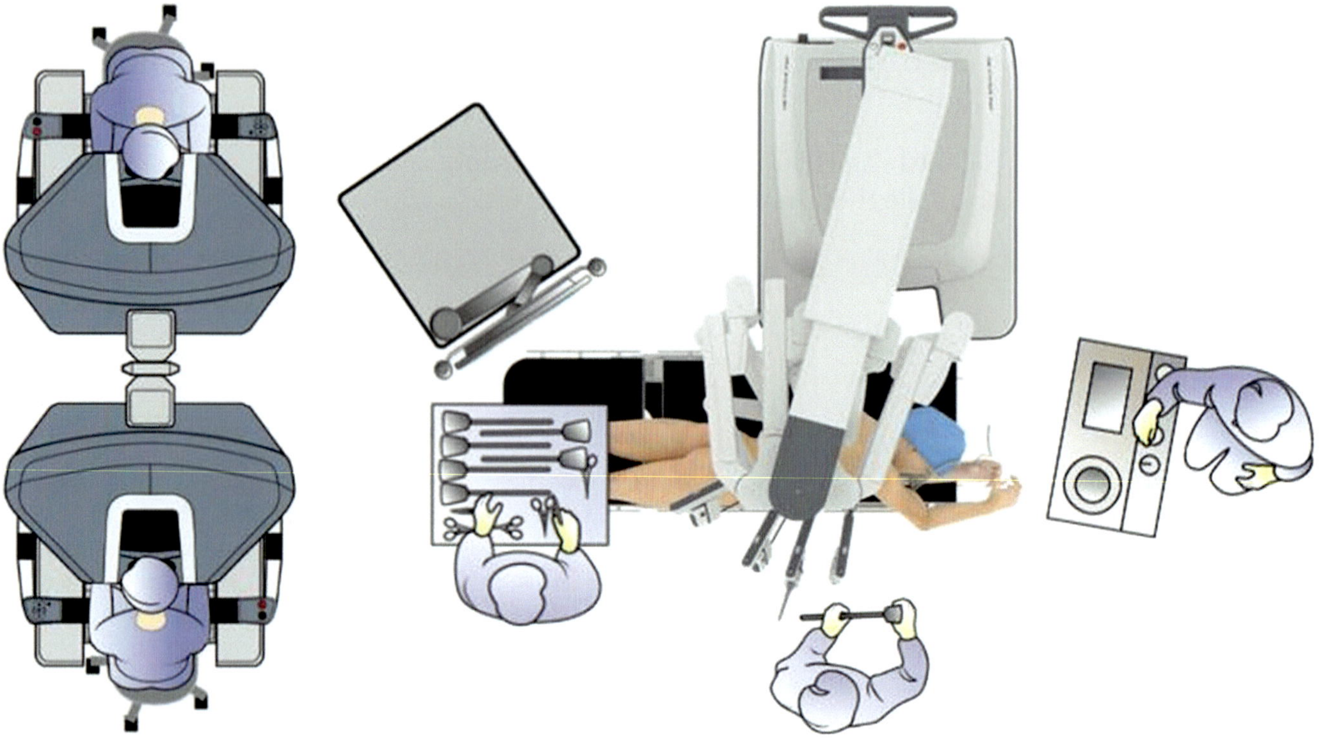

Fig. 14.1 The patient is positioned in a left-sided semi-prone position. The robotic system is placed at the dorsal side of the patient and the table assistant at the ventral side of the patient. (Reprinted from Kingma et al. [3]; with permission)

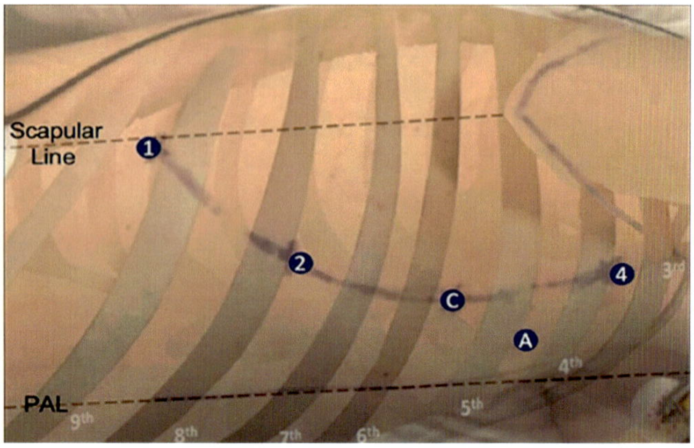

Fig. 14.2 Robotic arm 1 is placed in the tenth intercostal space, robotic arm 2 in the eighth intercostal space, robotic arm 3 which is used for the camera in the sixth intercostal space, and robotic arm 4 in the fourth intercostal space. The assistant port is placed in the fifth intercostal space. (Reprinted from Kingma et al. [3]; with permission of Oxford University Press)

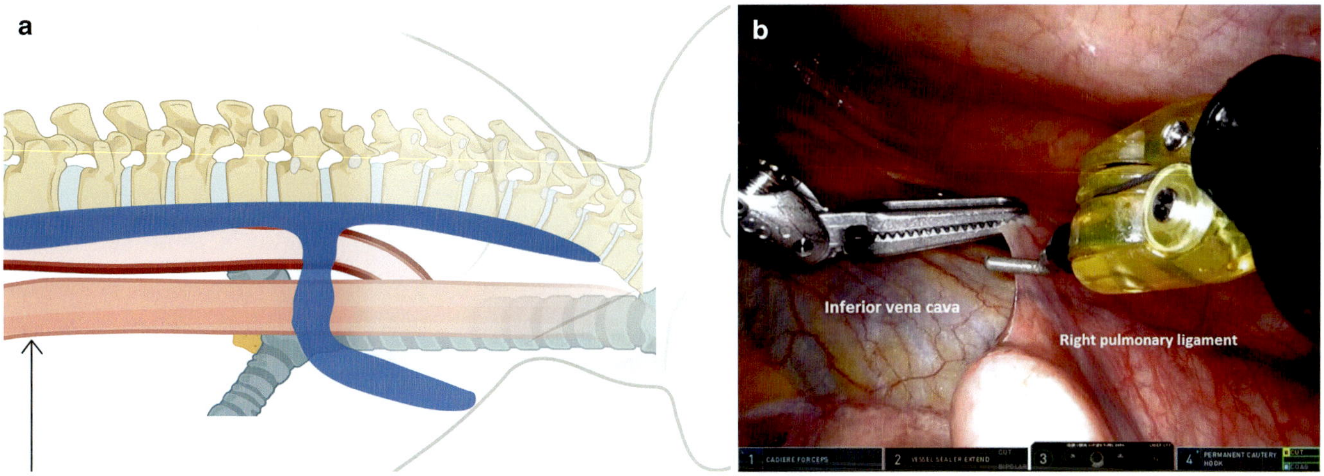

Fig. 14.3 The thoracic phase starts in the inferior mediastinum. At this point, the inferior pulmonary ligament will be mobilized, the azygos arch will be divided, and the dorsal side of the esophagus will be freed from the pericardium. The dissection starts with mobilizing the inferior pulmonary ligament up to the right pulmonary vein. In this way, a dissection plane between the esophagus and the pericardium is created. The right lower lobe of the lung is slightly retracted anteriorly to create an optimal plane. The cadiere forceps is placed in robotic arm 1, the vessel sealer in arm 2, the camera in arm 3, and the cautery hook in arm 4. (**a**, Created with BioRender.com)

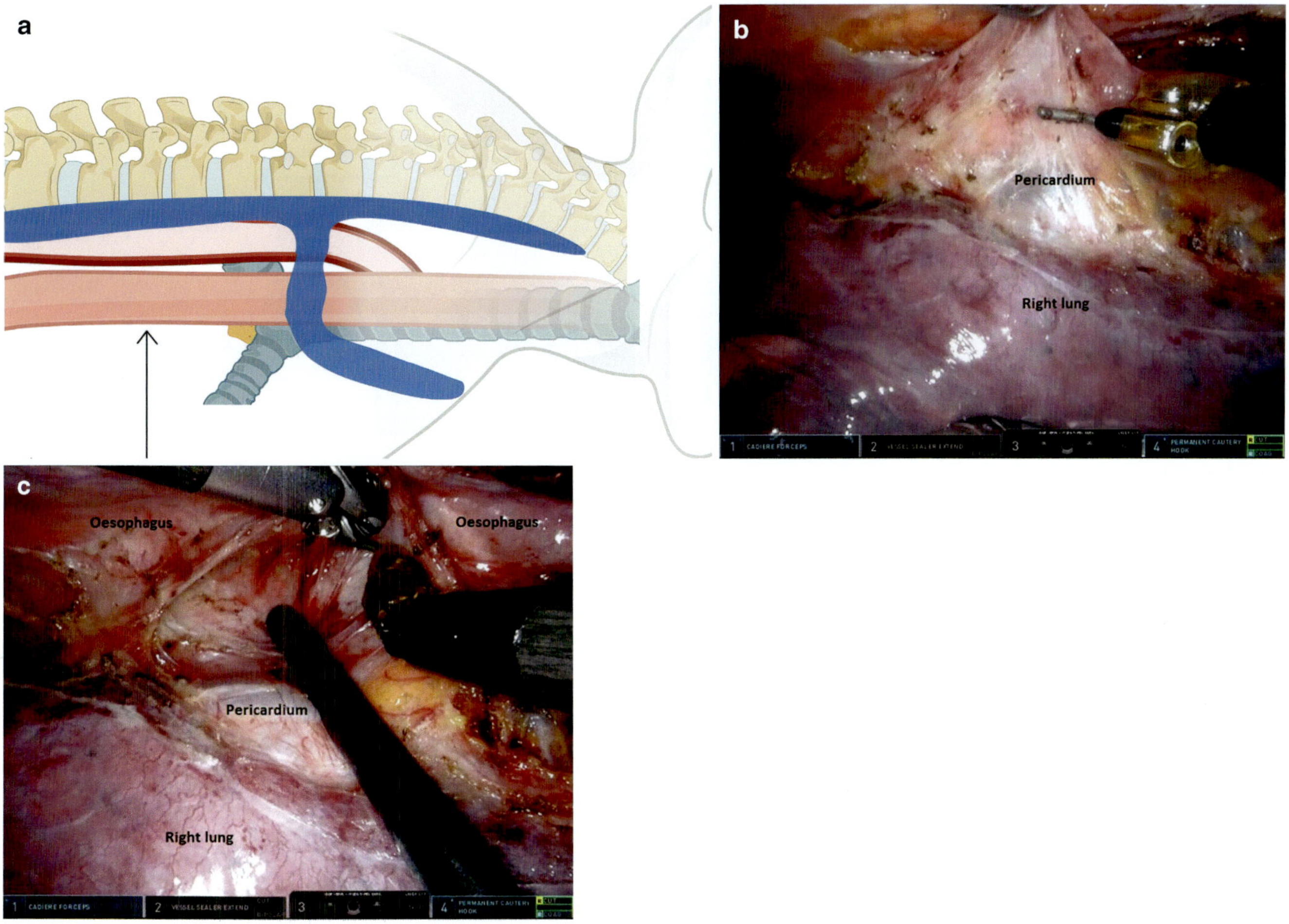

Fig. 14.4 After the pulmonary ligament is mobilized, opening the plane over the pericardium initiates mobilizing the ventral side of the esophagus in the inferior mediastinum. For this step the esophagus is lifted with robotic arm 1. This step is completed when the left pleura is reached. (**a**, Created with BioRender.com)

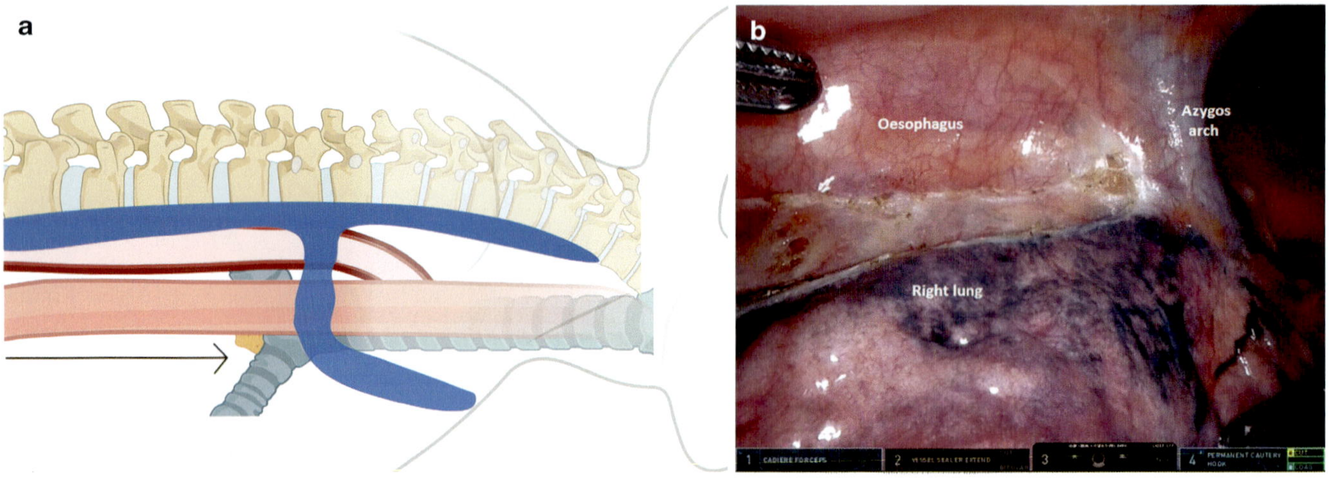

Fig. 14.5 Dissection of the parietal pleura at the right side towards the level of the arch of the azygos vein. Danger zones during this part of the dissection are the right pulmonary vein and right main bronchus. (**a**, Created with BioRender.com)

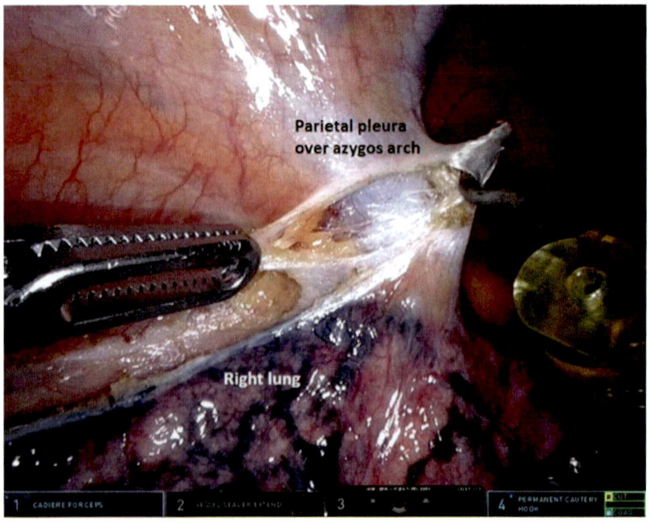

Fig. 14.6 Opening of the parietal pleura surrounding the azygos arch. This has to be done before the azygos arch is transected

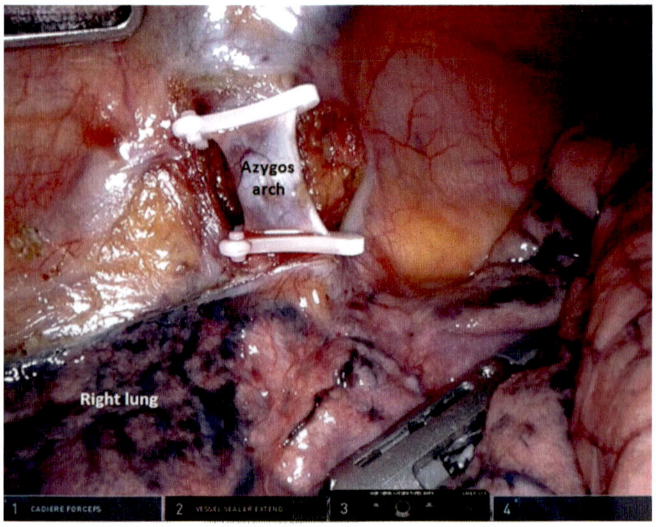

Fig. 14.7 Two Hem-o-lok clips are used after which the azygos vein is transected using the cutting function of the vessel sealer

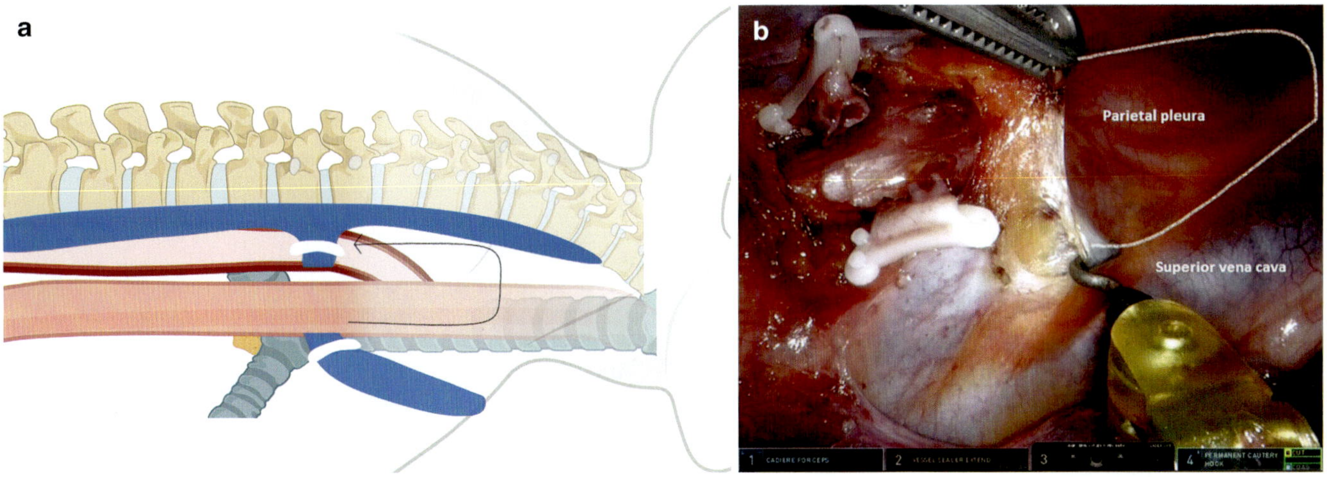

Fig. 14.8 The procedure continues to the superior mediastinum. Starting at the divided azygos arch, the parietal pleura is incised along the superior vena cava until the right subclavian vein and artery are reached. The dissection route is represented by the white line. The robotic arms are most of the time the same as in the inferior mediastinum with the cadiere forceps is in robotic arm 1, the vessel sealer in arm 2, the camera in arm 3, and the cautery hook in arm 4. (**a**, Created with BioRender.com)

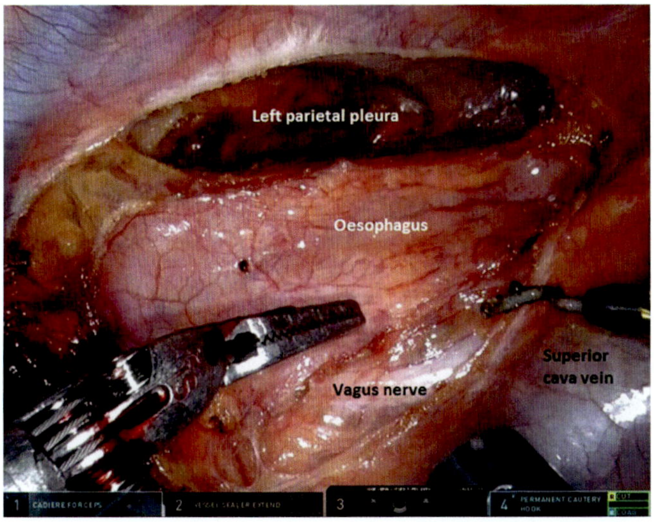

Fig. 14.9 Now that the parietal pleura at the left side is opened in the superior mediastinum, the esophagus is mobilized on its dorsal side towards the left pleura. At this step, it is of importance to include the meso-esophagus with the resection specimen including the thoracic duct. Be aware of the aortic arch and subclavian artery that runs at the level of the trachea to the left. Hereafter, the dissection continues at the ventral side of the esophagus over the trachea, where the right vagus nerve should be identified over the right rim of the trachea

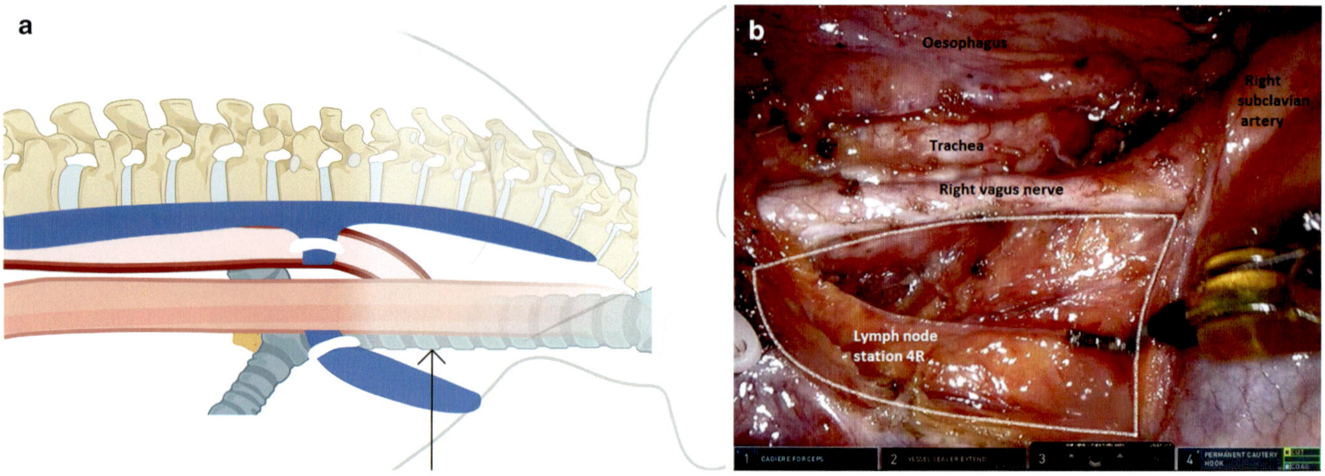

Fig. 14.10 After the right vagus nerve is freed, lymph node station 4R is harvested. Station 4R is located between the superior vena cava and the right border of the trachea (white line). Important landmarks during this part are the superior cava vein (lateral), the right subclavian artery and vein at its cross point with the right vagus (cranial), the right lateral rim of the trachea (medial), and the right azygos arch stump (caudal). (**a**, Created with BioRender.com)

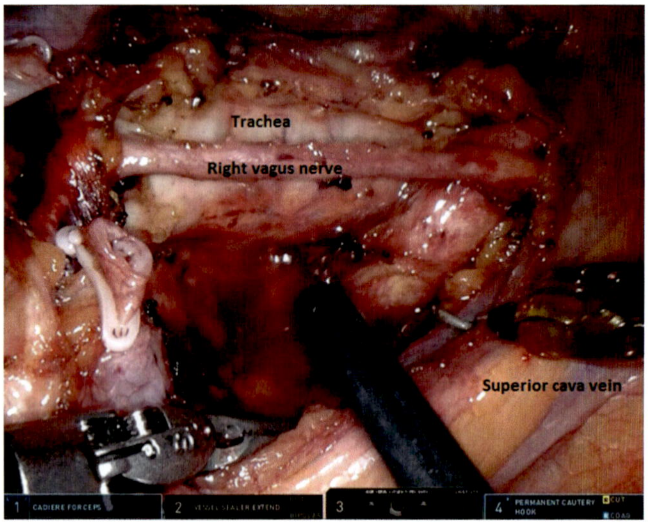

Fig. 14.11 Situation after lymph node station 4R is dissected

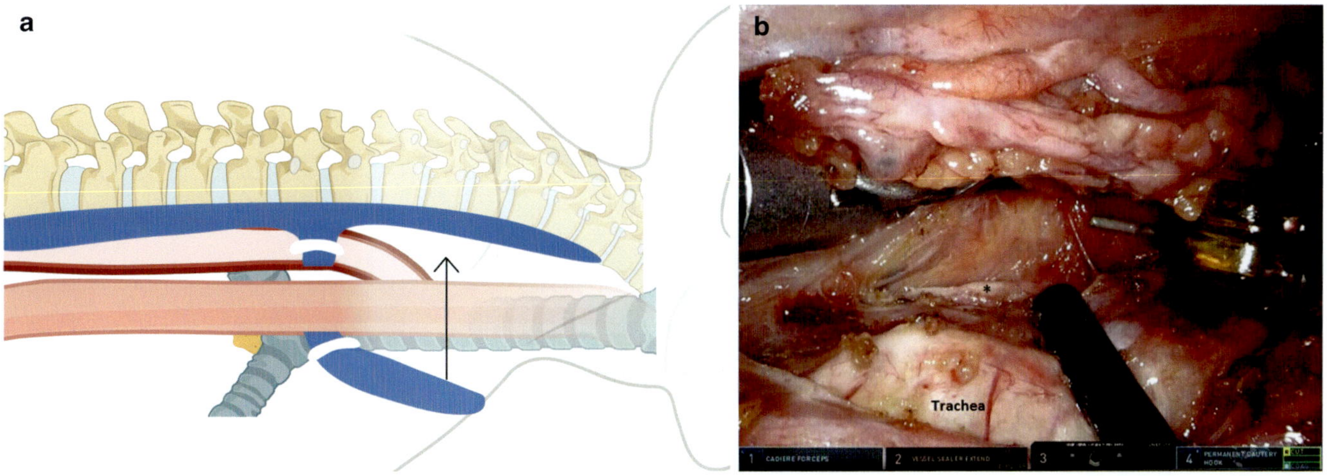

Fig. 14.12 The esophagus is slightly lifted with the cadiere (arm no. 1) to dissect it from the membranous part of the trachea and work towards the left paratracheal groove. Here, the left laryngeal recurrent nerve is identified at the left lateral rim of the trachea. The esophagus is now completely encircled. By lifting the esophagus upwards, the esophagus is further freed from the trachea towards the carina. *Left laryngeal recurrent nerve. (**a**, Created with BioRender.com)

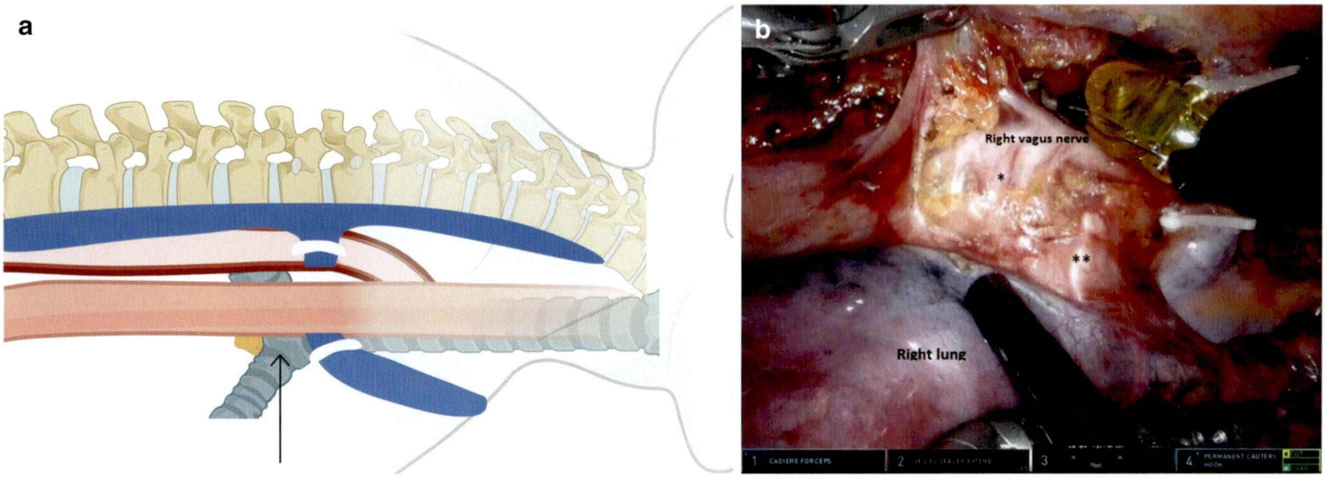

Fig. 14.13 The right vagus nerve is divided at the level of the inferior border of the right main bronchus to preserve the pulmonary vagus branches to the right main bronchus. *Pulmonary branches of the right vagus nerve. **Right main bronchus. (**a**, Created with BioRender.com)

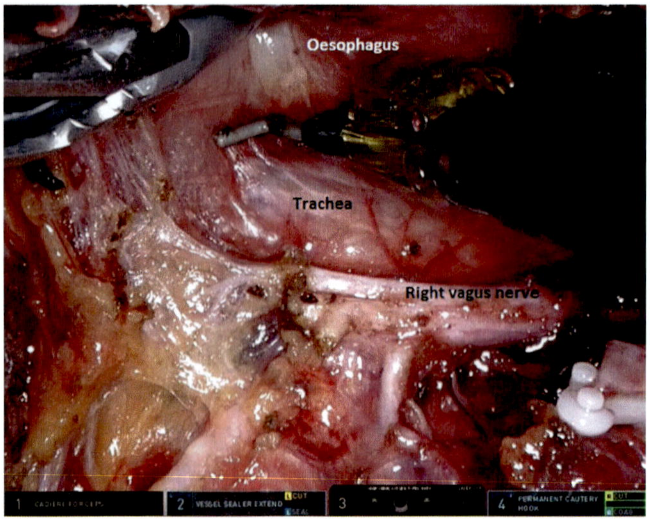

Fig. 14.14 After the right vagus nerve is divided, the inferior border of the right and left main bronchus is followed to expose the cranial aspect of the carinal nodes. A plane between the esophagus and trachea is created. To facilitate this step, the esophagus is lifted with the vessel sealer in robotic arm 2

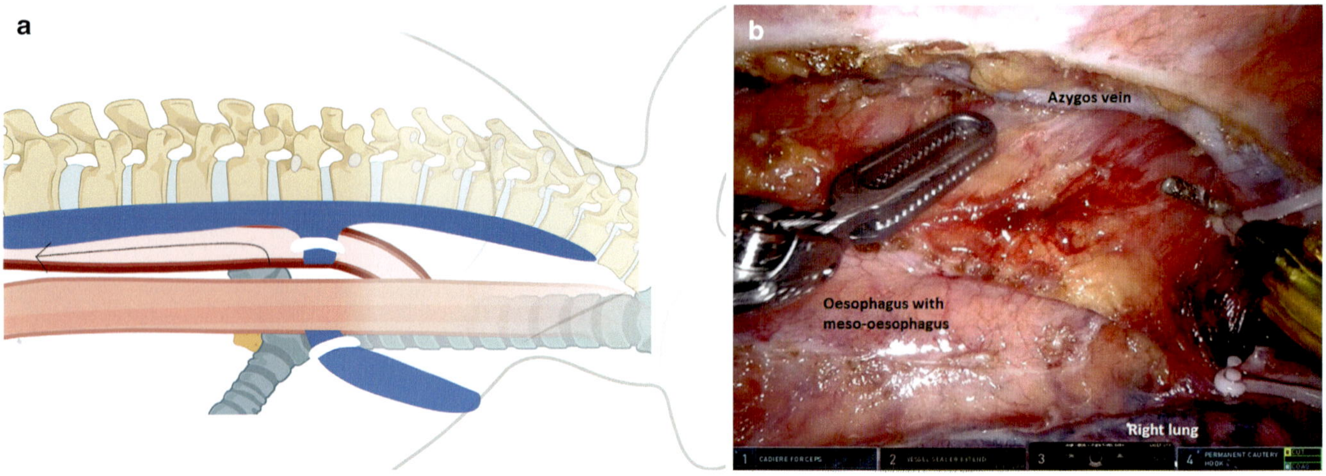

Fig. 14.15 The dissection continues at the level of the azygos vein towards the hiatus. The parietal pleura and lymphatic tissue over the aorta is dissected, guided by the inferior border of the azygos vein. (**a**, Created with BioRender.com)

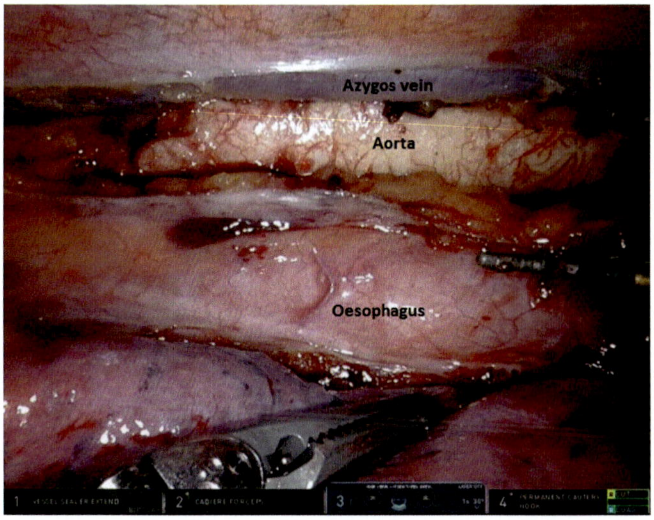

Fig. 14.16 The periesophageal lymphatic tissue, including the thoracic duct, is dissected en bloc with the specimen from the aorta to expose the meso-esophageal plane. At the level of the pericardium, the dissection continues until the left pleura is reached that should be kept intact

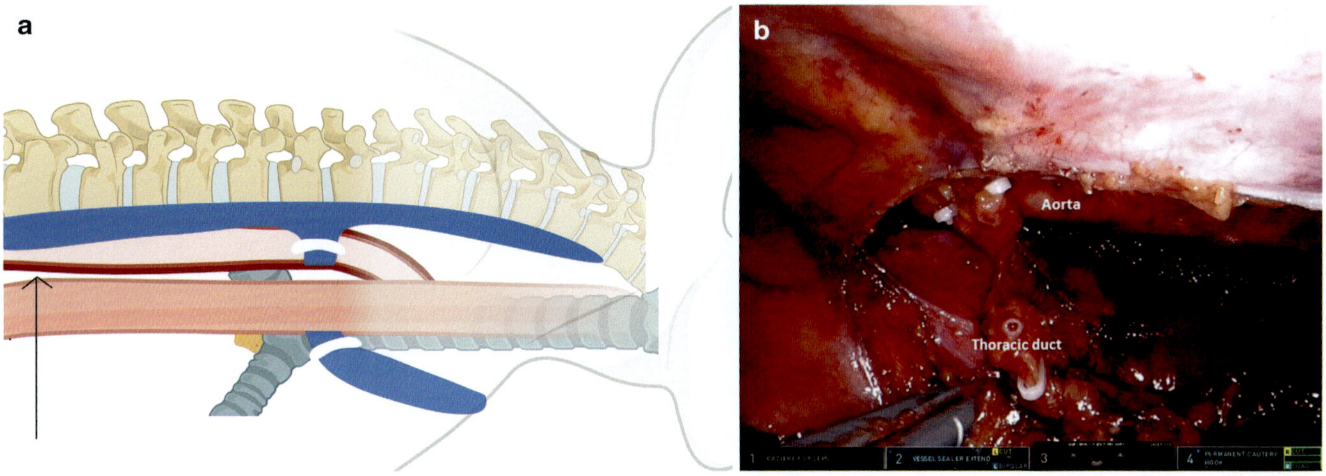

Fig. 14.17 At 5–7 centimeters cranial from the hiatus, the thoracic duct including its fatty sheath and fascia is encircled and divided using Hem-o-lok clips. The level above the hiatus is chosen to avoid the separate ductal branches that may cause chylothorax. (**a**, Created with BioRender.com)

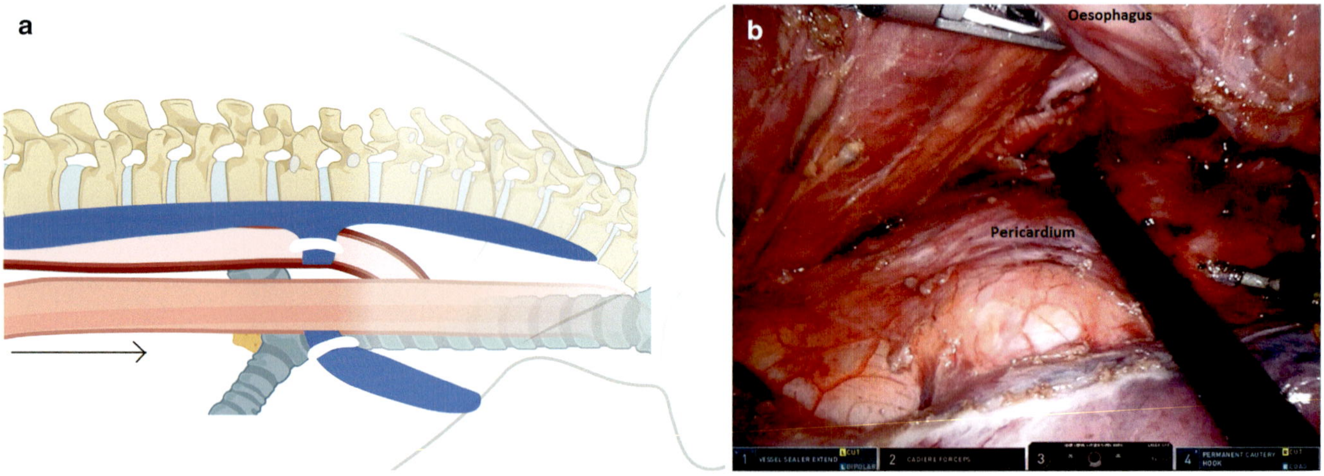

Fig. 14.18 The esophagus is encircled and lifted with the vessel sealer. The dissection continues cranially, to the carina over the plane between the pericardium and the esophagus. The suction device provides contra-traction towards the pericardium. (**a**, Created with BioRender.com)

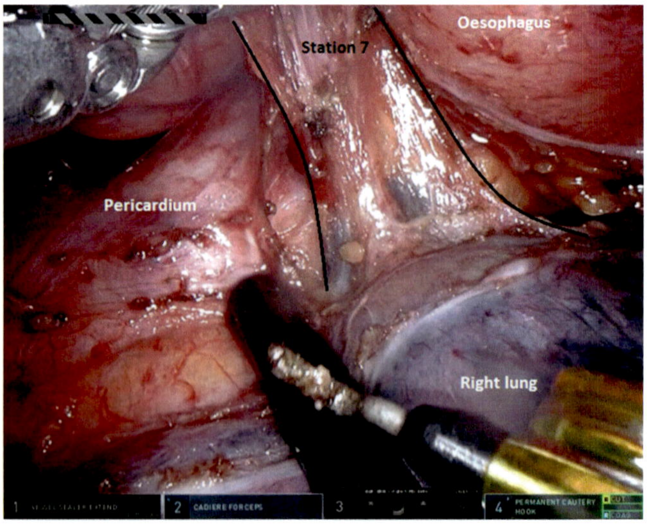

Fig. 14.19 The subcarinal lymph nodes (station 7) are surrounded by an enveloping fascia which is demonstrated in this photo. This surrounding fascia is incised to allow the subcarinal nodes to be lifted away from the superior pulmonary vein using the attachment to the esophagus that is lifted up. The carinal nodes are dissected from caudal to cranial and from the right towards the left bronchus

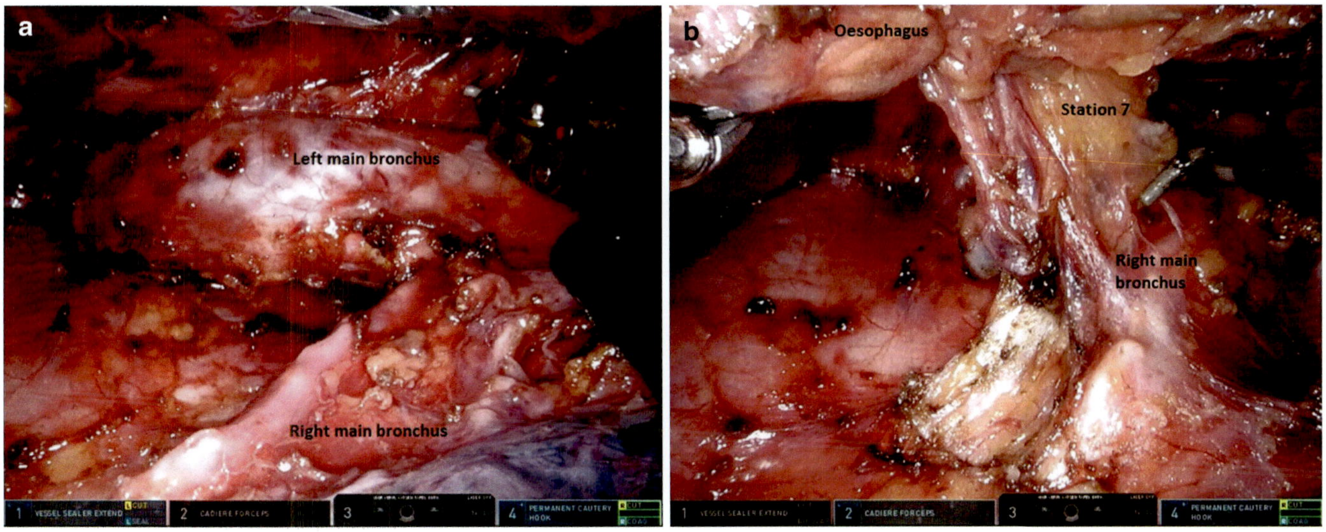

Fig. 14.20 The enveloping fascia around station 7 is dissected in Panel (**a**) so the lymph nodes could be collected. The feeding artery at the apex of the carina is sealed with the vessel sealer. In Panel (**b**) the result after lymph node station 7 is removed is shown

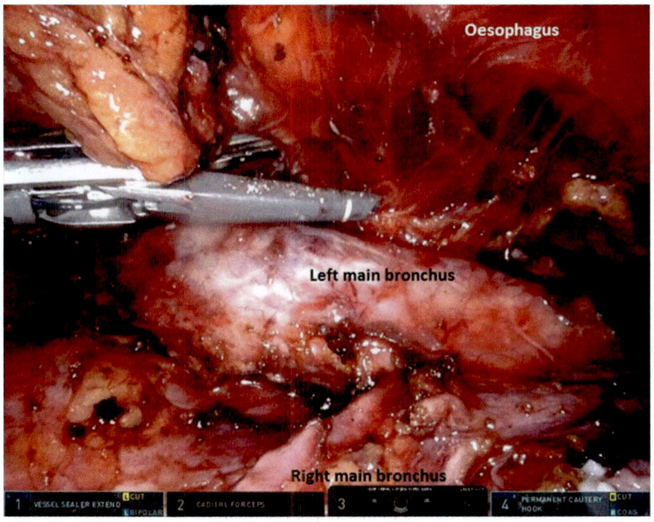

Fig. 14.21 Now that station 7 is resected en bloc with the esophagus, the left main bronchus is optimally exposed. At this point, the next step is to dissect the attachments between the dorsal side of the esophagus and the left main bronchus at the level of the aortic arch with the vessel sealer. The esophagus remains lifted to facilitate the dissection

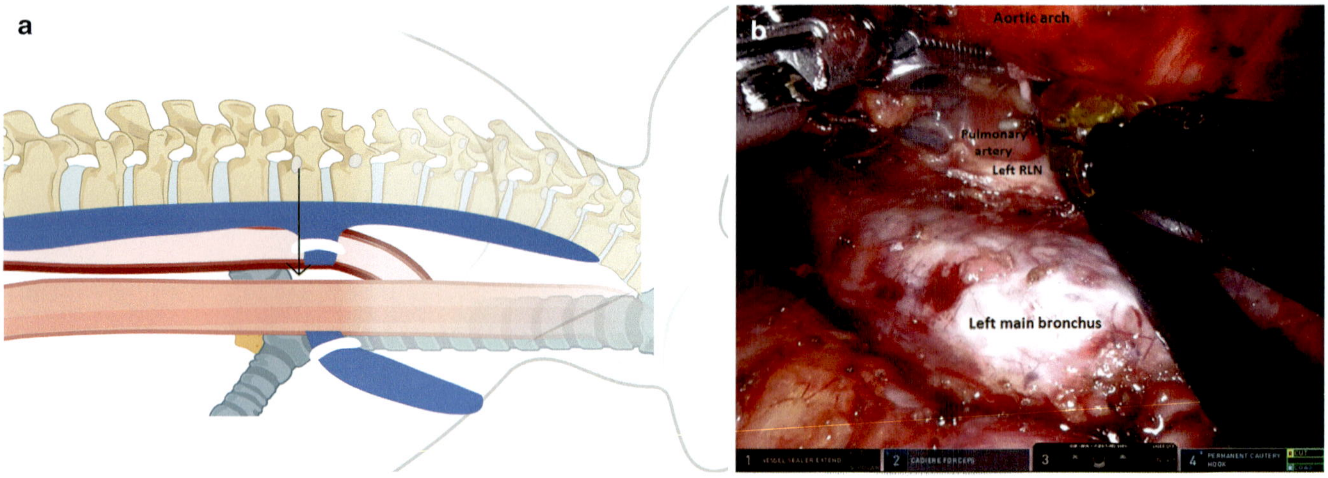

Fig. 14.22 The lymph node dissection in the mediastinum is completed when the aortopulmonary nodes of station 5 are retrieved. The nodes are located between the trachea/left main bronchus and the aortic arch along the left recurrent laryngeal nerve. (**a**, Created with BioRender.com)

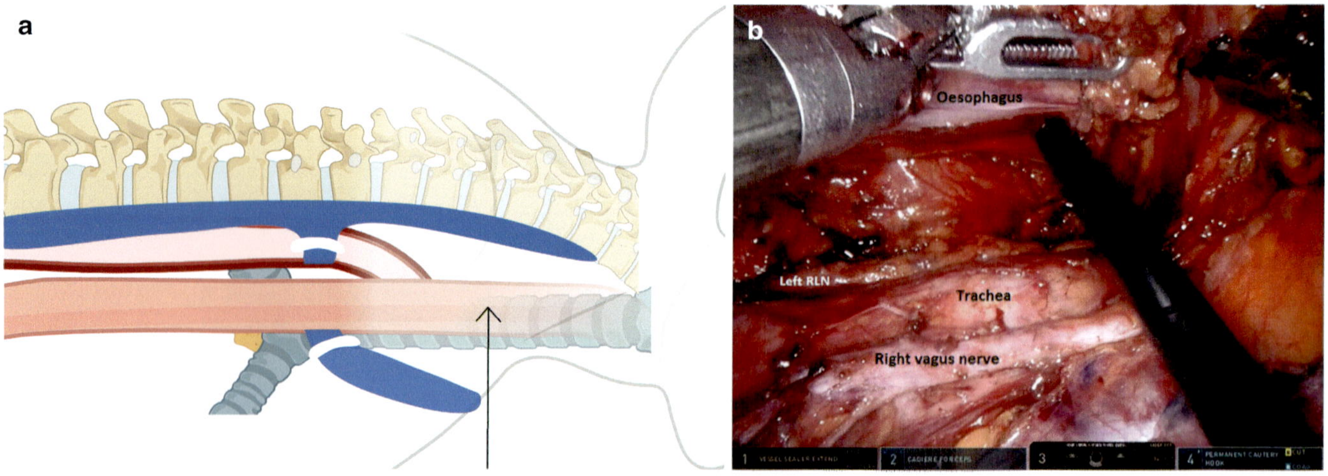

Fig. 14.23 The last step of the thoracic phase is the lymph node dissection around the left recurrent laryngeal nerve taking advantage of the maximal lifting of the esophagus, which is now possible after complete mobilization. (**a**, Created with BioRender.com)

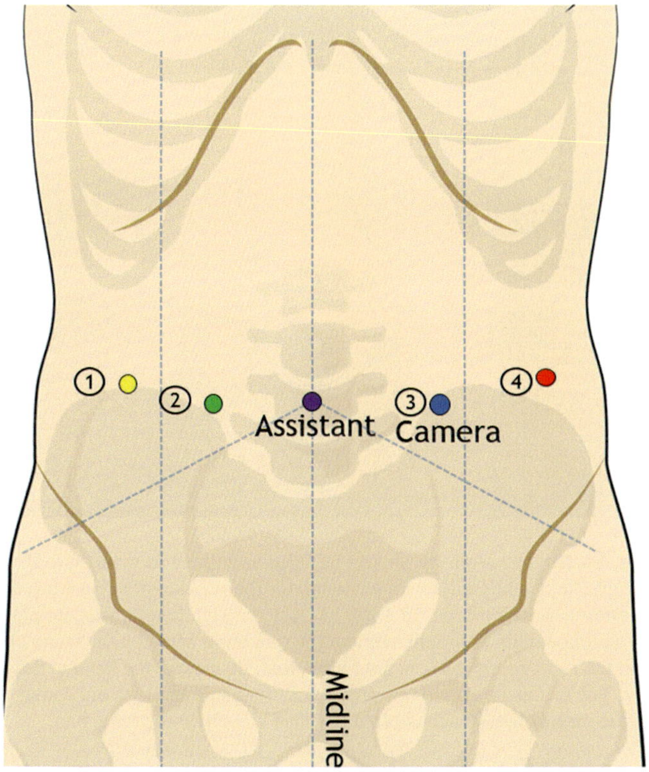

Fig. 14.24 For the abdominal phase, the patient is placed in supine position after which six incisions are made for the surgical instruments. Four incisions are for the robotic ports (4 × 8 mm); one incision is for the Nathanson to retract the liver (5 mm) and one incision for the assistant port (12 mm). (**a**, Created with BioRender.com)

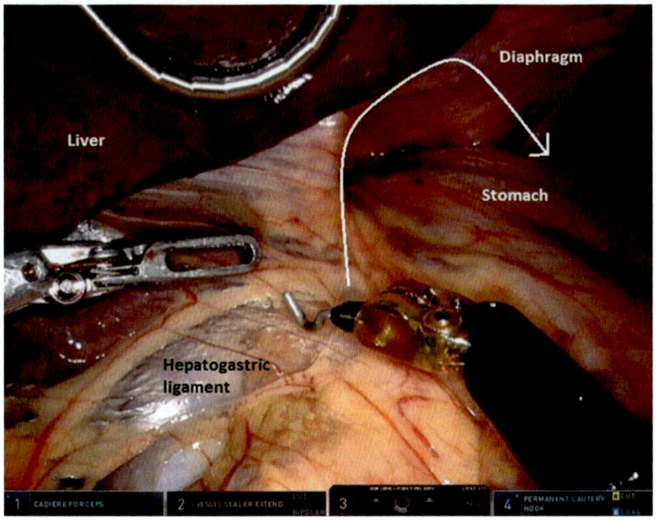

Fig. 14.25 The liver retractor is placed under the left liver lobe. The cadiere is placed in robotic arm 1, the vessel sealer in arm 2, the camera in arm 3, and the cautery hook in arm 4. The abdominal phase starts with opening the hepatogastric ligament which creates access to the omental bursa. The stomach is retracted caudally by the robotic arm. The dissection follows the white line in the photo and continues to the crus to mobilize the right side of the stomach. Grasping of the stomach should be avoided during the entire procedure to avoid damage of the future gastric tube

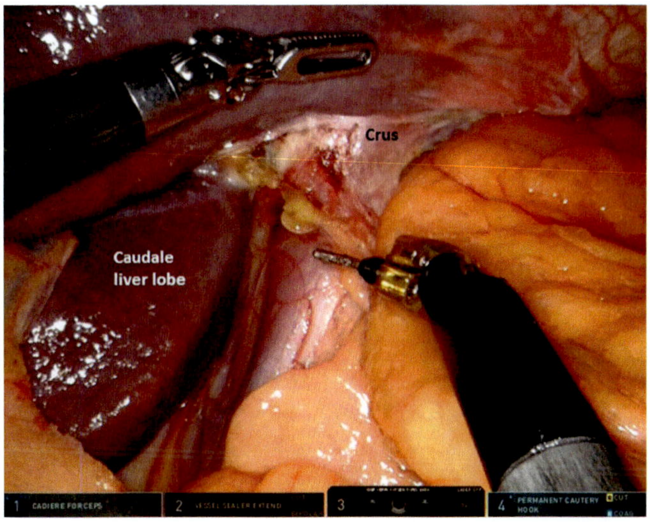

Fig. 14.26 The right crus is visualized and dissected until the hiatus is reached

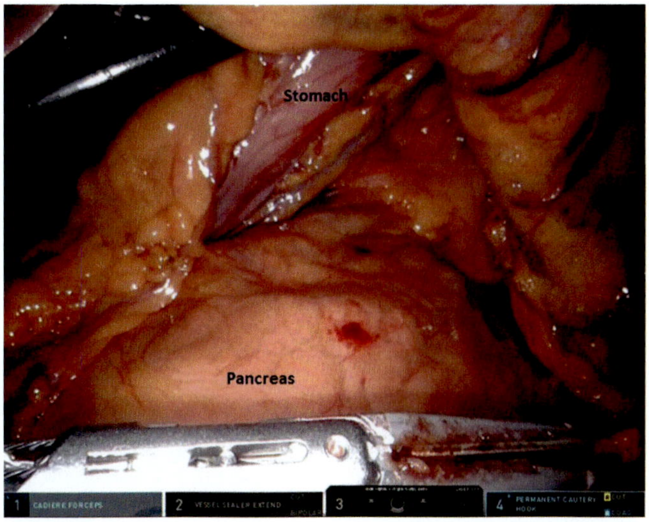

Fig. 14.27 The procedure continues to the greater curve of the stomach. The gastrocolic ligament is opened above the transverse colon. Caution should be taken to keep the right gastroepiploic artery undamaged as it provides the vascularization of the gastric conduit. The stomach is lifted with the cardiere, and the dissection is performed with the hook and vessel sealer

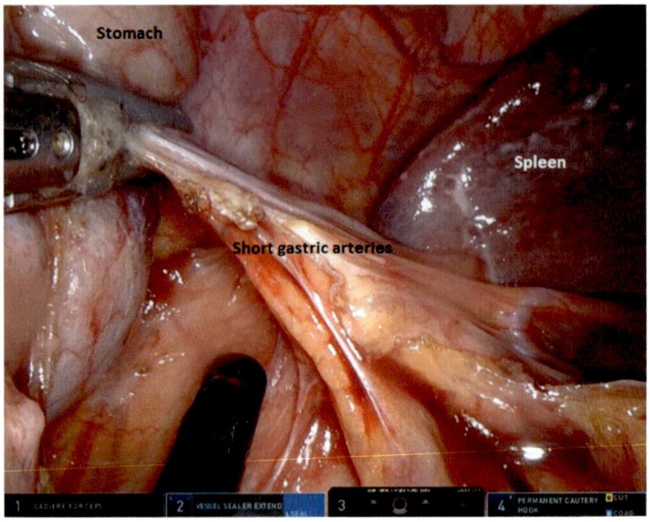

Fig. 14.28 The dissection of the greater curvature continues to the left upper quadrant. The table surgeon retracts the tissue laterally to the left, protecting the colon and enabling the formation of a tunnel between spleen and stomach. The short gastric arteries between the fundus and the spleen are then ligated with the vessel sealer. This part of the procedure ends by releasing the stomach from the left side of the crus

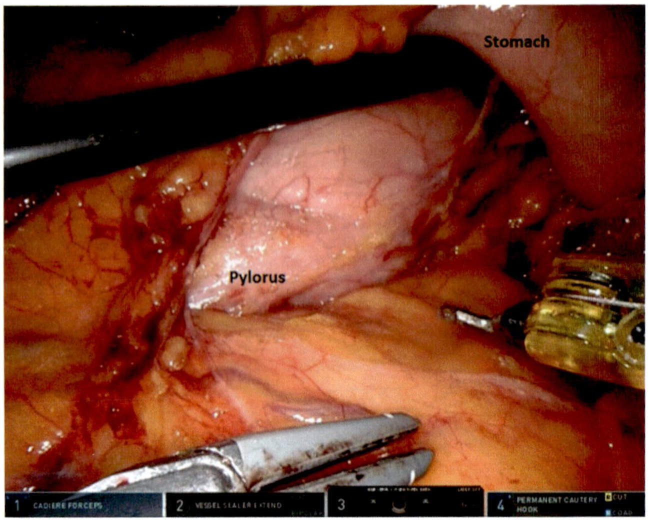

Fig. 14.29 The dissection continues to the posterior and distal side of the stomach. The greater curve of the stomach is mobilized towards the gall bladder as the main landmark. The stomach is lifted and dissected free from the pancreas towards the pylorus until the gastroduodenal artery is reached. The hepatic flexure is mobilized free from the duodenum (Kocher maneuver) to facilitate the mobilization of the future gastric tube. One of the robotic instruments is used to lift the stomach upwards

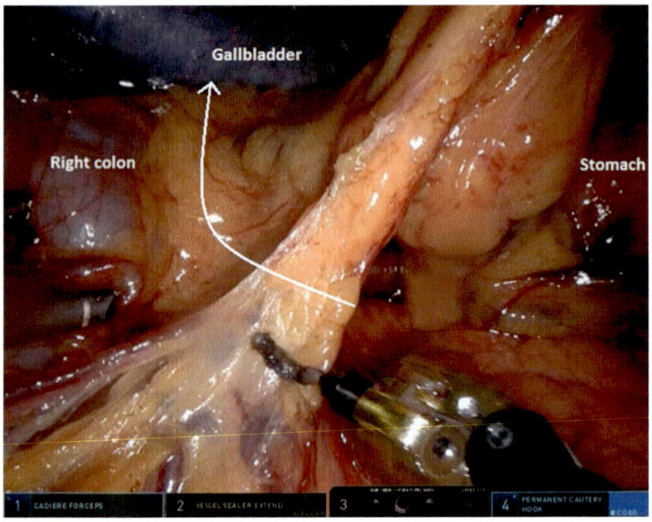

Fig. 14.30 The stomach should be fully mobilized to make sure that the gastric conduit will be long enough for the creation of a tension-free anastomosis in the neck. In order to create enough length, the first part of the duodenum is mobilized, and the omentum between the stomach and the right colon is dissected (white line) dissecting the hepatic flexure. The stomach is lifted upwards to facilitate this and to avoid damage to the mesocolon, which is often attached closely to the omentum

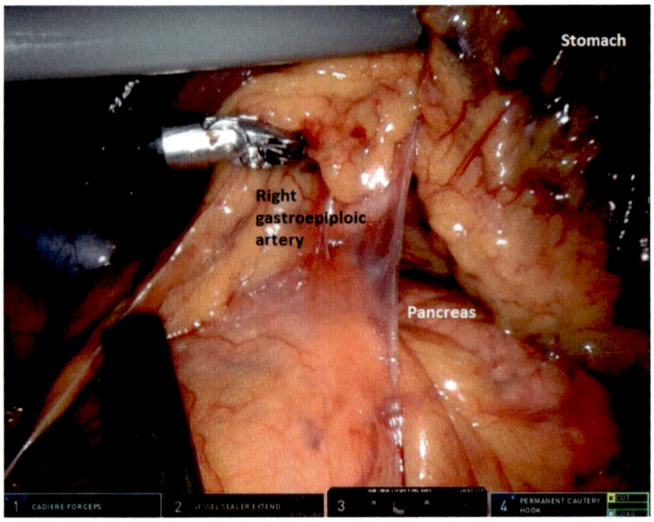

Fig. 14.31 Care should be taken to follow the plain over the mesogastrium, containing the gastroepiploic artery and vein. During this phase, the stomach is also lifted

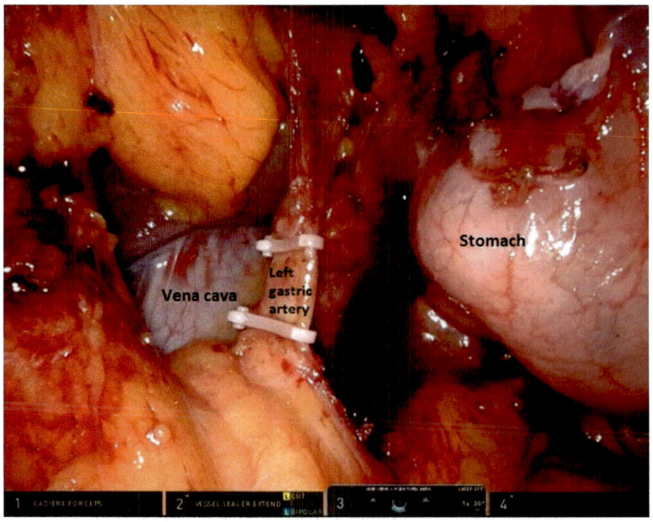

Fig. 14.32 Now that the most part of the stomach is mobilized, the dissection continues to the lymph node dissection. The stomach is lifted with the vessel sealer to expose the retrogastric region. Generally, the gastric vein is identified and divided with the vessel sealer before the gastric artery is encountered. The gastric artery is clipped with two Hem-o-loks and dissected with the cutting part of the vessel sealer. The Hem-o-lok clips are placed as proximal as possible to collect Station 7 en bloc. Lymph nodes stations of the celiac trunk (9), splenic artery (11), and hepatic artery (8) are collected separately. In general, the lymph nodes along the lesser curve and hiatus (1, 2, 3) are resected en bloc

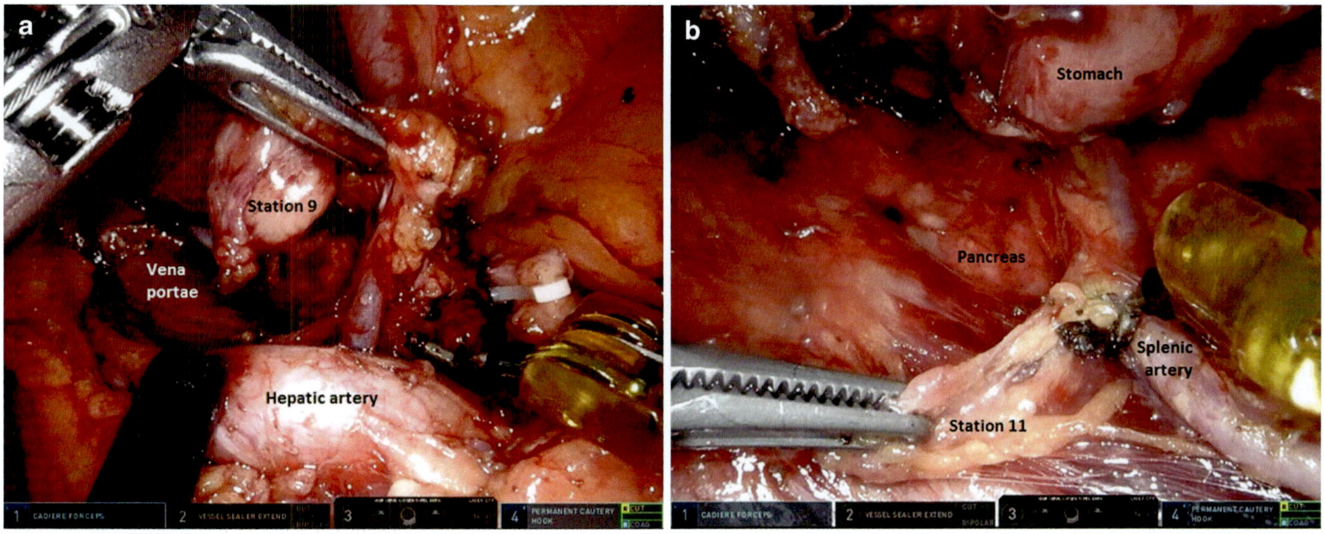

Fig. 14.33 After the left gastric artery is clipped, the lymphadenectomy continues to the celiac trunk (station 9), the splenic artery (station 11), and the hepatic artery (station 8) which ends the abdominal phase

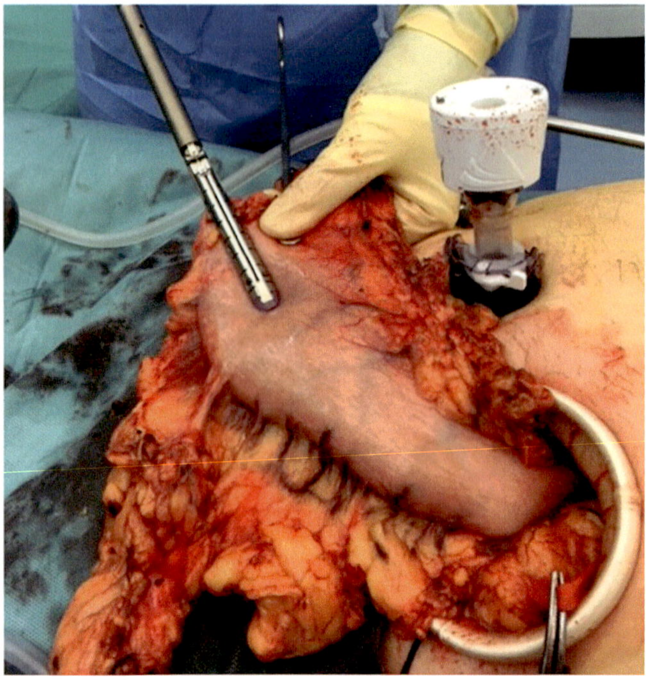

Fig. 14.34 After the lymphadenectomy, a vertical incision is made at the left side of the neck along the sternocleidomastoid muscle. The esophagus is encircled and transected at this level. A lace band is connected to the specimen. Under laparoscopic view the specimen is retracted through the hiatus towards the abdomen. A 7 cm transverse incision is made by connecting the incisions at the level of the ports of arm 3 and 4. A wound protector is used to retrieve the specimen. A gastric conduit is created which extracorporeal using an Endo GIA stapler. The gastric conduit is 3–4 centimeters in width. Special care should be taken to not damage the gastric conduit by excessive touching or grasping. As a routine a jejunal tube feeding is made in the first loop after Treitz ligament using the transverse incision

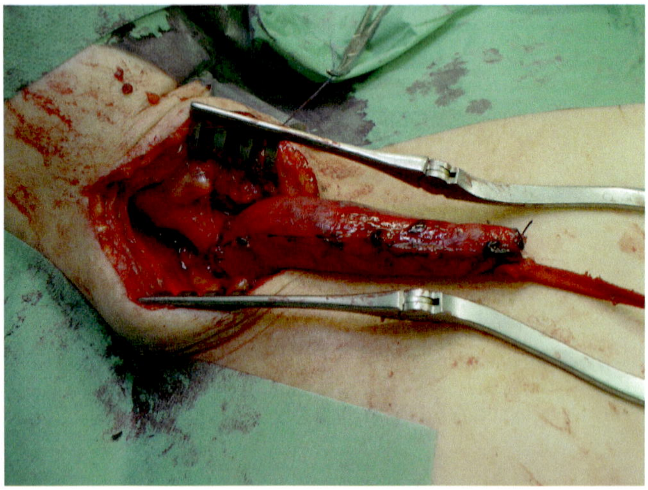

Fig. 14.35 The tube is connected to the lace band and mobilized to the neck through the mediastinum to land in the esophageal bed. A plastic bag surrounding the tube facilitates the sliding through the mediastinum. A hand-sewn end-to-side esophagogastrostomy is created, and the surplus of the gastric conduit is removed with the Endo GIA stapler. This concludes the McKeown procedure

References

1. van der Sluis PC, et al. Robot-assisted minimally invasive thoraco-laparoscopic esophagectomy versus open transthoracic esophagectomy for resectable esophageal cancer: a randomized controlled trial. Ann Surg. 2019; https://doi.org/10.1097/SLA.0000000000003031.
2. van der Sluis PC, Ruurda JP, van der Horst S, Goense L, van Hillegersberg R. Learning curve for robot-assisted minimally invasive thoracoscopic esophagectomy: results from 312 cases. Ann Thorac Surg. 2018; https://doi.org/10.1016/j.athoracsur.2018.01.038.
3. Kingma BF, Read M, van Hillegersberg R, Chao YK, Ruurda JP. A standardized approach for the thoracic dissection in robotic-assisted minimally invasive esophagectomy (RAMIE). Dis Esophagus. 2020;33(Supplement_2):doaa066. https://doi.org/10.1093/dote/doaa066.

Robotic Transcervical and Transhiatal Esophagectomy (RACE Procedure)

15

Peter P. Grimminger, Giovanni Capovilla, Carolina Froiio, and Hubert Stein

Introduction

The surgical treatment of intrathoracic esophageal cancer requires an esophageal resection with a radical mediastinal lymphadenectomy. This is normally achieved through a transthoracic approach. However, transthoracic esophagectomy requires one-lung ventilation, and the incidence of pulmonary postoperative complications is increased after both open and minimally invasive transthoracic procedures, mainly due to postoperative pneumonia. This is associated with an increased postoperative morbidity and mortality and requires a prolonged intensive care unit management and hospital stay. The transthoracic approach is therefore hardly recommendable to patients with low pulmonary function and previous thoracic surgery or infections, causing adhesions in the pleural space. Esophagectomy using a transhiatal approach has been proposed as an alternative to avoid opening the chest cavity; however concerns have been raised regarding its surgical radicality. A combined transhiatal and transcervical approach to perform esophagectomy without accessing the thorax and maintaining an adequate mediastinal lymphadenectomy has been described [1]; however the procedure was technically demanding as it implied the use of non-articulating conventional laparoscopic instruments in a narrow surgical space. In this context, the technical limitations of conventional laparoscopy might be overcome by the application of robotic systems such as the da Vinci Xi (Intuitive Surgical Inc., Sunnyvale, California, United States). The articulating instruments and the magnified field of vision may offer consistent advantages during the dissection and the lymphadenectomy in confined surgical spaces, as it is required during the transcervical mediastinal dissection. Our group recently demonstrated the feasibility of a robotic-assisted combined transhiatal and transcervical approach for esophagectomy (Robotic Assisted trans Cervical Esophagectomy – RACE) using the da Vinci Xi robotic system in a preclinical setting [2, 3]. The same approach was proved safe and feasible in a first case series [4]. We present here our technique for performing the RACE procedure (Figs. 15.1, 15.2, 15.3, 15.4, 15.5, 15.6, 15.7, 15.8, 15.9, 15.10, 15.11, 15.12, 15.13, 15.14, 15.15, 15.16, 15.17, 15.18, 15.19, 15.20, 15.21, 15.22, 15.23, 15.24, 15.25, 15.26, 15.27, 15.28, 15.29, 15.30, 15.31, 15.32, 15.33, 15.34, 15.35, 15.36, 15.37, 15.38, 15.39, 15.40, 15.41, 15.42, 15.43, 15.44, 15.45, 15.46, 15.47, 15.48, 15.49, 15.50, and 15.51).

P. P. Grimminger (✉) · G. Capovilla · C. Froiio
Department of General-, Visceral- and Transplant Surgery, University Medical Center Mainz, Mainz, Germany
e-mail: peter.grimminger@unimedizin-mainz.de

H. Stein
Department of Clinical Development Engineering, Intuitive Surgical Inc, Sunnyvale, CA, USA

O. Y. Kudsi, P. P. Grimminger (eds.), *Atlas of Robotic Upper Gastrointestinal Surgery*,
https://doi.org/10.1007/978-3-030-86578-8_15

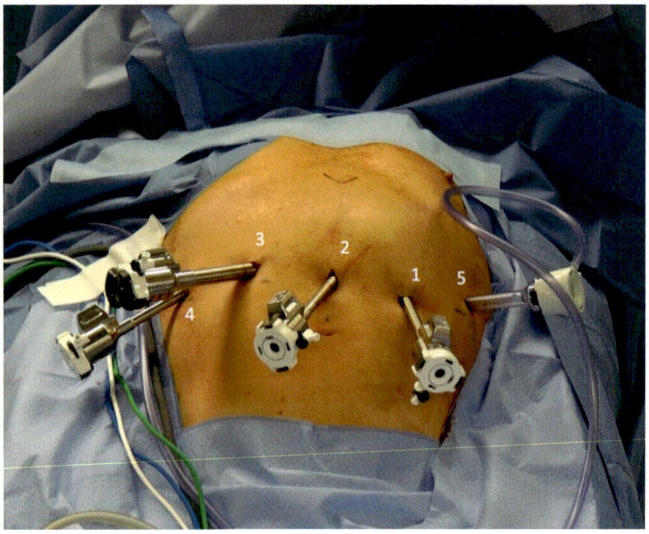

Fig. 15.1 Trocar position: the patient is placed in supine position with a 15° reverse Trendelenburg. Pneumoperitoneum is applied with a Veress needle in the upper left abdominal quadrant, 2–3 cm above the umbilical line. Upon removal of the Veress needle, a 8 mm trocar is placed to be used for the energy dissection device [1] (Synchroseal, Vessel Sealer Extend, or Monopolar Cautery Hook). The 8 mm midline camera trocar is placed about 3–4 cm above the umbilicus [2]. A 12 mm trocar used for the Fenestrated Bipolar Forceps and the Stapler is placed in the upper right quadrant [3]. A fenestrated Tip-Up grasper is introduced on the third arm, through another 8 mm trocar placed in the right lateral subcostal area [4]. Finally, a 12 mm assistant trocar is placed in the left lateral subcostal area and used for retraction, suction, and introduction/removal of any material during the dissection [5]. The da Vinci® Xi robotic system is positioned on the right side of the patient. The position of the assistant is on the patient's left side

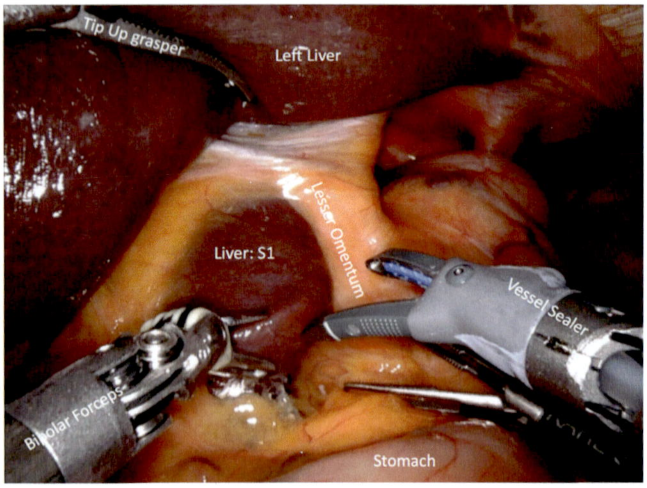

Fig. 15.2 The initial setting includes the use of the Fenestrated Bipolar Forceps on the left arm and a Vessel sealer (SynchroSeal, Intuitive, Sunnyvale, California, USA) on the right arm. The third robotic arm is equipped with a Tip-Up grasper and used to retract the left liver lobe

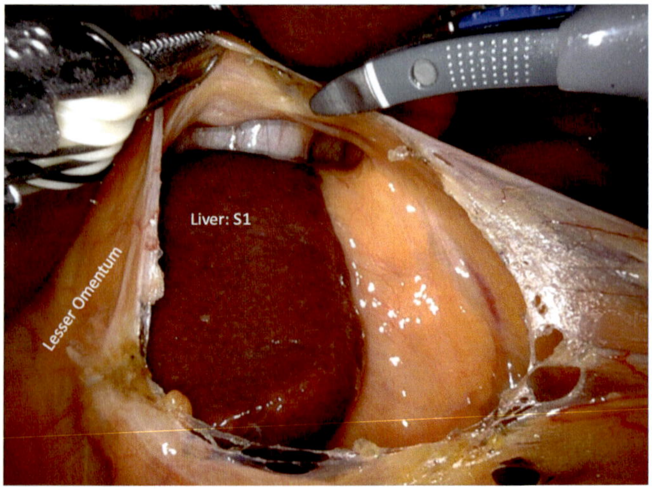

Fig. 15.3 The lesser omentum is opened, and the dissection is carried out toward the right diaphragmatic crus

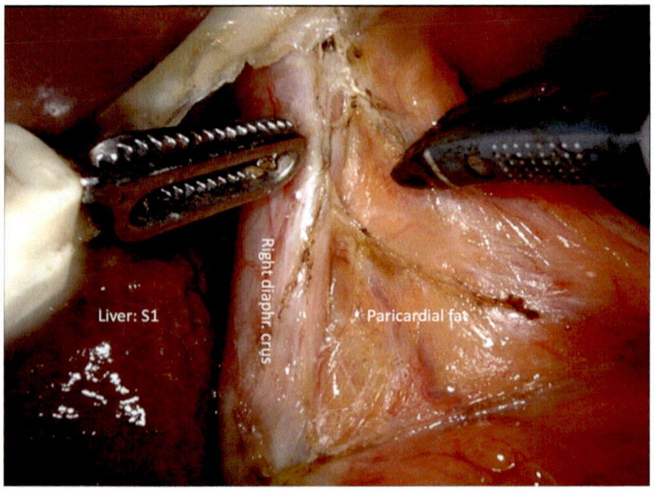

Fig. 15.4 The space between the right diaphragmatic crus and the pericardial fat is developed. The pericardial fat tissue is retracted to the left to provide tension and improve the field vision. The lower esophagus is completely freed on the right side. During this phase the lymph nodes of station 1 are collected and will be retrieved en bloc with the specimen

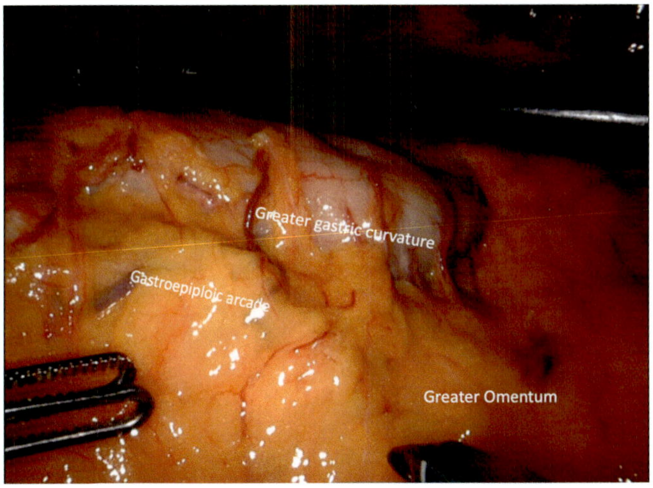

Fig. 15.5 In the next step the greater omentum is retracted caudally, and the gastroepiploic arcade is identified along the greater curvature

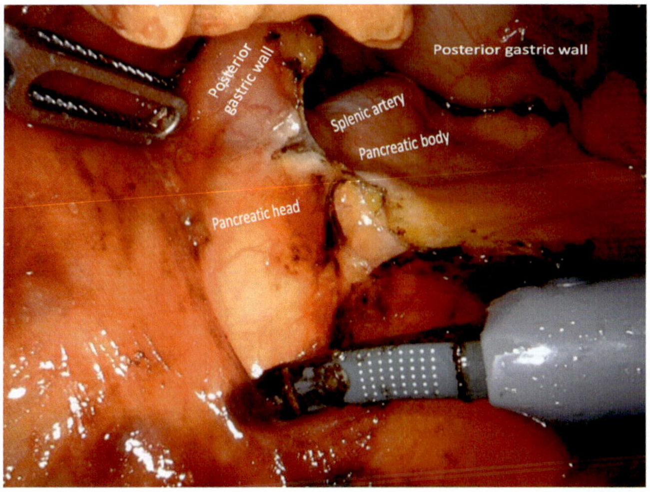

Fig. 15.7 During this phase any residual gastropancreatic ligament or adhesions with the transverse mesocolon are divided to achieve complete mobilization of the stomach

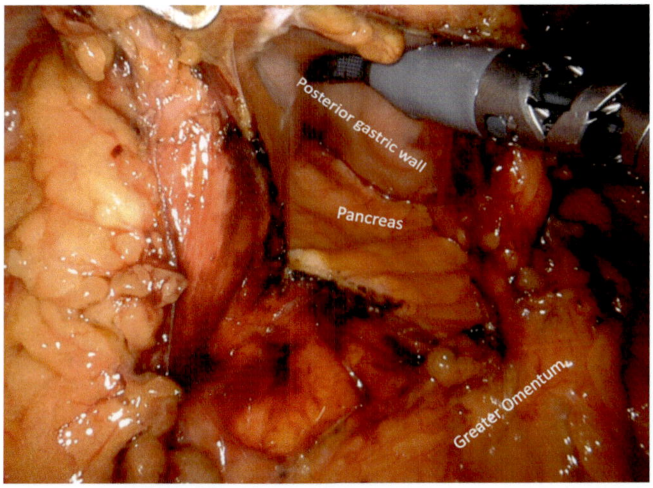

Fig. 15.6 The greater omentum is dissected, and a partial omentectomy is carried out along the greater curvature, toward the spleen. Direct vision of the gastroepiploic arcade can easily be acquired at the posterior aspect of the greater gastric curvature

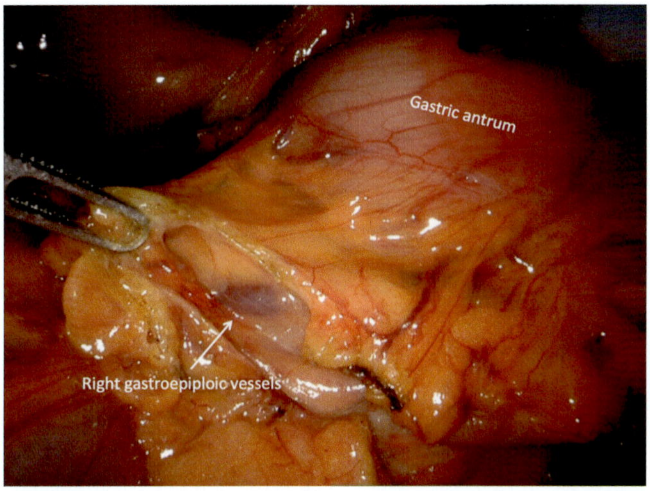

Fig. 15.8 The dissection is carried out toward the pylorus. The right gastroepiploic vessels are visualized and saved as they provide the vascularization to the gastric conduit

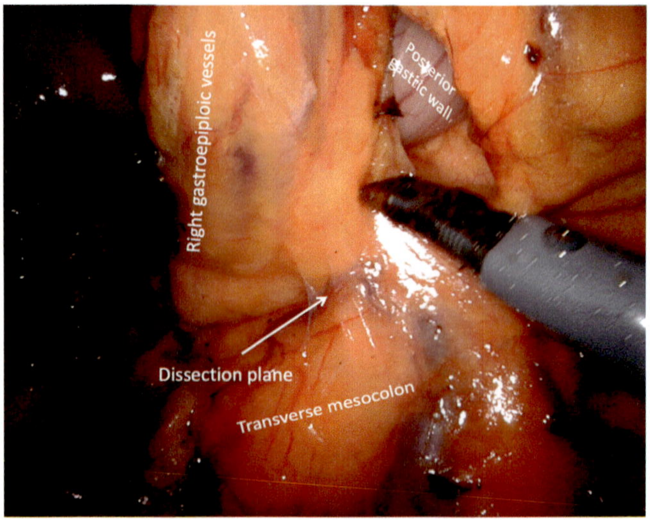

Fig. 15.9 Care should be taken in separating the posterior gastric wall from the transverse mesocolon in this phase. The antrum can be lifted up in order to bring the gastroepiploic vessels in orthogonal position and facilitate the dissection. The gastric mobilization should be extended toward the gallbladder until the postpyloric duodenum is visualized

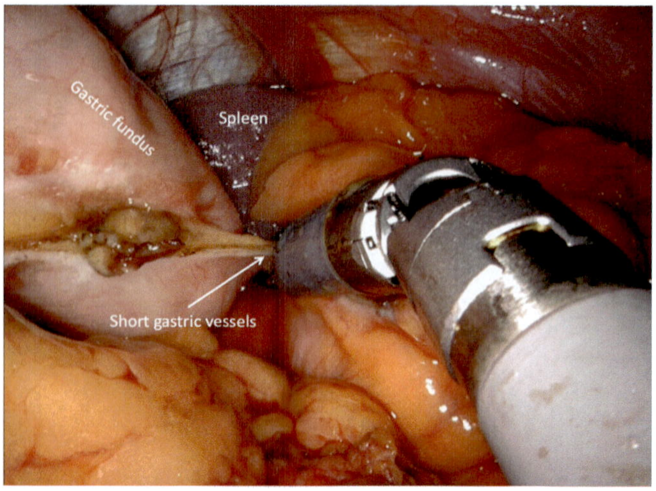

Fig. 15.11 The mobilization of the gastric fundus is completed by dividing the short gastric vessels. During this phase the stomach can be gently retracted toward the right using the third robotic arm (Tip-Up grasper); the assistant can retract the fat pad toward the left side to provide tension

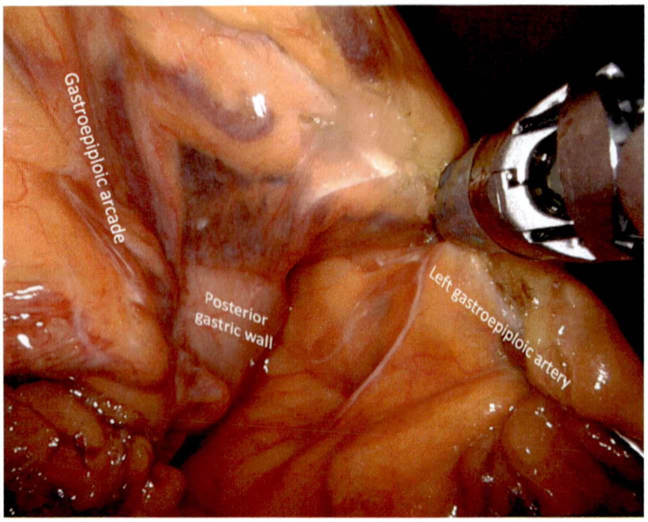

Fig. 15.10 The partial omentectomy is then continued toward the left. The left gastroepiploic vessels are encountered and transected. The gastroepiploic arcade is preserved to provide an adequate vascularization of the gastric conduit. Lymph nodes of station 4sb are retrieved during this phase and will be extracted en bloc with the specimen

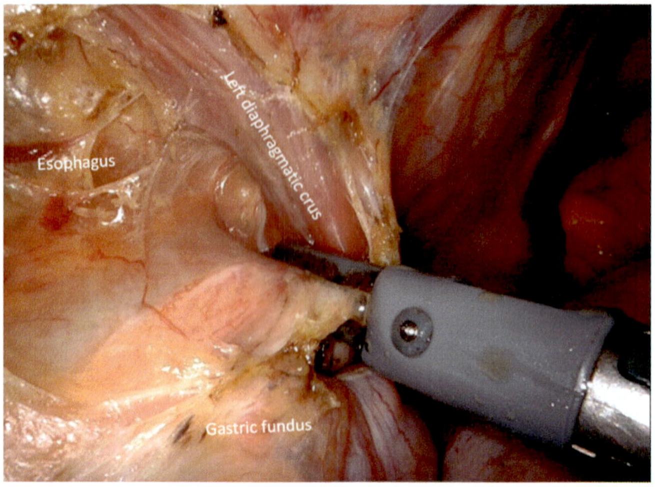

Fig. 15.12 The esophagus can be fully released from the left crus after complete dissection of lymph node station 2

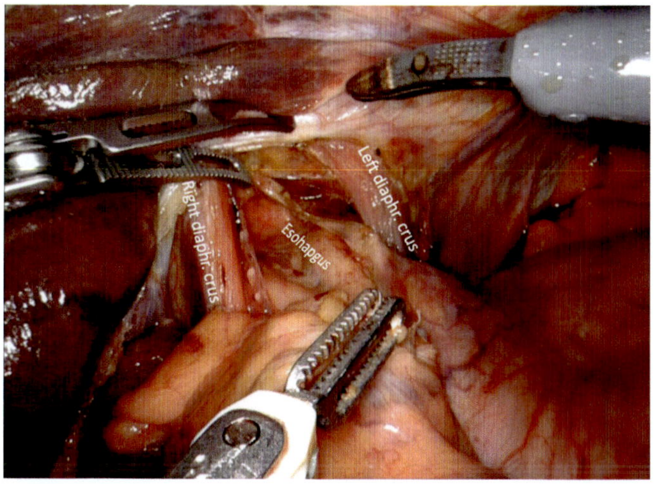

Fig. 15.13 The dissection plane is connected to the previously developed hiatal dissection plane on the right side

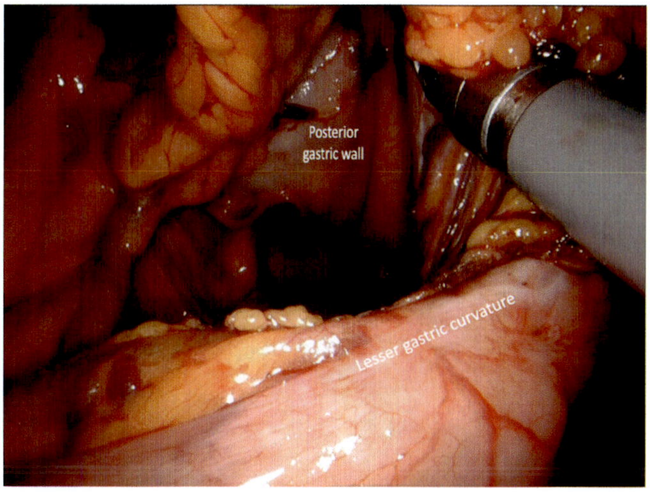

Fig. 15.15 The fat tissue is dissected from the lesser curvature to prepare the stomach for the gastric conduit creation

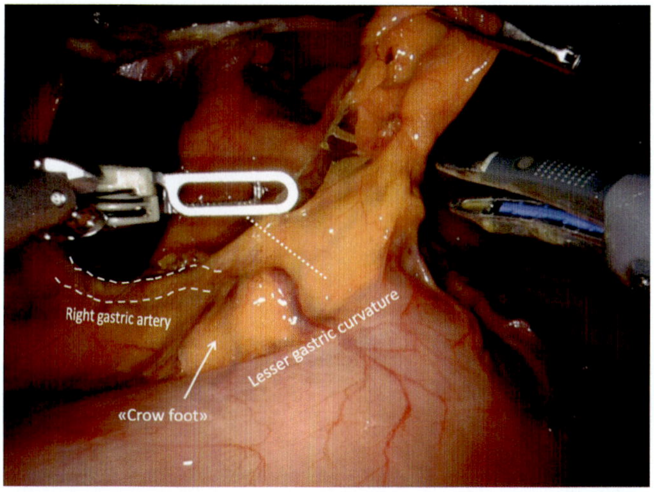

Fig. 15.14 The lesser curvature is prepared for the gastric conduit creation. We normally divide the vascular arcade at the lesser curvature left to the "crow foot" (dotted line) in order to preserve the vascular supply provided by the right gastric artery

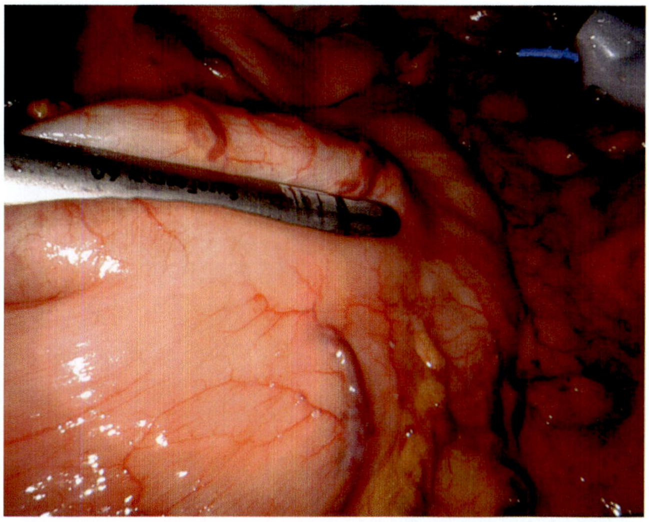

Fig. 15.16 The first stapler fire (SureForm™ Stapler, Intuitive, Sunnyvale, California, USA) is applied approximately between the distal third and the proximal two thirds of the lesser curvature

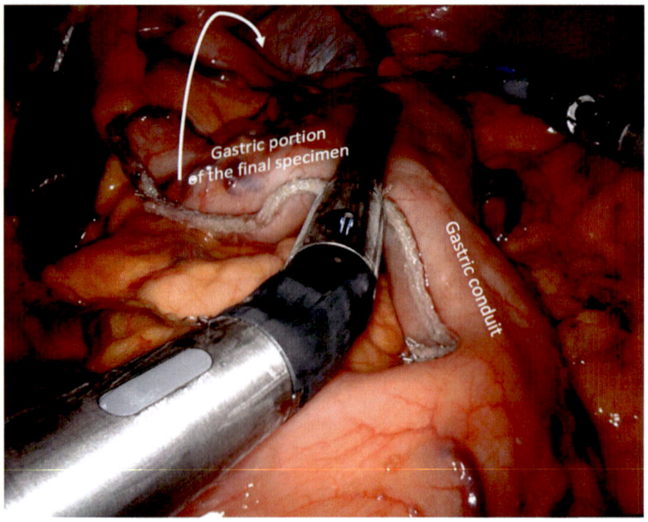

Fig. 15.17 Normally between 3 and 4 fires of the 60 mm stapler (blue or black reload) are used to complete the gastric conduit. This step differs from the normal Ivor Lewis procedure in that the gastric conduit will be completely separated from the fundus (see Fig. 15.34). After the creation of the gastric conduit, as normally done during RAMIE, the lesser curvature can be lifted cranially, thus improving the exposition for the subsequent lymphadenectomy (white arrow)

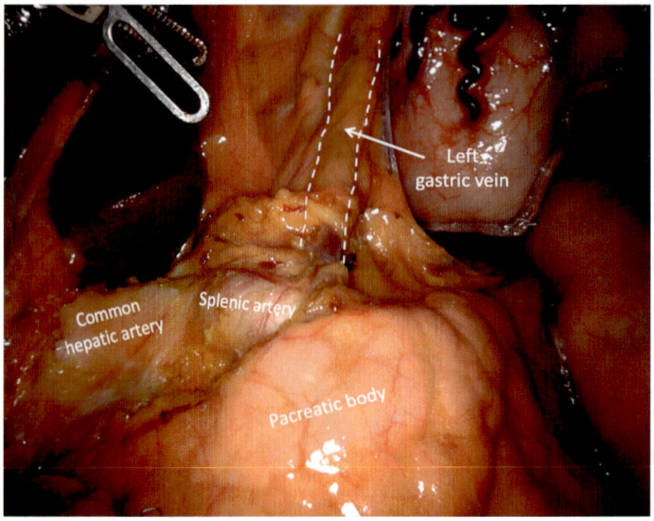

Fig. 15.19 Dissection of the anterior and posteromedial aspect of the common hepatic artery allows the retrieval of station 8 lymph nodes, which will be resected en bloc with the final specimen. The celiac trunk and the proximal portion of the splenic artery are identified. Gentle cranial traction on the lesser gastric curvature facilitates the exposure of the left gastric vein. Station 9 lymph nodes are collected during this phase

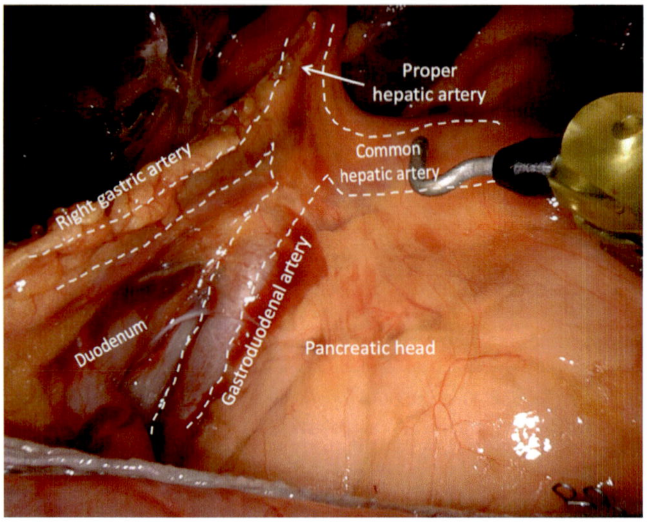

Fig. 15.18 The lymphadenectomy is started by dissecting the fat tissue medially from the right gastric artery. Following the right gastric artery, the proper hepatic artery is identified. Dissection of the surrounding fat tissue is carried out toward the celiac trunk medially. The origin of the gastroduodenal artery from the common hepatic artery is identified. In this phase we prefer to use the Permanent Cautery Hook (monopolar). Station 12 lymph nodes are collected during this phase and will be extracted en bloc with the final specimen

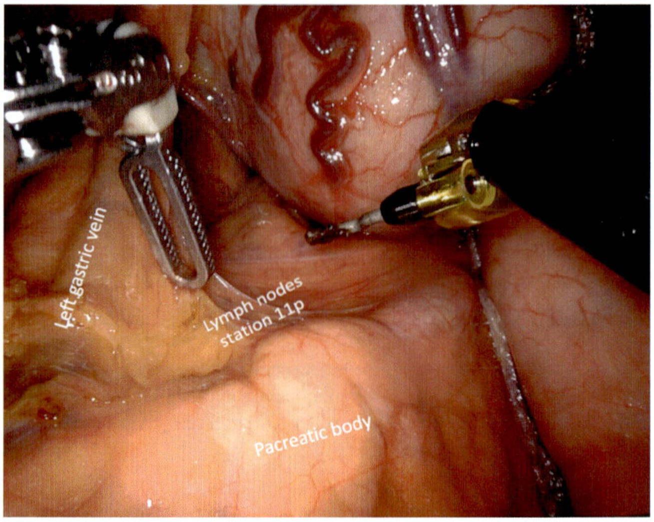

Fig. 15.20 The sovra-pancreatic fat is dissected medially along the superior border of the pancreatic body. Station 11p lymph nodes are retrieved during this phase

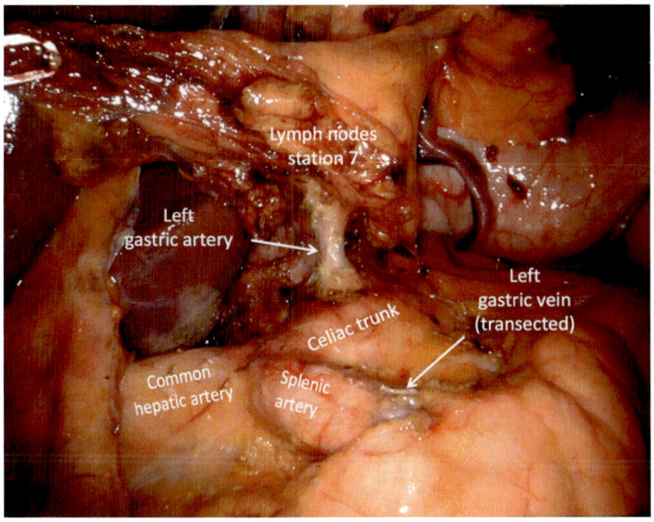

Fig. 15.21 After division of the gastric vein, the left gastric artery is identified and dissected posteriorly. During this phase the fat tissue surrounding the celiac trunk, the left gastric vessels, and the splenic artery is dissected and lifted cranially. This maneuver permits the retrieval of station 9, 7 and 11p lymph nodes that will be resected en bloc with the final specimen

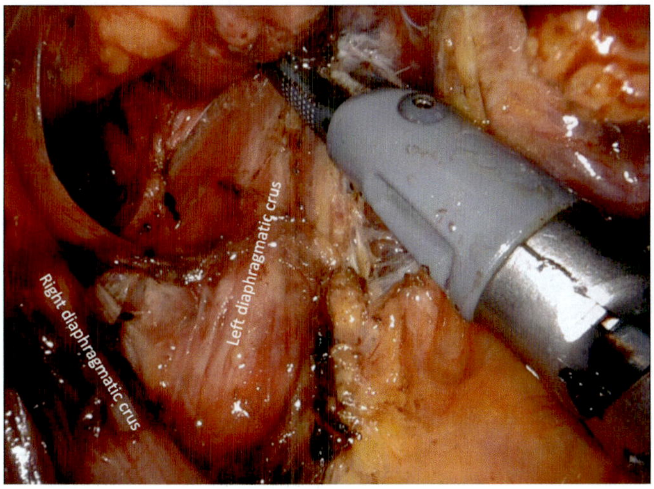

Fig. 15.22 After division of the left gastric artery, the dissection of the fat tissue is carried out posteriorly until the right and left diaphragmatic crura are reached

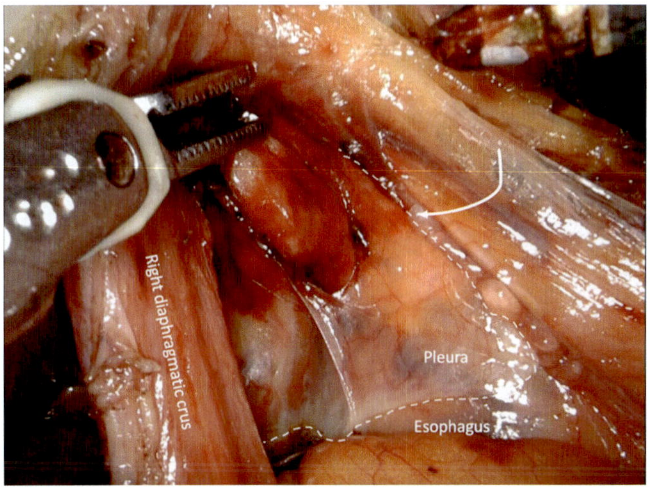

Fig. 15.23 The transhiatal dissection is initiated by developing the space between the esophagus and the right pleura laterally (arrow)

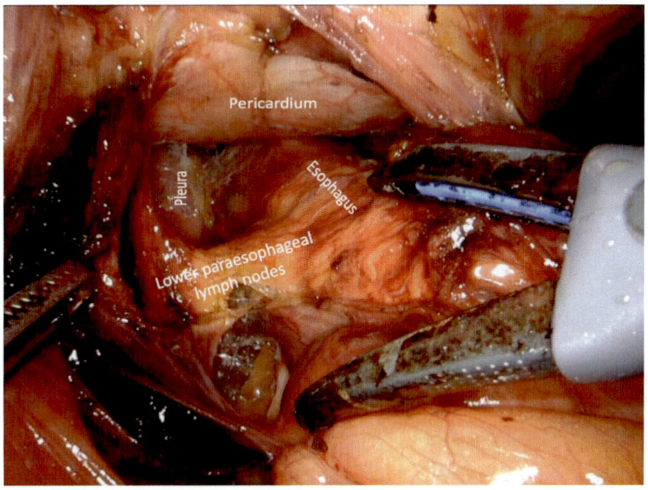

Fig. 15.24 The dissection is developed cranially, leaving the mediastinal pleura on the patient's right side intact. The avascular plane between the esophagus and the pericardium is developed anteriorly. The lower paraesophageal lymph nodes are encountered and can be dissected and resected en bloc with the specimen

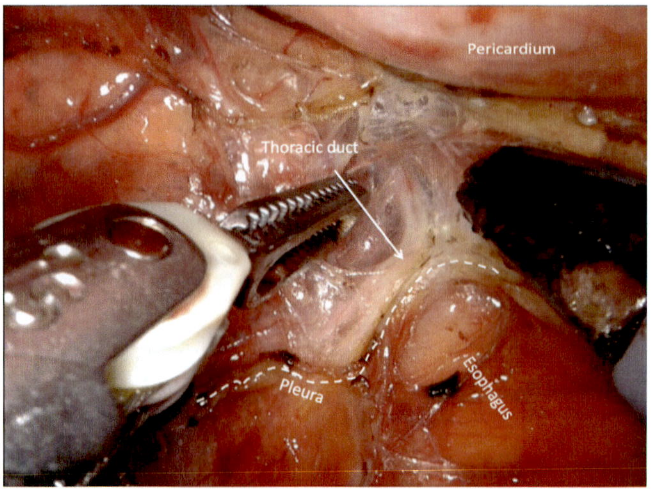

Fig. 15.25 While developing the right lateral plane in the lower mediastinum, the thoracic duct can be found under the mediastinal pleura 3–4 cm above the diaphragm and can be clipped and divided to prevent postoperative chylothorax

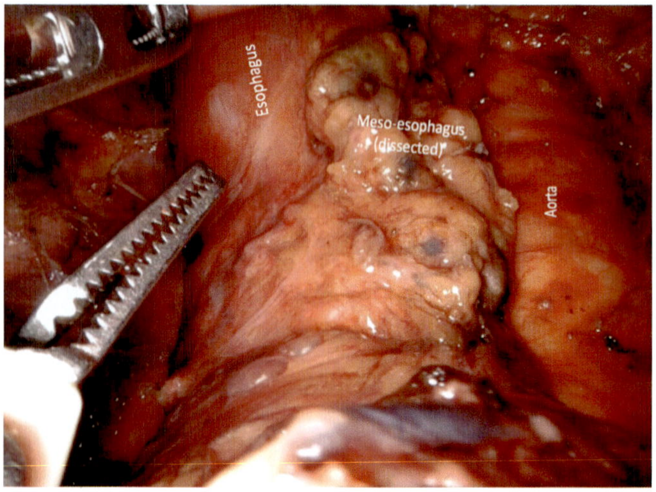

Fig. 15.27 By meticulous dissection of the meso-esophagus, the aortal plane should be visualized

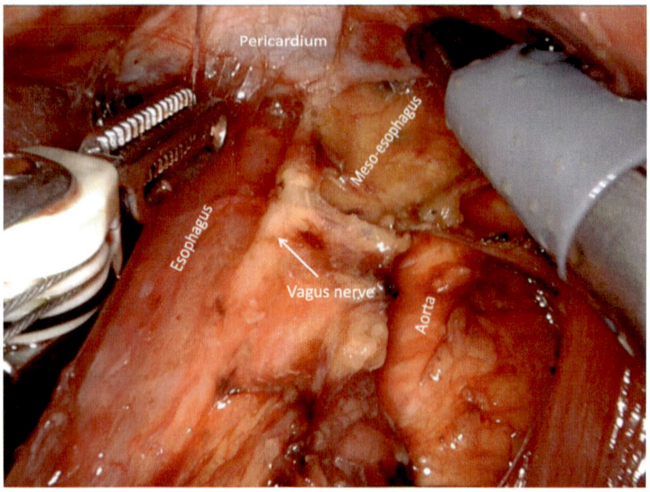

Fig. 15.26 On the left lateral side, the dissection plane is developed between the left pleura and the esophagus. The celluloadipose tissue comprising the mediastinal lymph nodes and the aortal branches directed to the esophagus (meso-esophagus) is readily accessible on this side during the transhiatal dissection. The left vagus nerve is also identified running along the left-anterior aspect of the esophagus

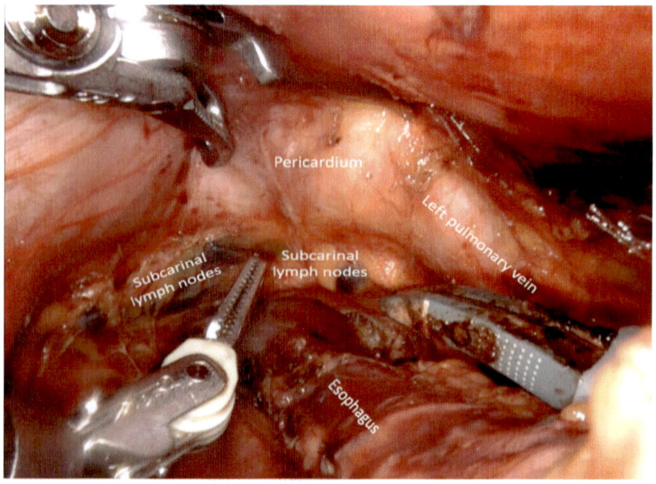

Fig. 15.28 Once the anterior aspect of the esophagus is completely freed from the pericardium, the dissection is extended cranially, thus exposing the subcarinal lymph nodes. Care should be taken to avoid inadvertent lesions to the left pulmonary vein while dissecting the left anterior aspect of the esophagus

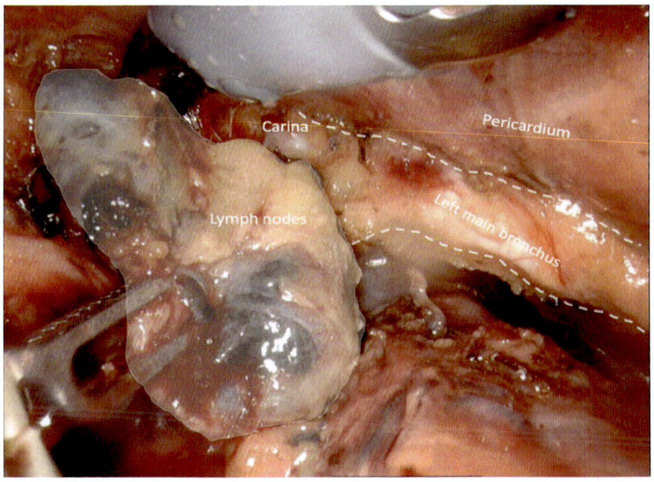

Fig. 15.29 Complete lymphadenectomy of the subcarinal and of the left and right main bronchus lymph nodes can be performed during this phase. Extreme care should be taken to avoid thermic injuries to the airways during the dissection

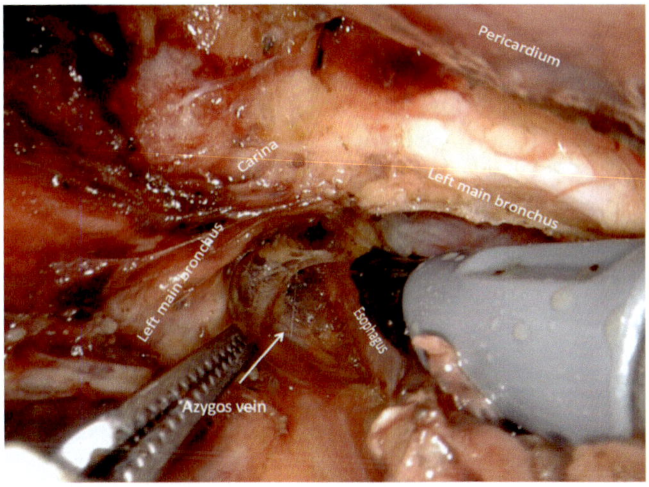

Fig. 15.31 The transhiatal dissection is normally concluded once the azygos vein is reached. The vein can be clipped and transected provided that adequate control of the vessel is acquired; however, since a bleeding would be difficult to control during the transhiatal or the transcervical phase, we normally prefer to dissect the vessel from the anterior aspect of the esophagus without attempting at clipping and transecting it

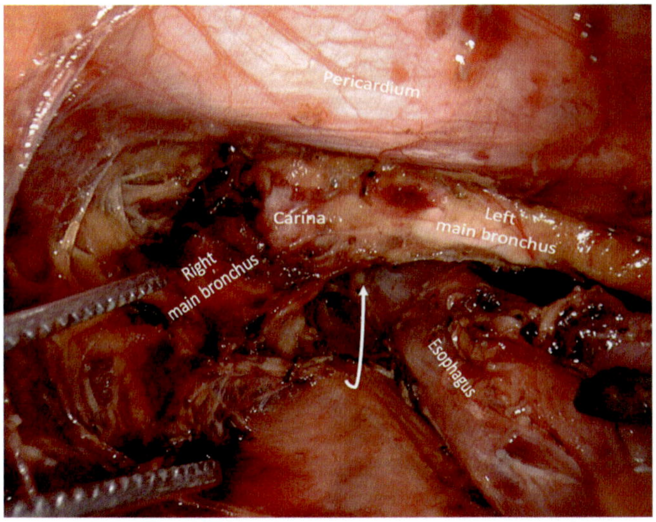

Fig. 15.30 Once the lymphadenectomy is completed, the carina and the two main bronchi are clearly visible. The dissection can be extended cranially to separate the esophagus from the pars membranacea of the trachea (arrow)

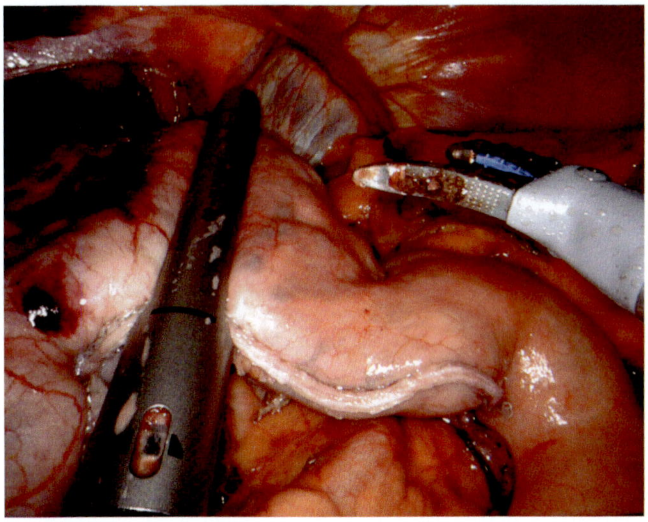

Fig. 15.32 The gastric conduit is then finalized by completely dividing the gastric fundus from the specimen

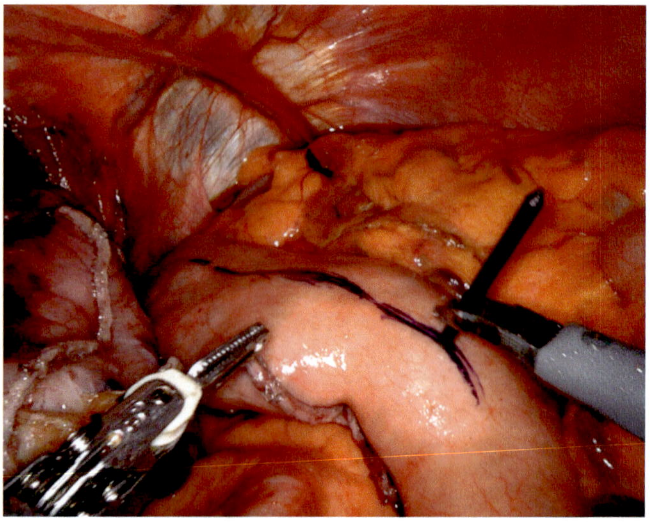

Fig. 15.33 The anterior surface of the gastric conduit is marked to assure its correct position during the cervical phase and to prevent twisting of the conduit during the cervical transposition

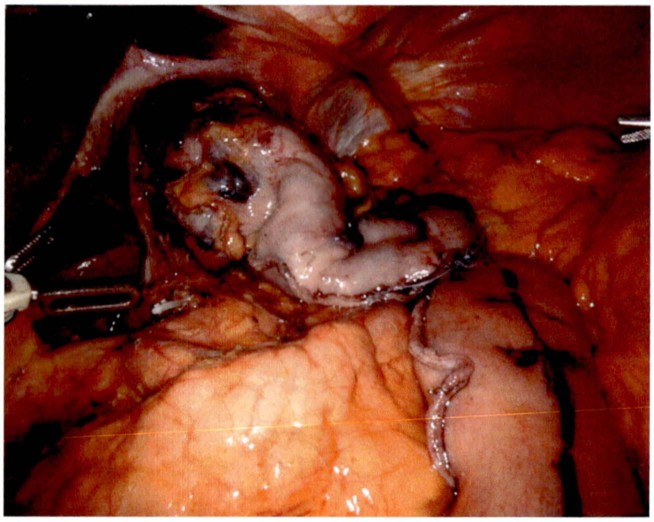

Fig. 15.35 The final appearance of the gastric conduit attached to the specimen is depicted in the figure. We meticulously check the apex of the conduit to evaluate the appearance of any ischemic demarcation zone

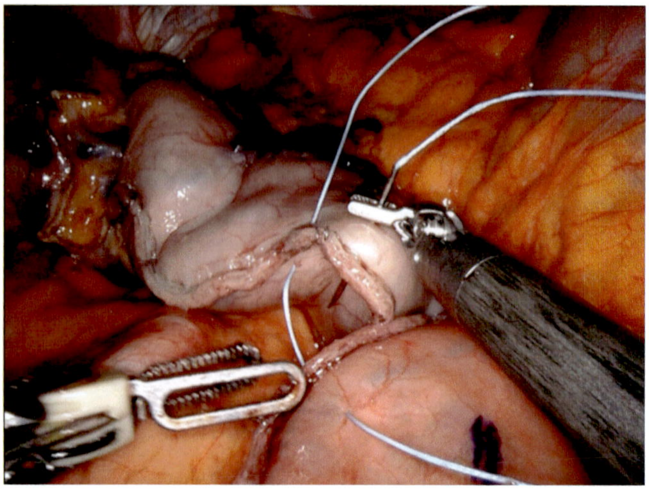

Fig. 15.34 While during RAMIE (transabdominal and transthoracic fully robotic esophagectomy) the gastric conduit is left attached to the specimen during the abdominal phase to facilitate the thoracic transposition, during RACE the conduit is completely separated from the specimen and approximated in an end-to-end fashion at its most apical point to the specimen's staple line using two or more interrupted cross stiches. This is done to reduce the bulkiness of the specimen and the gastric conduit to ease the cervical transposition

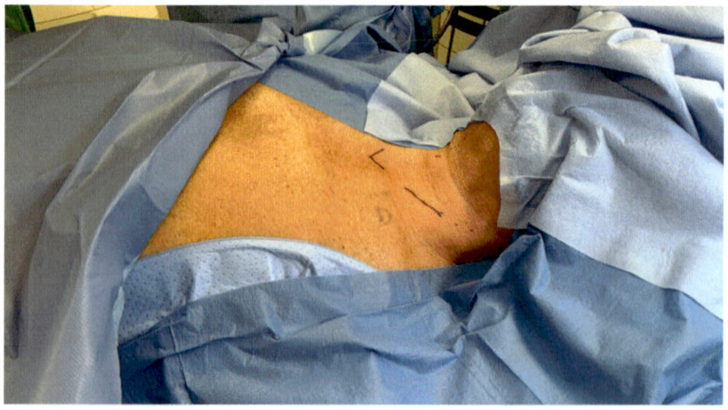

Fig. 15.36 For the transcervical phase, the patient's head is slightly stretched and turned to the right. A thick gastric intraluminal tube is placed, to facilitate the identification of the cervical esophagus. About two fingers above the left clavicle, a 3 cm skin incision was made at the anterior border of the sternocleidomastoid muscle

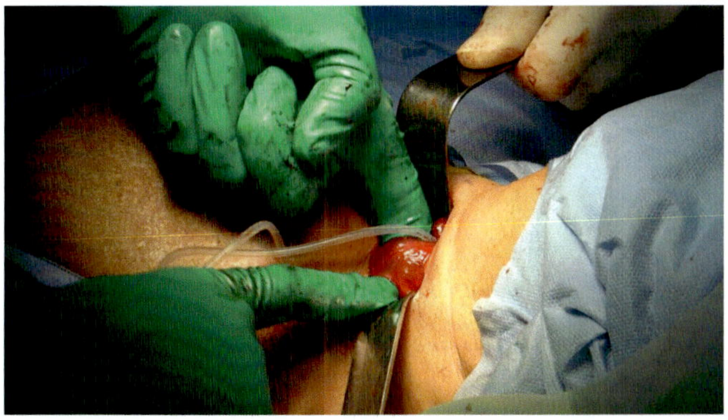

Fig. 15.37 The cervical esophagus is dissected and encircled using a silicon drain to retract the esophagus during the upper mediastinal preparation, as normally performed during a conventional open transcervical procedure. A blunt dissection is initially performed toward the thoracic inlet to facilitate the subsequent robotic dissection

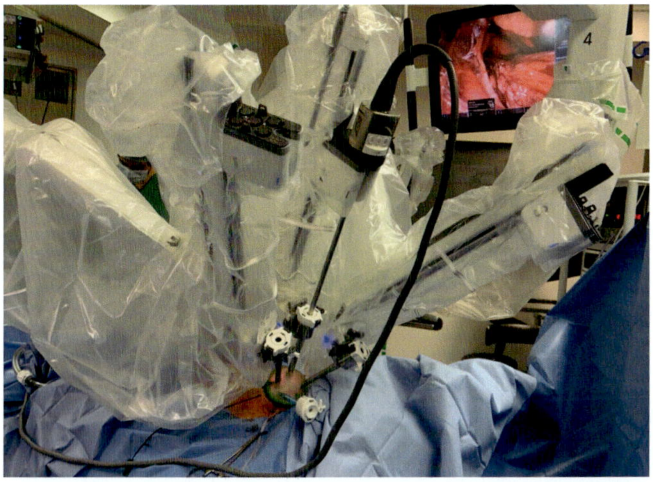

Fig. 15.38 The sternocleidomastoid muscle is lateralized, and an x-small Alexis Wound Retractor (Applied Medical, Rancho Santa Margarita, California, United States) is inserted. A GelPOINT Mini (Applied Medical, Rancho Santa Margarita, California, United States) is placed and a pressure of 5 mm Hg is applied. The da Vinci Xi surgical system is approaching the patient from the right side. The robotic arms are reaching over to the left and are docked in a cranial to caudal direction. The initial setting includes three 8 mm robotic trocars positioned as to form a triangle, with the central camera trocar as the apex. An energy dissection device (SynchroSeal or Vessel Sealer Extend) is placed on the right and a bipolar forceps on the left. A 5 mm assistant trocar is placed below to assist in the retraction and for suction

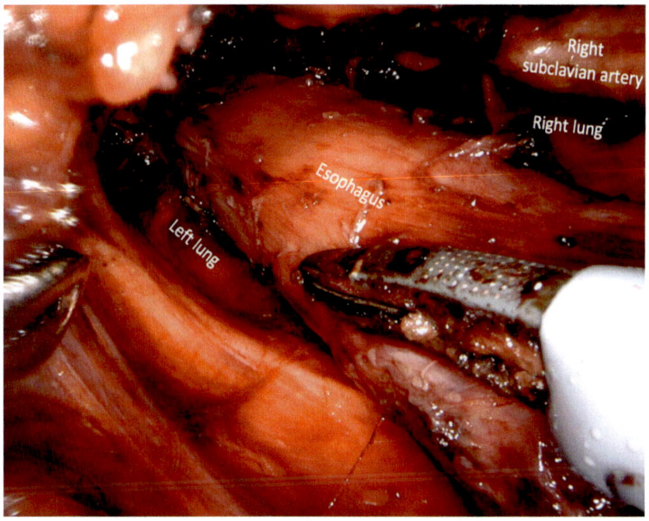

Fig. 15.39 The robotic dissection phase is initiated at the thoracic inlet. The left aspect of the esophagus was already prepared and dissected from the left common carotid artery and the left sternocleidomastoid muscle during the open transcervical phase

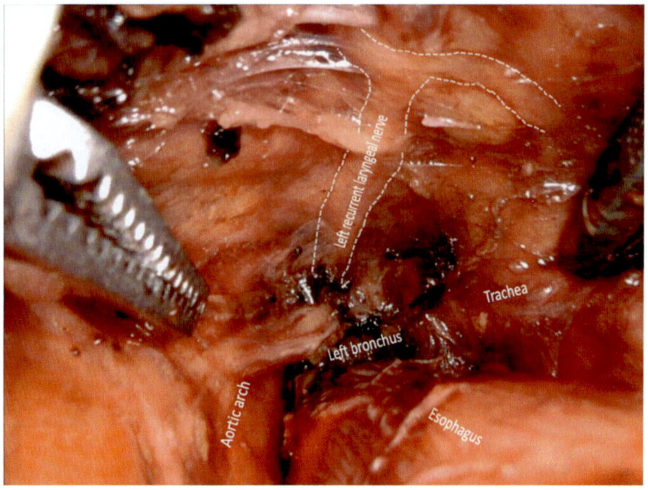

Fig. 15.40 The left side of the trachea is identified and gently pulled to the right to identify the left recurrent laryngeal nerve. The upper mediastinal esophagus with surrounding lymph nodes along the left recurrent nerve is dissected

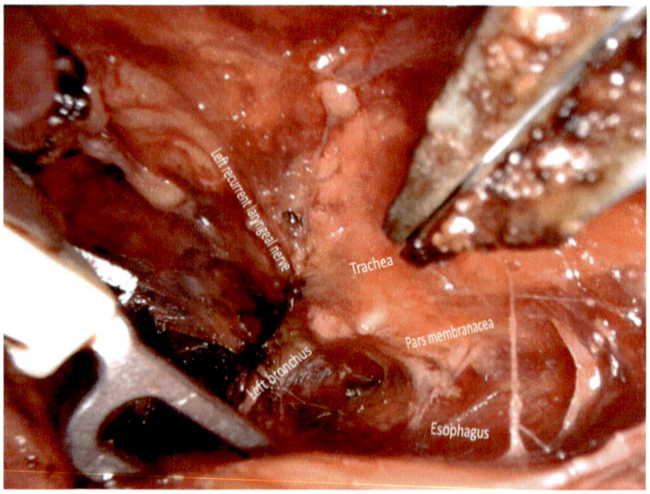

Fig. 15.41 Proceeding medially, the esophagus is dissected from the tracheal pars membranacea using the energy device and blunt dissection

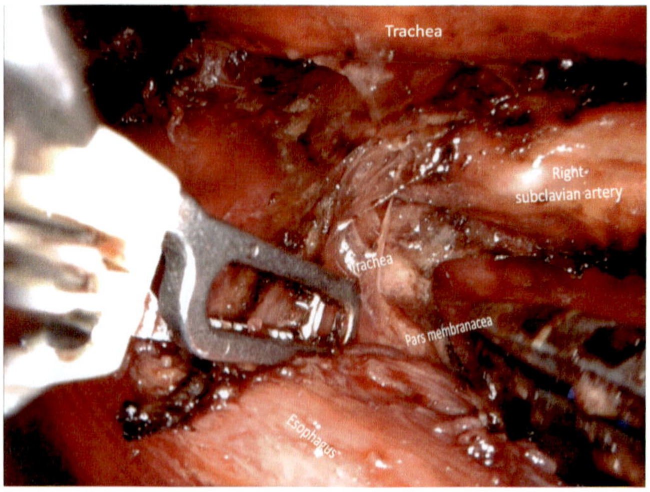

Fig. 15.42 After complete detachment of the anterior aspect of the esophagus from the pars membranacea, the right lateral plane is dissected. The right subclavian artery can be identified on the right side and should be carefully dissected from the right lateral aspect of the esophagus

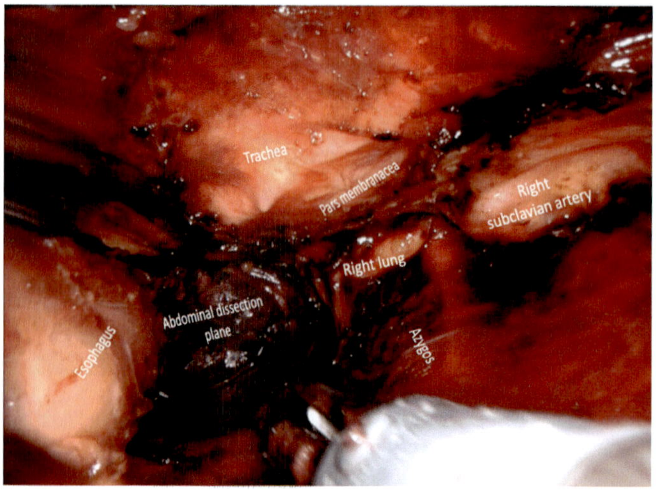

Fig. 15.43 After completing the dissection on the anterolateral aspect of the esophagus, the subclavian artery and the mediastinal pleura underneath are visible on both sides, the pars membranacea is completely freed from the anterior esophageal wall. The transcervical and the transabdominal dissection planes are connected. On the right side, the azygos vein is identified

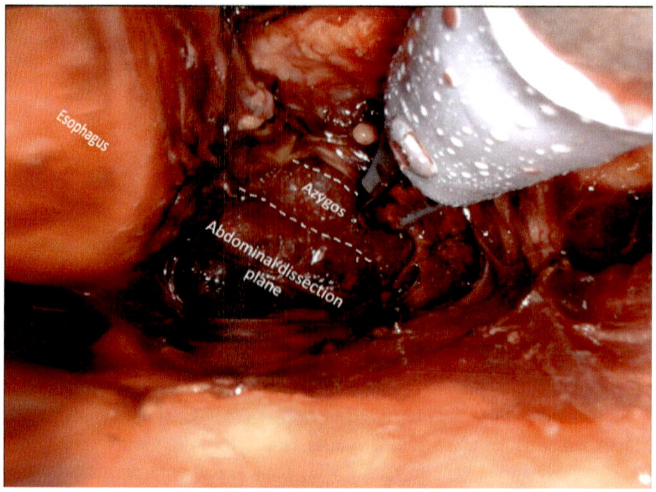

Fig. 15.44 The azygos vein is dissected laterally and preserved, thus connecting the transcervical and the transhiatal dissection planes

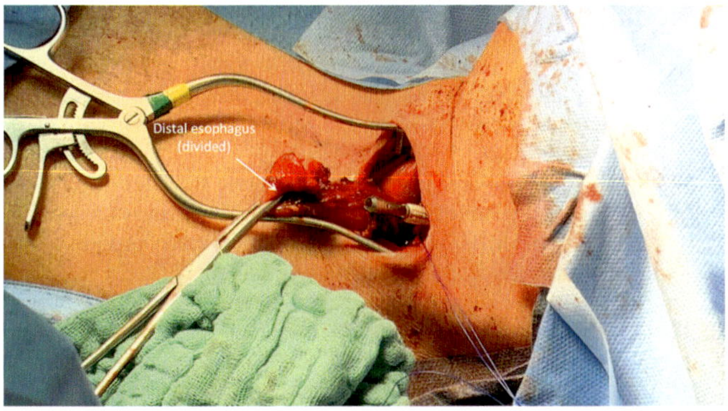

Fig. 15.45 The esophagus is then divided through the cervical incision. The head of the circular stapler is placed at the proximal esophageal stump using a purse-string suture. We normally use a 25 mm circular stapler (CEEA™, Covidien, Mansfield, MA, USA)

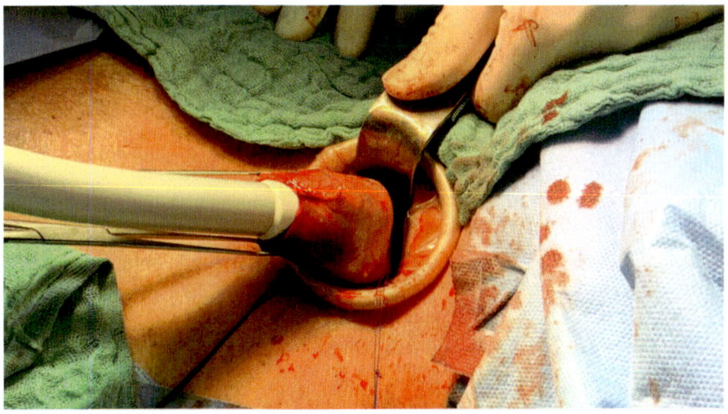

Fig. 15.48 The 25 mm circular stapler (CEEA™, Covidien, Mansfield, MA, USA) is inserted through the incision and connected to the head at the proximal esophageal stump to create an end-to-side circular stapled cervical anastomosis

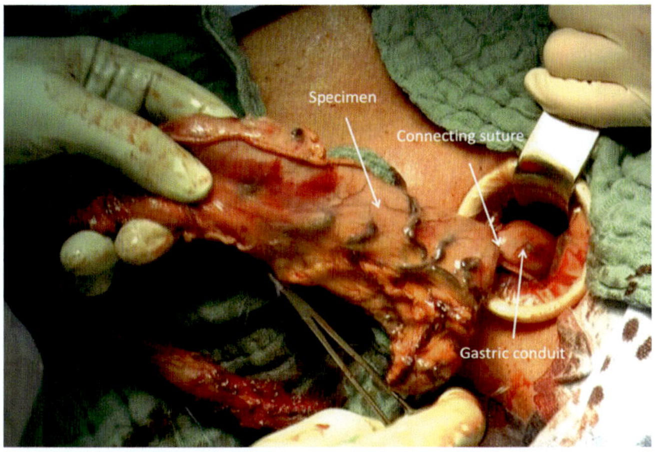

Fig. 15.46 The specimen and the attached gastric conduit are then pulled to the neck and exteriorized through the cervical incision. The connecting suture is removed, and the specimen is extracted

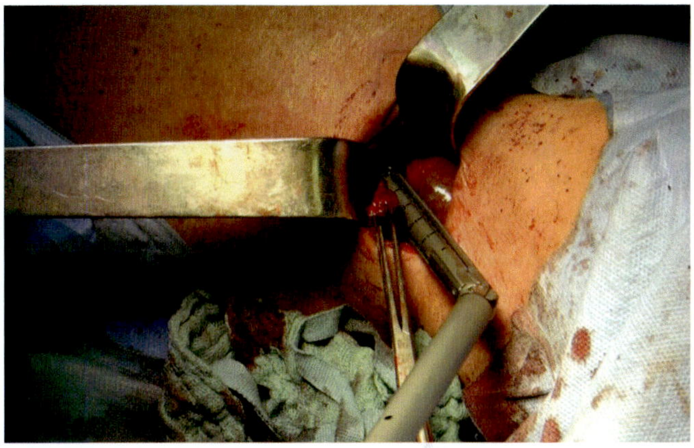

Fig. 15.49 The circular stapler entry site is closed using a linear stapler (Endo GIA™, Covidien, Mansfield, MA, USA)

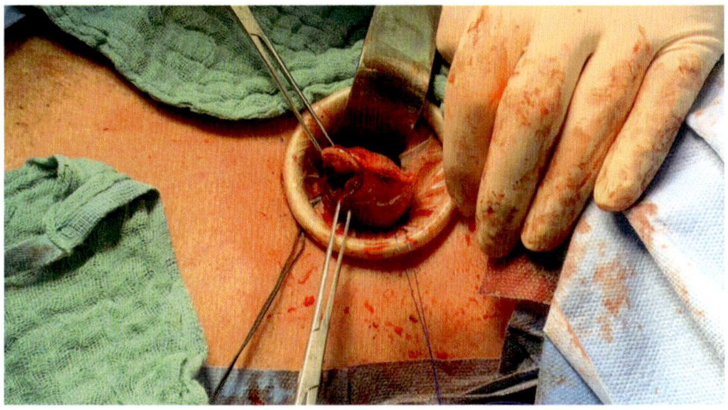

Fig. 15.47 The proximal portion of the gastric conduit is once again meticulously checked to evaluate the appearance of any ischemic demarcation zone. The conduit is opened proximally at the staple line

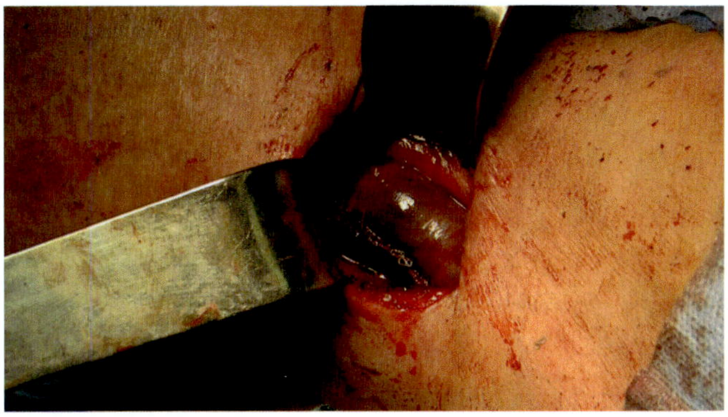

Fig. 15.50 The linear staple line is checked for bleeding. We normally avoid oversewing the linear stapler line to prevent narrowing of the proximal conduit

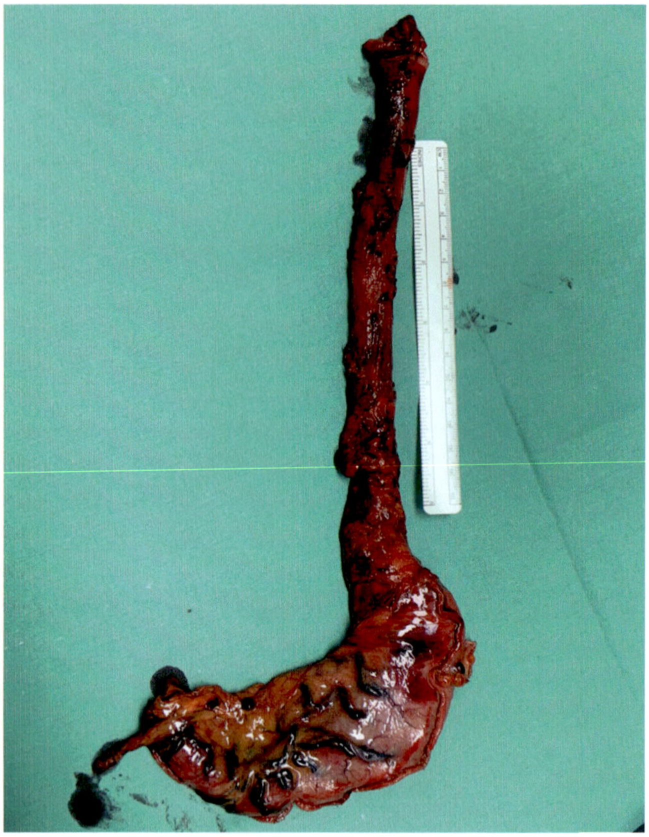

Fig. 15.51 The specimen is dissected at the back-table. The collected lymph node stations have been mentioned during the previous description

References

1. Fujiwara H, Shiozaki A, Konishi H, et al. Single-port mediastinoscopic lymphadenectomy along the left recurrent laryngeal nerve. Ann Thorac Surg. 2015;100:1115–7.
2. Grimminger PP, van der Sluis PC, Stein H, Lang H, van Hillegersberg R, Egberts JH. Feasibility of transcervical robotic-assisted esophagectomy (TC-RAMIE) in a Cadaver study—a future outlook for an extrapleural approach. Appl Sci (Basel). 2019;9:3572.
3. van der Sluis P, Egberts JH, Stein H, Sallum R, van Hillegersberg R, Grimminger PP. Transcervical (SP) and transhiatal DaVinci robotic esophagectomy: a cadaveric study. Thorac Cardiovasc Surg. 2021;69(3):198–203. https://doi.org/10.1055/s-0040-1716323. Epub 2020 Sep 8. PMID: 32898893.
4. Nakauchi M, Uyama I, Suda K, et al. Robot-assisted mediastinoscopic esophagectomy for esophageal cancer: the first clinical series. Esophagus. 2019;16(01):85–92.

Robotic-Assisted Proximal Gastrectomy with Double Tract Reconstruction

16

Peter P. Grimminger, Giovanni Capovilla, and Felix Berlth

Introduction

The incidence of cancer of the upper third of the stomach (proximal gastric cancer) and particularly of proximal early gastric cancer has increased worldwide in the recent years, probably as a consequence of the improvement of the endoscopic screening. Total gastrectomy is the most frequently performed surgical procedure for the treatment of proximal EGC, when endoscopic resection is not feasible. However, this technique shows considerable disadvantages, in that it may severely affect patients' feeding capacity and nutritional status. Proximal gastrectomy has been proposed as an alternative to total gastrectomy for the surgical treatment of proximally located EGC, with the potential advantage of improving the long-term functional outcome. However, the use of such technique was limited by its technical demand, the lack of standardization and the considerable incidence of postoperative esophagitis and stenosis of the gastrojejunal anastomosis [1]. In this context, proximal gastrectomy with "double tract" reconstruction has been proved to overcome the complications related to the other reconstructive techniques for proximal gastric resection [2]. Finally, a recent meta-analysis comparing laparoscopic proximal gastrectomy and laparoscopic total gastrectomy demonstrated the superiority of proximal gastrectomy in preventing vitamin B12 deficiency, with no increased risk of anastomotic stricture and reflux esophagitis and comparable clinical effect [3].

We present here our technique for Robotic-Assisted proximal gastrectomy with "double tract" reconstruction using the da Vinci Xi® Surgical System (Intuitive Surgical, Sunnyvale, CA, USA). Briefly, the proximal stomach is resected, leaving an adequate residual antral portion. The circular stapler anvil is trans-orally inserted and exteriorized through the distal esophageal stump using a dedicated device (OrVil™; Covidien, Mansfield, MA, USA). The specimen is then retrieved through a median mini-laparotomy. A proximal jejunal loop, at circa 30 cm from the Treitz ligament, is exteriorized through the mini-laparotomy and divided using a linear stapler (Endo GIA™, Covidien, Mansfield, MA, USA). An end-to-side hand-sewn single-layer anastomosis is performed at 50 cm from the proximal end of the distal jejunal loop. A circular stapler (CEEA™, Covidien, Mansfield, MA, USA) is introduced through the proximal end of the distal jejunal loop. Upon restoration of the pneumoperitoneum, the distal jejunal loop is transposed cranially in an antecolic position, after connection with the anvil the CEEA is fired, thus configuring an end-to-side esophago-jejunal anastomosis. A side-to-side gastrojejunal anastomosis is finally intracorporeally hand-sewn on the same bowel loop, thus leaving a 15-cm-long jejunal segment between the esophago-jejunal and the gastrojejunal anastomoses.

The use of the robotic platform provides undeniable advantages while performing this technique. The tridimensional stable view offers a clearer visual field during the lymphadenectomy. The EndoWrist considerably favors the far advanced precise dissection in narrower spaces such as the hiatus and the intracorporeal hand-sewing during the gastrojejunal anastomosis (Figs. 16.1, 16.2, 16.3, 16.4, 16.5, 16.6, 16.7, 16.8, 16.9, 16.10, 16.11, 16.12, 16.13, 16.14, 16.15, 16.16, 16.17, 16.18, 16.19, 16.20, 16.21, 16.22, 16.23, 16.24, 16.25, 16.26, 16.27, 16.28, 16.29, 16.30, 16.31, 16.32, 16.33, 16.34, 16.35, 16.36, 16.37, 16.38, 16.39, 16.40, 16.41, 16.42, 16.43, 16.44, 16.45, 16.46, 16.47, 16.48, 16.49, and 16.50).

P. P. Grimminger (✉) · G. Capovilla
Department of General-, Visceral- and Transplant Surgery, University Medical Center Mainz, Mainz, Germany
e-mail: peter.grimminger@unimedizin-mainz.de

F. Berlth
Department of General, Visceral and Transplant Surgery, University Medical Center of the Johannes Gutenberg University, Mainz, Germany

O. Y. Kudsi, P. P. Grimminger (eds.), *Atlas of Robotic Upper Gastrointestinal Surgery*,
https://doi.org/10.1007/978-3-030-86578-8_16

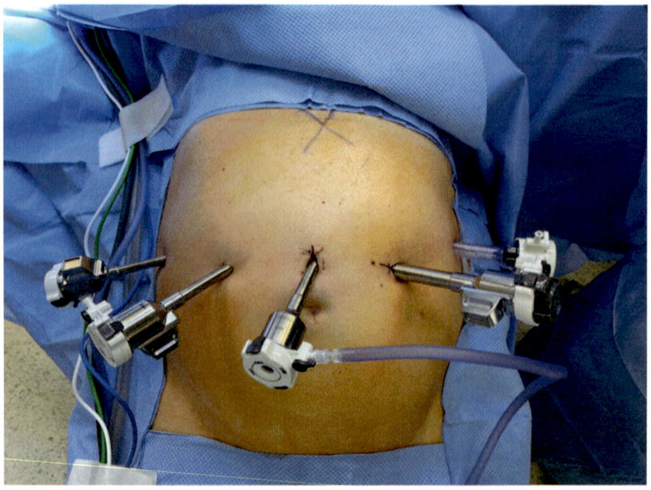

Fig. 16.1 Trocar position: the patient is placed in a normal supine position with a 15° reverse Trendelenburg. Pneumoperitoneum is applied with a Veress needle in the upper left abdominal quadrant. Upon removal of the Veress needle, a 12 mm trocar is placed to be used for the energy dissection device (Vessel Sealer Extend or Monopolar-Hook) and the Stapler. The 8 mm midline camera trocar is placed above the umbilicus; the distance from the umbilicus depends on the location of the gastric antrum in the computer tomography. An 8 mm trocar used for the Fenestrated Bipolar Forceps is placed in the upper right quadrant. A fenestrated Tip-Up grasper is introduced with the third arm, through another 8 mm trocar placed in the right lateral subcostal area. Finally, a 12 mm assistant trocar is placed in the left lateral subcostal area and used for retraction, suction, and introduction/removal of any material during the dissection and for the linear stapler

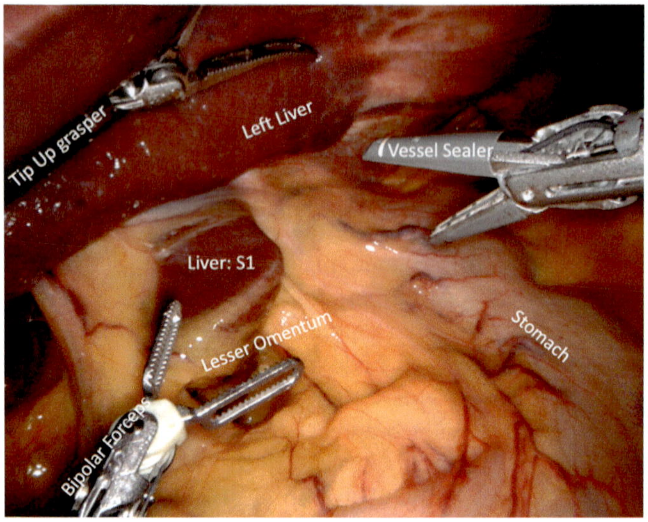

Fig. 16.2 The initial setting includes the use of the fenestrated bipolar forceps on the left arm and the Vessel Sealer on the right arm. The third robotic arm is equipped with a Tip-Up grasper and used to retract the left liver lobe

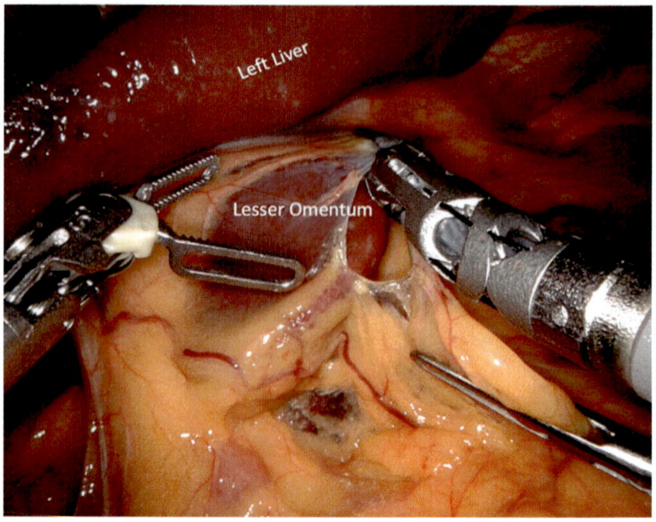

Fig. 16.3 The lesser omentum is opened, and the dissection is carried out toward the right diaphragmatic crus

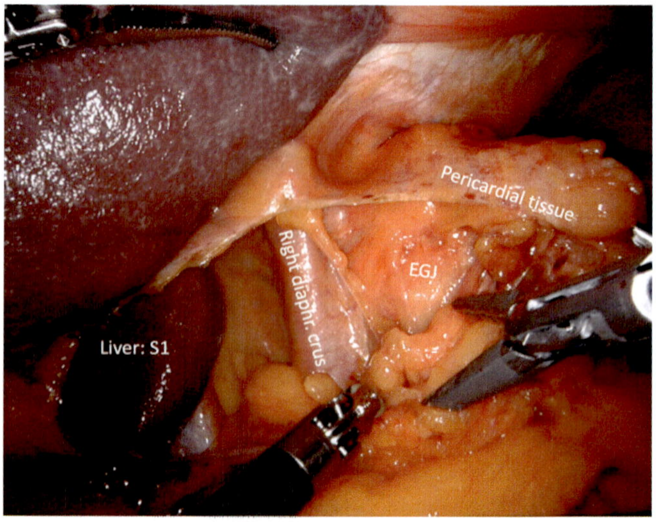

Fig. 16.4 The space between the right diaphragmatic crus and the pericardial fat is developed. During this phase the assistant surgeon can gently retract the pericardial tissue to the left to provide tension and improve the field vision

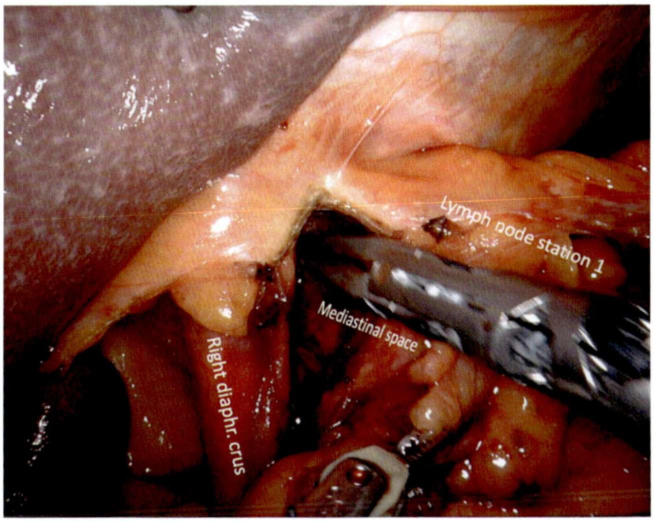

Fig. 16.5 The plane is developed deeper into the mediastinum in order to completely free the lower esophagus on the right side. During this phase the lymph nodes of station 1 are collected and will be retrieved en bloc with the specimen

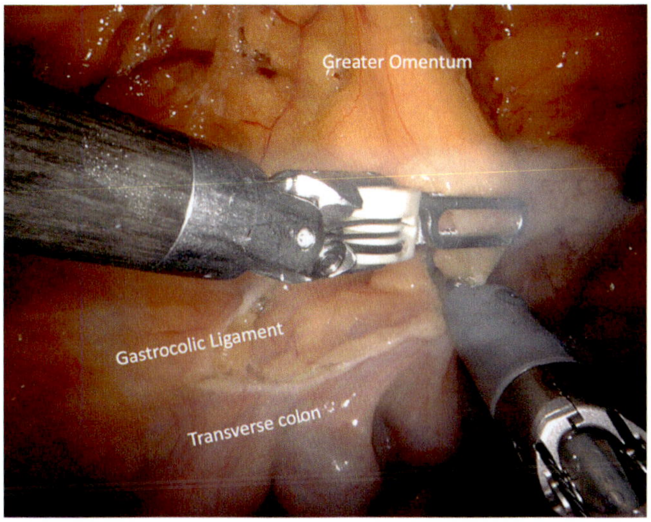

Fig. 16.7 The gastrocolic ligament is incised at the level of the mid-transverse colon. The greater omentum is dissected from the transverse mesocolon

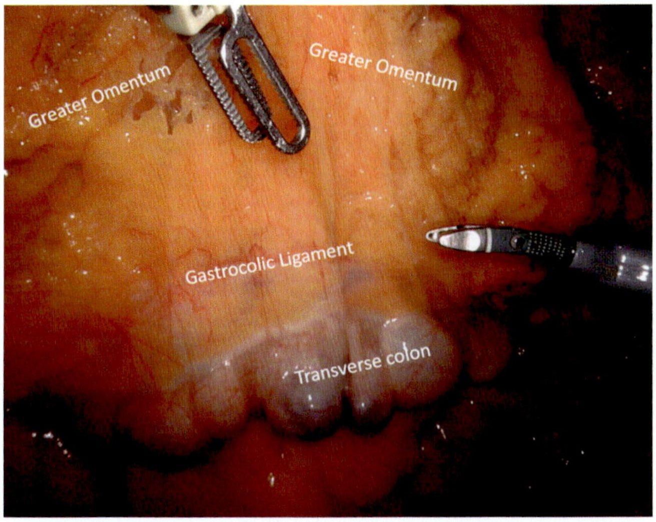

Fig. 16.6 The greater omentum is cranially retracted; the transverse mesocolon and the gastrocolic ligament are exposed

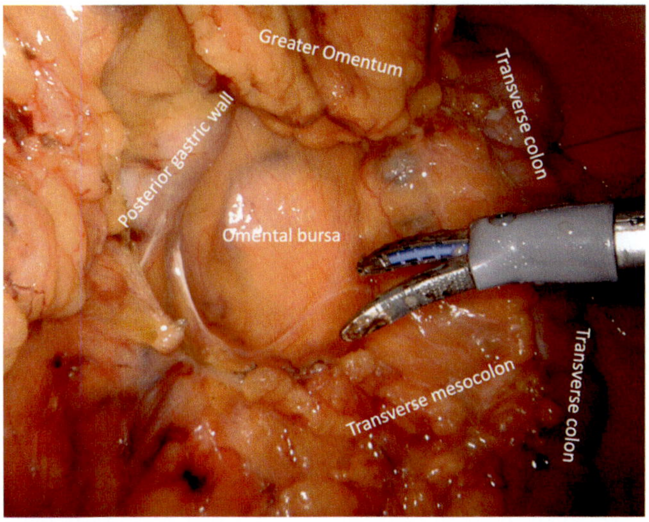

Fig. 16.8 Further dissection of the greater omentum from the transverse mesocolon gives access to the omental bursa. Visualization of the posterior gastric wall must be achieved

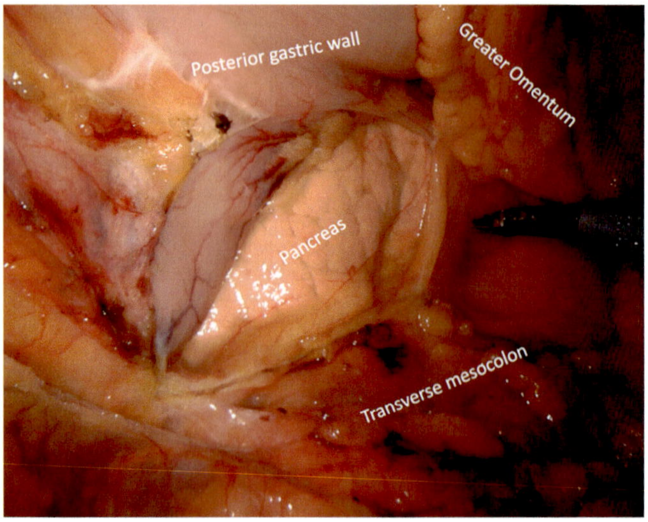

Fig. 16.9 To achieve complete mobilization of the greater curvature, the greater omentum and the posterior gastric wall are completely dissected from the anterior surface of the pancreas

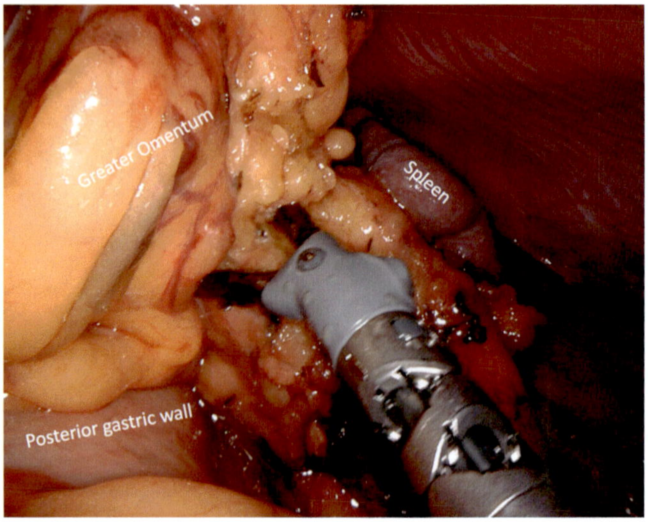

Fig. 16.10 The dissection is extended toward the spleen in order to completely mobilize the gastric fundus

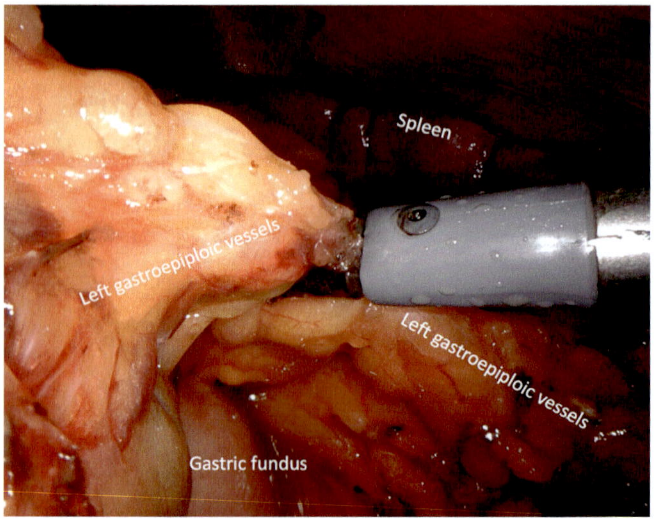

Fig. 16.11 The left gastroepiploic vessels are encountered and divided to achieve complete mobilization of the gastric fundus. During this phase the stomach can be gently retracted toward the right using the third robotic arm (Tip-Up grasper); the assistant can retract the fat pad toward the left side to provide tension. Lymph nodes of station 4sb and, above the left gastroepiploic artery, 4sa are retrieved during this phase and will be extracted en bloc with the specimen

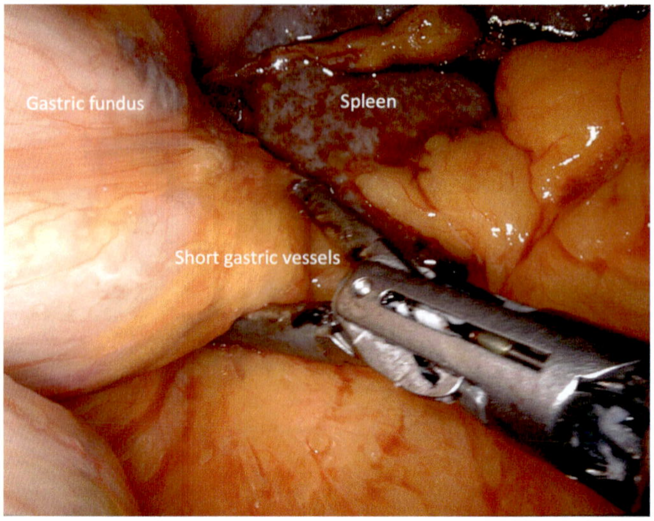

Fig. 16.12 The mobilization of the gastric fundus is completed by dividing the short gastric vessels. Lymph nodes of station 4sa are retrieved during this phase and will be extracted en bloc with the specimen

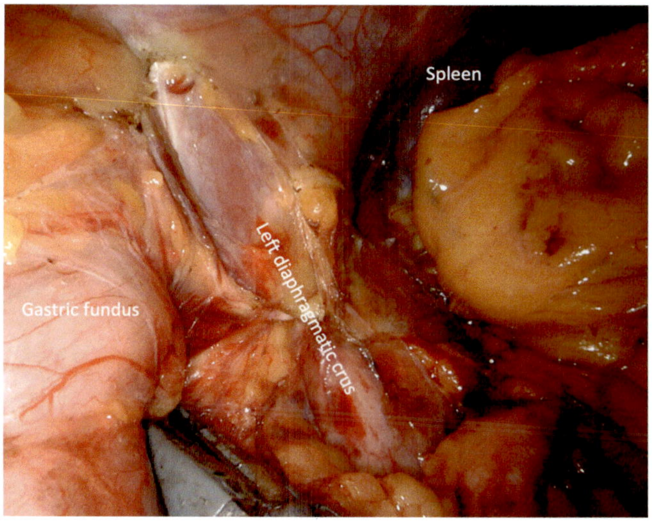

Fig. 16.13 After complete mobilization of the gastric fundus, the left diaphragmatic crus is visualized. The fundus, the cardias, and the distal esophagus are completely freed from the left crus. Lymph node station 2 is retrieved during this step and will be extracted en bloc with the specimen

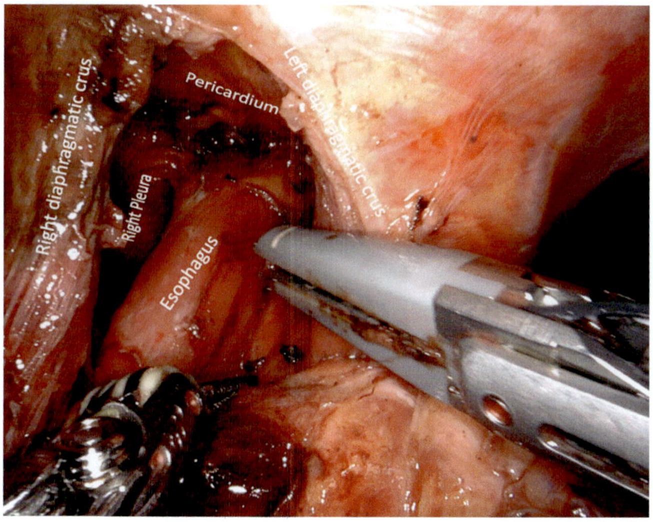

Fig. 16.14 The dissection plane is further developed toward the mediastinum, and complete mobilization of the lower esophagus is achieved

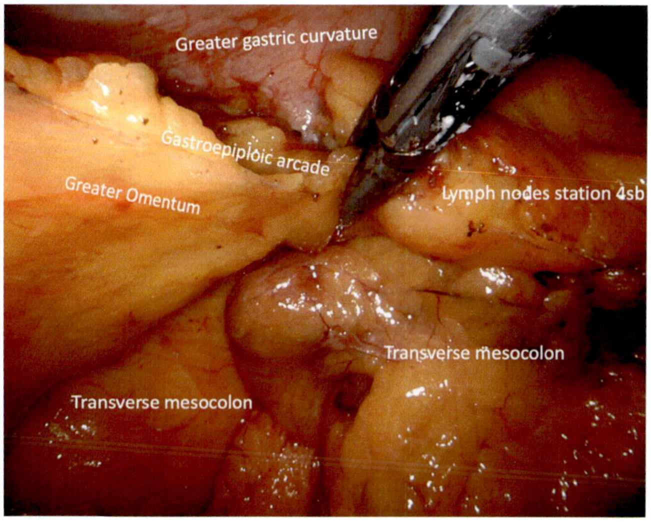

Fig. 16.15 The greater omentum is brought to the specimen side by separating it from the right transverse colon and distal stomach under preservation of the arcade. The arcade is then approached in the desired location of transection of the stomach. The proximal gastrectomy can be carried out as a hemigastrectomy or as a 2/3 proximal gastrectomy just by leaving the gastric antrum as a remnant

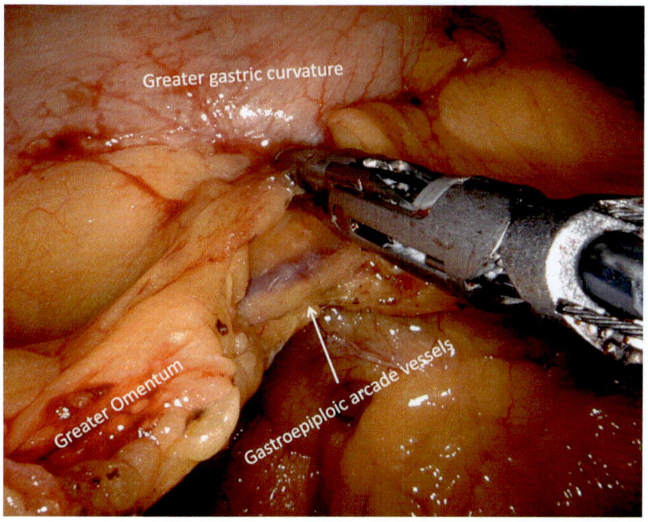

Fig. 16.16 The gastroepiploic arcade vessels are identified and dissected. The dissection is carried out at the transition zone between lymph nodes of station 4d and lymph nodes of station 4sb. Lymph nodes of station 4sb and, if desired, partly 4d, depending on the transection line, are dissected during this phase and will be resected en bloc with the specimen

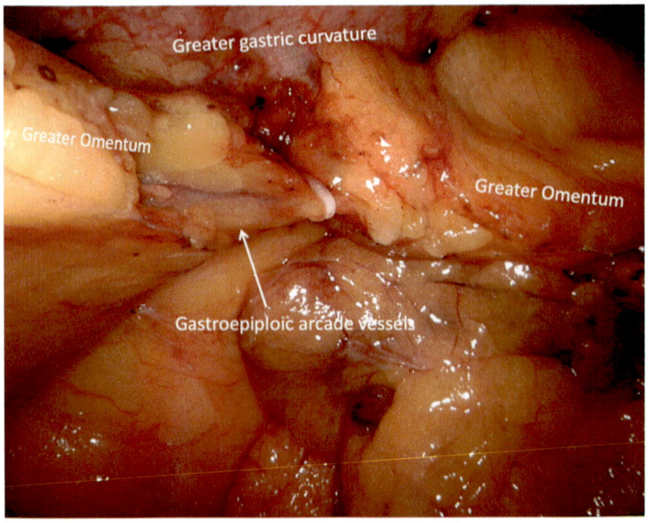

Fig. 16.17 The gastroepiploic arcade vessels are then clipped at the desired location and selectively divided

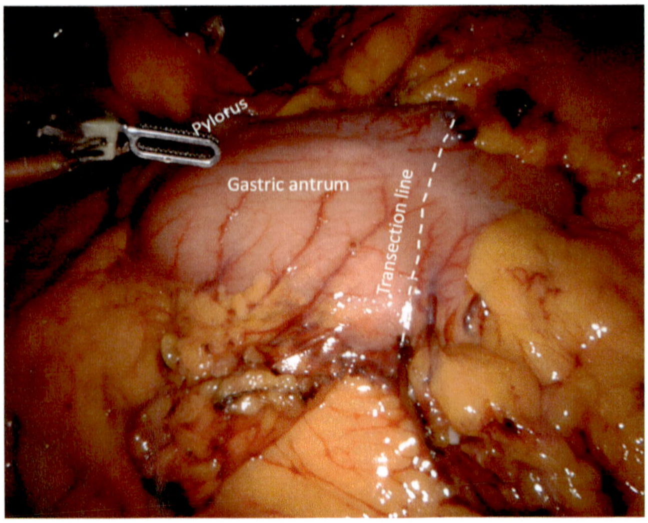

Fig. 16.18 The greater curvature is exposed for subsequent transection

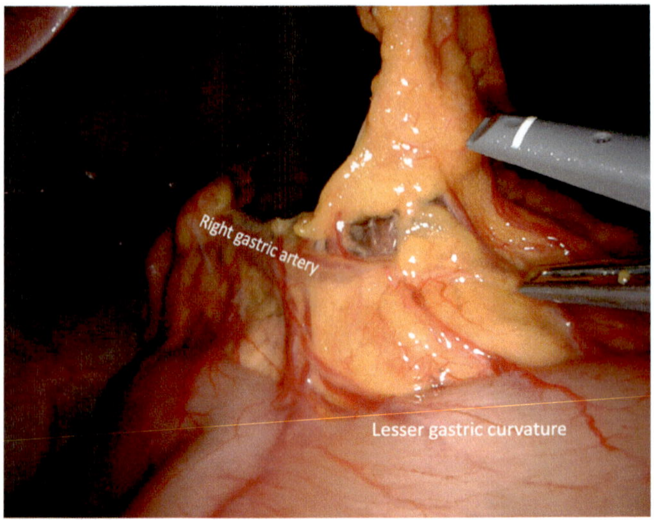

Fig. 16.19 As a next step, the lesser curvature is dissected: the right gastric artery is identified and isolated

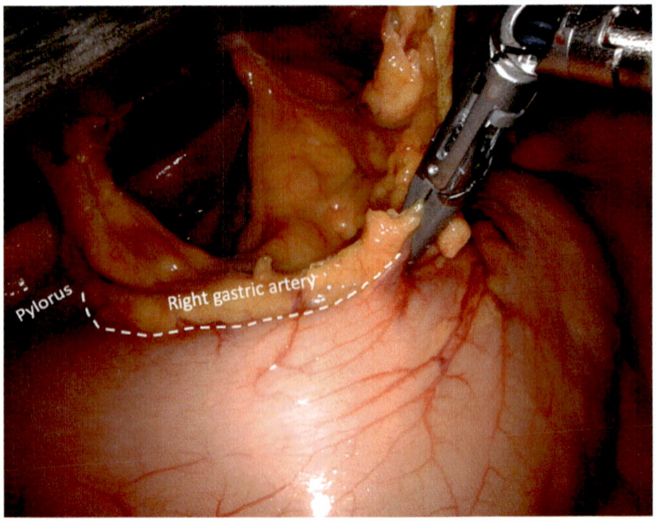

Fig. 16.20 The right gastric artery arcade can be divided using the vessel sealer

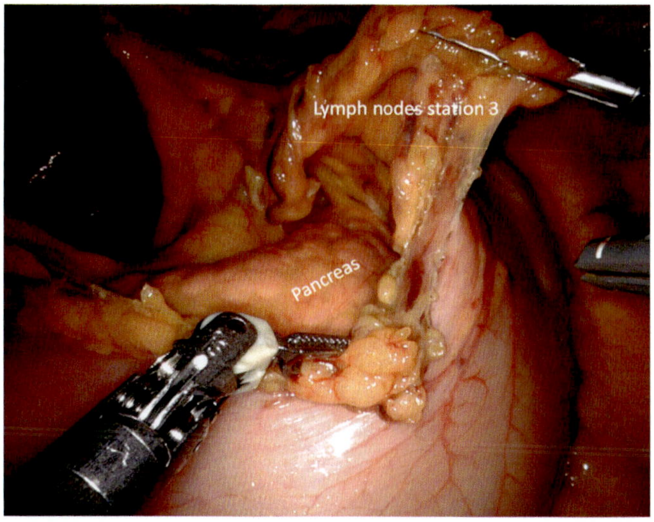

Fig. 16.21 The lesser curvature is freed at the resection site. During this phase the station 3 lymph nodes are dissected and will be retrieved en bloc with the final specimen

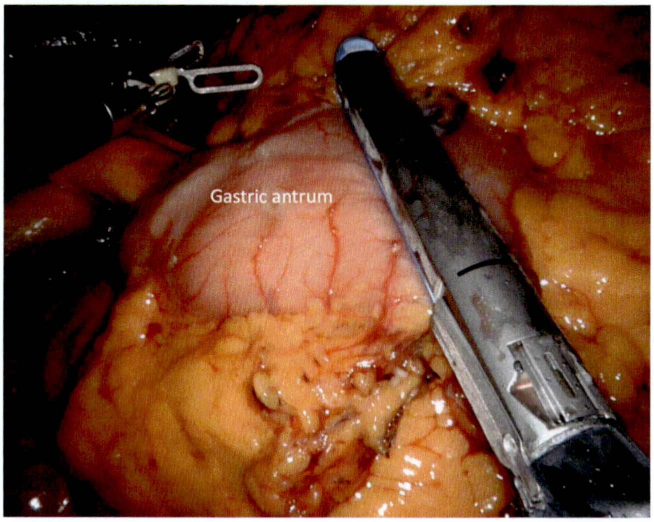

Fig. 16.22 The stomach is then resected so that a remnant antral portion of adequate length is left in place. We usually use a 60 mm Endo GIA Blue cartridge

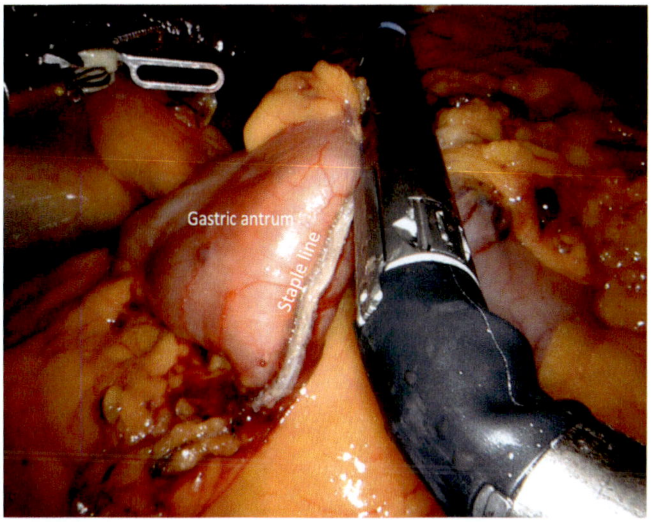

Fig. 16.23 The resection normally requires up to two fires of the linear staple

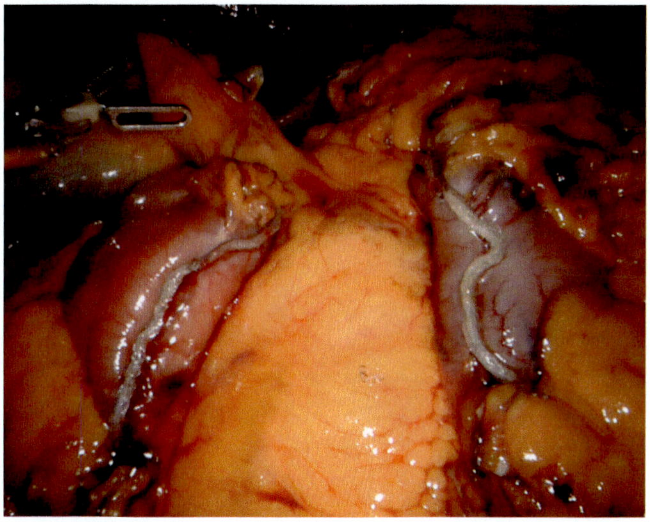

Fig. 16.24 The resected residual antrum is checked for adequate vascularization; in case of bleeding from the staple line, hemostasis is performed using the bipolar forceps

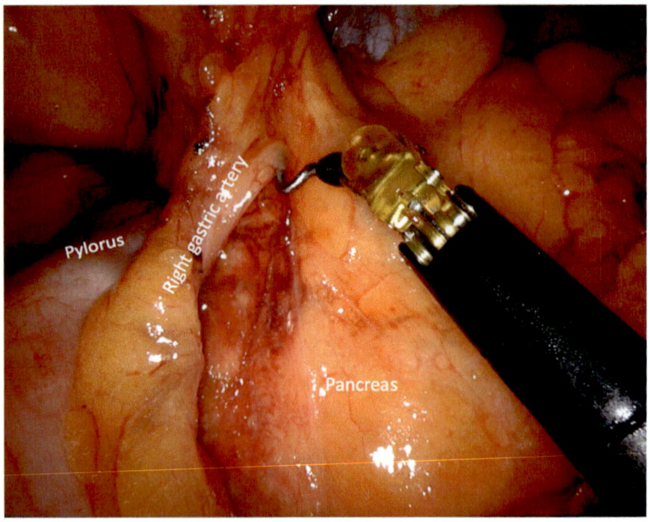

Fig. 16.25 Next the lymphadenectomy is preceded by dissecting the tissue medially from the right gastric artery

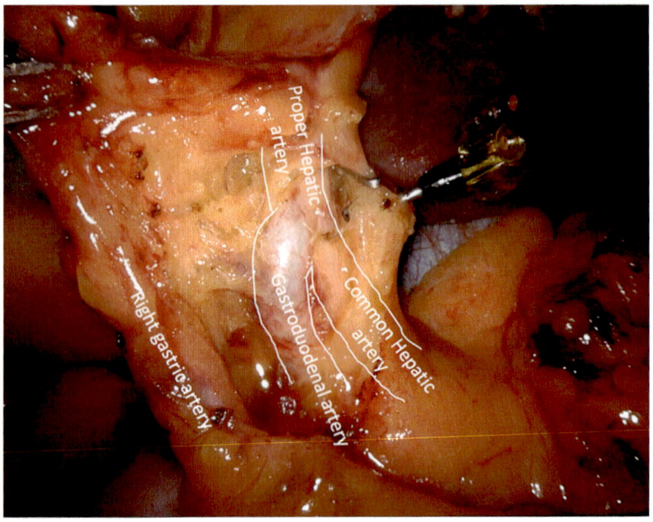

Fig. 16.27 The proper hepatic artery, lymph node station 12, is then followed and dissected from the surrounding tissue

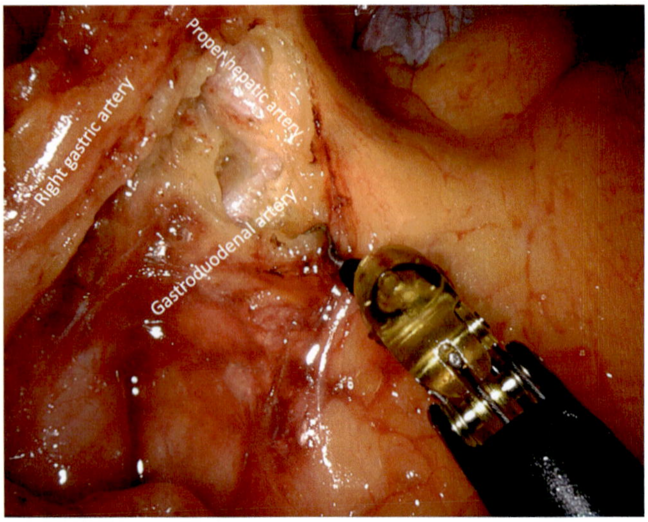

Fig. 16.26 Following the right gastric artery, the proper hepatic artery is identified. Dissection of the surrounding tissue is carried out toward the common hepatic artery medially. The origin of the gastroduodenal artery from the common hepatic artery is identified

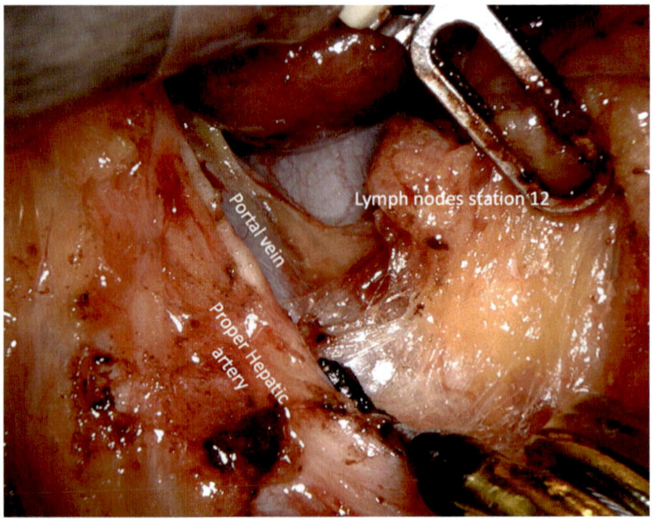

Fig. 16.28 The dissection can be extended posteriorly, identifying the lateral aspect of the portal vein

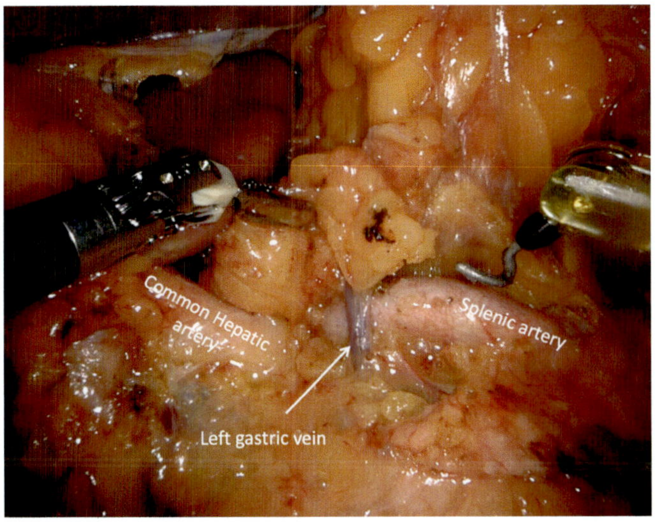

Fig. 16.29 Extending the dissection medially along the common hepatic artery, lymph node station 8 leads to the identification of the celiac trunk. The resected stomach can be gently uplifted by the assistant to provide tension and facilitate the identification of the left gastric vein

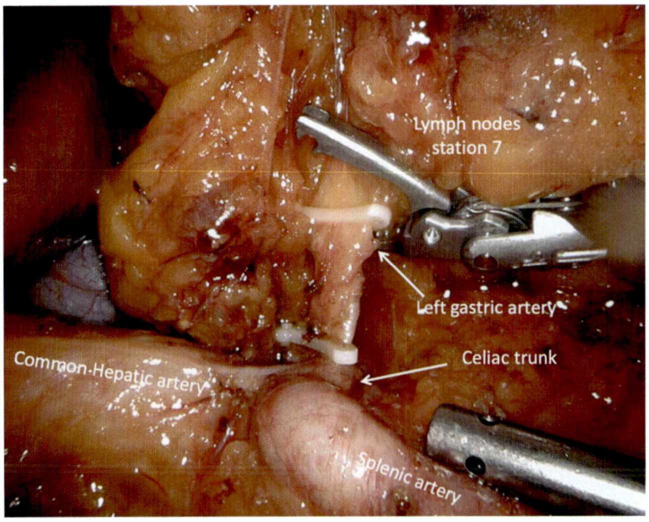

Fig. 16.31 After its complete exposure, the left gastric artery is clipped and divided

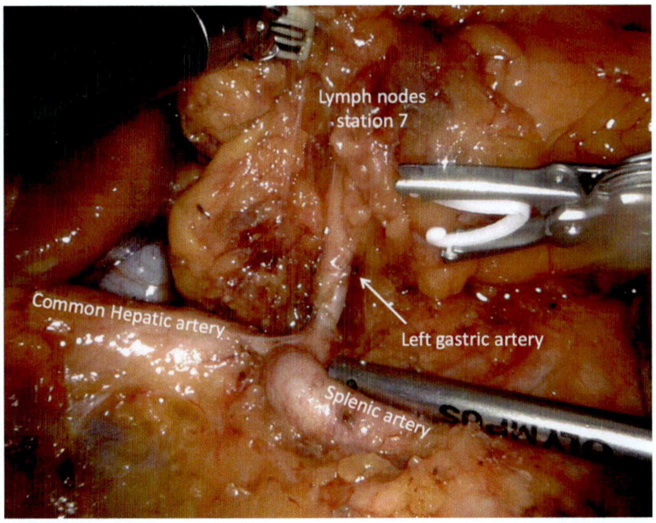

Fig. 16.30 After division of the gastric vein, the left gastric artery is identified and dissected anteriorly and posteriorly. During this phase the tissue surrounding the celiac trunk, the left gastric vessels, and the proximal splenic artery is dissected and lifted cranially. This maneuver permits the retrieval of station 9, 7 and 11p lymph nodes that will be resected en bloc with the final specimen

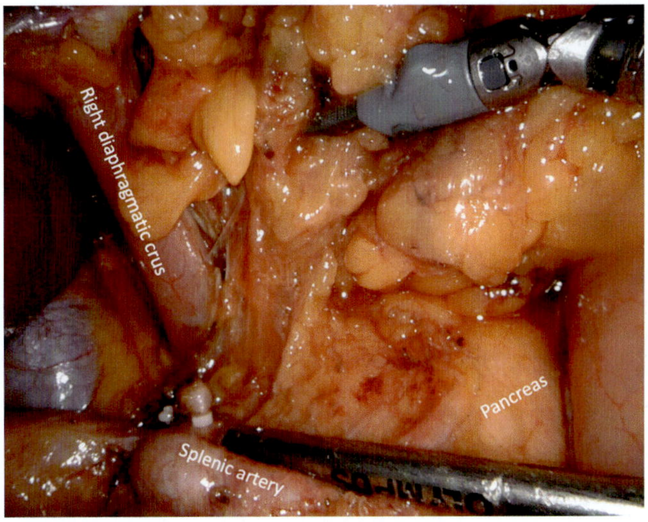

Fig. 16.32 After division of the left gastric artery, the dissection of the tissue is carried out posteriorly until the plane of the right and left diaphragmatic crura is reached

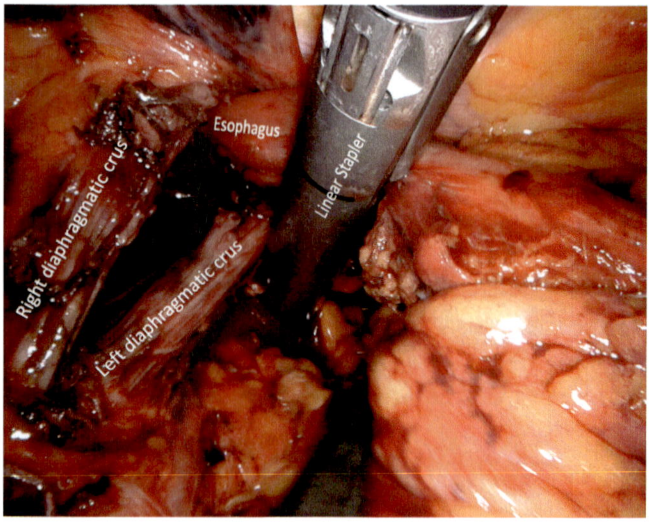

Fig. 16.33 The divided stomach is lifted and gently retracted to the left. The esophagus is divided using a 60 mm robotic linear stapler with a blue cartridge

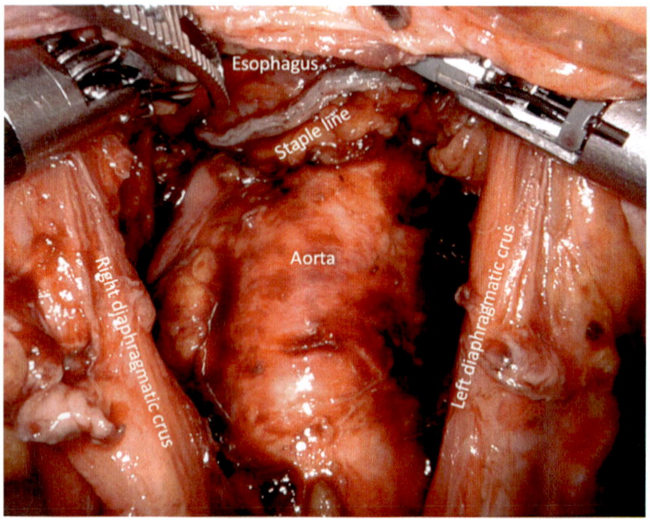

Fig. 16.34 After adequate mobilization of the lower esophagus and lymphadenectomy of pericardial lymph nodes, the esophageal resection and the retrieval of the specimen should allow the complete visualization of the left and right diaphragmatic crura and the aorta

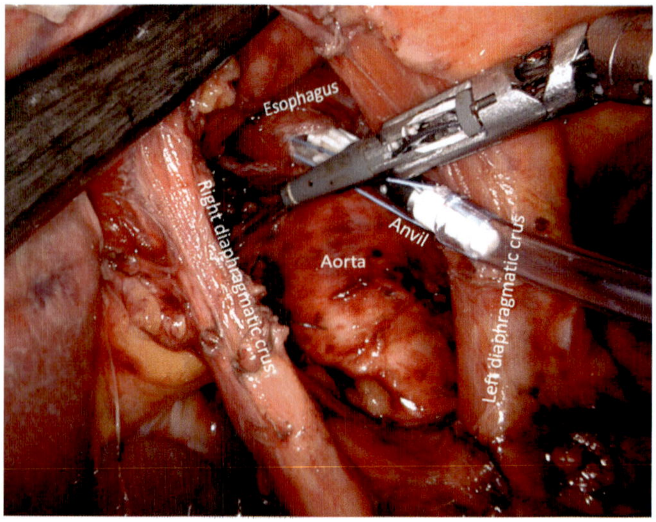

Fig. 16.35 Upon confirmation of a negative proximal margin at frozen section, the circular stapler's Anvil is placed in the distal esophageal stump trans-orally using a commercially available device (OrVil™; Covidien Mansfield, MA, USA). Different techniques can be used to introduce the anvil into the distal esophagus

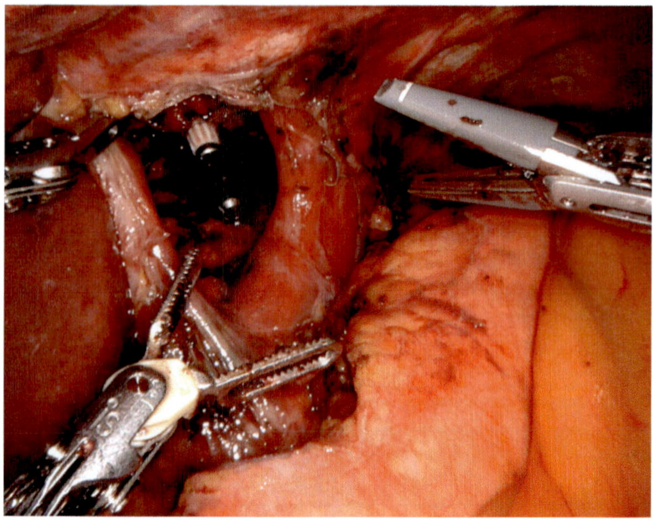

Fig. 16.36 The correct position of the Anvil and the hemostasis in the lymphadenectomy area are checked. In case of a "soft" esophageal wall or in case of excessive manipulation of the esophageal stump, a hand-sewn purse string may be used to reinforce the positioning of the Anvil

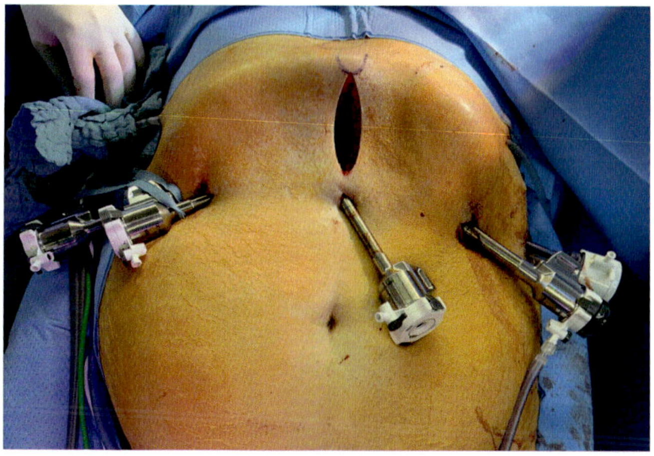

Fig. 16.37 A mini-laparotomy is performed on the midline, commonly above the camera trocar. The camera trocar position depends on the specific location of the stomach

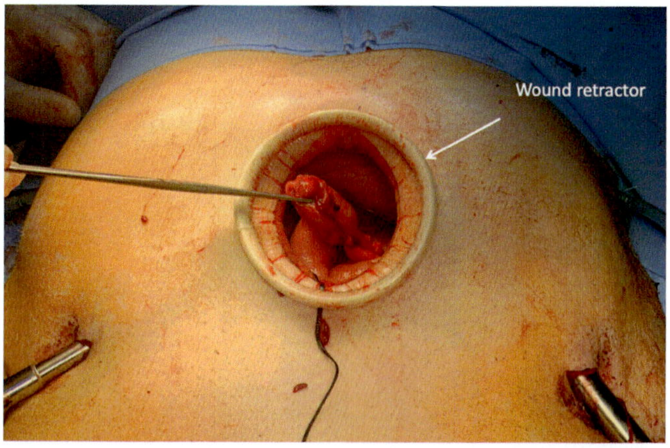

Fig. 16.38 The specimen extraction is facilitated by the use of a dual ring wound retractor (Alexis™, Applied Medical, Rancho Santa Margarita, CA)

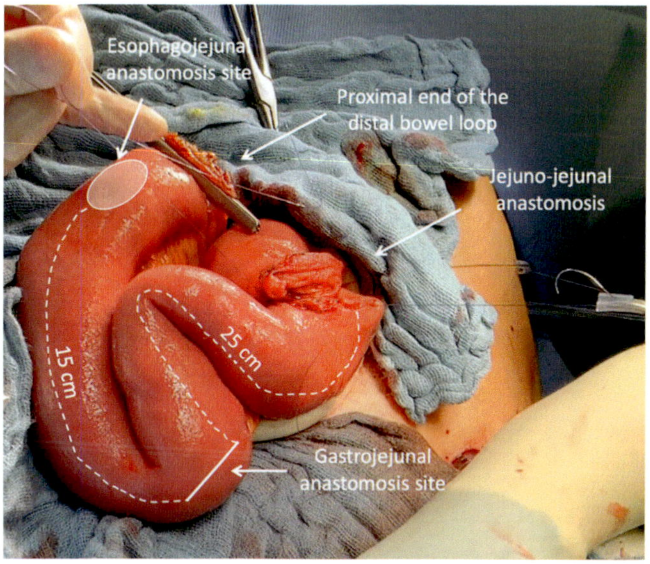

Fig. 16.39 A proximal jejunal loop, at circa 30 cm from the Treitz ligament, is exteriorized through the mini-laparotomy and divided using a linear stapler (Endo-GIA™, Covidien, Mansfield, MA, USA). An end-to-side hand-sewn single-layer anastomosis is performed at 35–40 cm from the proximal end of the distal jejunal loop using PDS 4-0. The length of the transposed jejunal loop should guarantee a distance of at least 10–15 cm between the esophago-jejunal anastomosis and the gastrojejunal anastomosis and a distance of at least 15–20 cm between the gastrojejunal anastomosis and the jejune-jejunal anastomosis

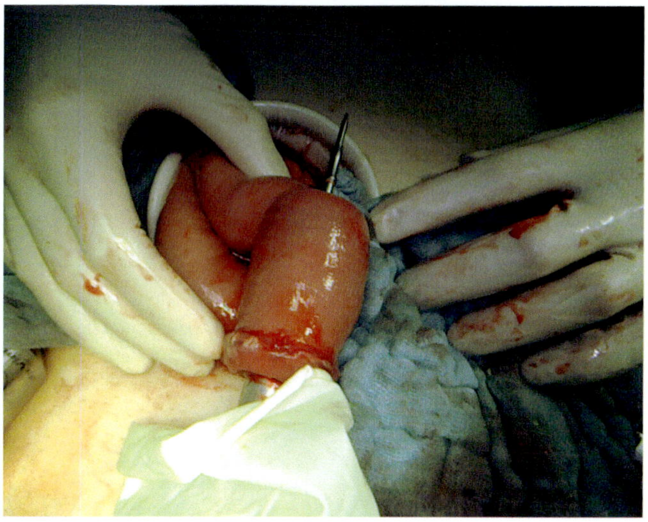

Fig. 16.40 The shaft of the circular stapler (CEEA™, Covidien, Mansfield, MA, USA) is inserted through the proximal margin of the distal bowel loop

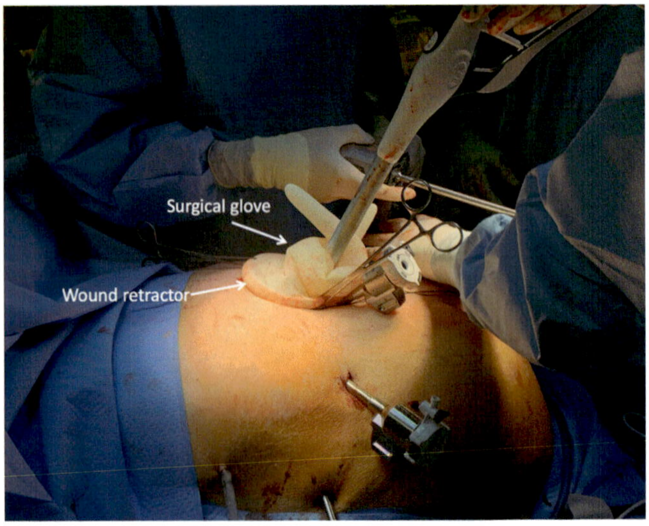

Fig. 16.41 The circular stapler is placed in the abdominal cavity, and the pneumoperitoneum is reestablished using a surgical glove and the wound retractor

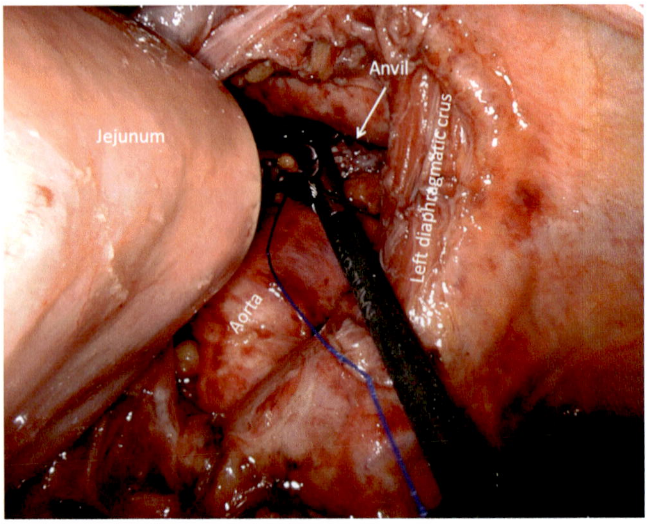

Fig. 16.42 The jejunal loop is transposed in an antecolic position. The head of the circular stapler and the anvil are connected under direct vision

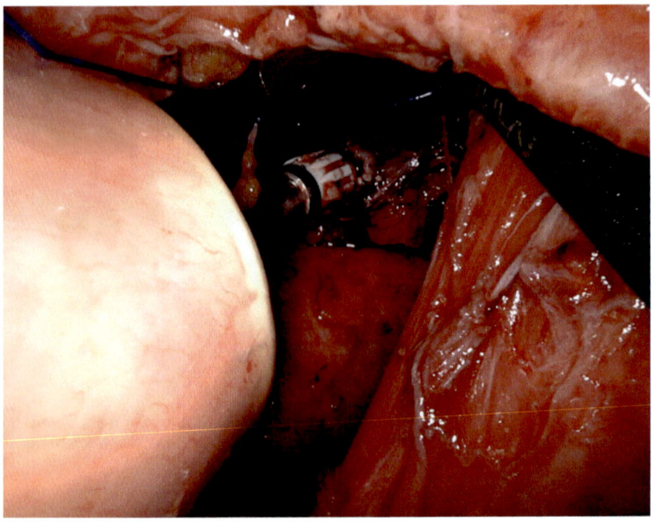

Fig. 16.43 When a reinforcement hand-sewn purse string is performed (blue thread), the suture tails are cut before firing the stapler. Care is taken to avoid the inclusion of any other structure except the esophagus and the jejunum in the stapler line

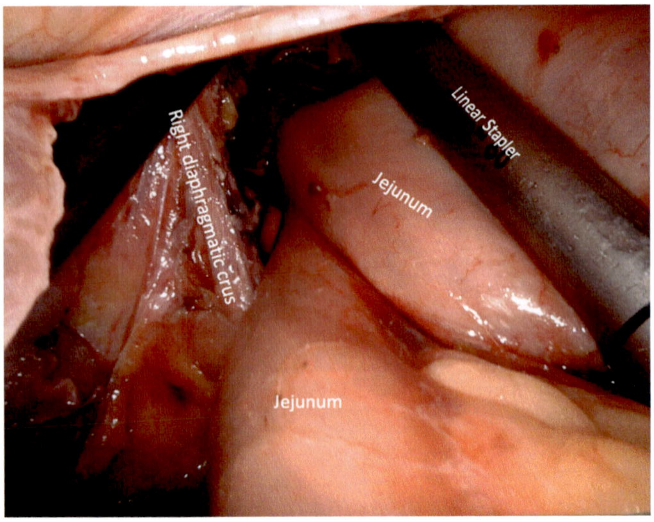

Fig. 16.44 The anastomosis is then completed by resecting the jejunal entry site of the circular stapler using a single fire of the linear stapler

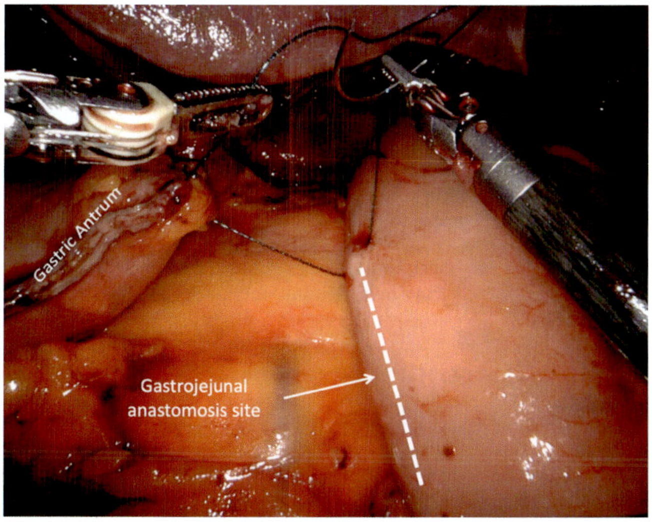

Fig. 16.45 The gastric remnant and the transposed jejunal loop are approximated using a barbed 3/0 reabsorbable suture

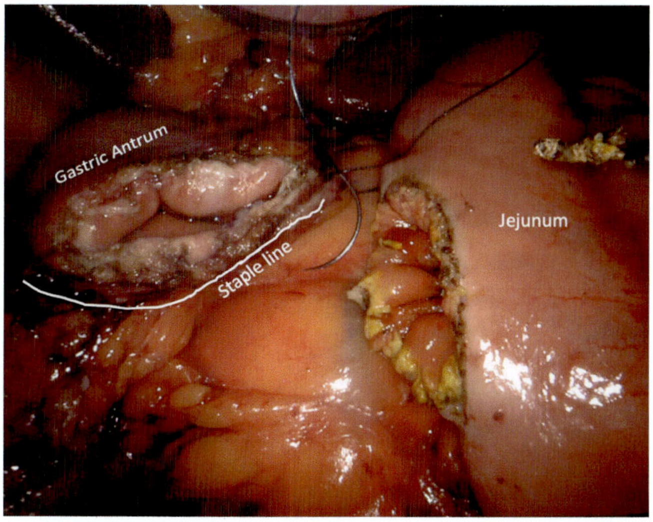

Fig. 16.46 The proximal end of the gastric remnant is opened anteriorly to the staple line. A corresponding opening is also performed in the jejunal lateral wall

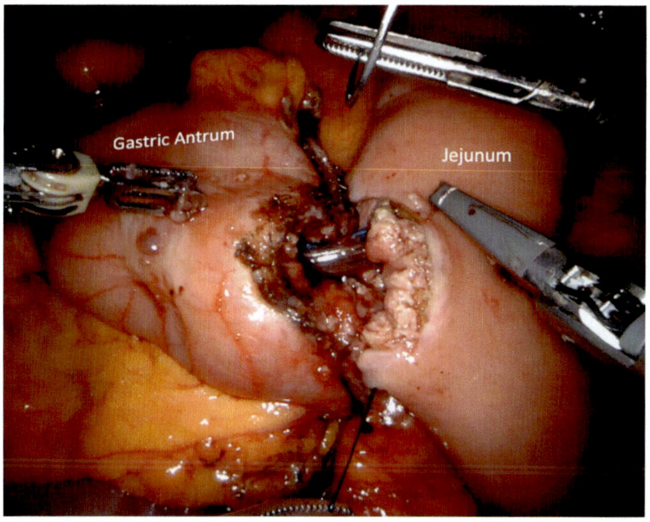

Fig. 16.47 Before completing the anastomosis, a gastric suction drain is passed through the anastomosis under direct vision

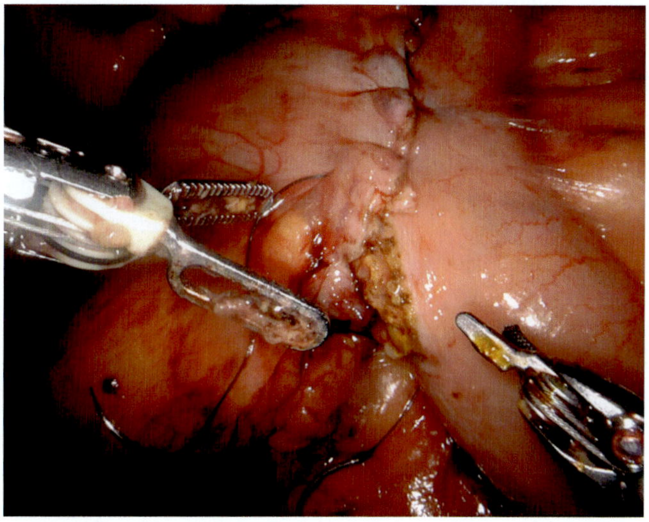

Fig. 16.48 A 6-cm-long hand-sewn single-layer side-to-end anastomosis is performed using a 3/0 reabsorbable barbed suture

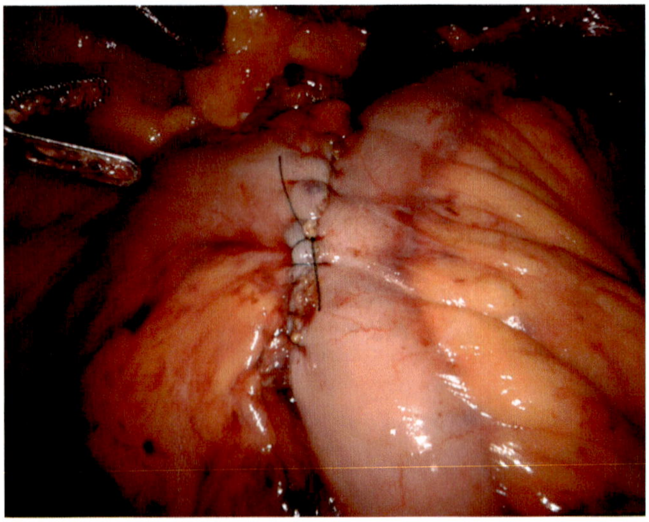

Fig. 16.49 Anastomotic spillage may be checked using methylene blue through the gastric tube

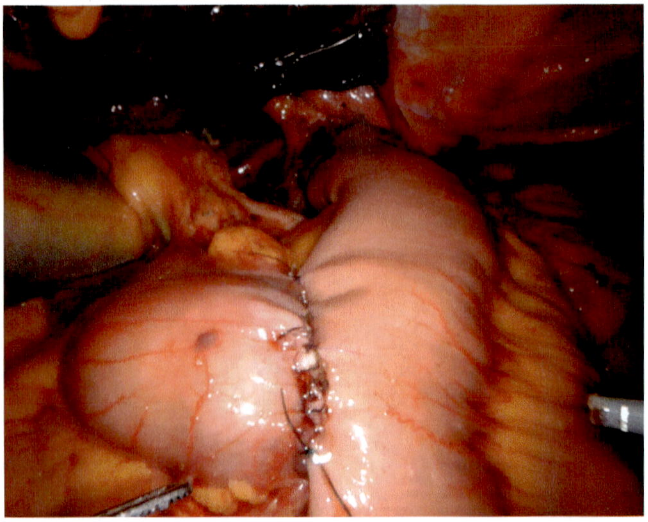

Fig. 16.50 The correct position of the transposed bowel loop is checked; any mesenteric defect is closed by intracorporeal sutures

References

1. Yoo CH, Sohn BH, Han WK, Pae WK. Long-term results of proximal and total gastrectomy for adenocarcinoma of the upper third of the stomach. Cancer Res Treat. 2004;36:50–5. https://doi.org/10.4143/crt.2004.36.1.50.
2. Nomura E, Kayano H, Lee SW, Kawai M, Machida T, Yamamoto S, Nabeshima K, Nakamura K, Mukai M, Uchiyama K. Functional evaluations comparing the double-tract method and the jejunal interposition method following laparoscopic proximal gastrectomy for gastric cancer: an investigation including laparoscopic total gastrectomy. Surg Today. 2019;49:38–48. https://doi.org/10.1007/s00595-018-1699-7.
3. Li S, Gu L, Shen Z, Mao D, Khadaroo PA, Su H. A meta-analysis of comparison of proximal gastrectomy with double-tract reconstruction and total gastrectomy for proximal early gastric cancer. BMC Surg. 2019;19(1):117. https://doi.org/10.1186/s12893-019-0584-7.

Robot-Assisted Total Gastrectomy and Roux-en-Y Reconstruction

17

Han-Kwang Yang and Felix Berlth

Introduction

Minimally invasive gastrectomy is on the rise since several prospective randomized trials provided evidence that it is oncologically safe compared to traditional open surgery, not only for early but also for locally advanced gastric cancer [1].

The large randomized trials were performed for distal gastrectomy and laparoscopic surgery; however it has been assumed that for the robot-assisted procedure, similar results could be achieved. This assumption was proved in a Korean multicenter comparative trial, which compared laparoscopic and robot-assisted procedures in terms of surgical radicality and postoperative morbidity [2]. For the subgroup of patients receiving a full D2 lymphadenectomy, a significantly lower blood loss could be shown in the robot-assisted gastrectomy group [3]. The benefits of robotic procedures, the angulating instruments, the magnified vision, and precise maneuvers, are illustrated in this chapter. Further technological progress and instrument development is supposed to significantly improve the robot-assisted gastrectomy procedure in the future.

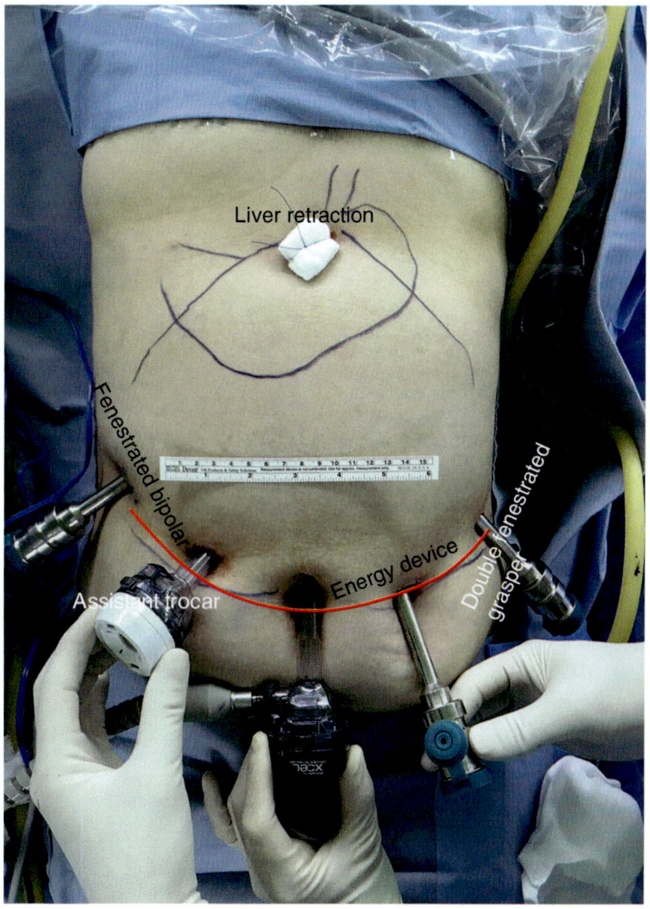

Fig. 17.1 The camera trocar is located infraumbilical; the other trocars are positioned in a slightly round shape. The 12 mm assistant trocar is put on the right side of the patient. The robotic instruments that are used for this procedure are: fenestrated bipolar on the left hand and energy device as well as double fenestrated grasper on the right hand

Robot-Assisted Total Gastrectomy

Preparation (Figs. 17.1 and 17.2)

H.-K. Yang
Department of Surgery, Seoul National University College of Medicine, Seoul, South Korea

F. Berlth (✉)
Department of General, Visceral and Transplant Surgery, University Medical Center of the Johannes Gutenberg University, Mainz, Germany
e-mail: felix.berlth@unimedizin-mainz.de

O. Y. Kudsi, P. P. Grimminger (eds.), *Atlas of Robotic Upper Gastrointestinal Surgery*,
https://doi.org/10.1007/978-3-030-86578-8_17

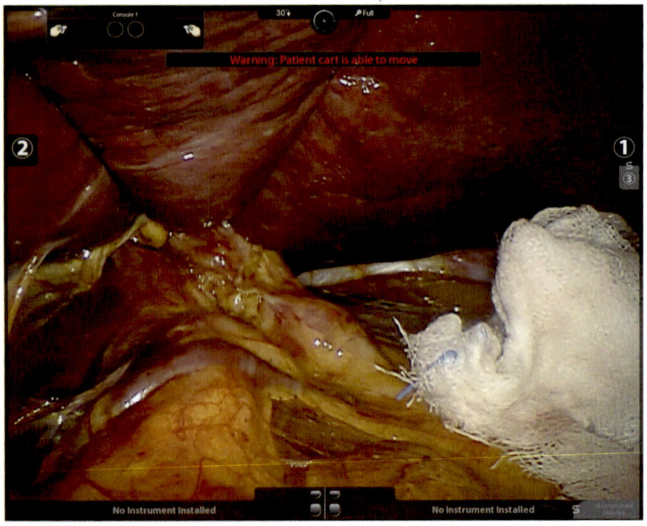

Fig. 17.2 Liver retraction is performed by monofil threat, which is anchored to soft tissue at the right crus with a clip. The threat is tied externally, the liver is gently retracted. Another threat can be used to retract the ligamentum teres hepatis in order to provide good exposure at the pyloric region

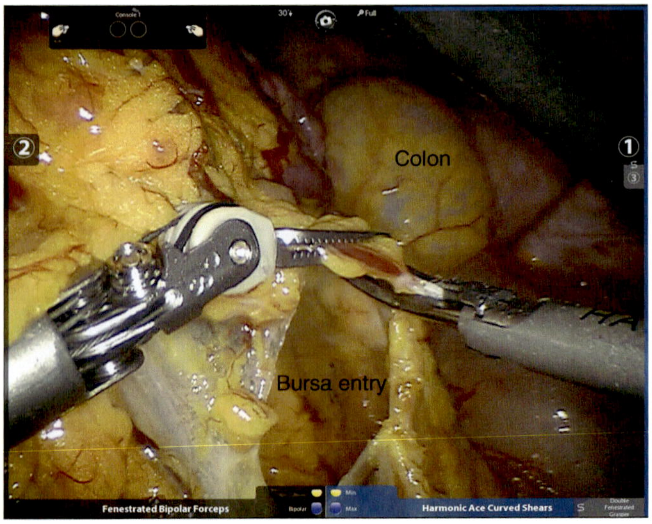

Fig. 17.3 The dissection begins with the omentectomy, and access to the bursa omentalis is achieved. In case of advanced gastric cancer, a total omentectomy is performed close to the transverse colon; in case of early gastric cancer, a partial omentectomy is indicated. In both cases, lymph node station 4sb remains at the specimen side

Omentectomy (Figs. 17.3, 17.4, and 17.5)

Left Gastroepiploic Vessels (Figs. 17.6 and 17.7)

Infrapyloric Area (Figs. 17.8, 17.9, 17.10, 17.11, 17.12, and 17.13)

Common Hepatic Artery (Figs. 17.14, 17.15, and 17.16)

Right Gastric Artery and Hepatoduodenal Ligament (Figs. 17.17, 17.18, 17.19, 17.20, 17.21, and 17.22)

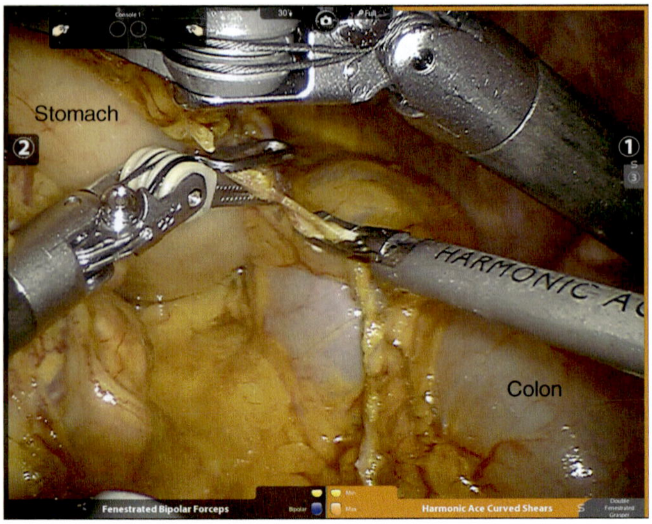

Fig. 17.4 The omentectomy is firstly directed toward the spleen and the left gastroepiploic vessels

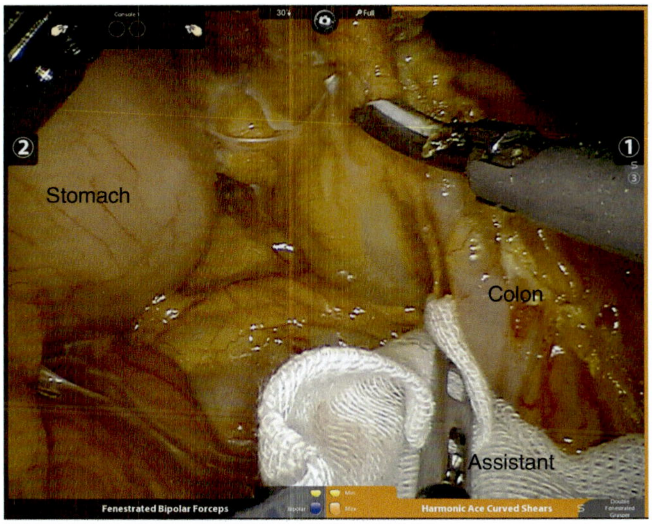

Fig. 17.5 The assistant can gently give countertraction by pushing the colon aside. This way, the dissection can follow the transverse colon toward the lower border of the spleen

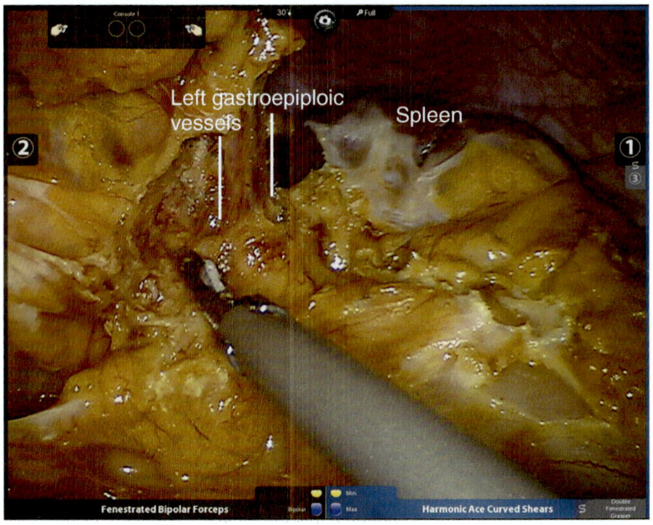

Fig. 17.6 The left gastroepiploic vessels are dissected and can be clipped. If access is not easy, the completion of the fundus region including lymph node station 4sa can be performed after complete mobilization of the stomach

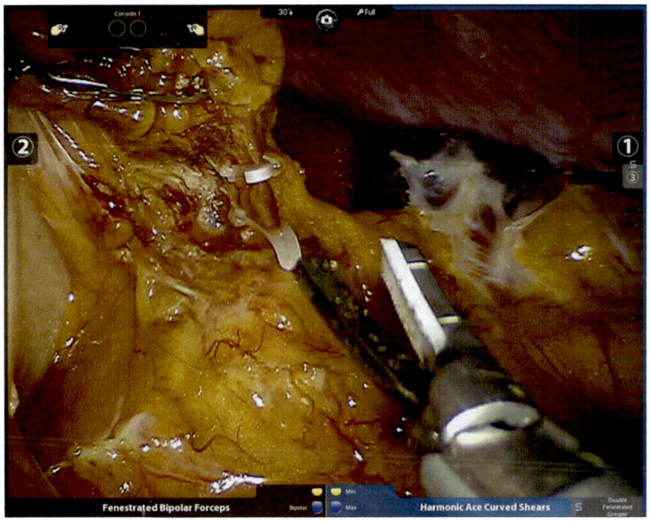

Fig. 17.7 Clipped left gastroepiploic vessels

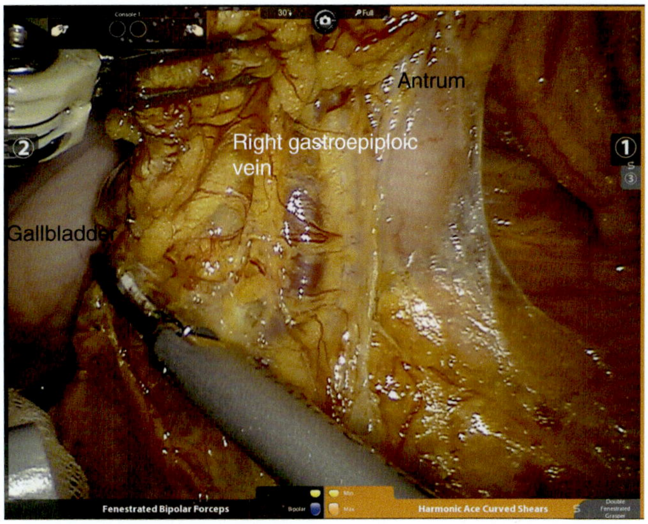

Fig. 17.8 The omentectomy is completed to the distal side, leaving lymph node station 4d at the specimen's side. Right after, the infrapyloric region is identified and dissected. The gallbladder is an important anatomical landmark to guide the dissection in direction of the post-pyloric duodenum

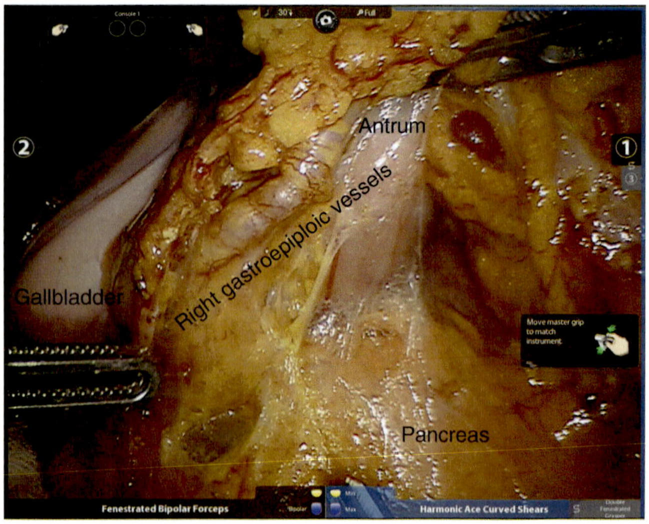

Fig. 17.9 The antrum can be lifted by the third robotic arm in order to separate the posterior pyloric region from the pancreas, until the gastroduodenal artery appears

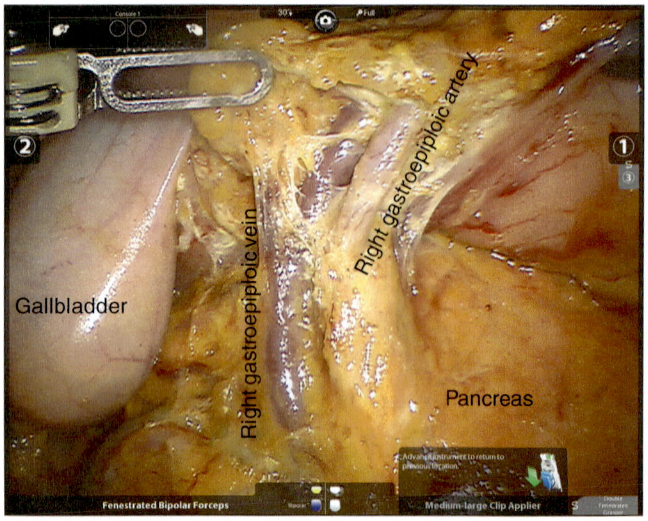

Fig. 17.10 The right gastroepiploic vessels are dissected, and lymph node station 6 remains with the specimen. Attention has to be paid not to injure the pancreas

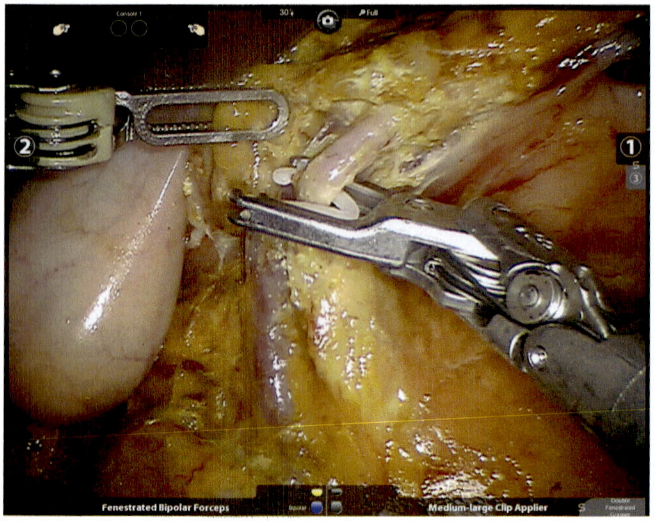

Fig. 17.11 The gastroepiploic vessels are clipped

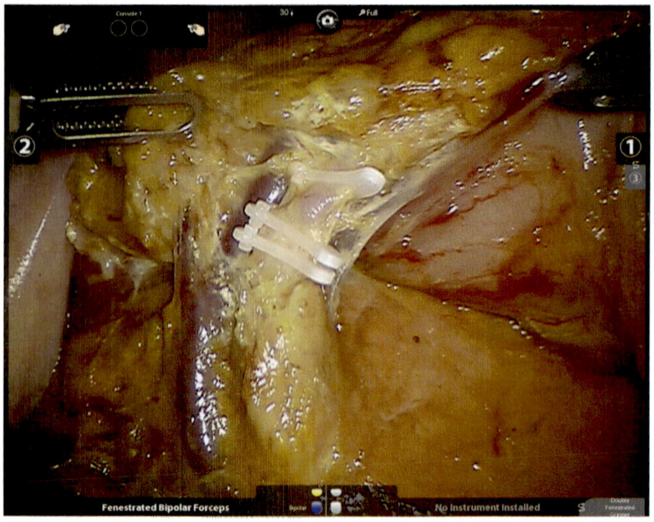

Fig. 17.12 The gastroepiploic vessels before being cut

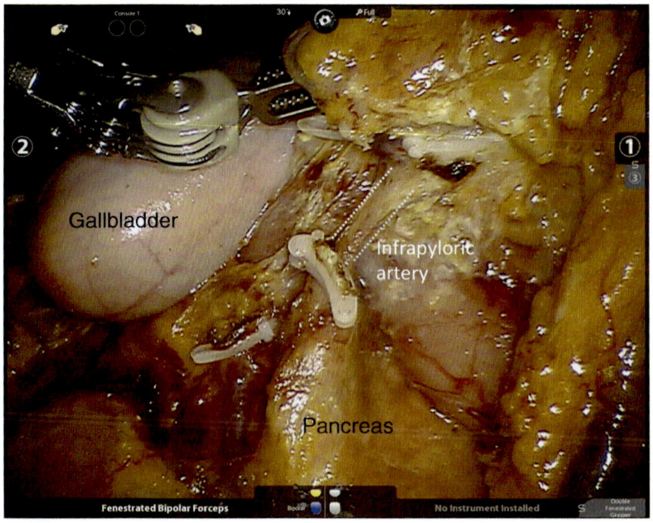

Fig. 17.13 Attention has to be paid to an infrapyloric artery, which can arise from the gastroduodenal artery. It often appears behind the right gastroepiploic artery and should be clipped separately

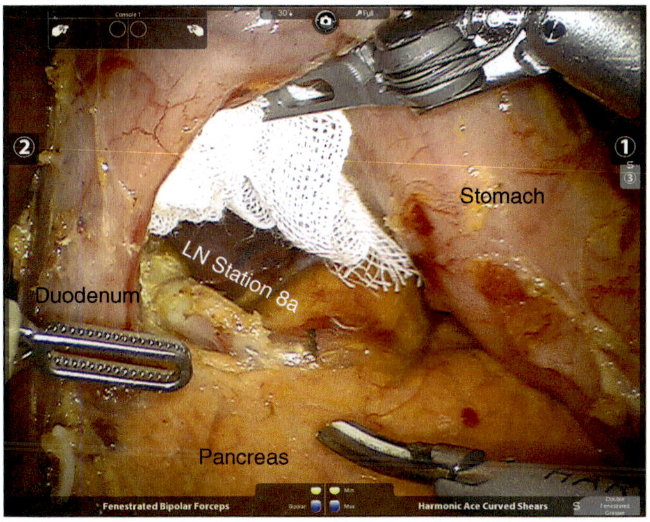

Fig. 17.15 The upper pancreatic border should be surely identified to safely dissection the lymphatic tissue above the common hepatic artery

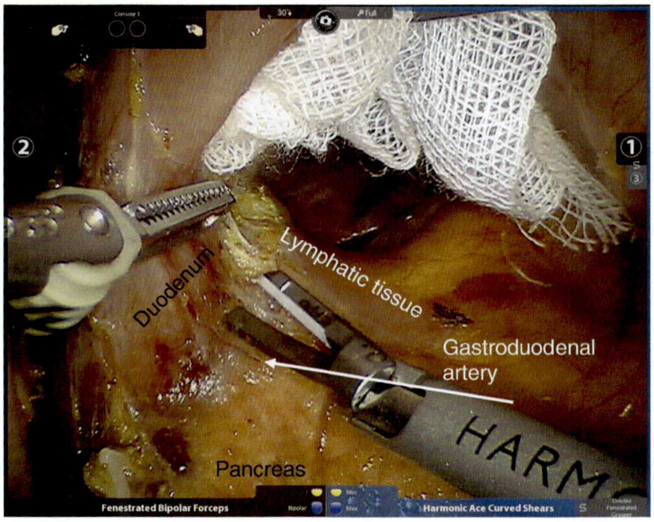

Fig. 17.14 The dissected lymph node station 6 is brought to the proximal side in order to receive a good distal transection line. By lifting the antrum, the dissection of lymph node station 8 can be already performed

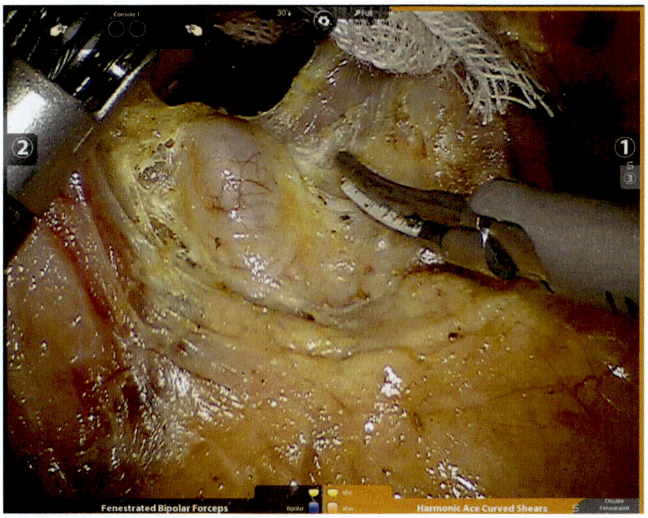

Fig. 17.16 By dissection the tissue in direction to the celiac trunk, lymph node station 8 (common hepatic artery) and lymph node station 12 (proper hepatic artery) are separated, lymph node station 8 remains with the celiac trunk tissue, and lymph node station 12 remains with the right gastric vessel tissue (lymph node station 5). An en bloc resection should be performed in any case

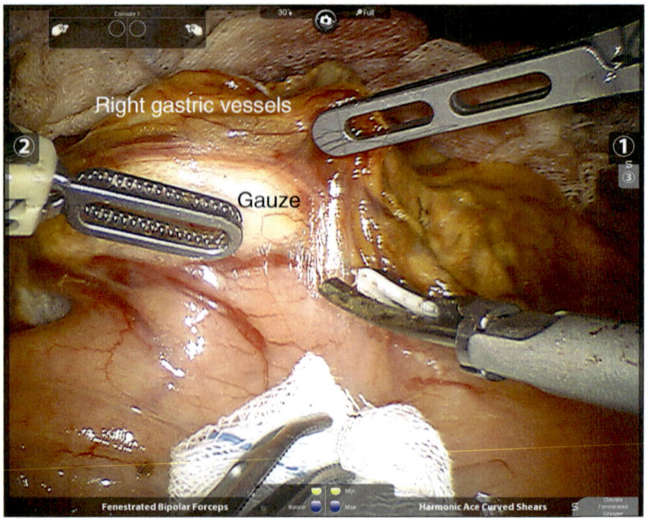

Fig. 17.17 By putting gauze in the lesser sac, the perigastric tissue on the lesser distal curvature side in direction to the hepatoduodenal ligament can be dissected

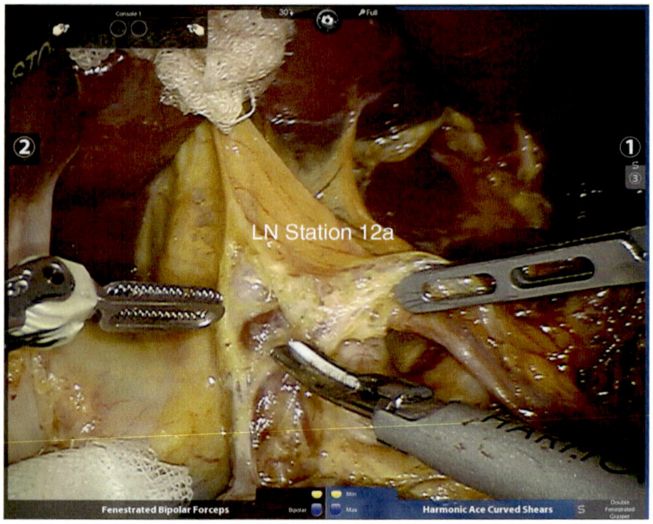

Fig. 17.19 The origin of the right gastric vessels is identified

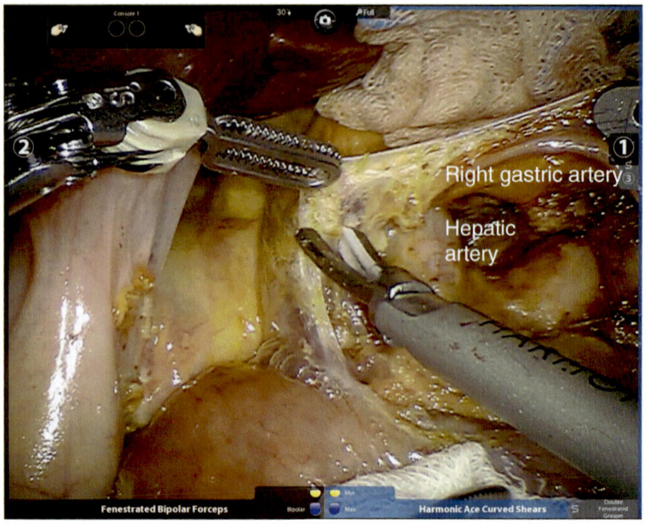

Fig. 17.18 Assof the dissection along the common hepatic artery, the planes can be identified more easily. Traction and countertraction can be performed by two robotic arms, while the assistant can triangulate by gently pushing the pylorus downward

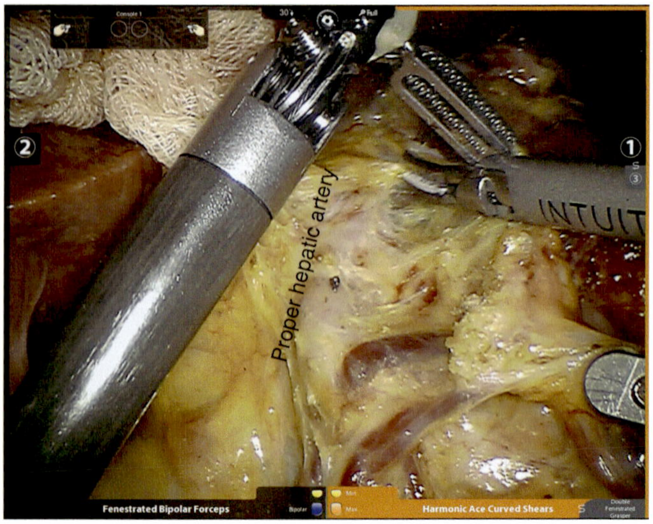

Fig. 17.20 Lymph node station 12 is harvested by dissecting the tissue on the proper hepatic artery

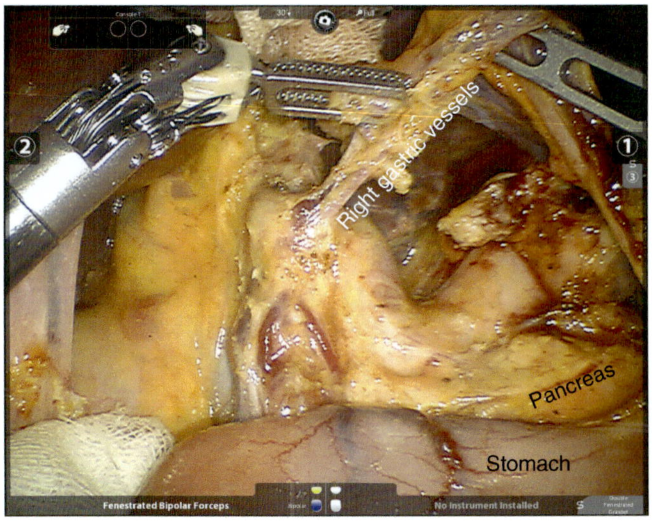

Fig. 17.21 The roots of the right gastric vessels are dissected at its roots

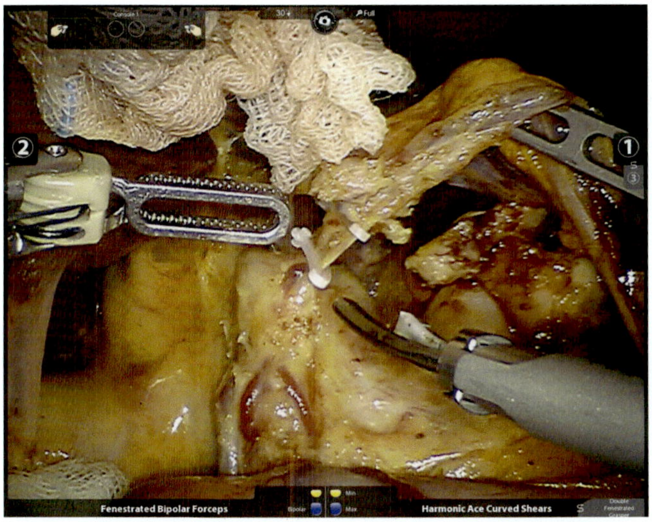

Fig. 17.22 The right gastric vessels are clipped and separated

Distal Transection (Figs. 17.23 and 17.24)

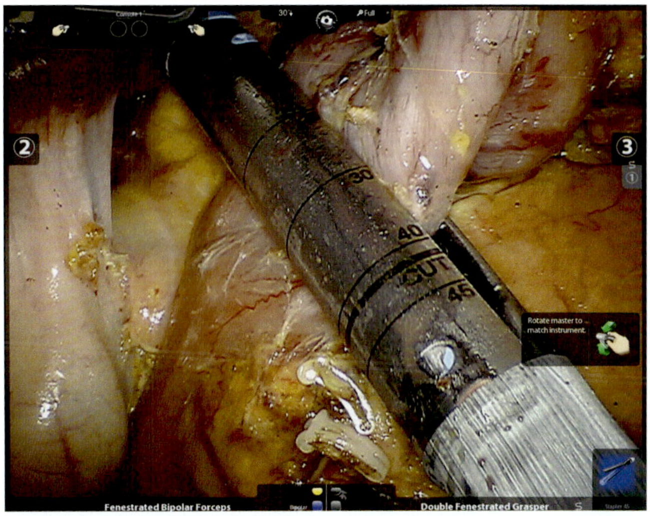

Fig. 17.23 Now the duodenal transection can be performed safely by linear stapler

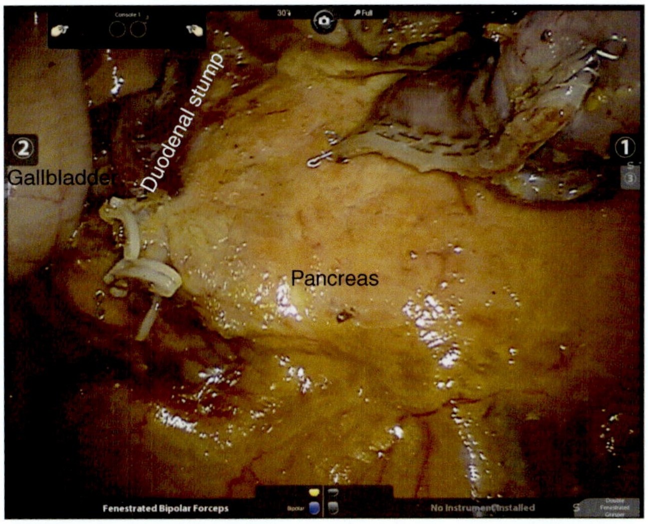

Fig. 17.24 View after distal transection

Celiac Trunk (Figs. 17.25, 17.26, 17.27, 17.28, 17.29, and 17.30)

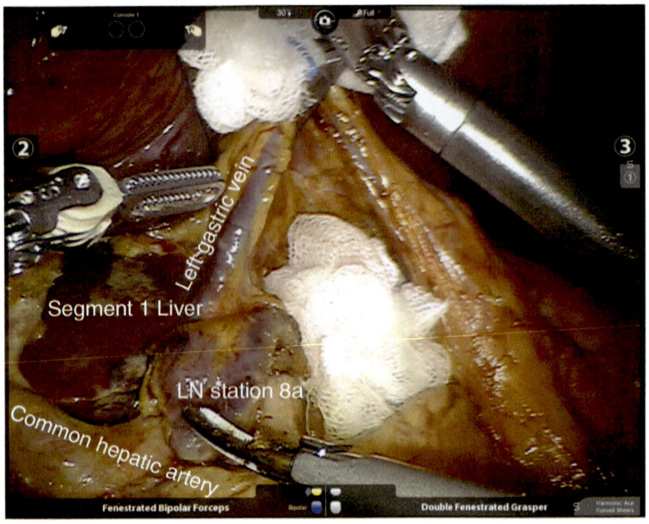

Fig. 17.25 After distal transection, the suprapancreatic lymph node dissection can be completed. The third robotic arm can hold the vascular pedicle of the left gastric artery and retract the liver at the same time

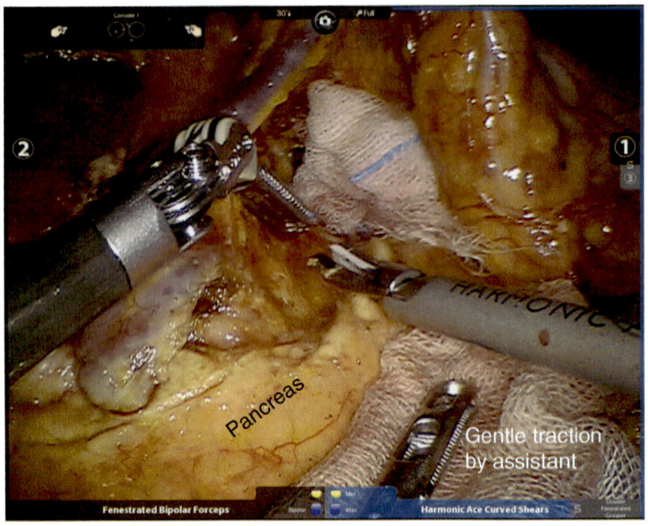

Fig. 17.26 The dissection is guided by the upper pancreatic border. The assistant can use a gauze to gently roll the pancreas and deliver countertraction

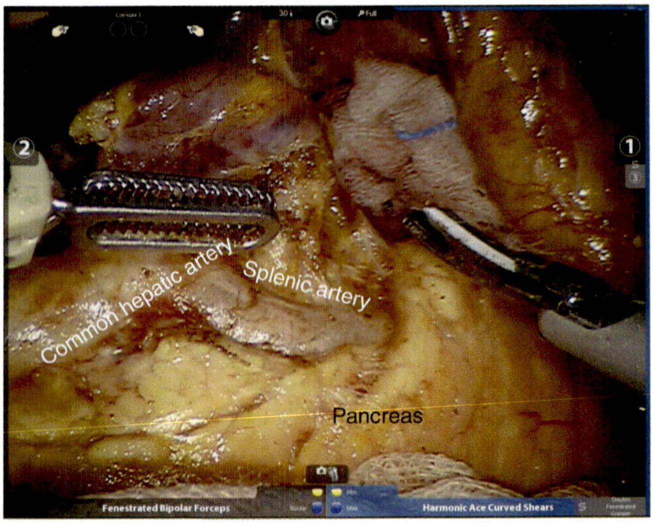

Fig. 17.27 The celiac trunk and splenic artery are identified before clipping the left gastric artery

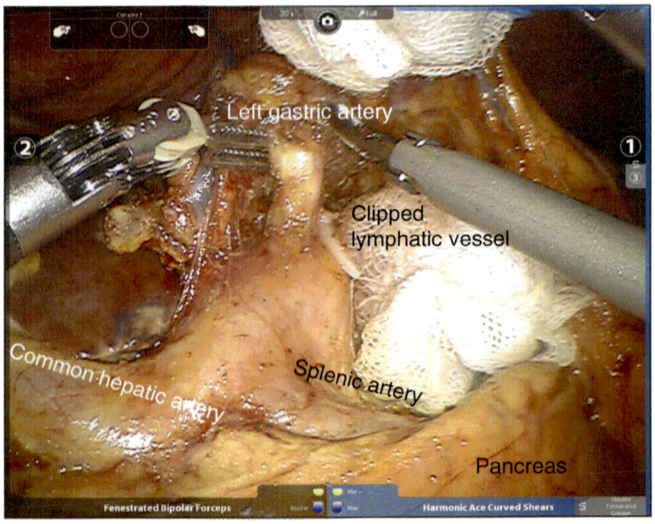

Fig. 17.28 If lymphatic vessel appears in the celiac trunk's region, it can be clipped as well in order to prohibit lymphatic leak

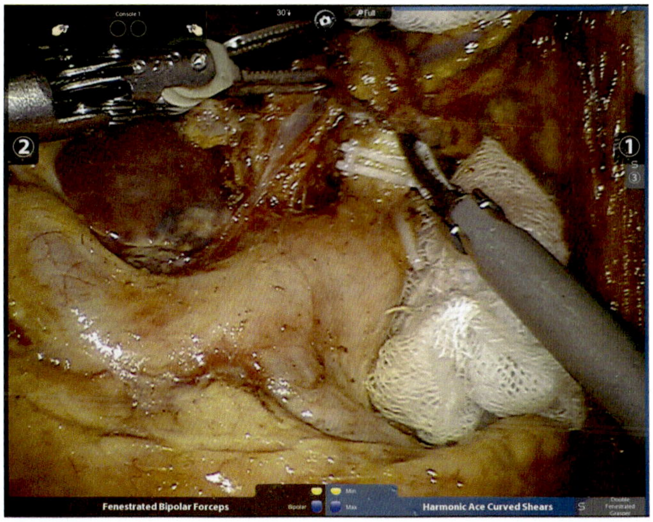

Fig. 17.29 The left gastric artery and the left gastric vain are clipped separately

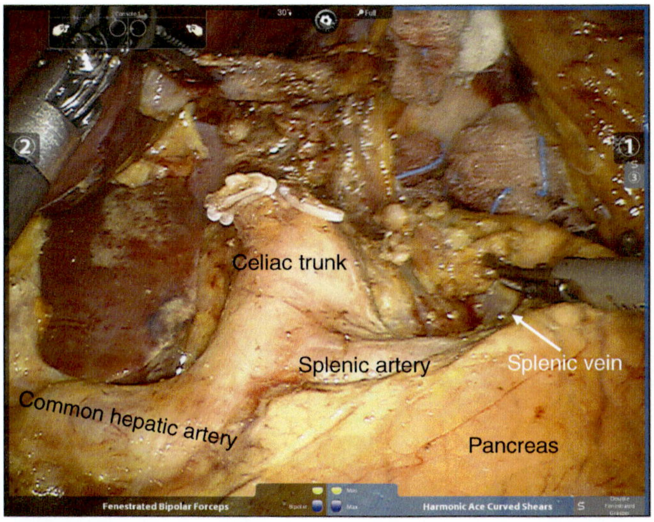

Fig. 17.30 View after the left gastric artery is cut

Splenic Vessels (Figs. 17.31, 17.32, 17.33, and 17.34)

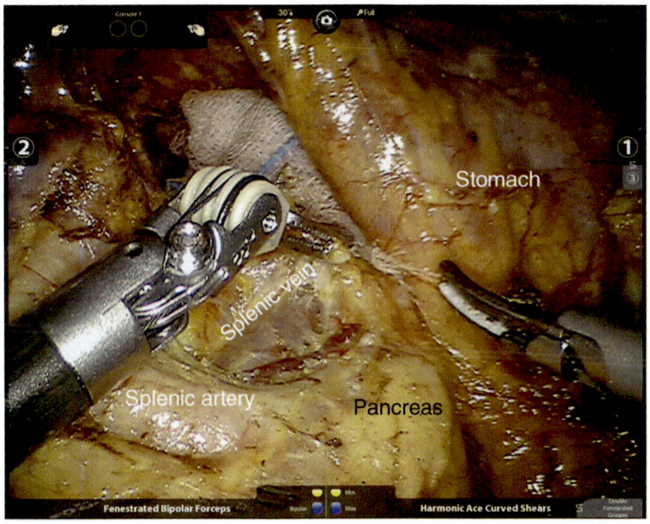

Fig. 17.31 The suprapancreatic dissection is completed by dissecting lymph node station 11 along the splenic vessels. For a radical dissection, the splenic vain is visualized

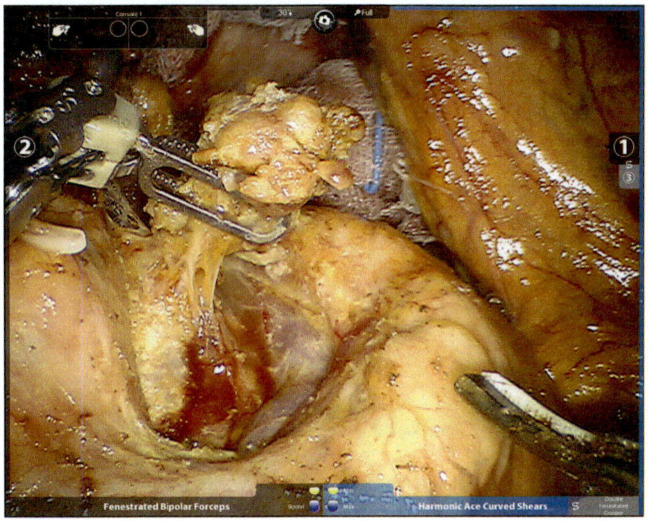

Fig. 17.32 For this step the countertraction of the assistant is of high importance in order to safely dissect on the pancreatic border without injure to the splenic vessels

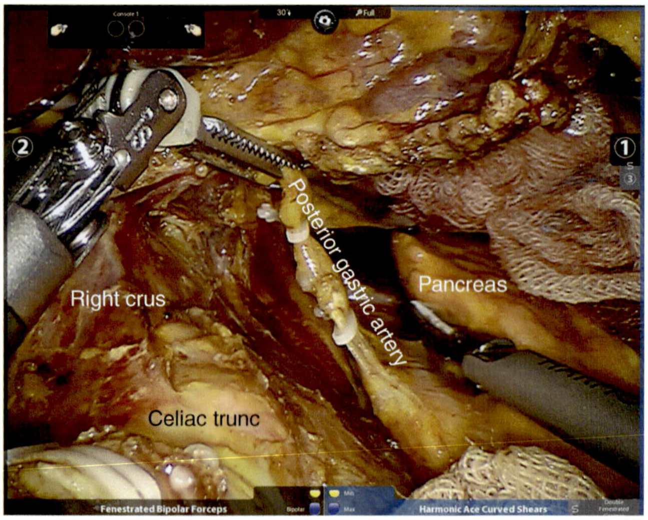

Fig. 17.33 Following the splenic artery on the suprapancreatic border, a posterior gastric artery can be identified, clipped, and separated. It appears on the level of hiatus and the border between lymph node stations 11p and 11d

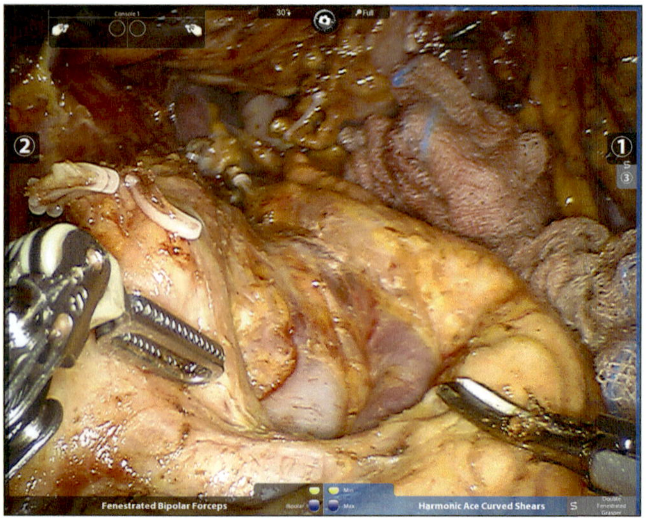

Fig. 17.34 The suprapancreatic lymph node dissection is completed. Sight from the celiac trunk in direction to the spleen

Fundus (Figs. 17.35 and 17.36)

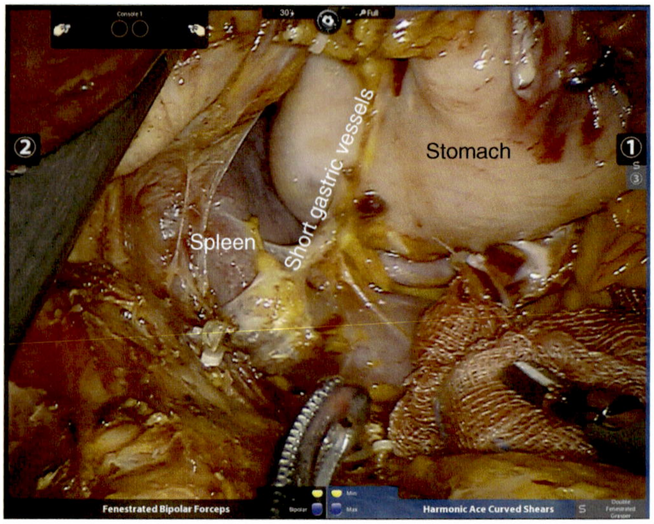

Fig. 17.35 Now the remnant short gastric vessels can be safely dissected from the upper side

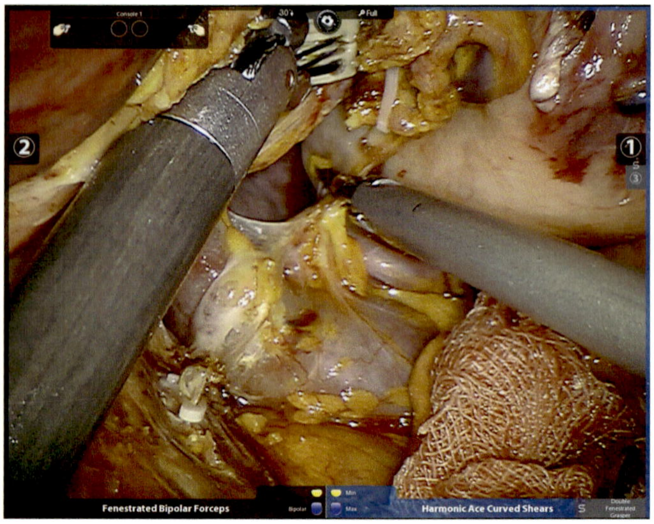

Fig. 17.36 The previous complete mobilization of the stomach provides good exposure of the area

Esophagus (Fig. 17.37)

Anvil and Proximal Transection (Figs. 17.38, 17.39, 17.40, 17.41, 17.42, 17.43, 17.44, 17.45, and 17.46)

Reconstruction (Figs. 17.47, 17.48, 17.49, and 17.50)

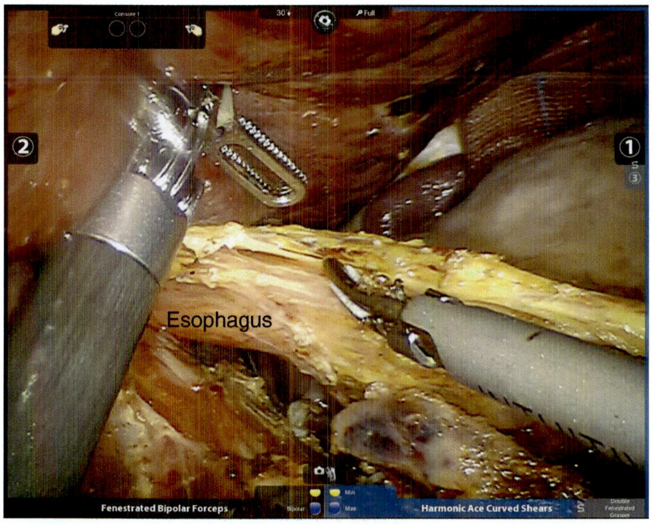

Fig. 17.37 The esophagus is cleared of tissue; the vagus nerves are cut which gives some extra length for reconstruction. This is the last step of the resection, and the robotic system is undocked afterward

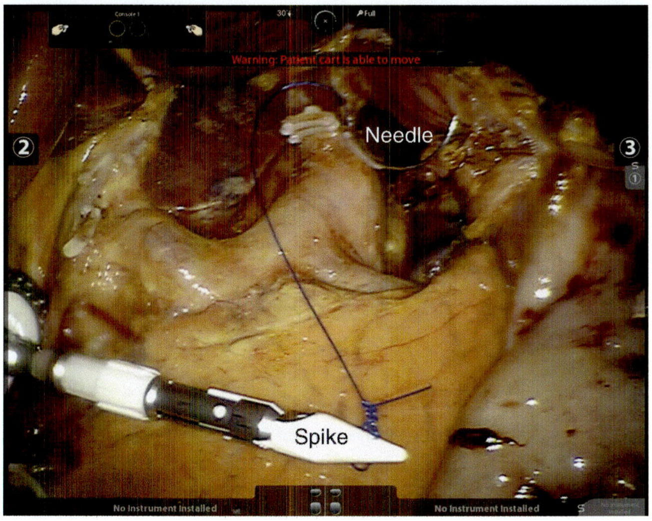

Fig. 17.38 The anvil is used with spike, which is connected to a 2-0 monofil threat with needle. The anvil is put intraabdominally through midline minilaparotomy, which will be used to also retrieve the specimen as well as perform the esophagojejunostomy later on

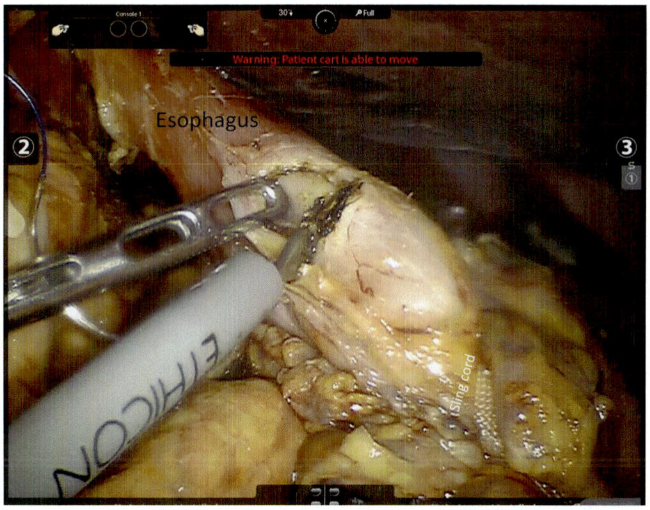

Fig. 17.39 Anterior esophagotomy is performed. The esophagus can be retracted by a sling cord that is pulled by the assistant

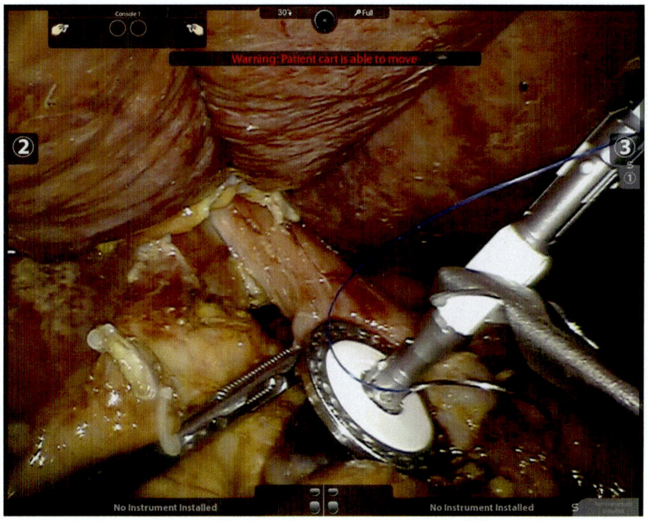

Fig. 17.40 The anvil is put into the esophagus. A 25 mm anvil is used

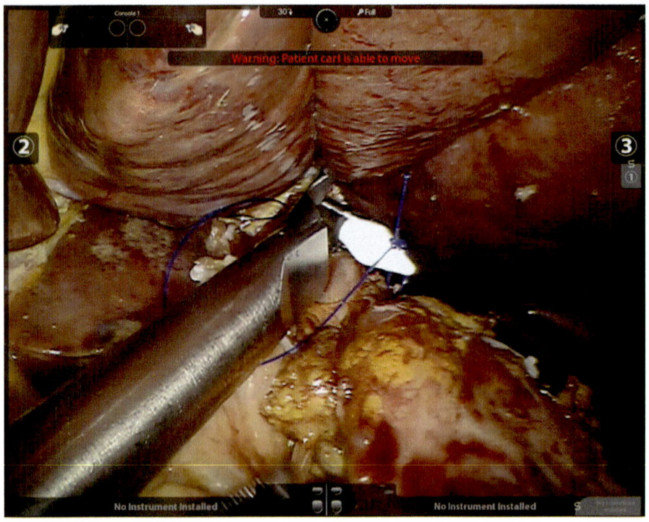

Fig. 17.41 The anvil needs to be pushed gently to the right direction

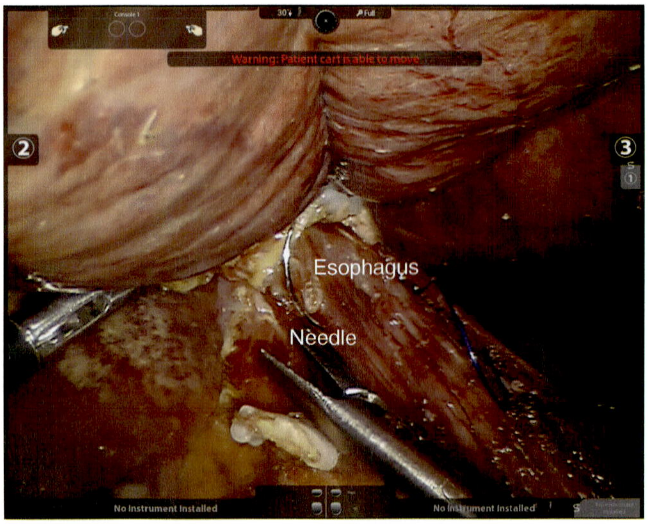

Fig. 17.42 After the anvil is pushed into the esophagus' lumen, the needle is stitched inside out to the right lateral esophagus wall above the level of esophagotomy

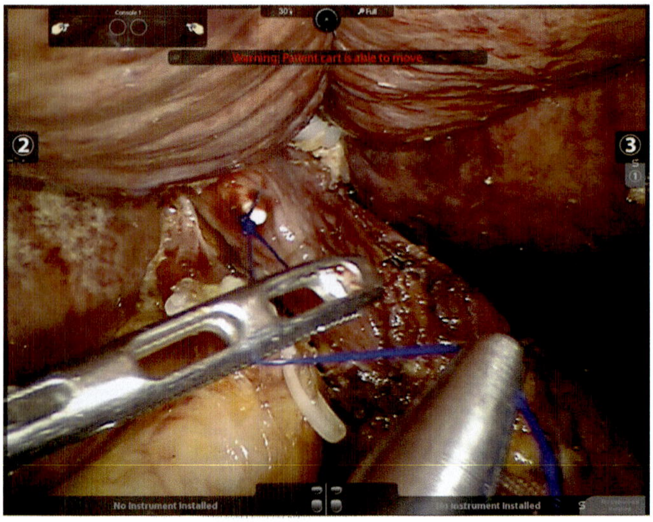

Fig. 17.43 The anvil is pulled through partly

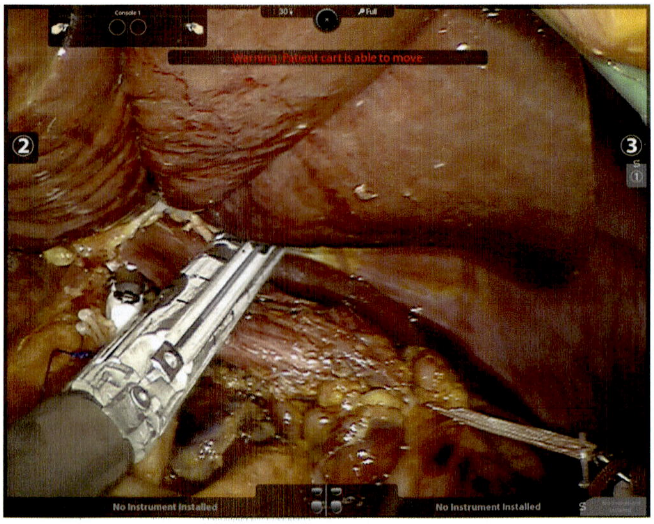

Fig. 17.44 The proximal transection can be performed, covering the esophagotomy. The esophagus is retracted again using the sling cord surrounding the cardia region

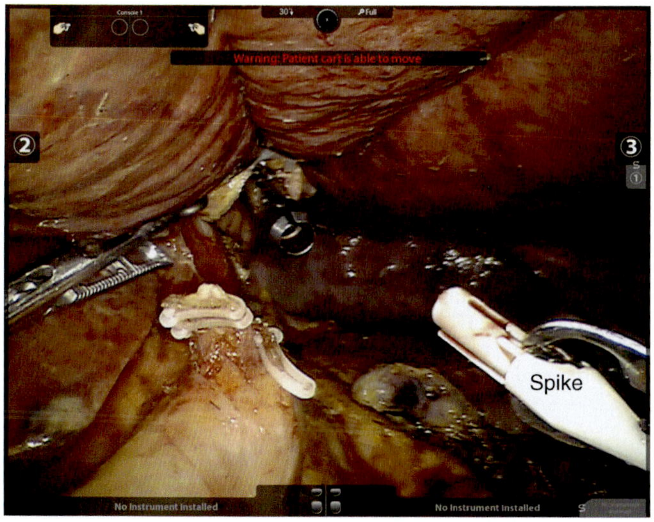

Fig. 17.45 The anvil is now pulled through and the spike is removed

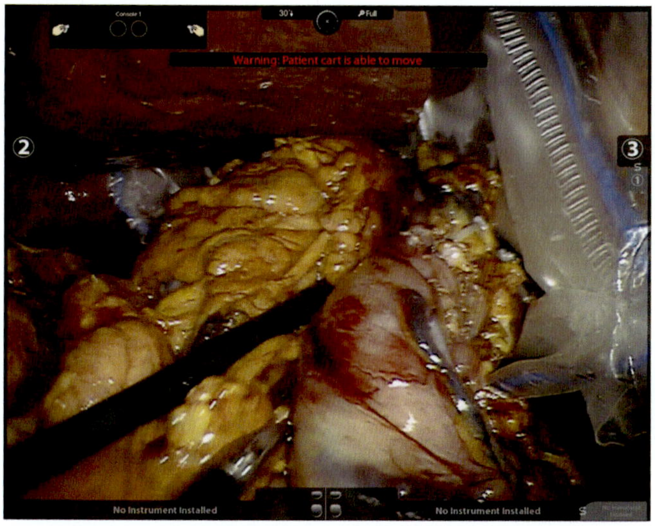

Fig. 17.46 The specimen is retrieved in a bag

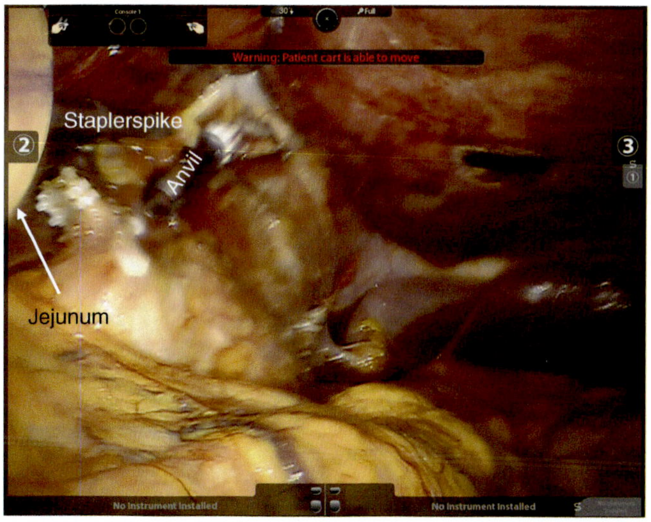

Fig. 17.47 After performing the jejunojejunostomy extracorporeally, the jejunum is fixed on the stapler with a vessel loop. The desired location of anastomosis is marked with a pen. For stapler entering, the mini-laparotomy at the location of former camera trocar is used

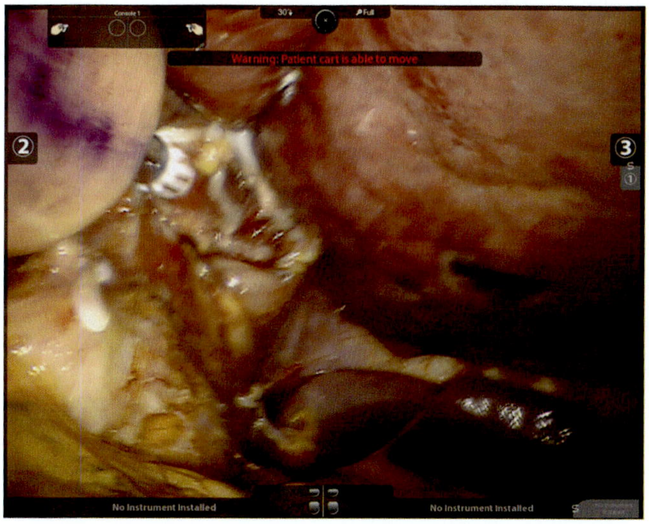

Fig. 17.48 After both ends are connected, the esophagus and jejunum are approximated

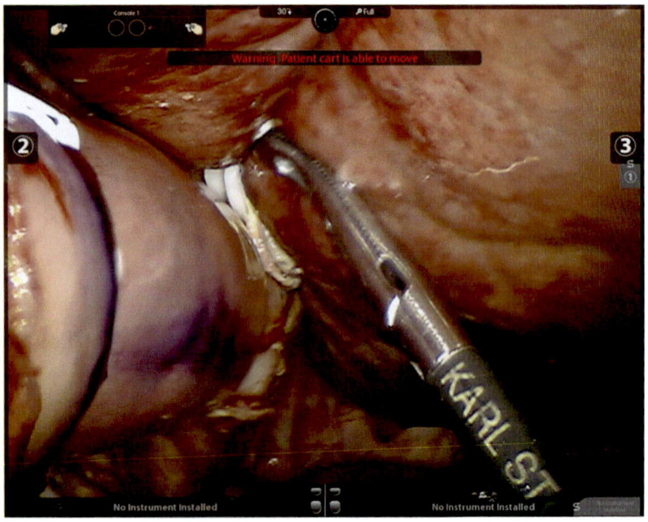

Fig. 17.49 The anastomosis is performed

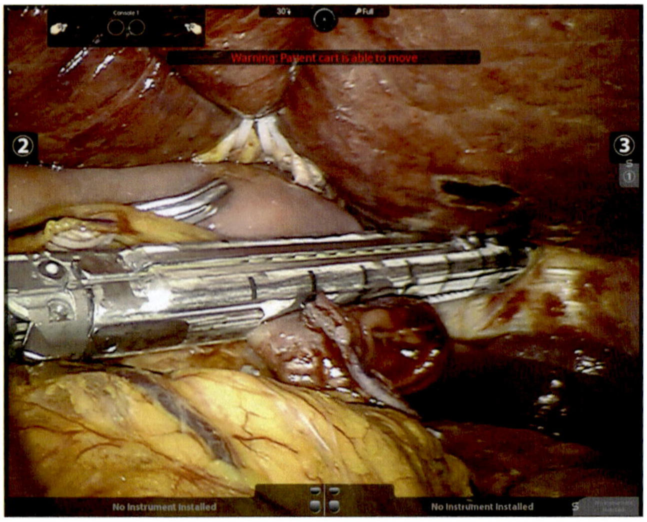

Fig. 17.50 The jejunum is closed by linear stapler. The total gastrectomy is finished

References

1. Hyung WJ, Yang HK, Park YK, et al. Long-term outcomes of laparoscopic distal gastrectomy for locally advanced gastric cancer: the KLASS-02-RCT randomized clinical trial. J Clin Oncol. 2020;38(28):3304–13. https://doi.org/10.1200/JCO.20.01210. Epub 2020 Aug 20.
2. Kim HI, Han SU, Yang HK, et al. Multicenter prospective comparative study of robotic versus laparoscopic gastrectomy for gastric adenocarcinoma. Ann Surg. 2016;263(1):103–9. https://doi.org/10.1097/SLA.0000000000001249.
3. Park JM, Kim HI, Han SU. Who may benefit from robotic gastrectomy?: a subgroup analysis of multicenter prospective comparative study data on robotic versus laparoscopic gastrectomy. Eur J Surg Oncol. 2016;42(12):1944–9. https://doi.org/10.1016/j.ejso.2016.07.012. Epub 2016 Jul 29.

Robot-Assisted Gastrectomy

18

Adrian Billeter, Martin Wagner, Manuela Capek, and Beat Peter Müller-Stich

Introduction

Gastrectomy remains the only curative treatment for gastric cancer. Minimally invasive surgery has convincingly shown to achieve similar oncologic outcomes as open surgery while reducing morbidity and length of hospital stay. While laparoscopic assisted gastrectomy has been widely established in recent years, robotic surgery may offer some additional benefits such as better visualization and better means for manipulating the tissue as well as the ability to perform complex reconstructions. Furthermore, the robotic platform may allow for a more complete lymphadenectomy compared to open or laparoscopic gastrectomy.

When performing robot-assisted gastrectomy, we suggest performing the resection in a clockwise fashion. We start with the dissection of the lesser omentum followed by dissection of the hiatus. This part is completed by the dissection of the gastrophrenic ligament followed by the dissection of the short gastric vessels until the splenic artery in the splenic hilum has been reached. Then, the greater omentum is dissected from the transvers colon. This step is completed by the lymphadenectomy above and around the splenic artery (lymph nodes of stations 10 and 11). The greater omentum is then completely dissected from the colon and hepatic flexure until the anterior duodenum can be seen. After this step, the lymphatic pedicle of the right epiploic vessels is dissected at the origin. After that, the duodenum is transected, and the lymphadenectomy around the common hepatic artery and hepatoduodenal ligament is performed until the portal vein is reached (lymph nodes of station 12).

During these steps, the right gastric artery is also cut at the base including the lymphatic vessels. Lastly, the lymphadenectomy is completed toward the coeliac axis with transection of the left gastric vessels including the coronary vein and left gastric artery (lymph nodes of station 12). This step is finalized by the lymphadenectomy toward the dorsal conjunction of the diaphragmatic crura. Next the esophagus is mobilized and transected. The reconstruction is performed by using a linear stapled side-to-side Roux-en-Y reconstruction as commonly used during bariatric surgery. The biliopancreatic limb is anastomosed using a linear stapler anastomosis with the esophagus followed by the jejunojejunostomy. Both anastomoses are performed about 50 cm from the duodenojejunal flexure and the esophagojejunostomy, respectively.

Lastly, the two anastomoses are divided by transection of the jejunum between the esophagojejunostomy and the jejunojejunostomy. Thereby, the candy cane is formed. The mesenteric defects of the jejunojejunostomy and the Peterson defect are closed to prevent internal hernias. Usually, we also remove the gallbladder although this step is not performed by all surgeons. The patency of the esophagojejunostomy can be tested by a large gastric calibration tube (42 French), and the esophagojejunostomy can be tested using a methylene blue leak test. The resected stomach is removed through a small Pfannenstiel incision for cosmetic reasons and to reduce postoperative pain and risk of incisional hernias. Frozen sections of the resection margins are performed before reconstruction.

A. Billeter · M. Wagner · M. Capek · B. P. Müller-Stich (✉)
Department for General, Visceral and Transplantation Surgery, Division for Minimally Invasive and Robot-Assisted Surgery, Division for Upper Gastrointestinal Surgery, Heidelberg University Hospital, Heidelberg, Germany
e-mail: beat.mueller@med.uni-heidelberg.de

O. Y. Kudsi, P. P. Grimminger (eds.), *Atlas of Robotic Upper Gastrointestinal Surgery*,
https://doi.org/10.1007/978-3-030-86578-8_18

Procedure

Positioning of Trocars and Diagnostic Laparoscopy (Fig. 18.1)

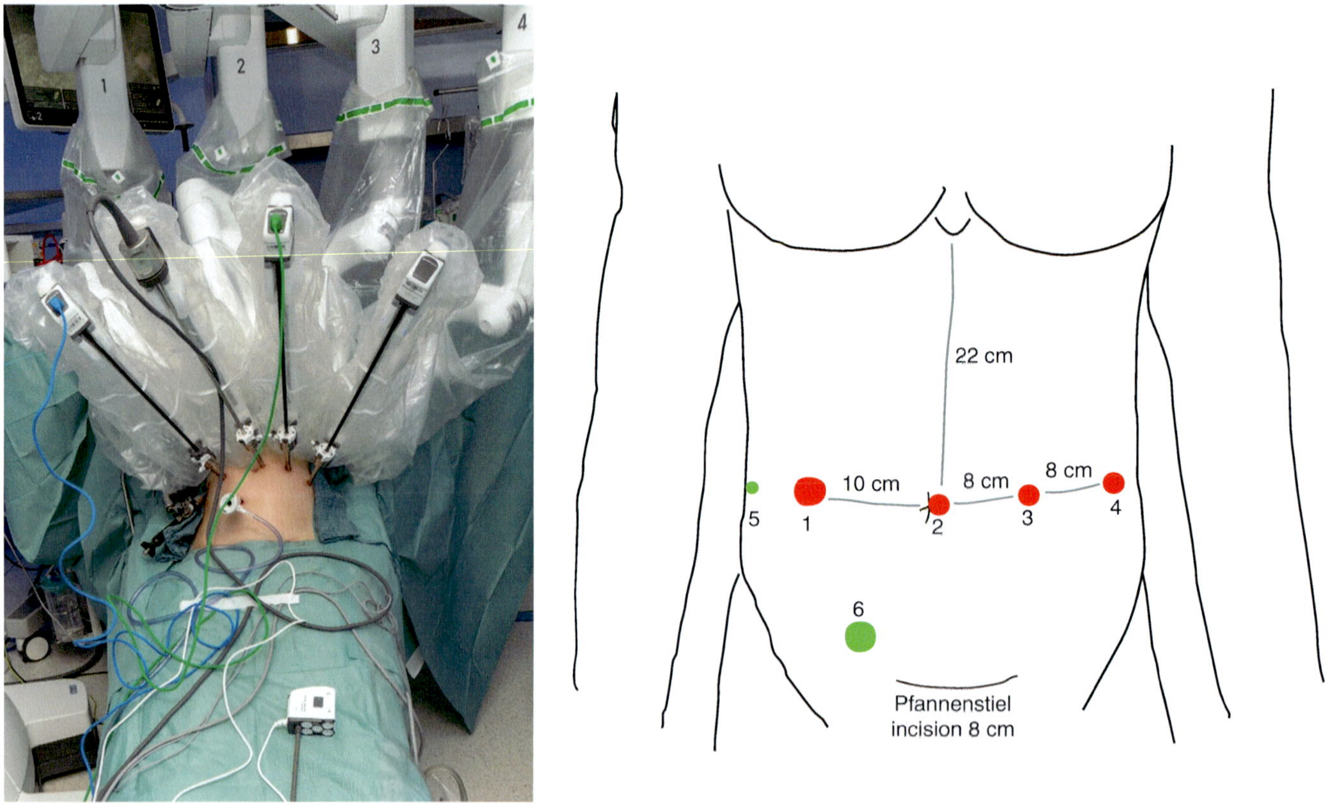

Fig. 18.1 Trocar positioning
1. 12 mm robotic trocar
2–4. 8 mm robotic trocar
5. 5 mm assistant trocar for the liver retractor
6. 12 mm assistant trocar
Distance between trocar 1 and 2 is 8–10 cm. Distance between trocars 2–4 is 7–8 cm. The line at the bottom marks the Pfannenstiel incision line

Dissection of the Lesser Omentum, Hiatus, and Gastrophrenic Ligament (Figs. 18.2, 18.3, 18.4, 18.5, 18.6, 18.7, 18.8, and 18.9)

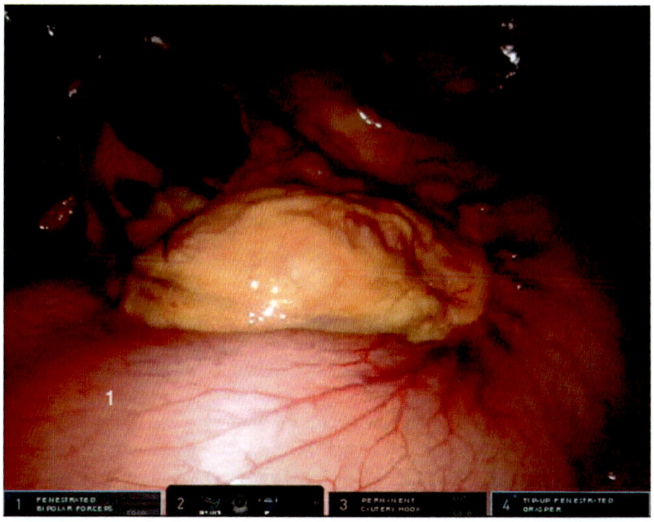

Fig. 18.2 Overview
1. Stomach

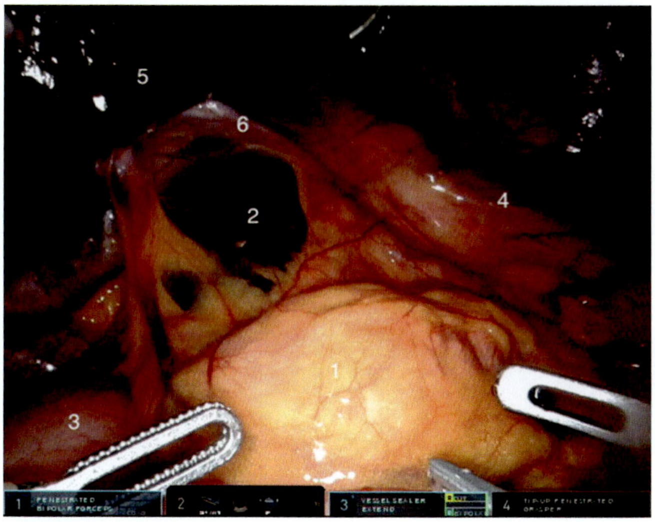

Fig. 18.3 Overview
1. Pancreas
2. Lesser omentum
3. Duodenum
4. Gastric cardia
5. Liver
6. Additional left hepatic artery

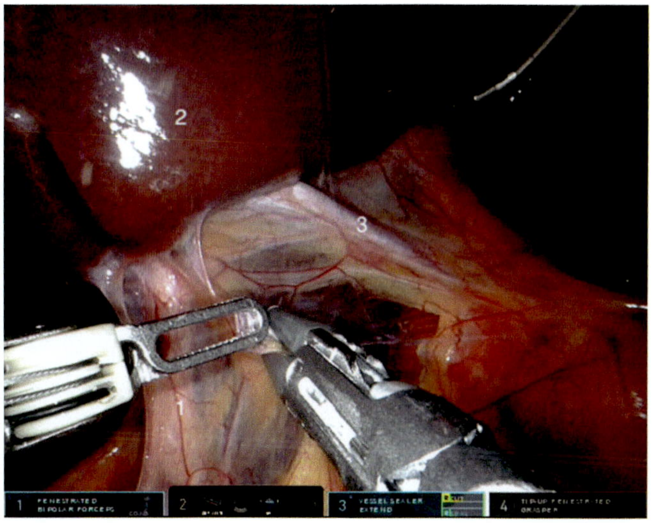

Fig. 18.4 Dissection of the lesser omentum close to the liver. Additional left hepatic artery running through the lesser omentum can be cut if it is not an aberrant left gastric artery (check in the arterial phase of a CT scan). Dissection of the lesser omentum to the right crus of the diaphragm (lymph node station 3)
1. Hepatoduodenal ligament
2. Liver
3. Additional left hepatic artery

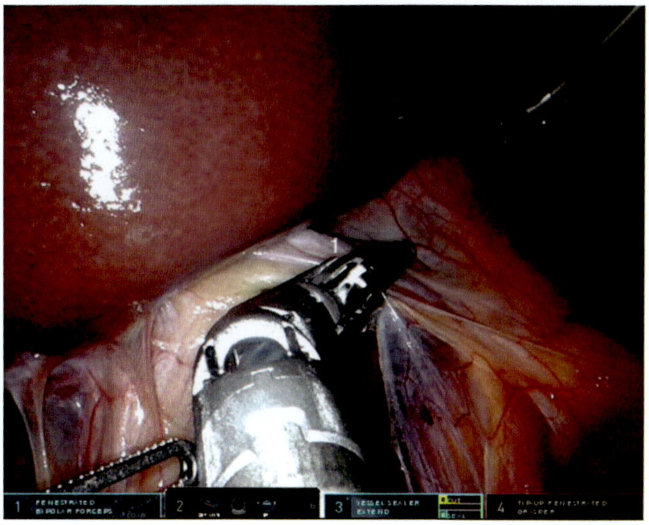

Fig. 18.5 Dissection of the additional hepatic artery using the vessel sealer. In patients with an aberrant left hepatic artery, the vessel must be preserved and the lymph nodes must be dissected from the left gastric artery and coeliac axis
1. Additional left hepatic artery

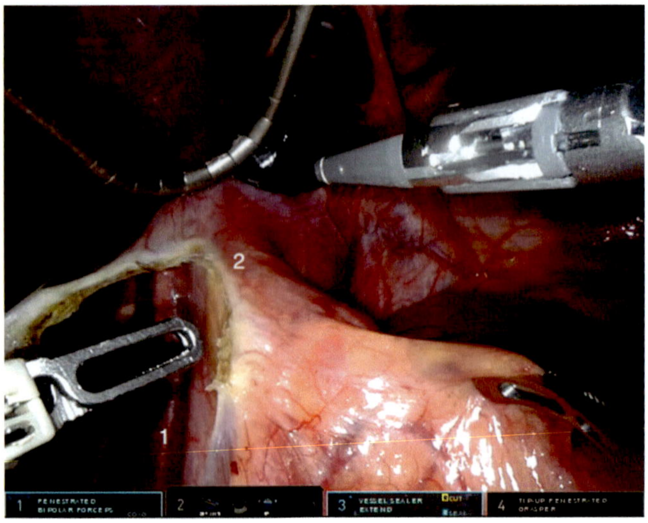

Fig. 18.6 Circular incision of the peritoneum around the hiatus and mobilization of the distal esophagus (lymph node station 1/2)
1. Right crus of the diaphragm
2. Esophagus

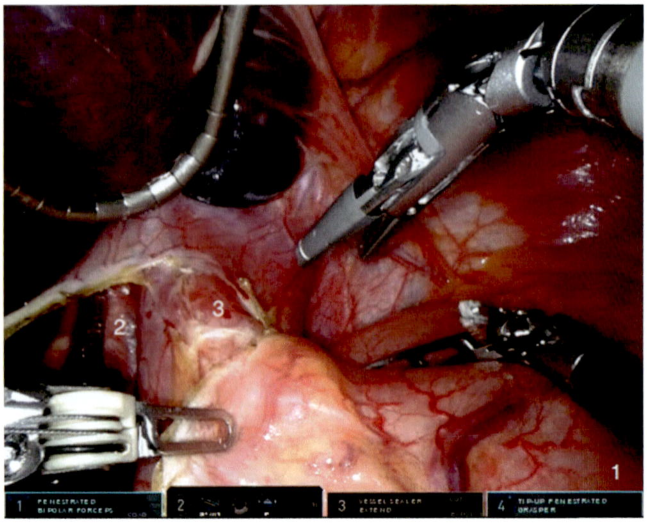

Fig. 18.7 Circular incision of the peritoneum around the hiatus and mobilization of the distal esophagus. The abdominal esophagus can be seen
1. Gastric fundus
2. Right diaphragmatic crus
3. Esophagus

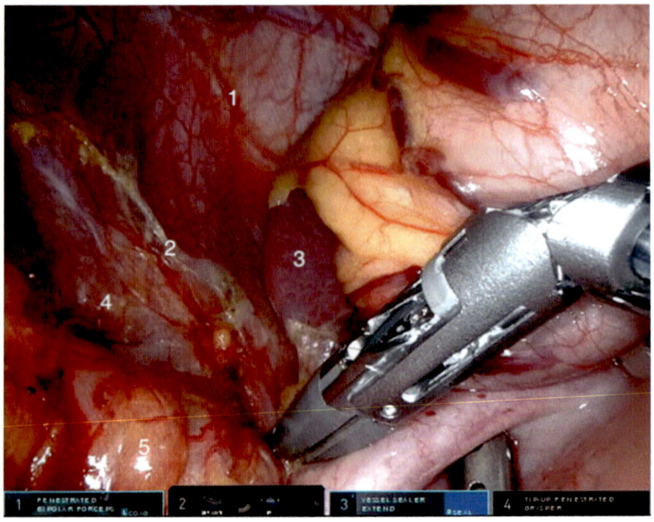

Fig. 18.8 Dissection of the gastrophrenic ligament and mobilization of the gastric fundus. Dissection of the short gastric vessels with the vessel sealer close to the spleen until the splenic artery and vein in splenic hilum
1. Left diaphragm
2. Partially dissected gastrophrenic ligament
3. Upper pole of the spleen
4. Left crus of the diaphragm
5. Gastric cardia

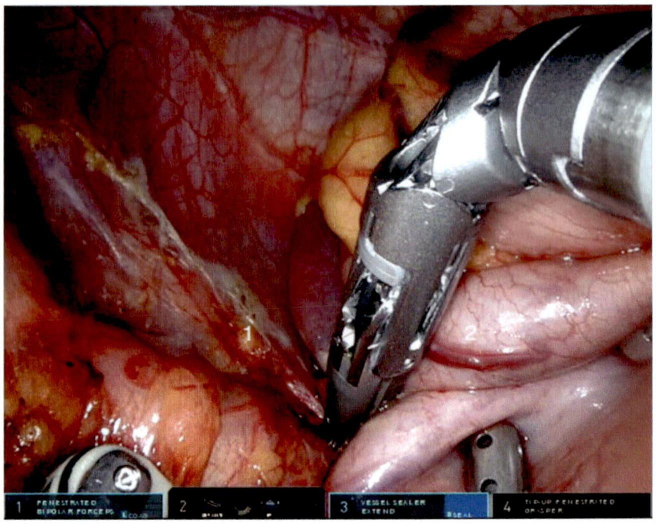

Fig. 18.9 Gastrophrenic ligament
1. Gastrophrenic ligament
2. Completely mobilized gastric fundus

Dissection of the Gastrocolic Ligament (Lymph Node Station 4d) (Figs. 18.10, 18.11, 18.12, 18.13, and 18.14)

Lymphadenectomy Along the Splenic Artery (Lymph Node Station 10/11) (Figs. 18.15, 18.16, 18.17, and 18.18)

Complete Dissection of the Greater Omentum and Mobilization of the Hepatic Flexure (Figs. 18.19, 18.20, and 18.21)

Lymphadenectomy of the Right Gastroepiploic Arcade (Lymph Node Station 6) (Figs. 18.22, 18.23, and 18.24)

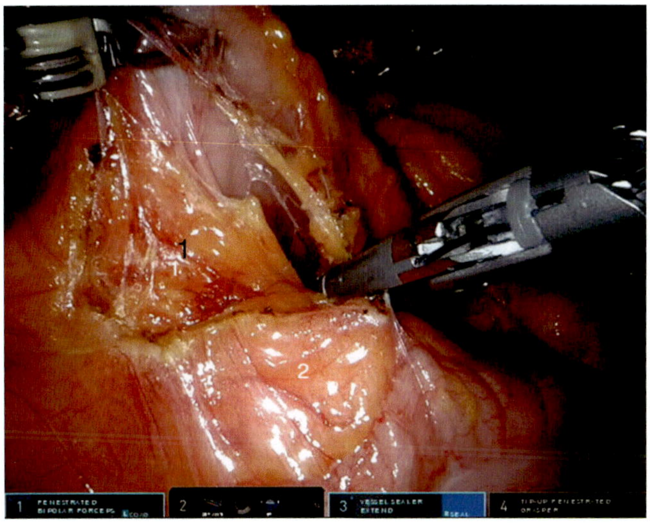

Fig. 18.11 Dissection of the gastrocolic ligament along the transverse colon (Lymph node station 4d)
1. Gastrocolic ligament
2. Transverse colon

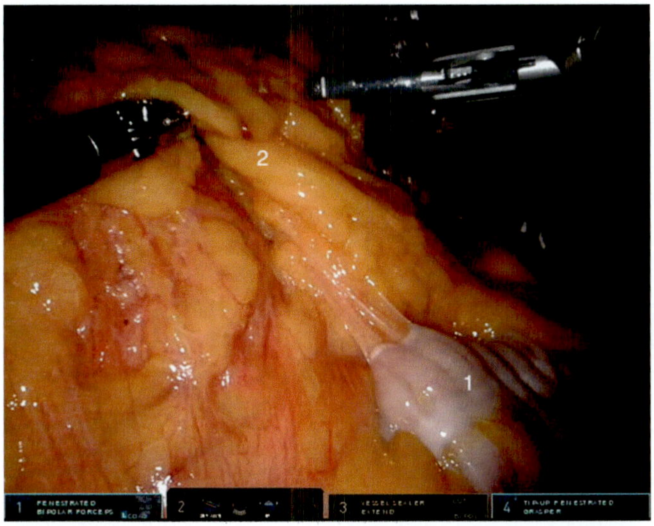

Fig. 18.10 The greater omentum is completely placed on top of the stomach
1. Transverse colon
2. Greater omentum

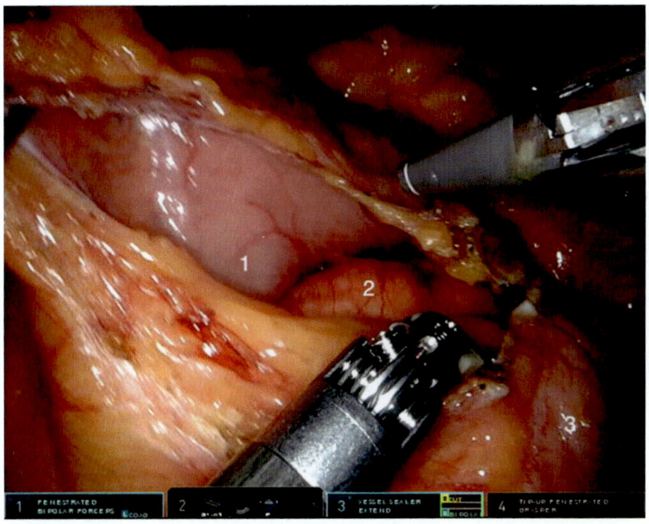

Fig. 18.12 Opening of the lesser sac (bursa omentalis)
1. Back wall of the stomach
2. Pancreas
3. Transverse colon

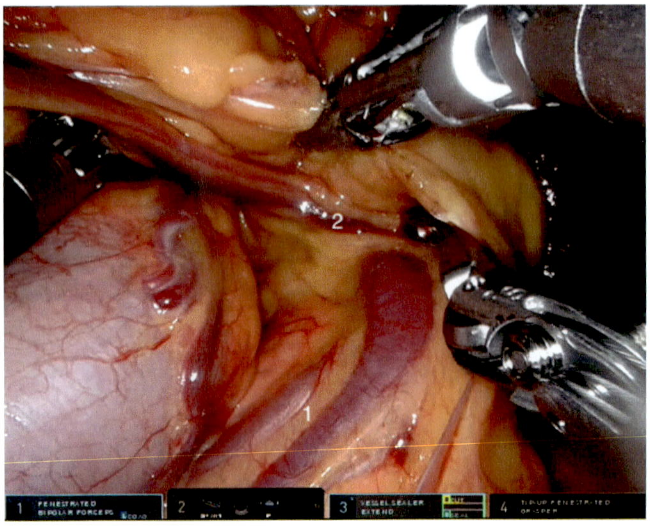

Fig. 18.13 Dissection of the left gastroepiploic vessels, which arise from the splenic vessels
1. Splenic vessels
2. Left gastroepiploic vessels

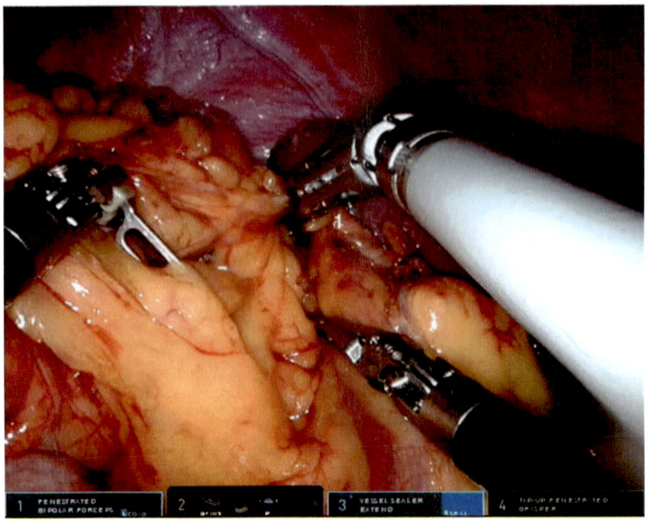

Fig. 18.14 Dissection of the remaining short gastric vessels from the spleen upward to the gastric fundus
1. Short gastric vessels

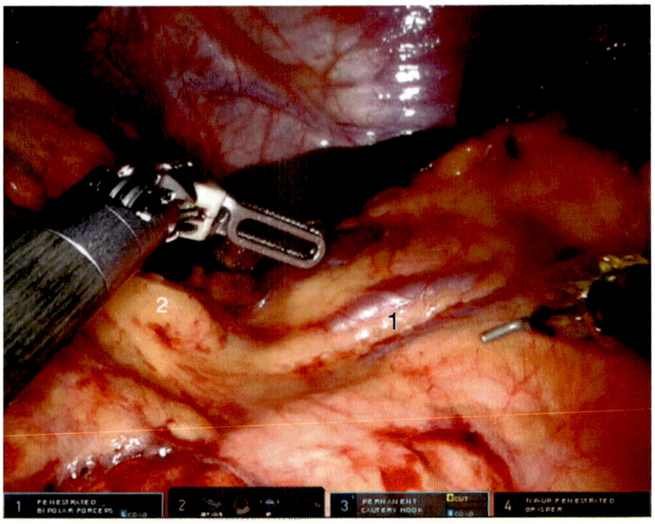

Fig. 18.15 Lymphadenectomy along the splenic vessels (lymph node station 10/11)
1. Splenic vessels
2. Lymph node station 10/11

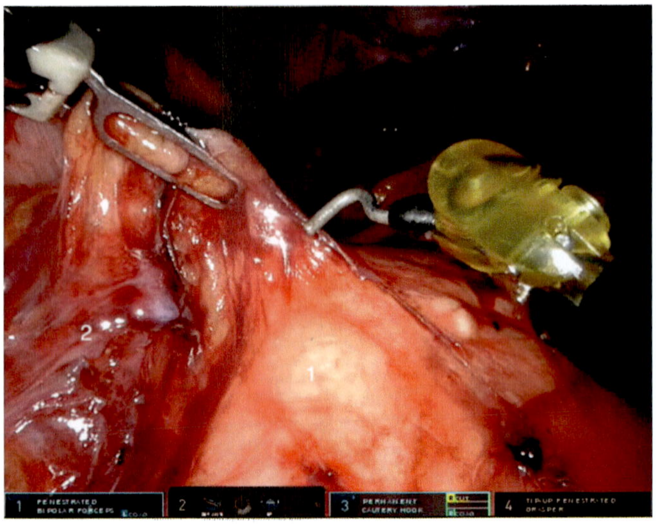

Fig. 18.16 Lymphadenectomy along the splenic vessels (lymph node station 10/11)
1. Pancreas
2. Lymph nodes

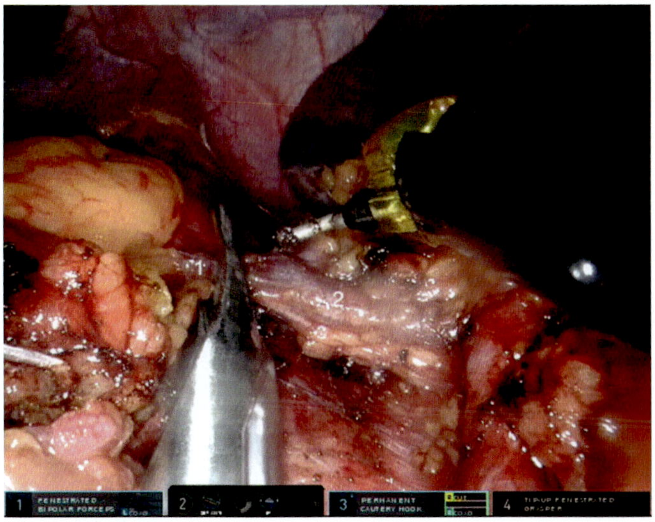

Fig. 18.17 Clipping and cutting of the posterior gastric artery
1. Posterior gastric artery
2. Upper pole artery of the spleen

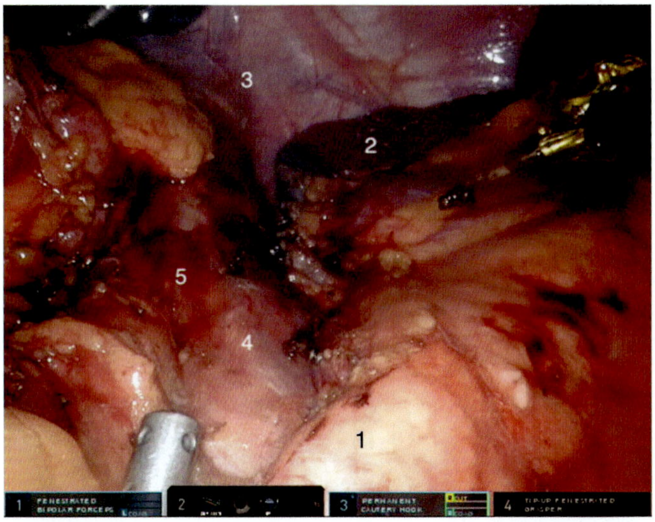

Fig. 18.18 Completed lymphadenectomy along the splenic vessels (lymph node station 10/11)
1. Pancreas
2. Spleen
3. Diaphragm
4. Gerota's fascia
5. Left diaphragmatic crus

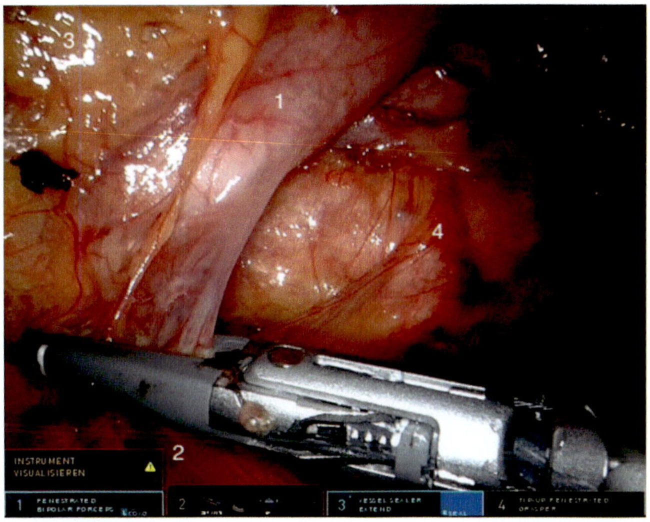

Fig. 18.19 Separation of the gastric meso from the colonic meso
1. Stomach
2. Meso of the transverse colon
3. Omentum
4. Pancreas

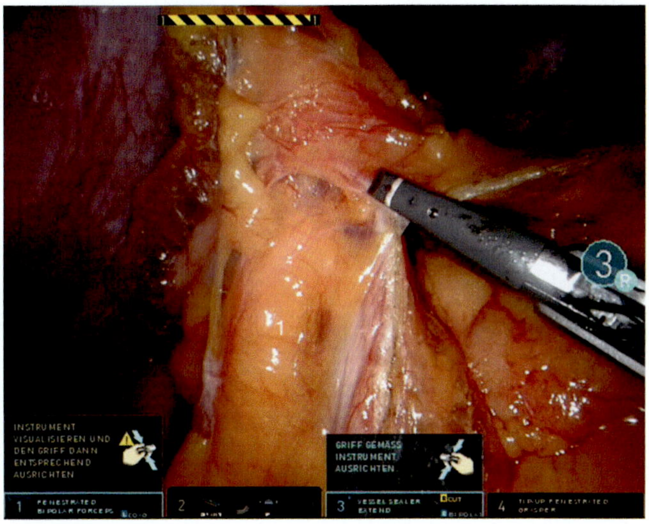

Fig. 18.20 Mobilization of the hepatic flexure
1. Hepatic flexure of the colon

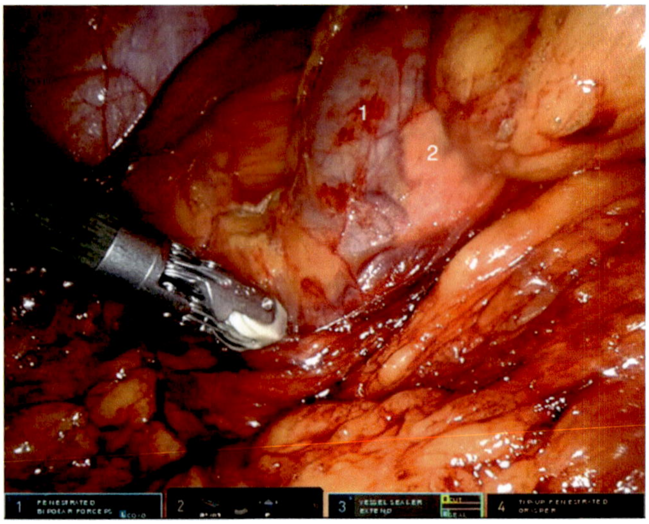

Fig. 18.21 Dissection of the hepatocolic ligament with visualization of the anterior part of the duodenum
1. Duodenum
2. Pancreas

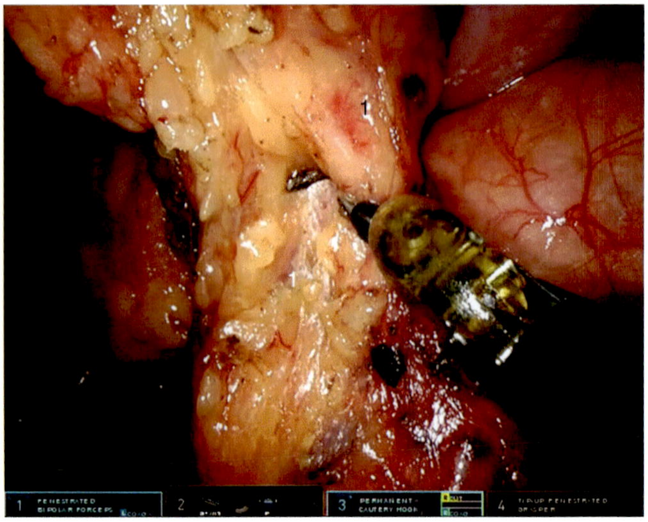

Fig. 18.22 Lymphadenectomy along the right gastroepiploic vessels (lymph node station 6)
1. Gastroepiploic pedicle

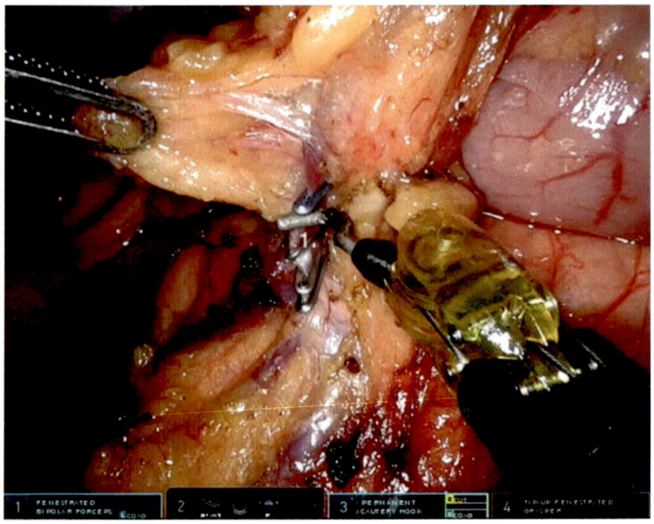

Fig. 18.23 Division of the right gastroepiploic vein
1. Right gastroepiploic vein

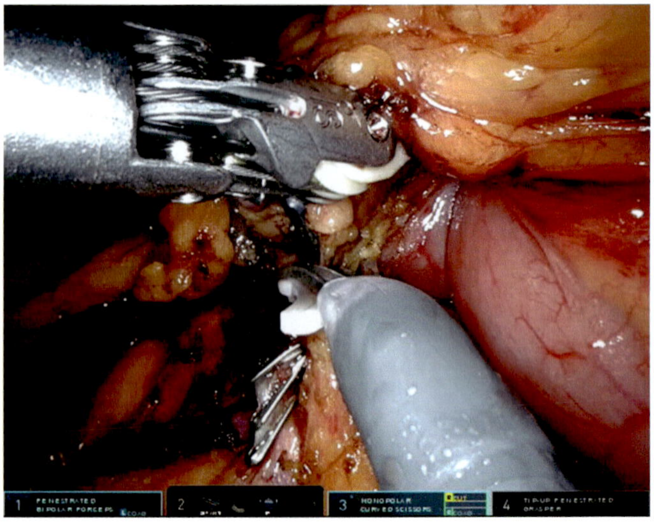

Fig. 18.24 Division of the right gastroepiploic artery

Lymphadenectomy Along the Right Gastric Artery and of the Hepatoduodenal Ligament and Transection of the Duodenum (Lymph Node Stations 5 and 12) (Figs. 18.25, 18.26, 18.27, 18.28, 18.29, and 18.30)

Lymphadenectomy Along the Common Hepatic Artery and Coeliac Axis (Lymph Node Station 8 and 9), Transsection of the Esophagus (Figs. 18.31, 18.32, 18.33, 18.34, 18.35, and 18.36)

Retrieval of the Stomach (Figs. 18.37 and 18.38)

Esophagojejunostomy with Roux-En-Y Reconstruction (Figs. 18.39, 18.40, 18.41, 18.42, 18.43, 18.44, 18.45, 18.46, 18.47, and 18.48)

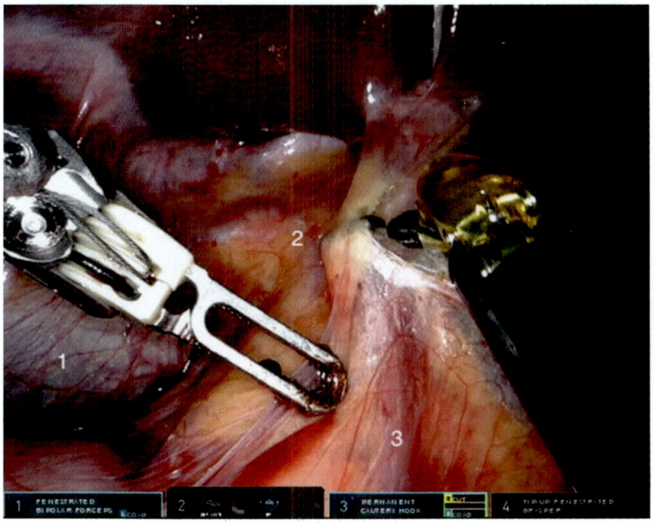

Fig. 18.25 Lymphadenectomy of the hepatoduodenal ligament (lymph node station 12)
1. Gallbladder
2. Right hepatic artery
3. Right gastric artery

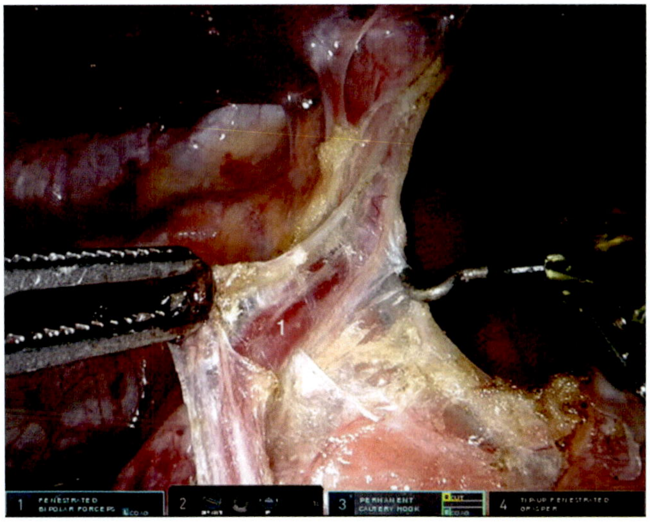

Fig. 18.26 Preparation of the right gastric artery (lymph node station 5)
1. Right gastric artery

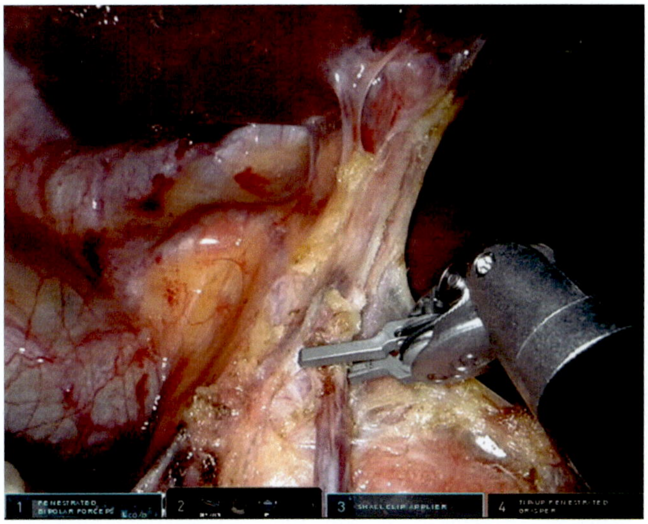

Fig. 18.27 Division of the right gastric artery

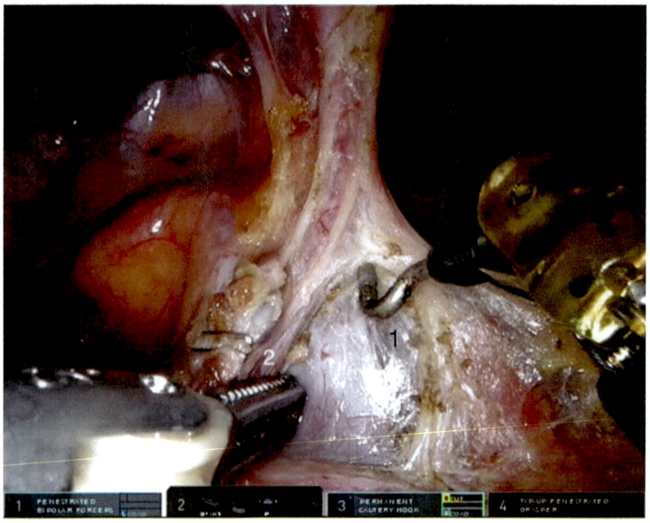

Fig. 18.28 Lymphadenectomy down to the left side of the portal vein
1. Portal vein
2. Proper liver artery

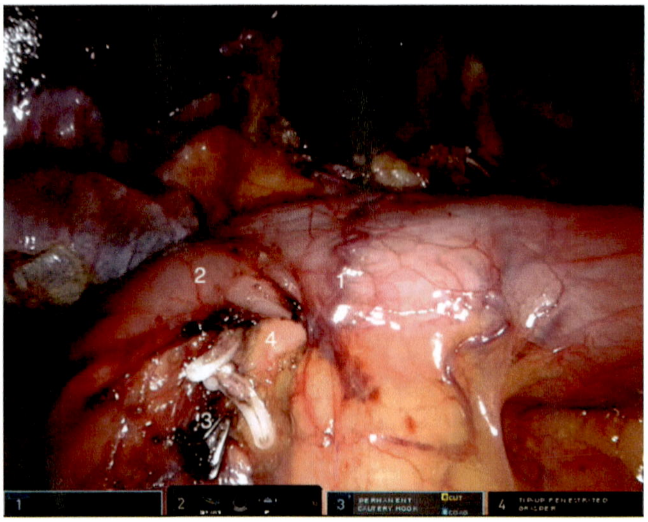

Fig. 18.29 Dissection of the pylorus and the duodenum
1. Pylorus
2. Duodenum
3. Clipped and transected right epiploic vessels
4. Pancreas

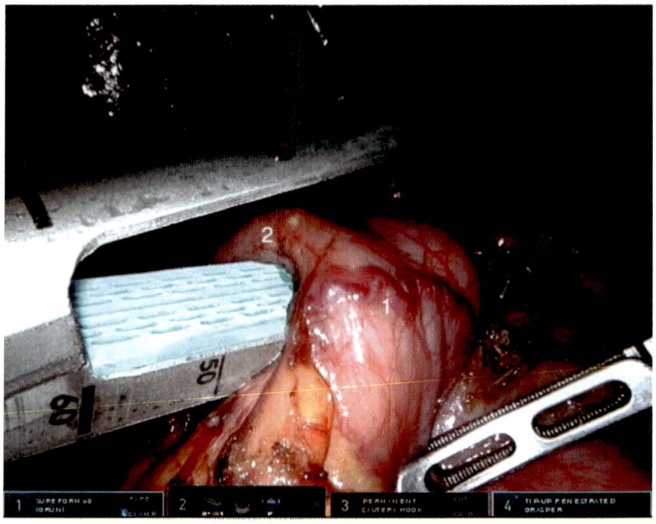

Fig. 18.30 Transection of the duodenum
1. Pylorus
2. Duodenum

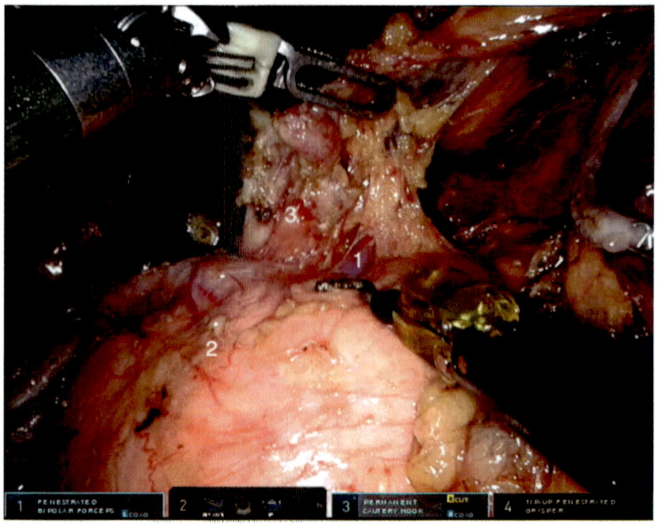

Fig. 18.31 Lymphadenectomy along the common hepatic artery (the lesser omentum is held upwards with the fourth arm)
1. Coronary vein
2. Pancreas
3. Lymph nodes surrounding the common hepatic artery

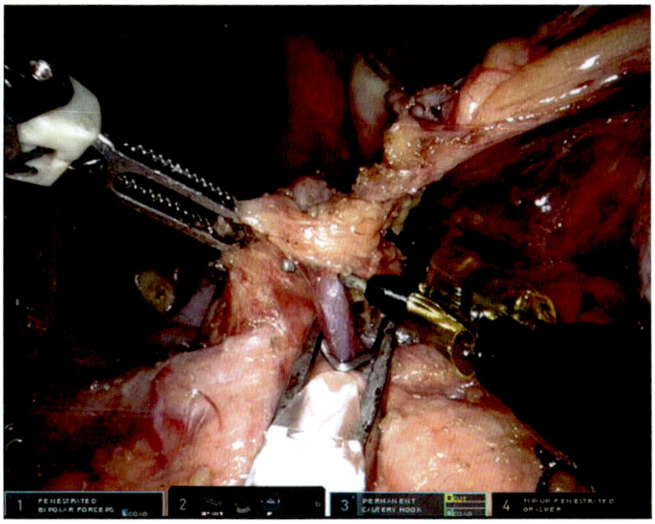

Fig. 18.32 Division of the coronary vein

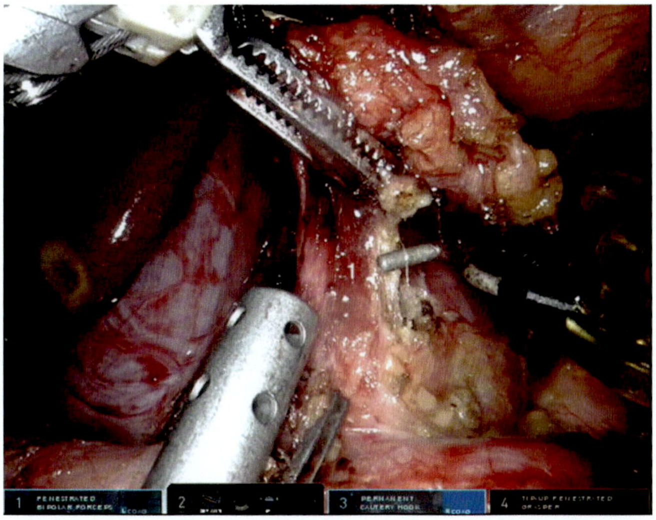

Fig. 18.33 Dissection of the left gastric artery (lymph node station 9)
1. Left gastric artery

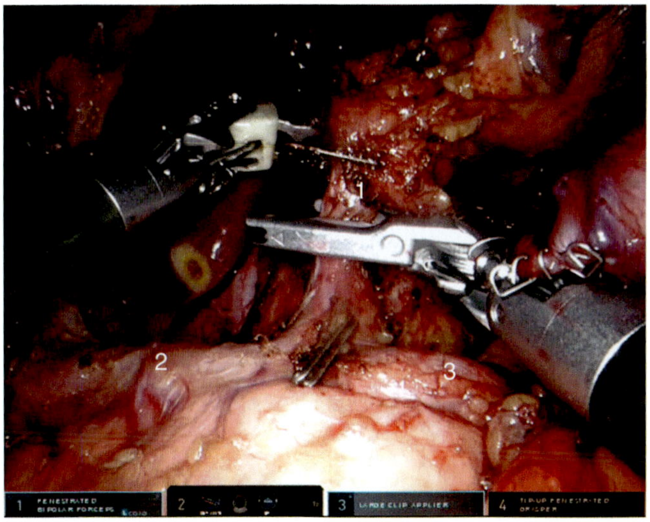

Fig. 18.34 Division of left gastric artery
1. Left gastric artery
2. Common hepatic artery
3. Splenic artery

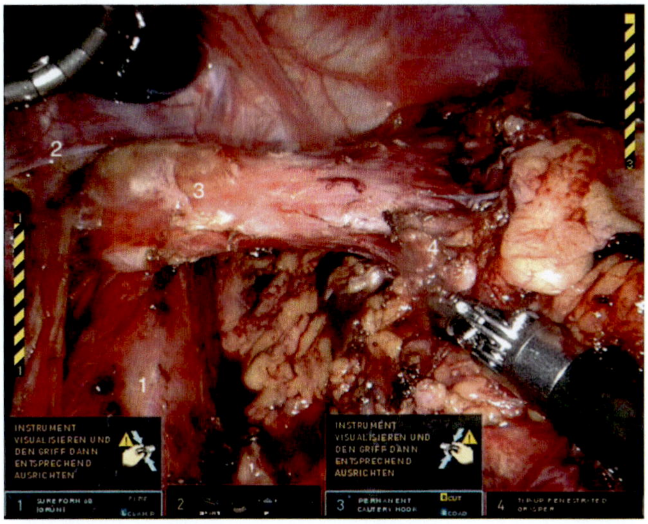

Fig. 18.35 Mobilization of the esophagus after completed lymphadenectomy
1. Left crus of diaphragm
2. Right crus of diaphragm
3. Esophagus
4. Paracardial lymph nodes (1/2)

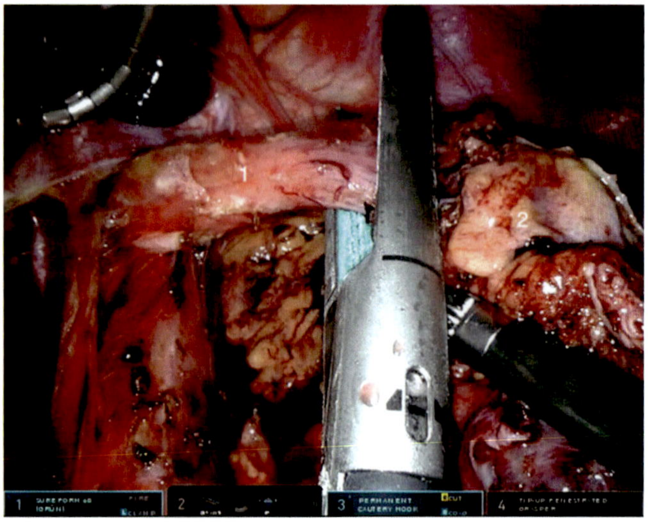

Fig. 18.36 Transection of the distal esophagus (first cut the vagal nerves separately!)
1. Esophagus
2. Stomach (cardia)

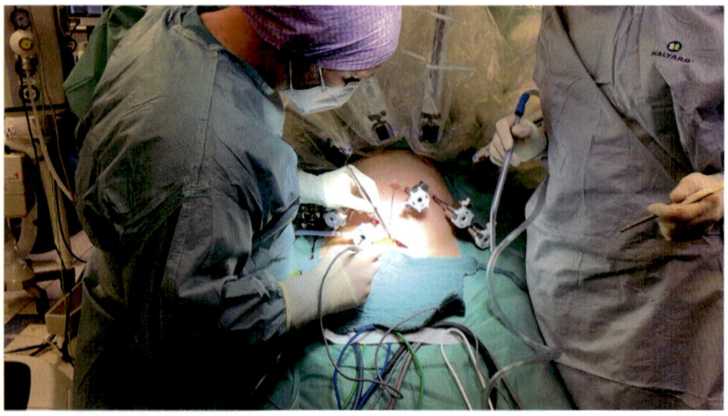

Fig. 18.37 Pfannenstiel incision

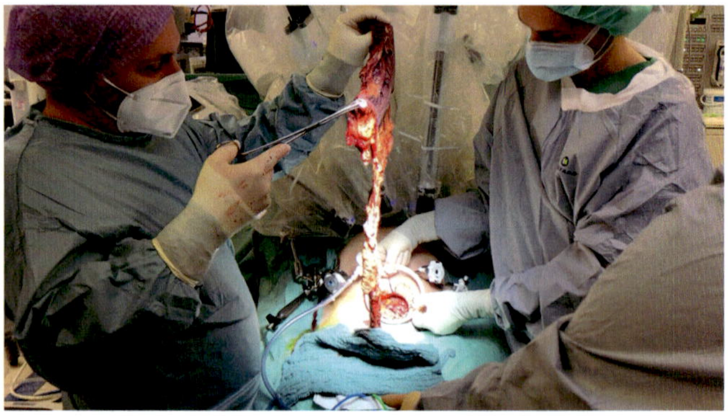

Fig. 18.38 Retrieval of the stomach

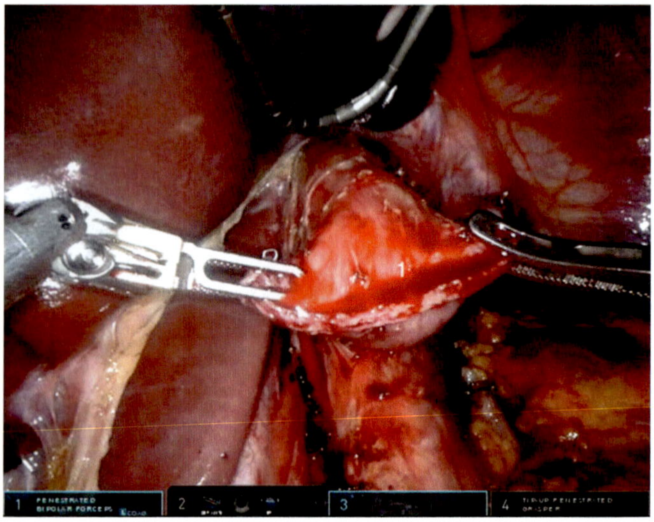

Fig. 18.39 Insertion of a 42 French calibration tube into the esophagus
1. Esophagus with calibration tube inside

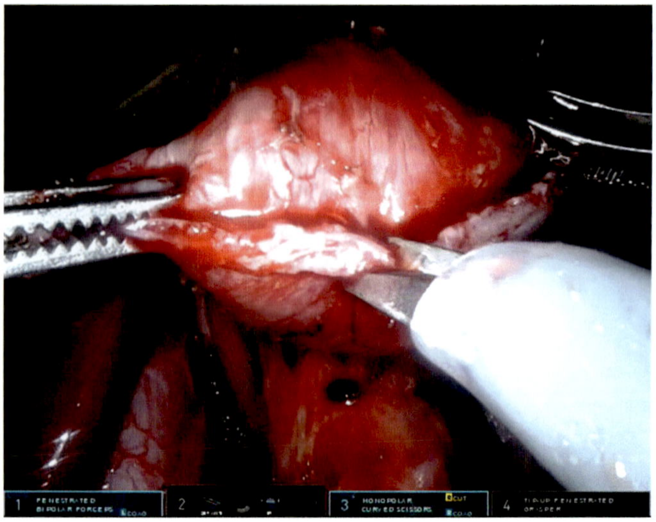

Fig. 18.40 Incision of the esophageal staple line (use cold scissors!)

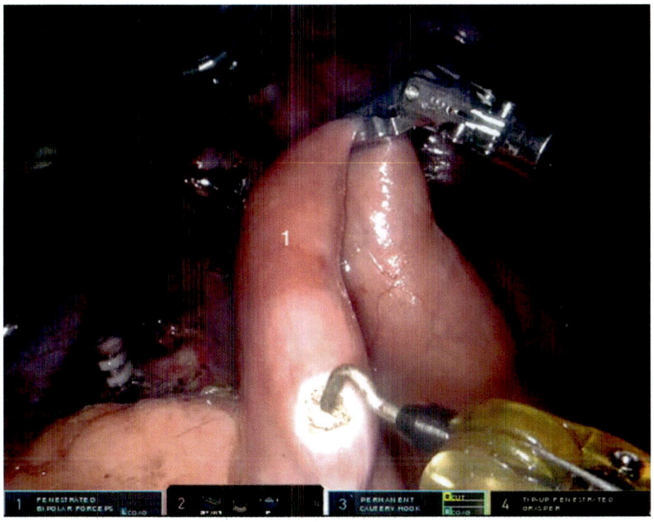

Fig. 18.41 Incision of the jejunum 50 cm from the duodenojejunal flexure
1. Jejunum

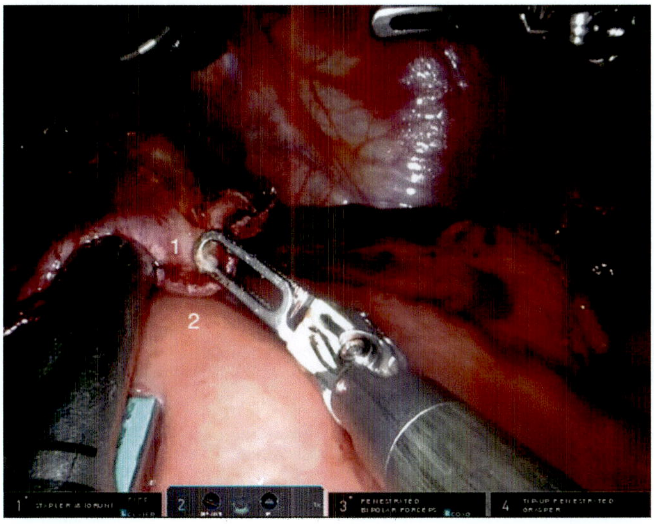

Fig. 18.42 Creation of a linear stapler side-to-side esophagojejunal anastomosis
1. Esophagus
2. Jejunum

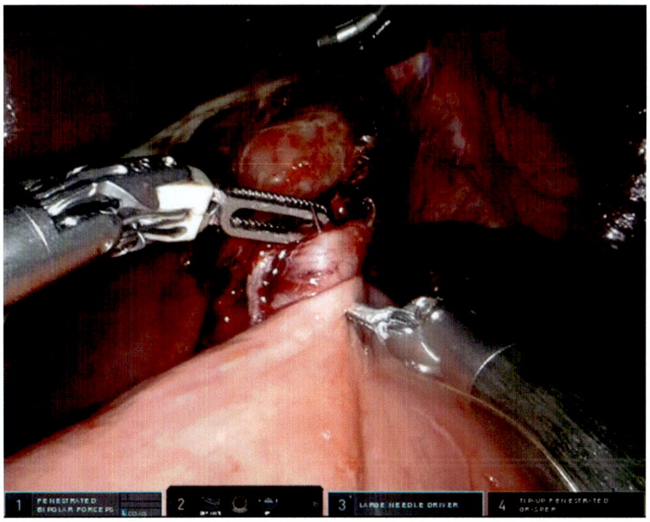

Fig. 18.43 Closure of the enterotomy with a modified double row technique

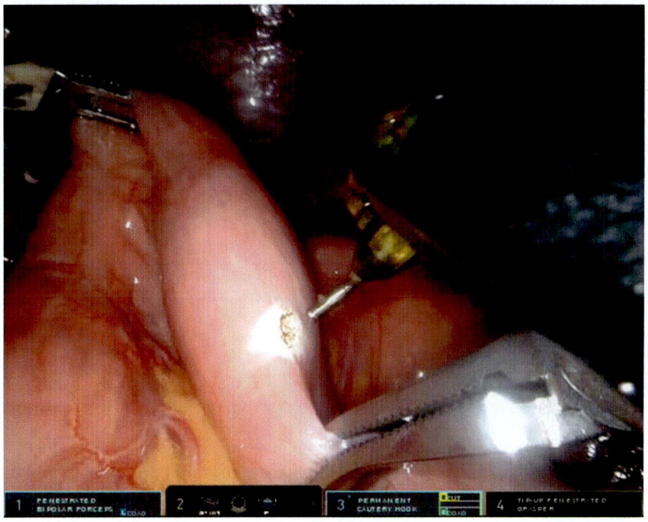

Fig. 18.44 Incision of the jejunum 50 cm from the esophagojejunostomy

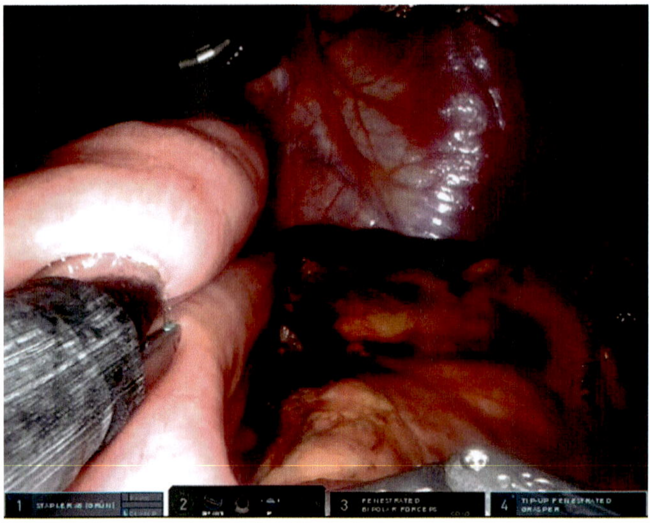

Fig. 18.45 Creation of a side-to-side jejunojejunostomy

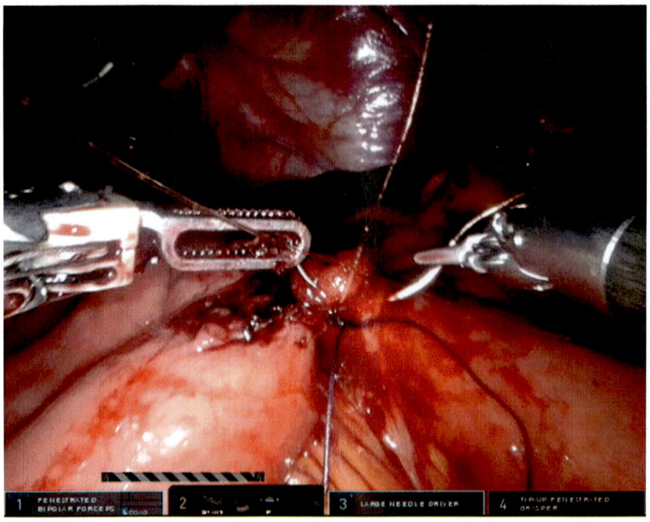

Fig. 18.46 Closure of the enterotomy with a modified double row technique

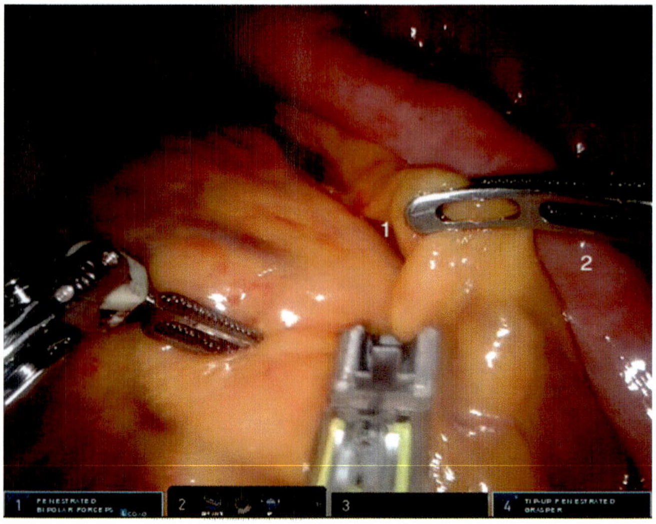

Fig. 18.47 Closure of the mesenteric defects with Endohernia clips
1. Mesenteric defect
2. Jejunum

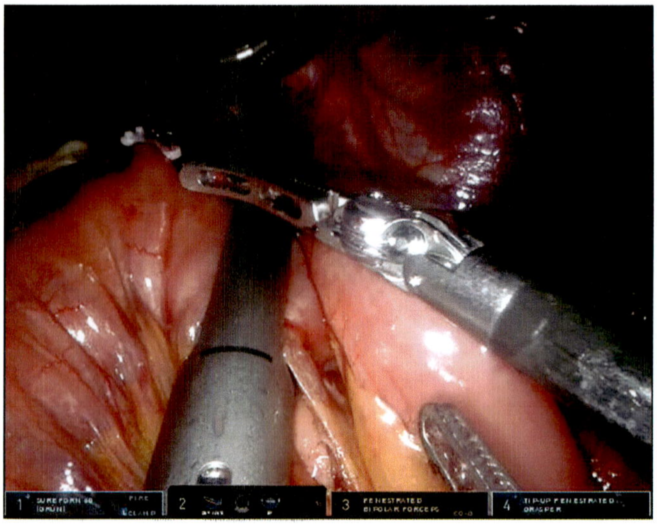

Fig. 18.48 Transection of the jejunum between the anastomoses

Suggested Reading

Aiolfi A, Lombardo F, Matsushima K, Sozzi A, Cavalli M, Panizzo V, et al. Systematic review and updated network meta-analysis of randomized controlled trials comparing open, laparoscopic-assisted, and robotic distal gastrectomy for early and locally advanced gastric cancer. Surgery. 2021;S0039–6060(21)00339–1.; https://doi.org/10.1016/j.surg.2021.04.014.

Choi S, Song JH, Lee S, Cho M, Kim YM, Hyung WJ, et al. Surgical merits of open, laparoscopic, and robotic gastrectomy techniques with D2 lymphadenectomy in obese patients with gastric cancer. Ann Surg Oncol. 2021; https://doi.org/10.1245/s10434-021-09952-6.

Kinoshita T, Sato R, Akimoto E, Tanaka Y, Okayama T, Habu T. Reduction in postoperative complications by robotic surgery: a case-control study of robotic versus conventional laparoscopic surgery for gastric cancer. Surg Endosc. 2021; https://doi.org/10.1007/s00464-021-08483-1.

Marano L, Fusario D, Savelli V, Marrelli D, Roviello F. Robotic versus laparoscopic gastrectomy for gastric cancer: an umbrella review of systematic reviews and meta-analyses. Updat Surg. 2021; https://doi.org/10.1007/s13304-021-01059-7.

Terashima M. The 140 years' journey of gastric cancer surgery: from the two hands of Billroth to the multiple hands of the robot. Ann Gastroenterol Surg. 2021;5(3):270–7. https://doi.org/10.1002/ags3.12442. eCollection 2021 May.

Robot-Assisted Distal Gastrectomy

19

Han-Kwang Yang and Felix Berlth

Introduction

The distal gastrectomy is the prototype of minimally invasive gastrectomy since all prospective randomized trials for early and advanced gastric cancer investigating the oncological safety and postoperative benefits of laparoscopic surgery were applied for distal gastrectomy.

As the history of robot-assisted procedures is somewhat younger, large randomized trials for the robot approach are pending, but since equal safety and radicality in comparison to the laparoscopic approach has been proven (see "Total Gastrectomy" chapter), the robotic approach is widely accepted. Indeed, studies suggest benefits of robot-assisted gastrectomy in terms of surgical precision in case of lymphadenectomy with vessel preservation or a low complication rate after suprapancreatic lymph node dissection [1]. As in oncological gastric cancer resection the technique itself would contribute to the success [2], the robotic approach for distal gastrectomy is believed to become a standard approach for distal gastric cancer resection, if a robotic system is in place (Figs. 19.1, 19.2, 19.3, 19.4, 19.5, 19.6, 19.7, 19.8, 19.9, 19.10, 19.11, 19.12, 19.13, 19.14, 19.15, 19.16, and 19.17).

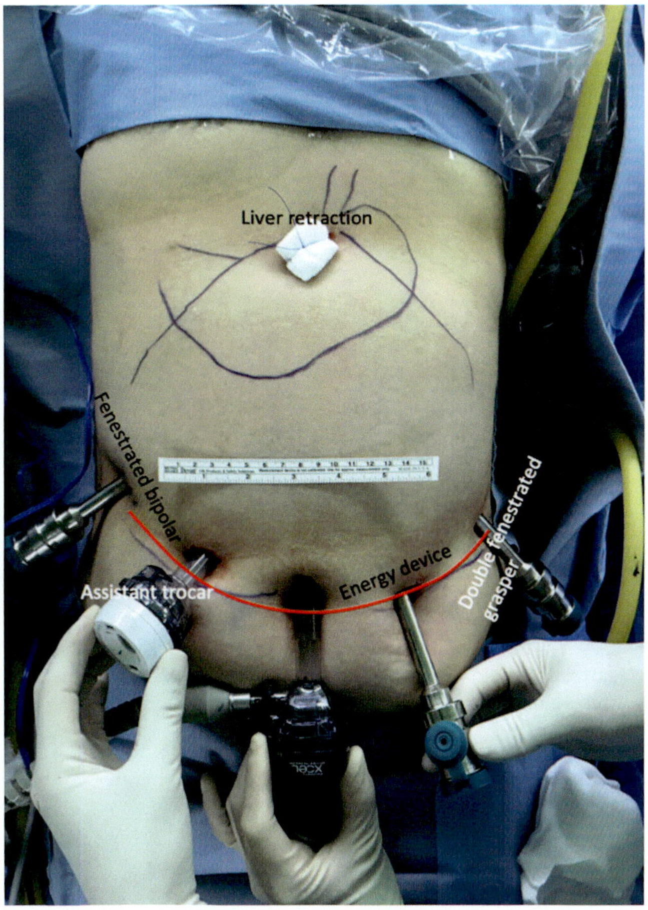

Fig. 19.1 The camera trocar is placed in infraumbilical position. The assistant trocar I placed on the patient's right side above the level of umbilicus, the distance to the camera trocar is 8 cm minimum. The trocars are positioned in a slightly round shape

H.-K. Yang
Department of Surgery, Seoul National University College of Medicine, Seoul, South Korea

F. Berlth (✉)
Department of General, Visceral and Transplant Surgery, University Medical Center of the Johannes Gutenberg University, Mainz, Germany
e-mail: felix.berlth@unimedizin-mainz.de

O. Y. Kudsi, P. P. Grimminger (eds.), *Atlas of Robotic Upper Gastrointestinal Surgery*, https://doi.org/10.1007/978-3-030-86578-8_19

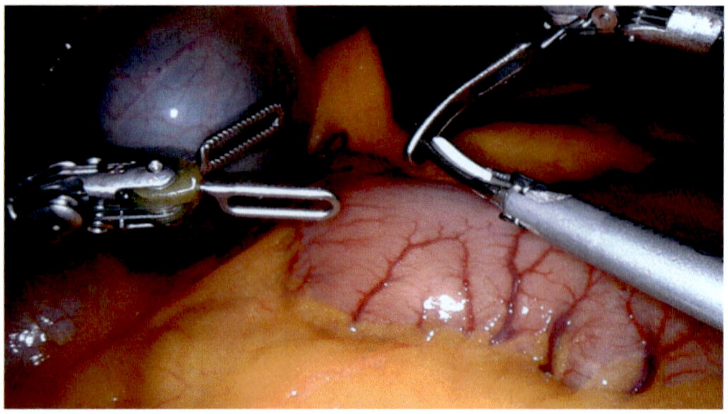

Fig. 19.2 The instruments that are used: energy device on right hand, fenestrated bipolar forceps on left hand, and double fenestrated grasper on the right lateral hand

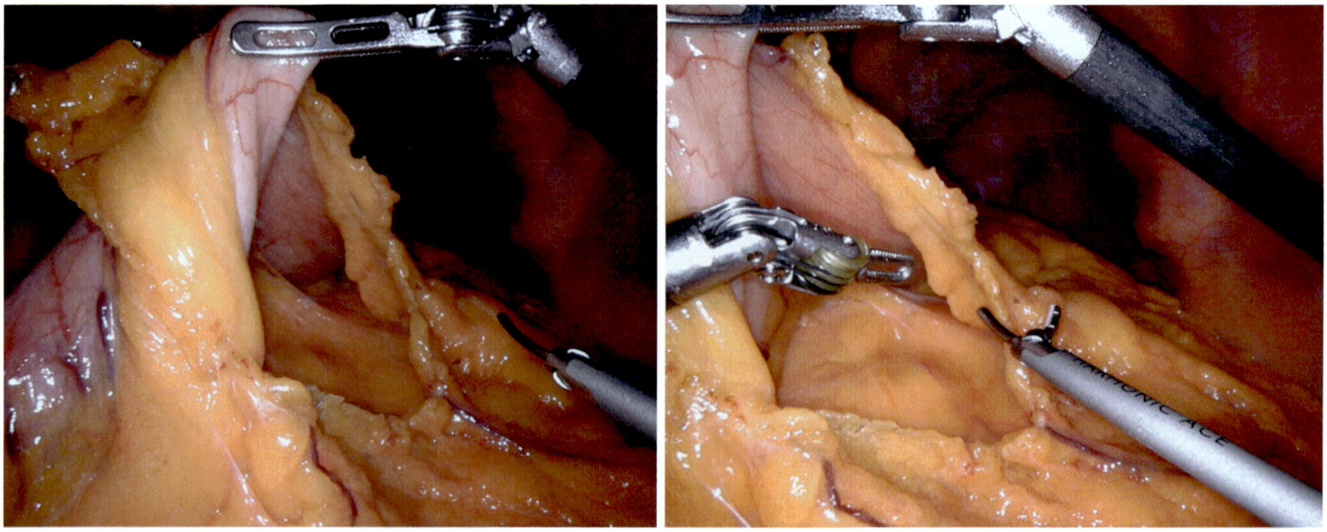

Fig. 19.3 The omentum is divided by energy device in direction to the splenic lower pole. There the left gastroepiploic vessels are divided between clips. For early gastric cancer, a partial gastrectomy is performed; for advanced gastric cancer, a total omentectomy is required. After having opened the bursa, the third robotic arm can gently grasp the stomach's posterior side for good exposure

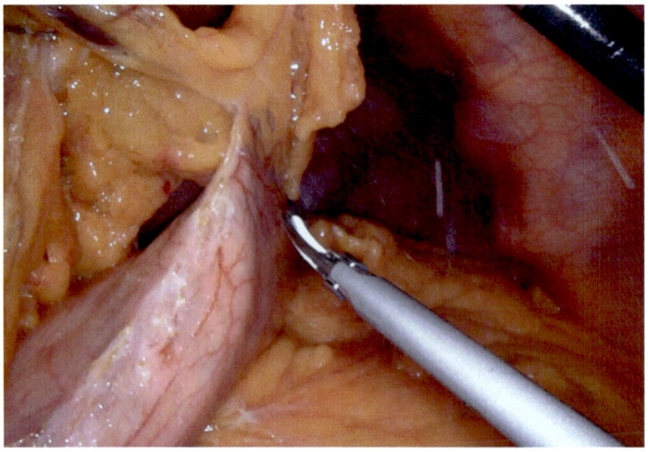

Fig. 19.4 The greater curvature is cleared by exposing the proximal vessel arcade. The lymph nodes of lymph node station 4sb are brought to the specimen's side, and the greater curvature is prepared for later transection

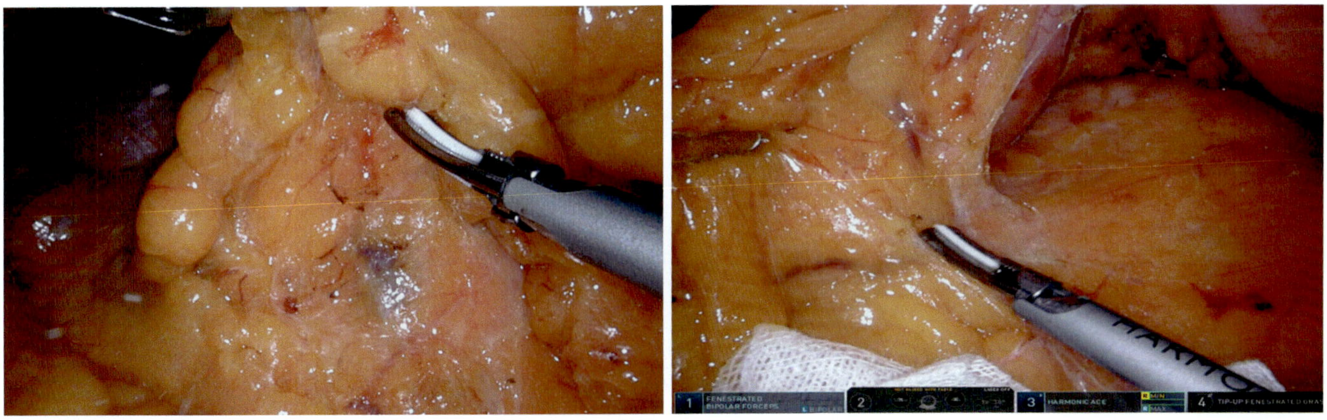

Fig. 19.5 The omentectomy is continued to the distal side of the stomach. Posterior side attachments to the pancreas need to be cut, and then the fusion plane of infrapyloric pedicle and transverse mesocolon is exposed. The plane is gently divided by blunt and sharp dissection

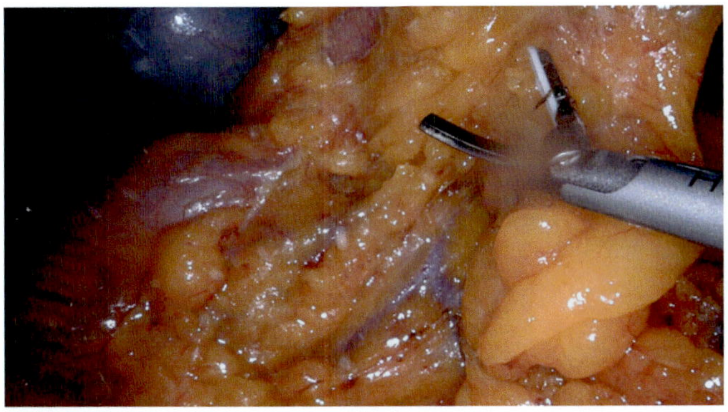

Fig. 19.6 The omentectomy is followed to the duodenum. The gallbladder can be a structure guiding the direction

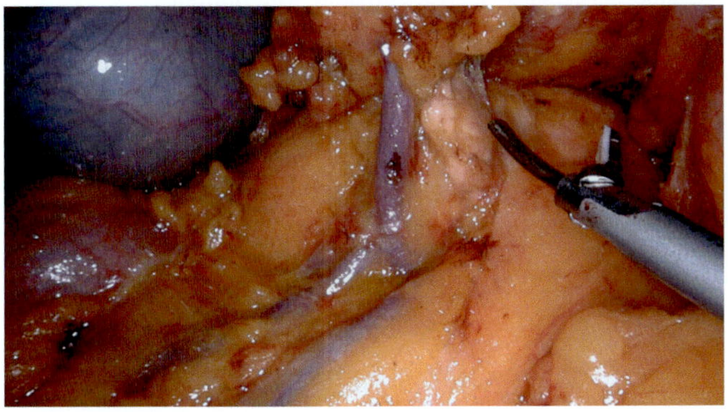

Fig. 19.7 The infrapyloric pedicle is dissected at its roots, and caution has to be taken to the pancreas

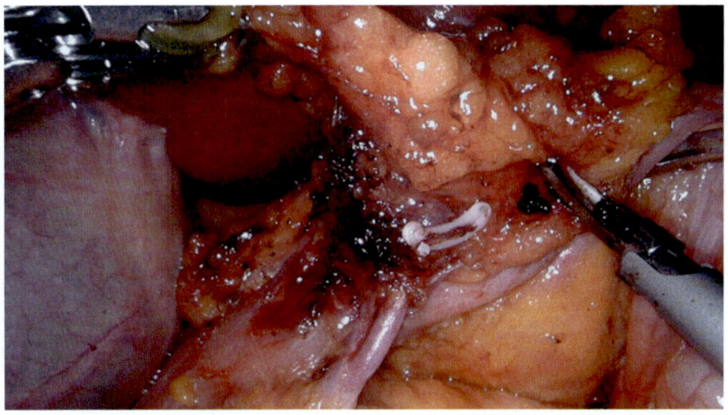

Fig. 19.8 The duodenum is cleared, so the whole lymph node station 6 is brought to the specimen's side, when the duodenum is transected

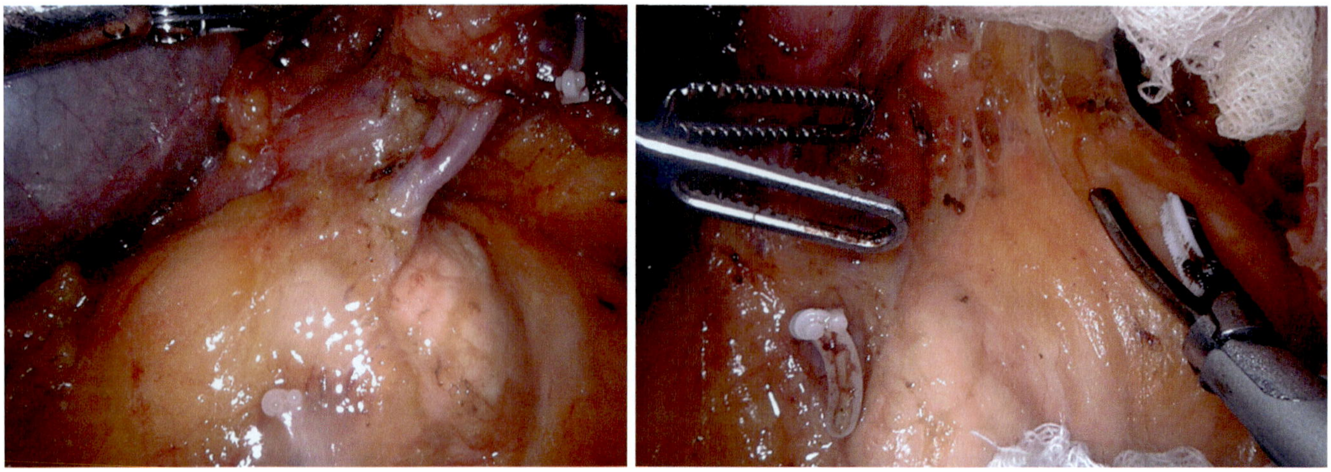

Fig. 19.9 The right gastroepiploic artery and vein are clipped and cut separately

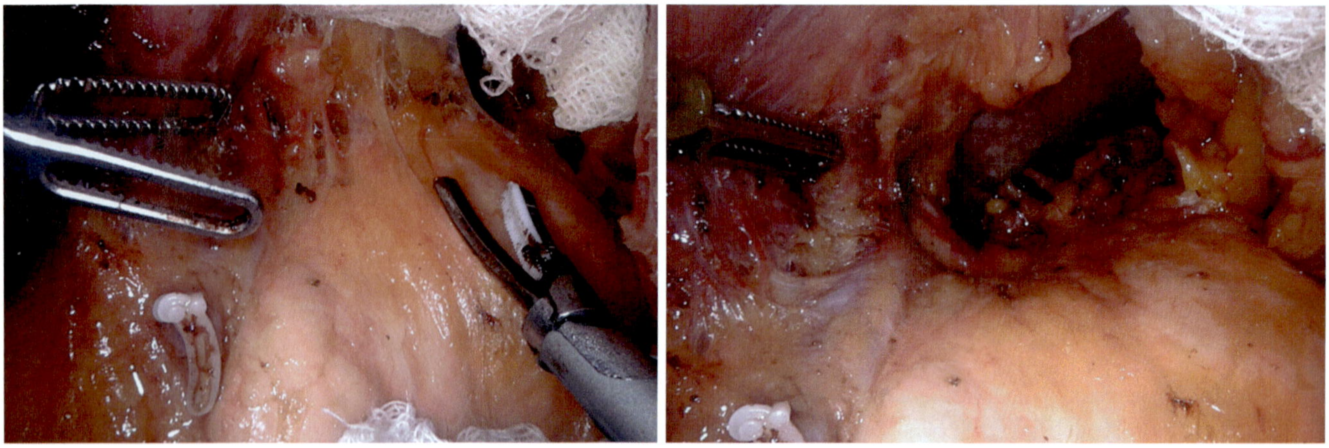

Fig. 19.10 On the duodenum's posterior side, the gastroduodenal artery is dissected, and small branches to the duodenum are cut with very small bites of the energy device in order to provide enough distal margin length and duodenal stump when reconstructing with Billroth I

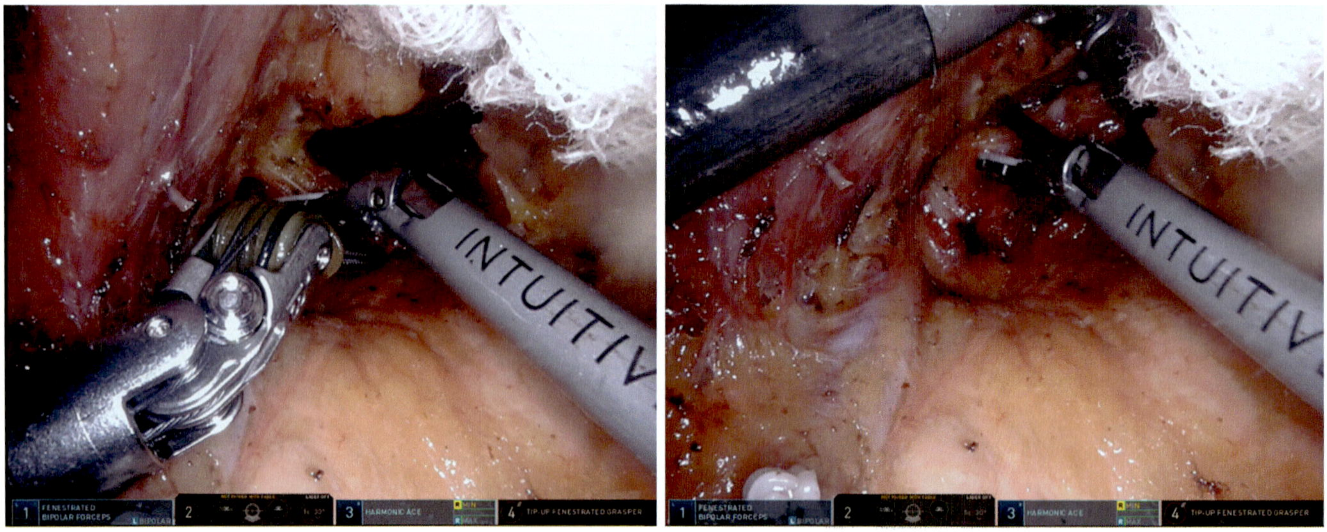

Fig. 19.11 The antrum is retracted to the patient's ventral side so dissection of the suprapancreatic area over common hepatic artery, lymph node station 8 can be partly performed. In this step lymph node station 5 and lymph node station 8 can be divided

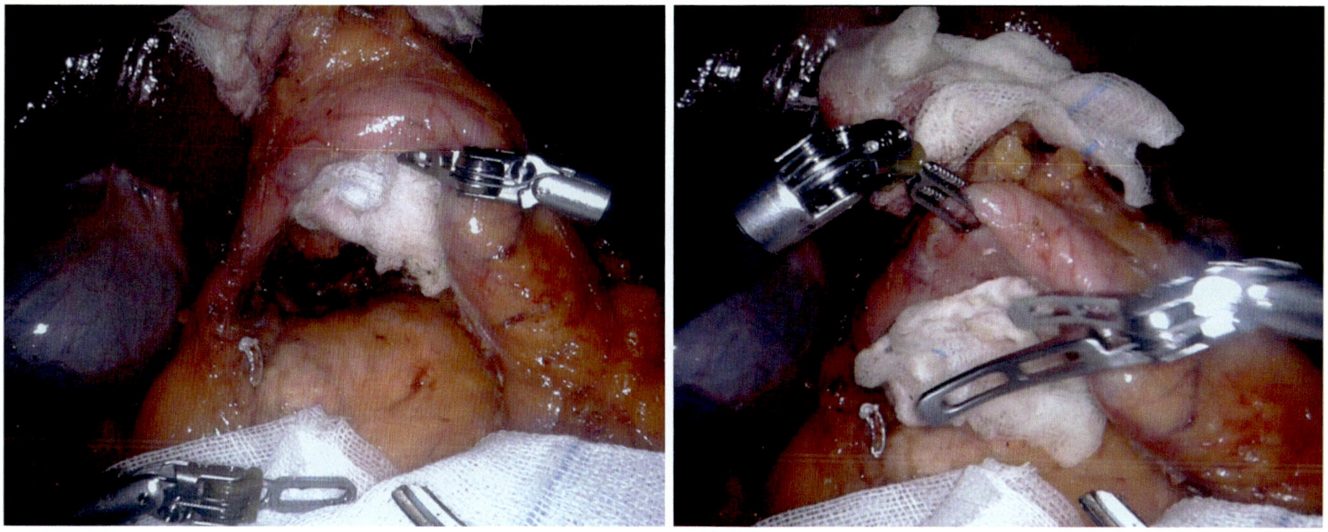

Fig. 19.12 Gauze is put in the bursa and dissection continues on the anterior side. The gauze pumps up the lesser sac and protects the common hepatic artery and the pancreas when approaching from anterior

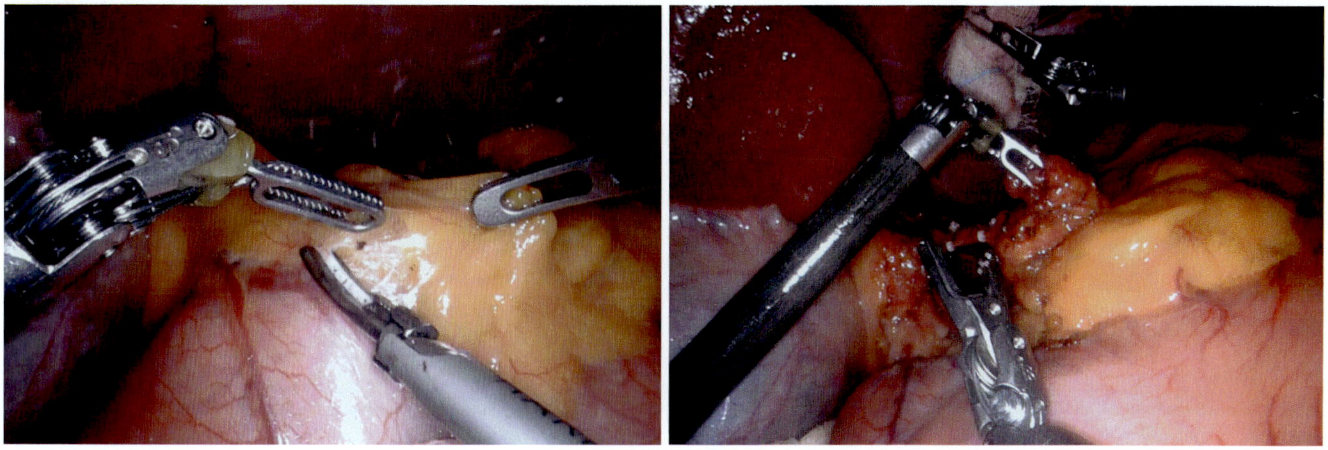

Fig. 19.13 The pylorus and proximal duodenum are dissected on the lesser curvature side, and then dissection follows common hepatic artery to the roots of the right gastric vessels, which are clipped and cut. Following that direction, the proper hepatic artery can be dissected. In this way, lymph node station 12a is connected to lymph node station 5 and is brought to the specimen's side

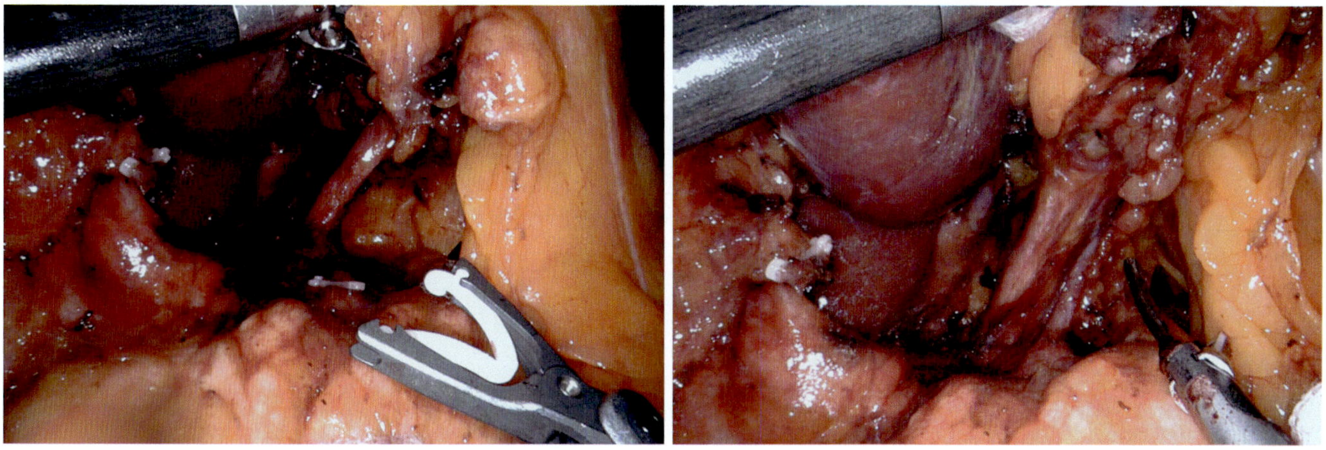

Fig. 19.14 The stomach is retracted in caudal direction in order to expose the suprapancreatic area. The dissection along the common hepatic artery is completed in direction to the celiac trunk. The left gastric vein is clipped and cut

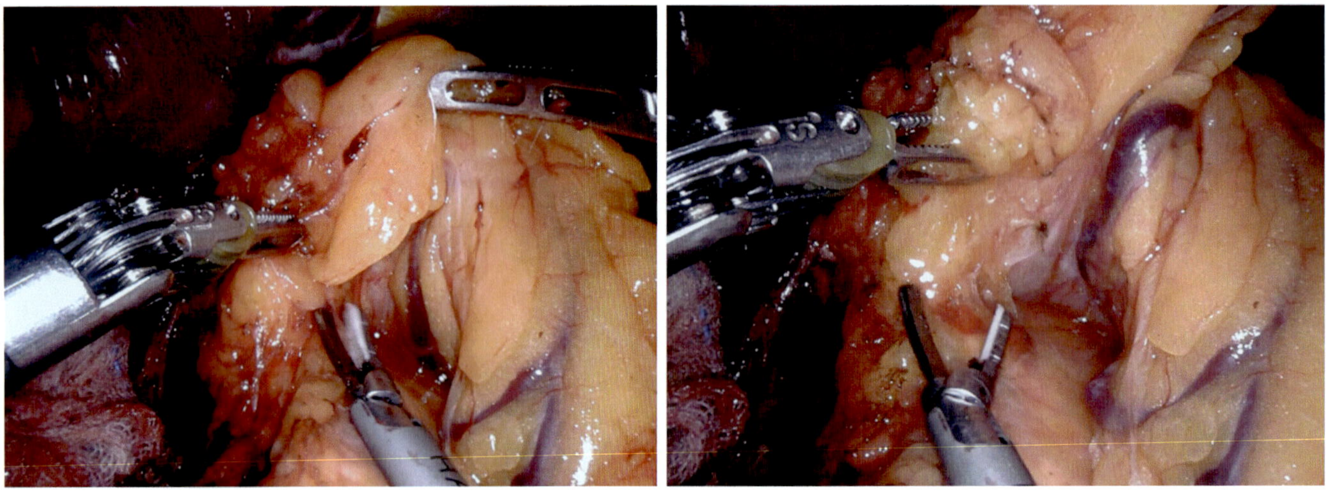

Fig. 19.15 Depending on the desired level of radicality, the splenic vessels can be followed close to the splenic hilum if complete lymph node station 11 dissection is necessary

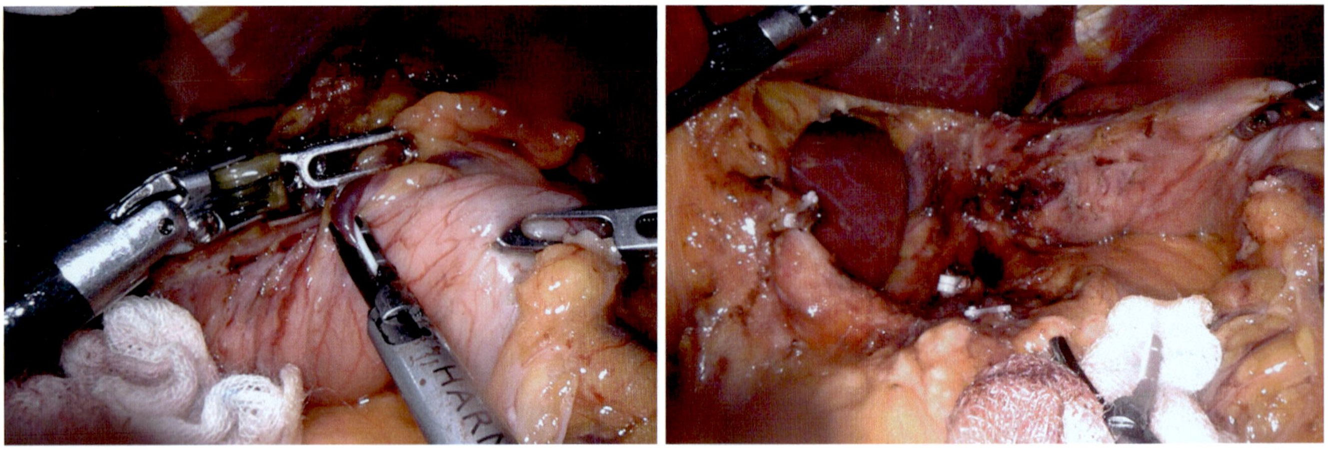

Fig. 19.16 The right crus and right side of the esophagogastric junction is dissected, and then the lesser curvature is cleared to the desired location of proximal transection. This way, lymph node station 1 and lymph node station 3 are brought to the specimen's side. The Lymph node dissection is completed, and transection and reconstruction can be performed. In case of Billroth I with circular stapler, both can be performed simultaneously through upper abdominal mini-laparotomy

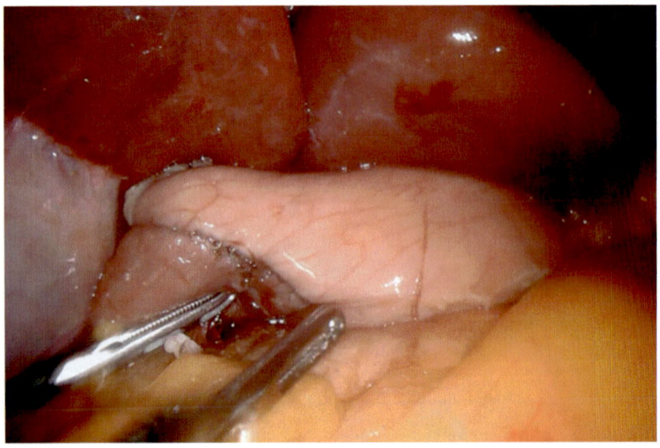

Fig. 19.17 After Billroth I reconstruction with circular stapler

References

1. Han DS, Suh YS, Ahn HS, Kong SH, Lee HJ, Kim WH, et al. Comparison of surgical outcomes of robot-assisted and laparoscopy-assisted pylorus-preserving gastrectomy for gastric cancer: a propensity score matching analysis. Ann Surg Oncol. 2015;22(7):2323–8. https://doi.org/10.1245/s10434-014-4204-6.
2. Yang HK, Berlth F. Gastric cancer surgery: the importance of technique and not only the extent of lymph node dissection. Lancet Oncol. 2019;20(3):329–31. https://doi.org/10.1016/S1470-2045(19)30073-7.

Robotic Partial Gastrectomy for GIST Tumors

20

Matthias Biebl, Christian Denecke, Tomasz Dziodzio, Robert Öllinger, and Johann Pratschke

Introduction

Gastrointestinal stromal tumors are mesenchymal tumors of the gastrointestinal tract that potentially can be malignant. Although GIST tumors have been detected in all age groups, the predominant number of cases are found in individuals in their 60s [1], with a prevalence of around 13 per 100,000 and an incidence of 1–1.5 per 100,000 per year [2]. The stomach seems to be the leading location (around 60%) for this type of tumor, and often, very small tumors of less than 1 cm are incidental findings in individuals older than 50 years [3]. Surgical R0 resection is the only potentially curative treatment, which in larger tumors may also include multivisceral resection. The natural history of small asymptomatic GISTs is largely unknown, but generally, resection is recommended for symptomatic tumors, tumors with high-risk criteria such as ulceration, irregular borders, internal heterogeneity, growth during follow-up or enlargement of regional lymph nodes, as well as any tumor exceeding 2–5 cm in diameter [3].

Surgical treatment aims at complete tumor resection, and care has to be taken to avoid tumor rupture during the procedure. With the evolution of minimally invasive surgery, this approach has been increasingly advocated, following the same principles as open resection. Consequently, minimally invasive resection of gastric GIST tumors has gained popularity and is currently the most commonly used approach, regardless of tumor location [4, 5]. As dorsally located tumors especially of the corpus or antrum are often fixed to the retroperitoneal structures and sometimes be located close to the pylorus, which may preclude from classical wedge resection and require direct suturing for reconstruction, a robotic approach has been introduced for such indications as a safe and feasible way of minimally invasive tumor resection [6, 7].

Case Presentation

We present the case of a 78-year-old male patient with a biopsy-proven 5 cm gastric GIST tumor located at the dorsal prepyloric antrum (Fig. 20.1). The patient had a medical history remarkable for arterial hypertension, type II diabetes mellitus, hyperlipidemia, and post acute liver failure status due to paracetamol intoxication 1 year ago and suffered from metastasized prostate cancer under medical treatment. The gastric tumor itself was asymptomatic and discovered during CT scan for prostate cancer staging.

Operating Room Setup, Patient Positioning, and Instruments Used

The patient was placed in supine position with spread legs and the table tilted upward 30 degrees (Fig. 20.2). The standard robotic setup for upper GI procedures was chosen, using four robotic trocars in a horizontal line about 20 cm below the xiphoid process, and the camera positioned in the midline. In order to get good view to the gastric antrum from both above and below, care was taken not to place the trocars too caudally. Two robotic trocars were located left to the umbilicus (mid-clavicular line and at the costal margin) and one at the right costal margin. One 12 mm assist trocar was positioned right to the camera trocar (Fig. 20.3).

The da Vinci robot was approximated to the table from the patient's left side. The table-side surgeon was positioned between the patient's legs. Robotic instruments used included a tip-up fenestrated forceps introduced from the left lateral trocar, an articulated bipolar sealing device introduced

M. Biebl (✉) · C. Denecke · T. Dziodzio · R. Öllinger
J. Pratschke
Department of Surgery, Campus Charité Mitte|Campus Virchow Klinikum, Charité – Universitätsmedizin Berlin, Corporate Member of Freie Universität Berlin, Humboldt-Universität zu Berlin, and Berlin Institute of Health, Berlin, Germany
e-mail: matthias.biebl@charite.de

O. Y. Kudsi, P. P. Grimminger (eds.), *Atlas of Robotic Upper Gastrointestinal Surgery*,
https://doi.org/10.1007/978-3-030-86578-8_20

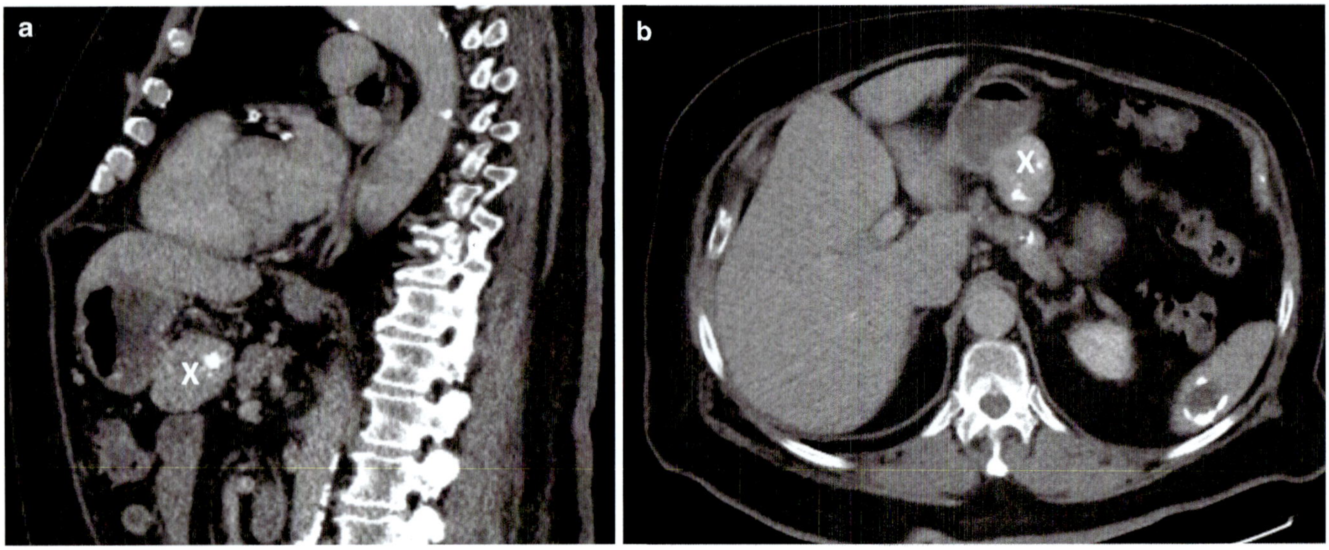

Fig. 20.1 CT scan showing location of the GIST (x) at the dorsal side of the gastric antrum: (**a**) Sagital view (**b**) transverse view

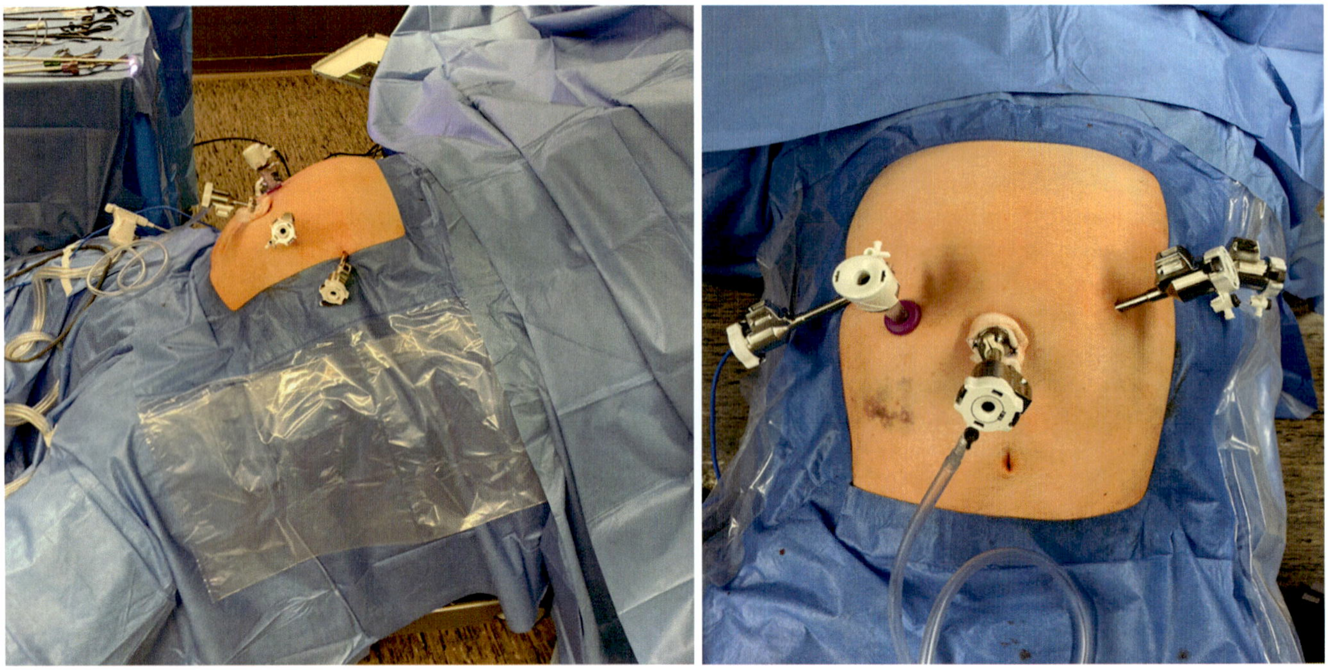

Fig. 20.2 Patient positioning and trocar setup

through the medial left trocar, and a fenestrated bipolar forceps through the right lateral trocar.

Gastric Mobilization and Identification of the Tumor

In order to be able to mobilize the tumor enough to assess resectability, the gastric antrum was mobilized from above through the lesser omentum as well as from below through the gastrocolic ligament. First, the lesser omentum was divided and the tumor visualized from above. Along the right gastric artery, several enlarged lymph nodes were noted and resected for pathological analysis (Fig. 20.4).

After mobilization of the accessible parts of the tumor from above, the approach was switched to from below in order not to compromise tumor integrity through excessive manipulation from above (Fig. 20.5).

Using the tip-up fenestrated forceps, the ventral side of the stomach was lifted ventrally, and the gastroomental arcade was safely identified. Next, the gastroomental ligament was broadly divided with the vessel sealer and the

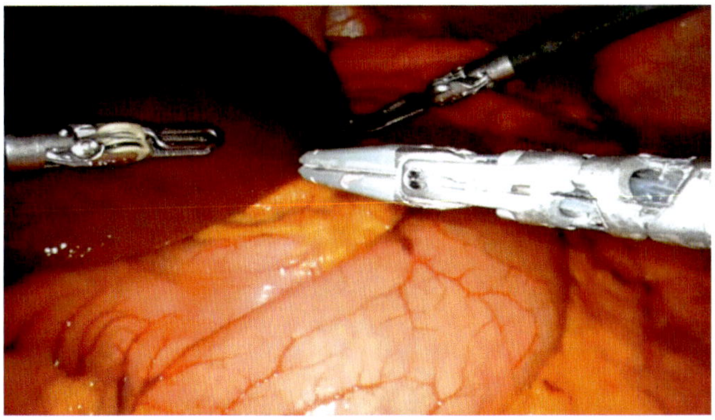

Fig. 20.3 Instrument placement and view at the beginning of the procedure

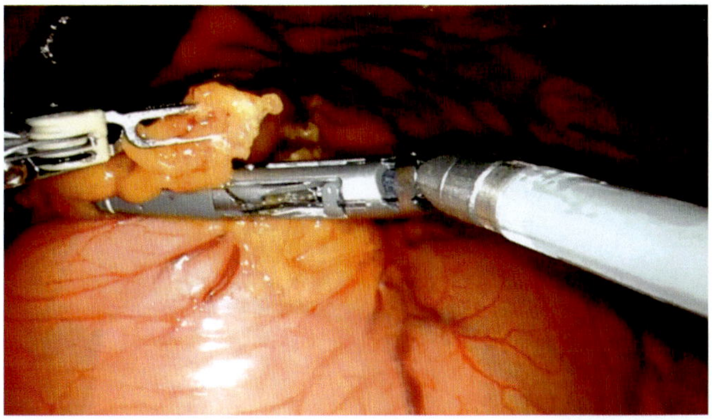

Fig. 20.4 Resection of lymph nodes along the right gastric artery

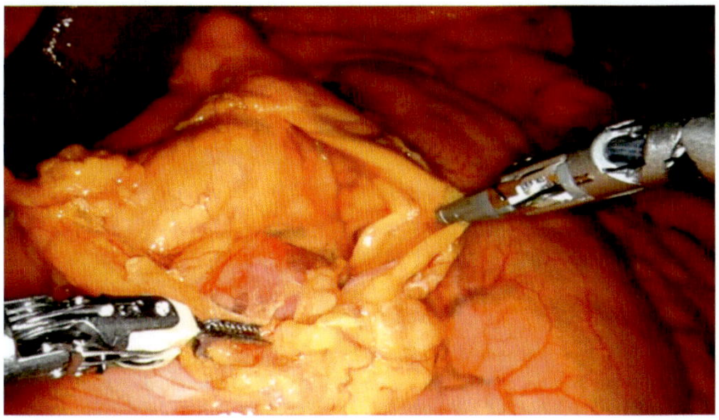

Fig. 20.5 Identification of the tumor from above. Note that without excessive mobilization, the tumor could not be further mobilized, and, therefore, the approach was switched to from below

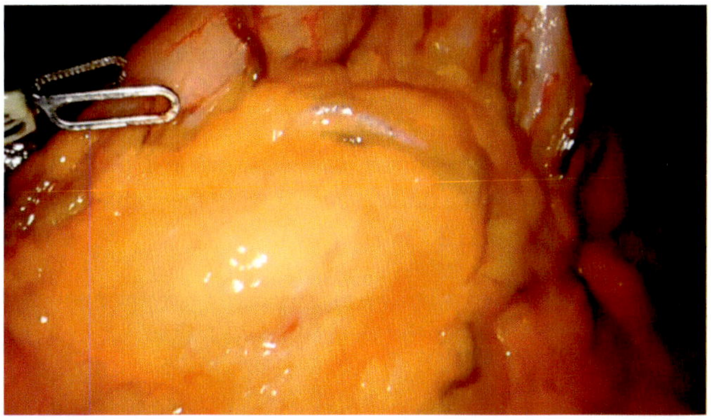

Fig. 20.6 Visualization of the gastroomental arcade for safe access to the omental bursa

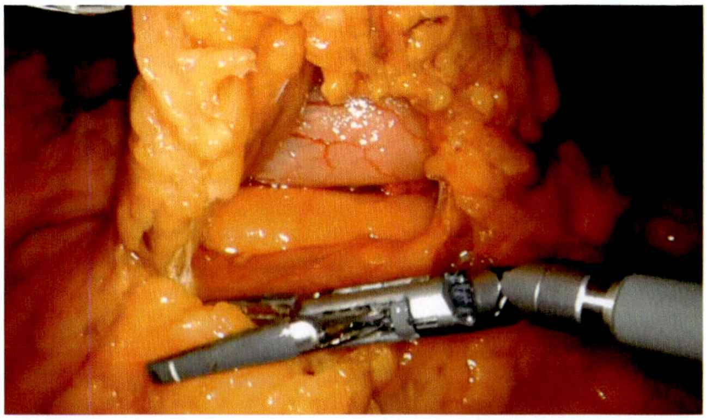

Fig. 20.7 Access of the bursa omentalis through the gastrocolic ligament using the articulated bipolar Vessel Sealer

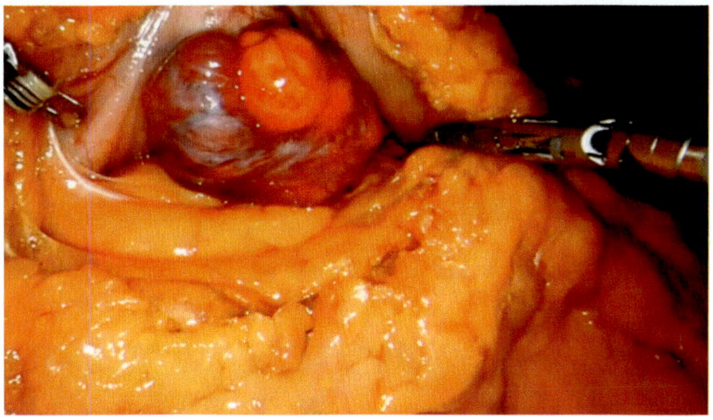

Fig. 20.8 Identification of the tumor and completion of the mobilization from above

tumor identified from below. Some dorsal adhesions of the tumor with the retroperitoneum were identified and taken down (Figs. 20.6, 20.7, and 20.8).

Following complete mobilization of the gastric antrum, the resection strategy was evaluated. In this situation, a dorsal rotation of the antrum was possible and the basis of the tumor completely visualized from above. Therefore, a transverse wedge resection of the tumor using an endoscopic stapler without compromise of the antral passage seems feasible and was therefore aimed at. Resection was performed using two 60-mm-thick (green) linear endoscopic stapler loads. In order to ensure a constant safe resection margin, it is not advisable to staple as much as possible with one load, but rather to use several small bites under direct vision (Figs. 20.9 and 20.10).

The tumor was positioned in a retrieval bag and meticulous hemostasis along the staple line obtained. At the end of the procedure, the specimen was retrieved and the trocars removed and a silicone drain placed next to the staple line for 24 h (Figs. 20.11 and 20.12).

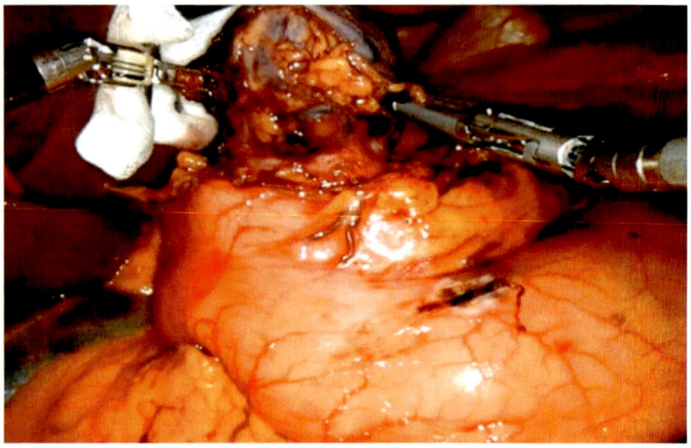

Fig. 20.9 The tumor (blue) is rotated from dorsal to cranial. Note the sharp line of the tumor and the healthy stomach. Atypical wedge resection using endoscopic linear stapler seems meaningful

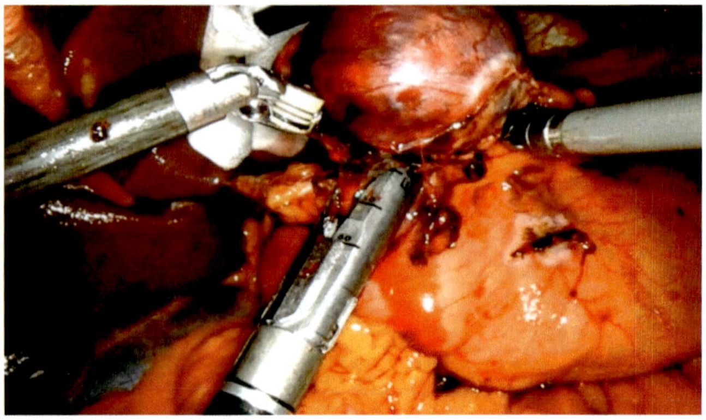

Fig. 20.10 First staple line in a transverse way from ventral to dorsal

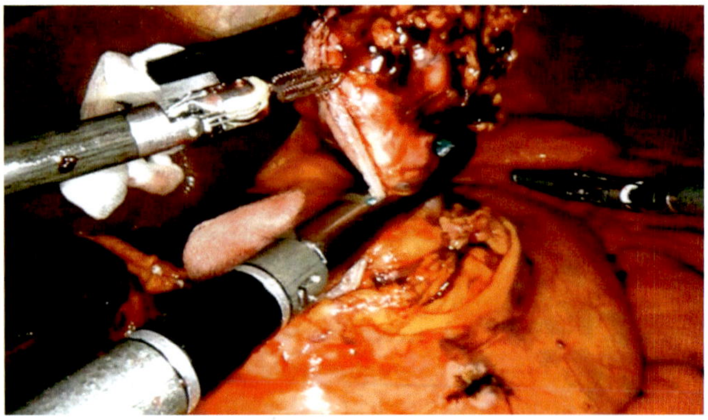

Fig. 20.11 Completion of stapler resection under direct visualization of the cranial resection margin

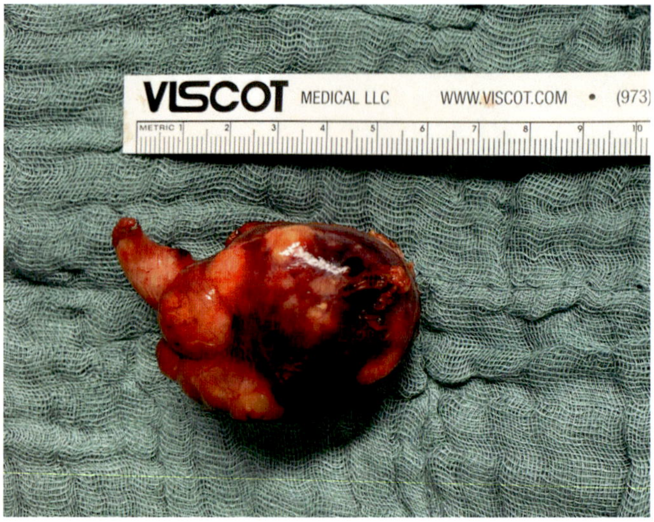

Fig. 20.12 Macroscopic view of specimen

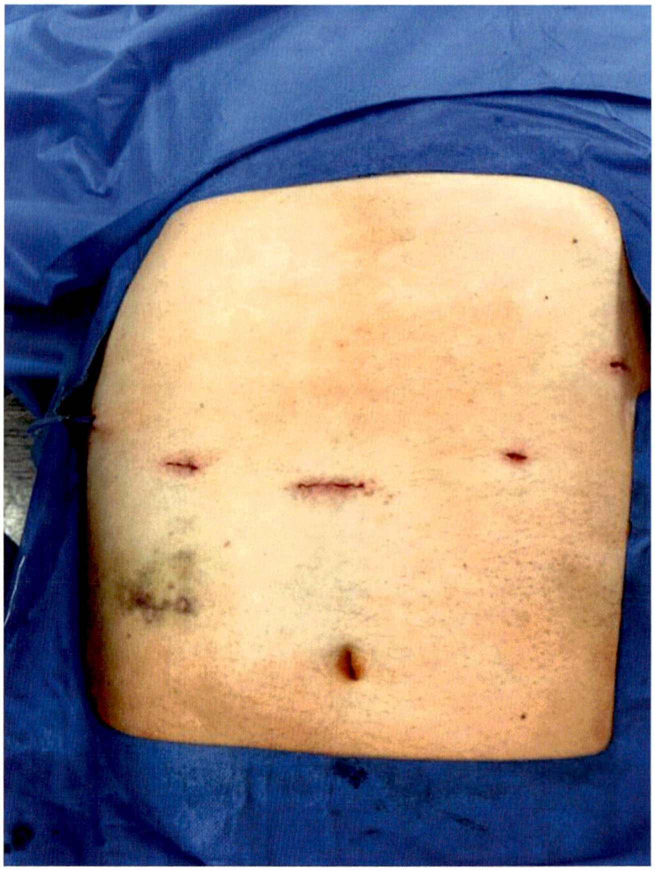

Fig. 20.13 Situs and trocar position after robotic resection

Total procedure time was 42 min, and the patient was discharged after an uneventful postoperative course on postoperative day 6. Figure 20.13 depicts the postoperative situs and the positioning of the incisions after wound closure.

Tumor histology revealed a 49 mm pT2pN0(0/3) R0L0V0Pn0 GIST with an intermediate risk with a mitosis rate of 7/50 HPF.

References

1. Ma GL, Murphy JD, Martinez ME, Sicklick JK. Epidemiology of gastrointestinal stromal tumors in the era of histology codes: results of a population-based study. Cancer Epidemiol Biomark Prev. 2015;24:298–302.
2. Nilsson B, Bümming P, Meis-Kindblom JM, Odén A, Dortok A, Gustavsson B, et al. Gastrointestinalstromal tumors: the incidence, prevalence, clinical course, and prognostication in the preimatinib mesylate era—a population-based study in western Sweden. Cancer. 2005;103:821–9.
3. Nishida T, Blay J-Y, Hirota Y, Kang Y-K. The standard diagnosis, treatment, and follow-up of gastrointestinal stromal tumors based on guidelines. Gastric Cancer. 2016;19:3–14.
4. Hagerty BL, Torres MB, Drake J, Hernandez JM, Mullinax JE, Blakely AM, et al. Trends and predictors of failure of minimally invasive surgery for gastric GIST. J Gastrointest Surg. 2021;25:1319–22.
5. Xiong Z, Wan W, Zeng X, Wang T, Zhang R, Li C, et al. Laparoscopic versus open surgery for gastric gastrointestinal stromal tumors: a propensity score matching analysis. J Gastrointest Surg. 2020;24:1785–94.
6. Solaini L, Cavaliere D, Fico V, Milone M, De Pascale S, Desiderio J, et al. Open versus laparoscopic versus robotic gastric gastrointestinal stromal tumour resection: a multicentre cohort study. Int J Med Robot. 2021;17(2):e2198.
7. Winder A, Strauss DC, Jones RL, Benson C, Messiou C, Chaudry MA, et al. Robotic surgery for gastric gastrointestinal stromal tumors: a single center case series. J Surg Oncol. 2020; https://doi.org/10.1002/jso.26053. Online ahead of print.

21 Robotic Vertical Sleeve Gastrectomy

Hany Takla and Augustus Gleason

Introduction

Sleeve gastrectomy has become the most widely performed bariatric operation in recent years. While the laparoscopic sleeve gastrectomy (LSG) remains the gold standard, the increasing accessibility to robotic surgical systems as well as advances in robotic surgical technology including robotic stapling and energy devices points to the robotic sleeve gastrectomy (RSG) becoming more of a standard practice in different parts of the world [1]. In our experience the added benefit of better visualization and wristed instruments in higher BMI patients offer better ergonomics for the operating surgeon which in turn reflects on achieving better exposure, better hemostasis, and safer dissection during this procedure.

Data comparing the laparoscopic sleeve gastrectomy to the robotic counterpart suggests that the RSG is associated with longer operating time and a higher rate of postoperative complications [2]. However, other studies exist that account for learning curves and involvement of residents/fellows that do not demonstrate a negative impact on outcomes [3]. Furthermore, it is suggested that having the stapler in the operating surgeon's control from the console will mitigate these differences. Using a standardized approach and steps and understanding the advantages the robotic platform offers are the keys to success to implement robotic sleeve gastrectomy in your practice.

The robotic sleeve gastrectomy setup and approach is similar to that of the laparoscopic version of the operation. It is important to obtain good exposure of the hiatus, GE junction, and stomach anatomy before proceeding with your dissection. Identification of the pylorus and incisura and takedown of the gastrocolic ligament are enhanced with three-arm coordination. Care must be taken at the dissection of the short gastric arteries and fundus to ensure appropriate setup for stapling. With proper mobilization of the stomach and insertion of a bougie tube, stapling can begin. Vertical stapling along the greater curvature tubularizes the stomach. Again, care must be taken at the fundus and angle of His with three-arm exposure. This setup ensures good stapling technique and avoidance of retained fundus. We advise using the firefly technology liberally to check for the blood supply especially at the angle of His which is the most common site for staple line leaks mainly due to poor blood supply.

Procedure: Illustrated Steps

Figures 21.1, 21.2, 21.3, 21.4, 21.5, 21.6, 21.7, 21.8, 21.9, 21.10, 21.11, 21.12, 21.13, 21.14, 21.15, 21.16, 21.17, 21.18, 21.19, 21.20, 21.21, 21.22, 21.23, 21.24, 21.25, 21.26, 21.27, 21.28, 21.29, 21.30, 21.31, 21.32, 21.33, 21.34, 21.34, 21.35, 21.36, 21.37, 21.38, 21.39, 21.40, 21.41, 21.42, 21.43, 21.44, and 21.45 illustrate a robotic vertical sleeve gastrectomy and hiatal hernia repair.

H. Takla (✉)
Departments of General and Bariatric Surgery, Beth Israel Lahey Health Winchester Hospital, Winchester, MA, USA
e-mail: hany.m.takla@lahey.org

A. Gleason
Surgical Simulation and Education Research Fellow, Lahey Hospital and Medical Center Department of Surgery, Burlington, MA, USA

O. Y. Kudsi, P. P. Grimminger (eds.), *Atlas of Robotic Upper Gastrointestinal Surgery*,
https://doi.org/10.1007/978-3-030-86578-8_21

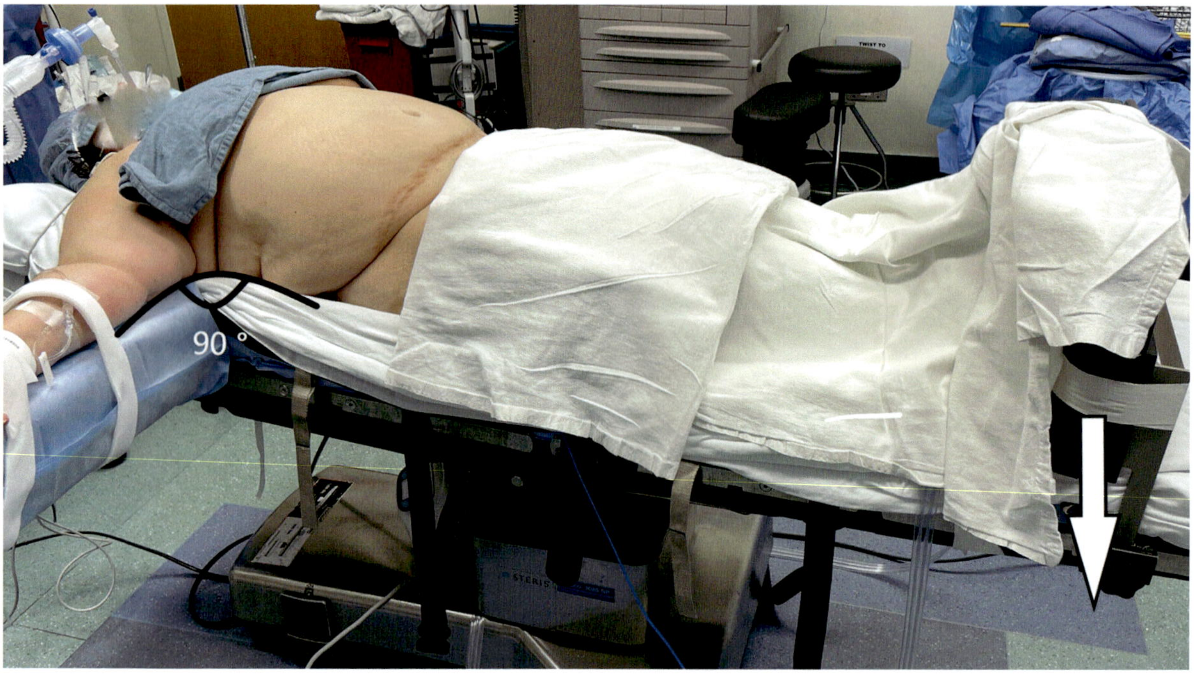

Fig. 21.1 Patient is placed supine, arms out at 90 degrees, foot board placed for steep reverse Trendelenburg

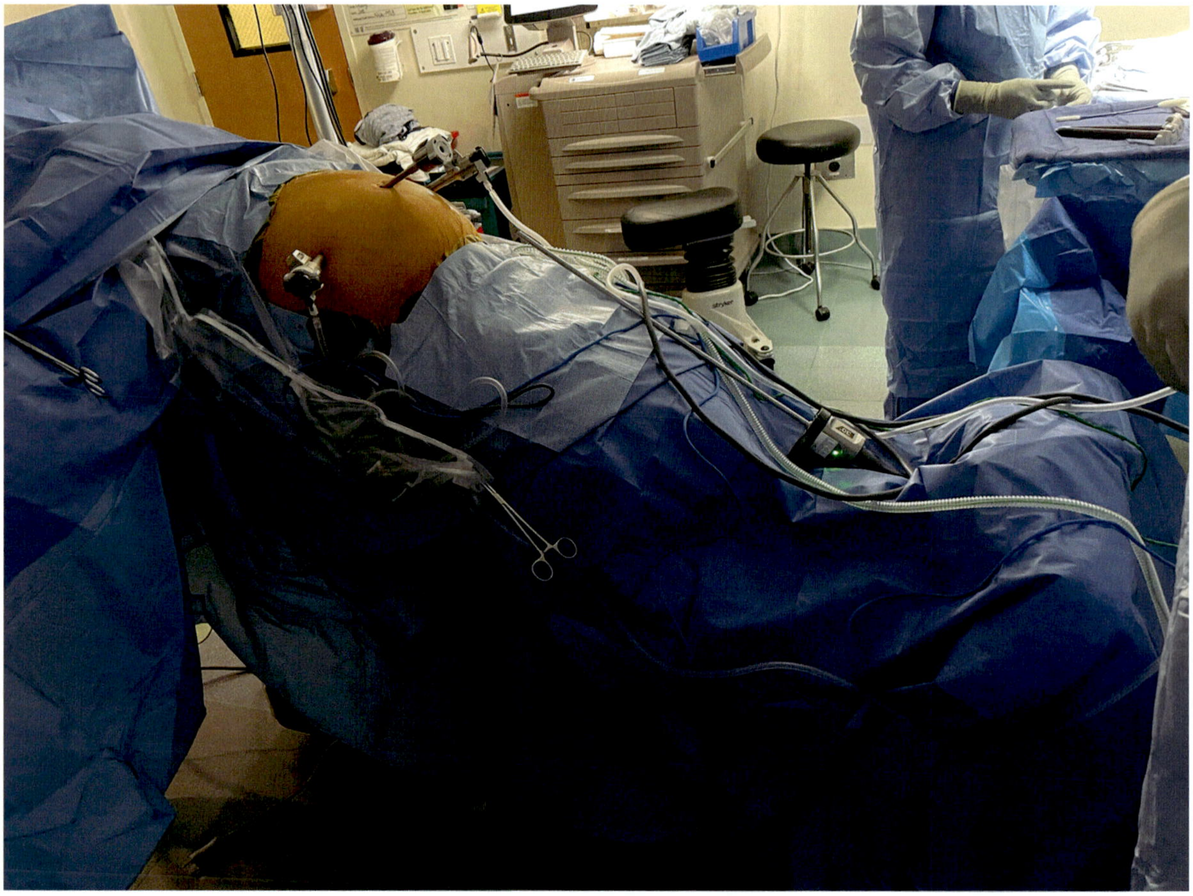

Fig. 21.2 Preparation and draping of the abdomen with robot trocar placement. Robot will be docked on the right side of the patient

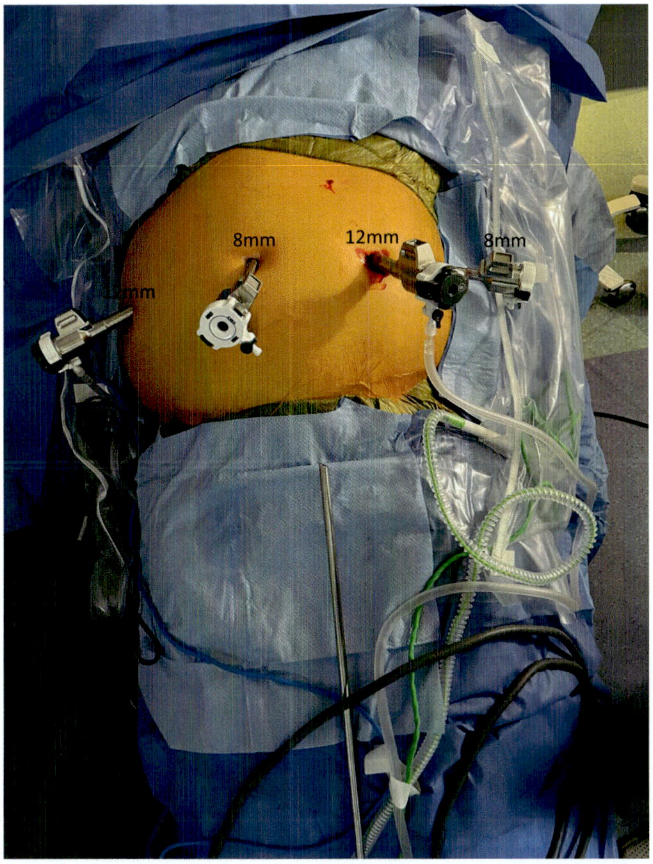

Fig. 21.3 Four robotic trocars are placed in linear fashion supraumbilical across the abdomen. We prefer to use two 12 mm ports for stapling and two 8 mm ports

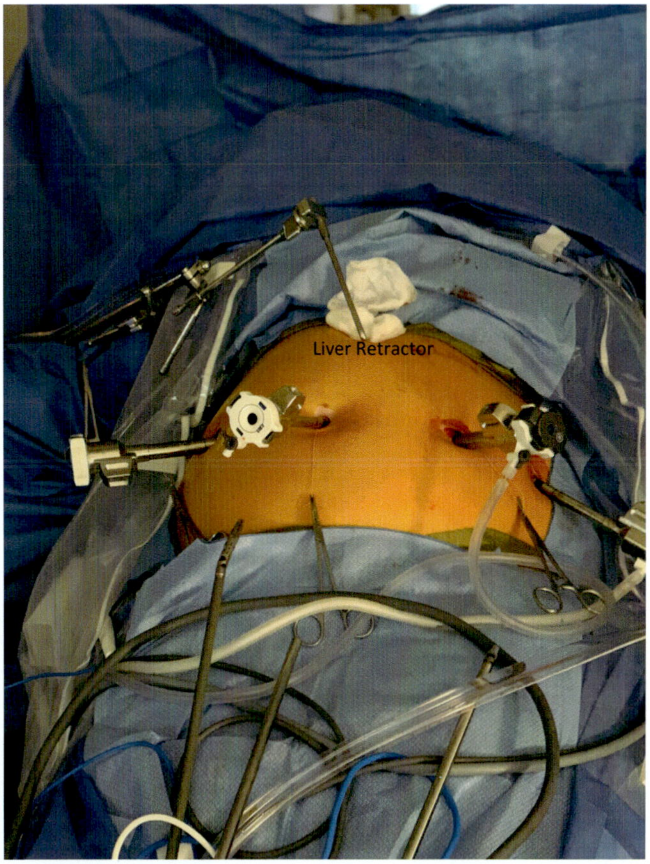

Fig. 21.4 A Nathanson liver retractor can be placed in the subxiphoid position. Intracorporeal liver retraction using a suspension barbed suture will be demonstrated as well

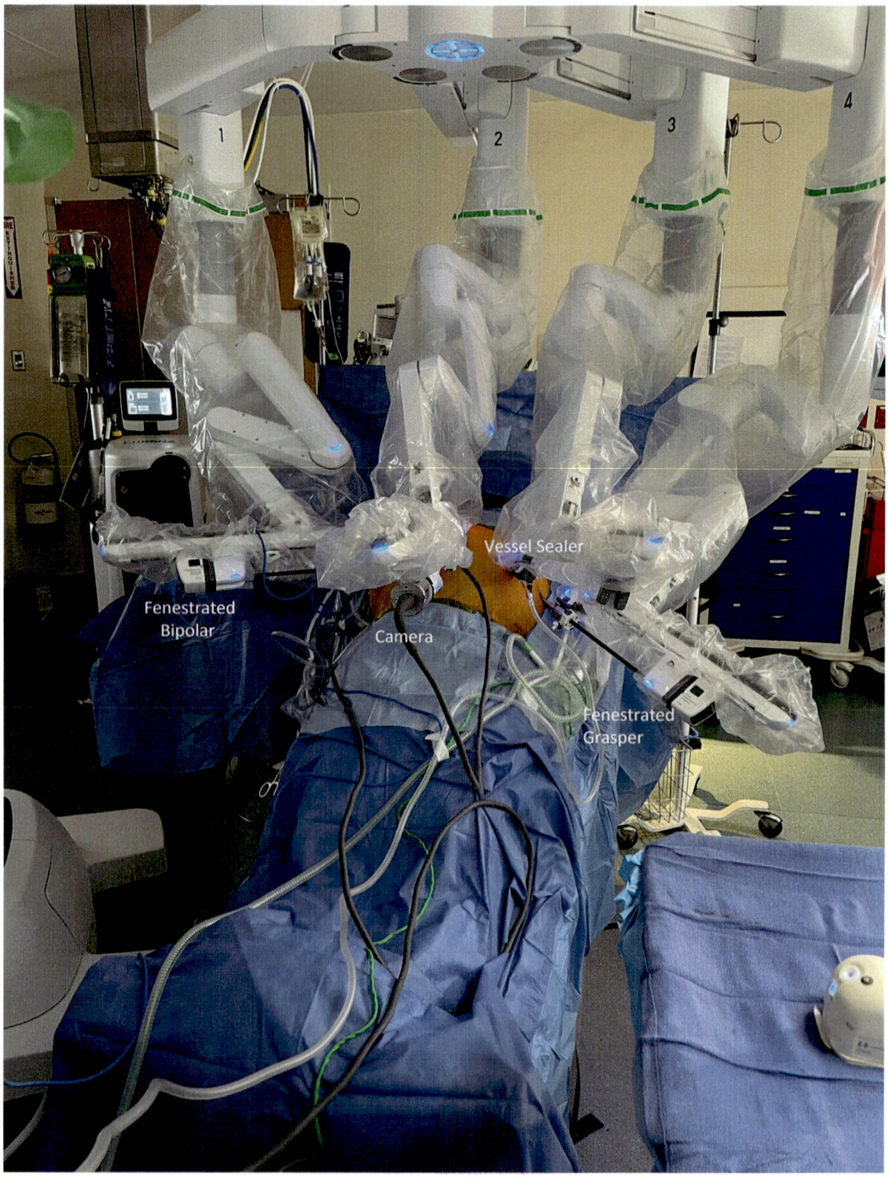

Fig. 21.5 The robot is docked from the right side. Arm 1 (far right): fenestrated bipolar. Arm 2 (right medial): 30 degree camera. Arm 3 (left medial): Vessel sealer or needle driver. Arm 4 (far left): fenestrated grasper

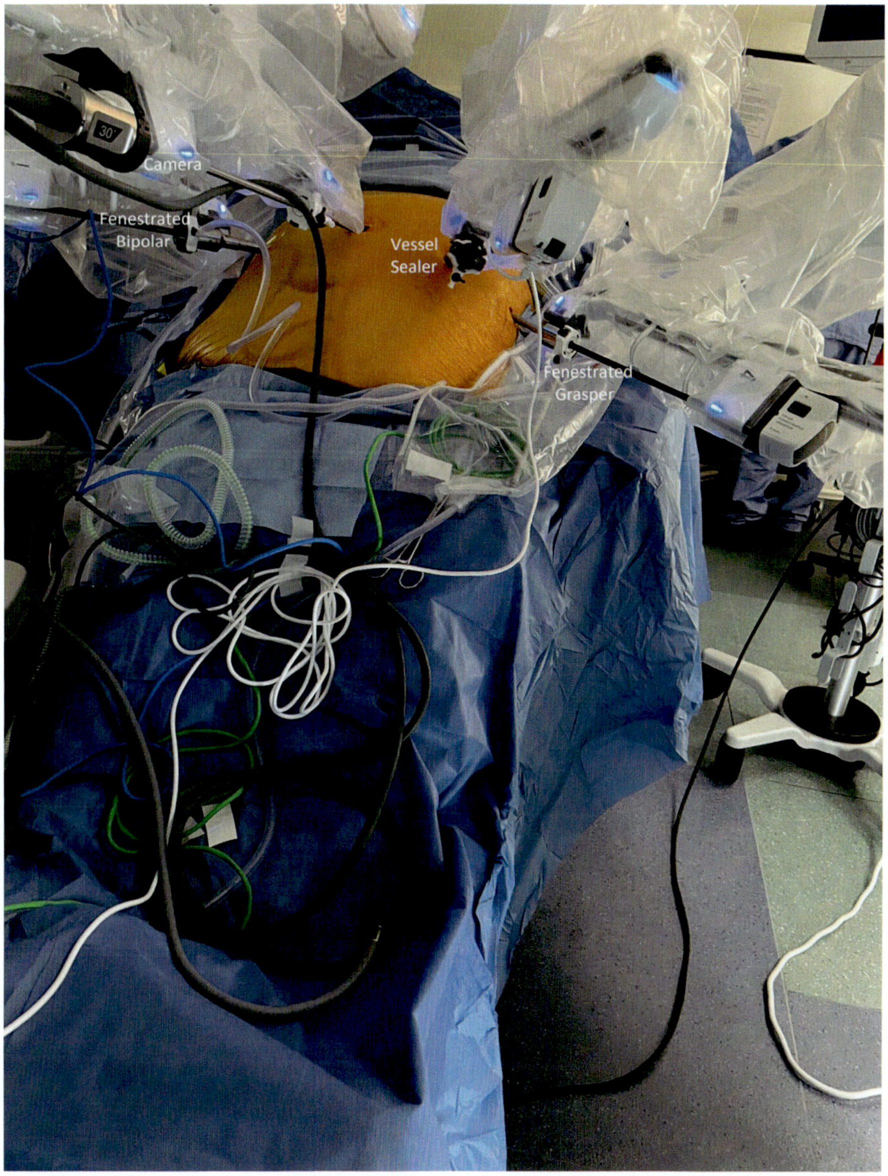

Fig. 21.6 Demonstrating appropriate spacing of the trocars and robotics arms

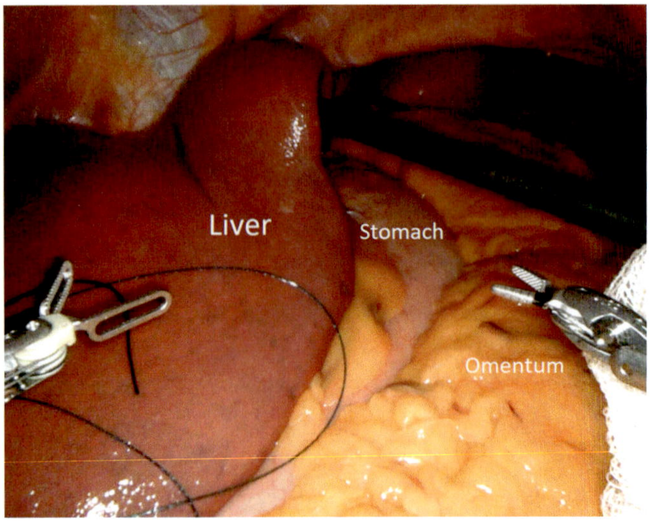

Fig. 21.7 Initial insufflation and inspection reveals the stomach mostly concealed by the liver and omentum. The omentum is swept laterally, and the liver is retracted anterior and cephalad. This case will demonstrate the use of a temporary suspension suture for liver retraction

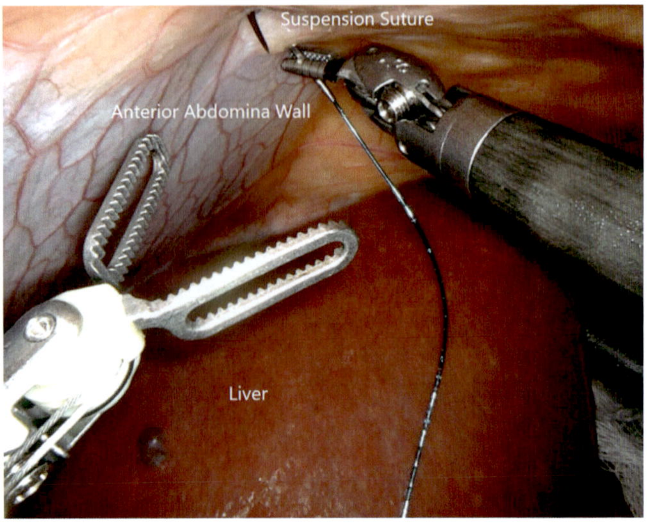

Fig. 21.8 Liver retraction is performed using a 2–0 barbed suture which will create a temporary sling to keep the liver edge out of the operative field and provide excellent hiatal exposure

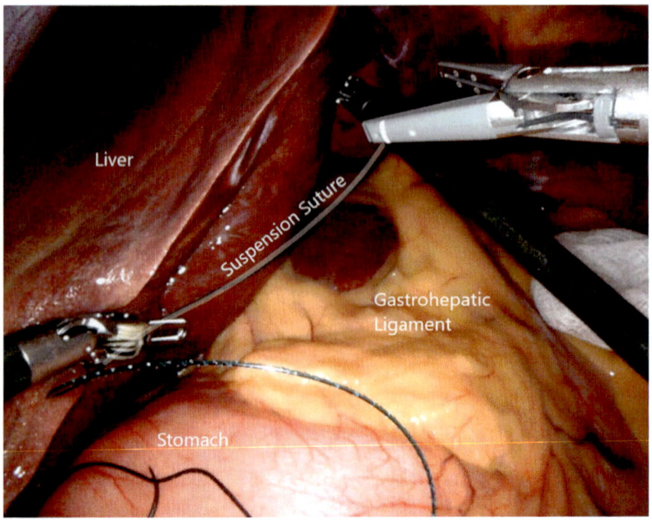

Fig. 21.9 Optimizing liver retraction and exposure

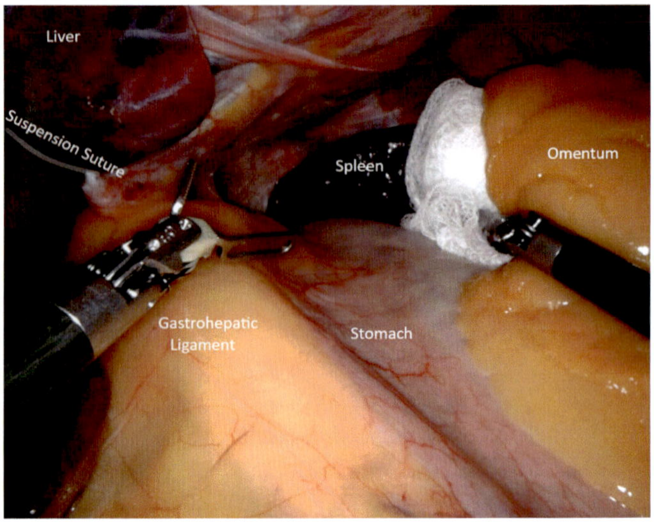

Fig. 21.10 The operative field is now exposed demonstrating the gastrohepatic ligament, stomach, and spleen. The omentum is further swept laterally and caudad

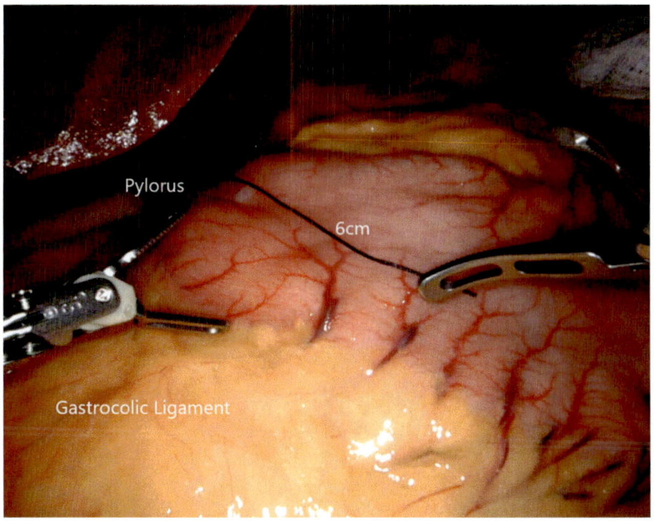

Fig. 21.11 Attention is turned to the distal stomach. The pylorus and incisura angularis are identified. A 6 cm silk tie is used to aid in measuring the distance from the pylorus as a guide for dissection and avoid excessive narrowing at the incisura

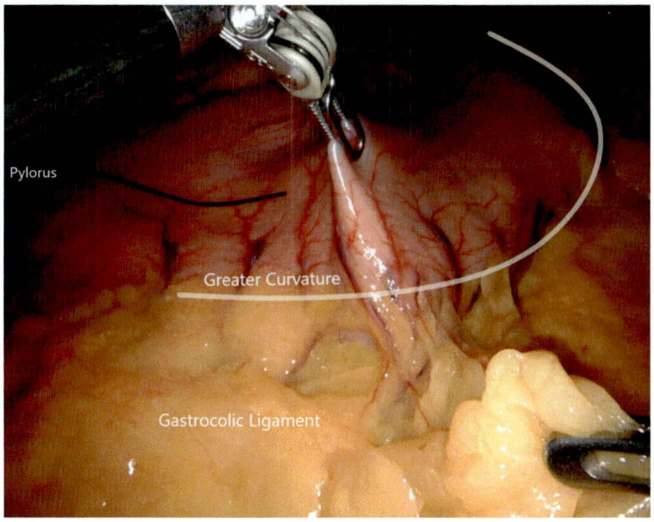

Fig. 21.12 The dissection of the gastrocolic ligament along the greater curvature begins using the vessel sealer

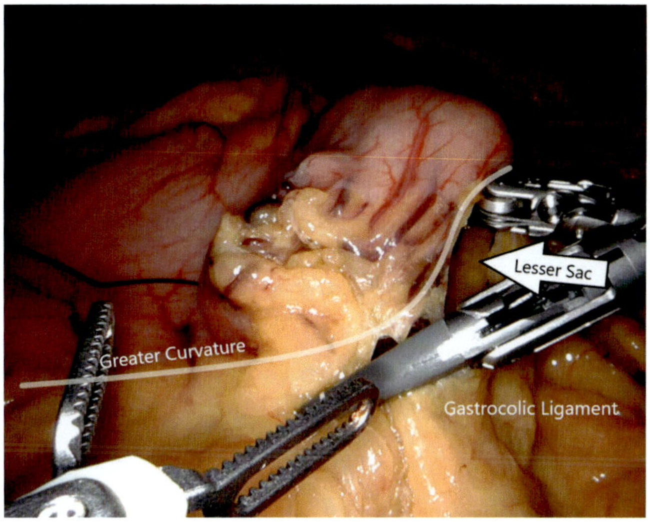

Fig. 21.13 The lesser sac is exposed, and retraction of the stomach anteriorly provides a good view of the dissection plane along the greater curvature

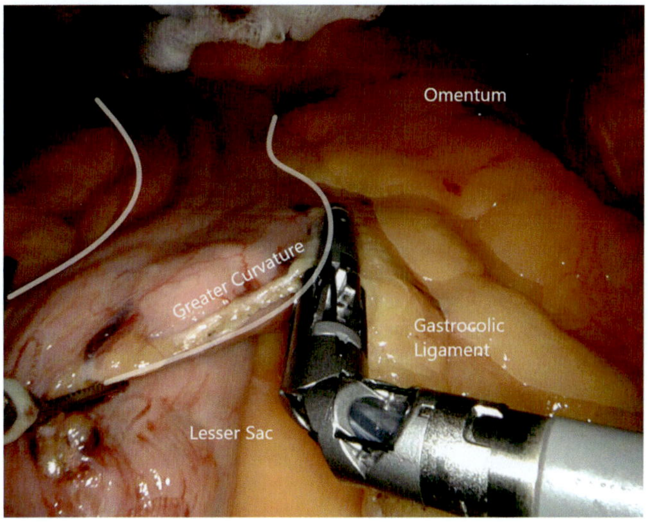

Fig. 21.14 Three-arm coordination provides good exposure and allows for easy dissection of the gastrocolic ligament while remaining close to the greater curvature

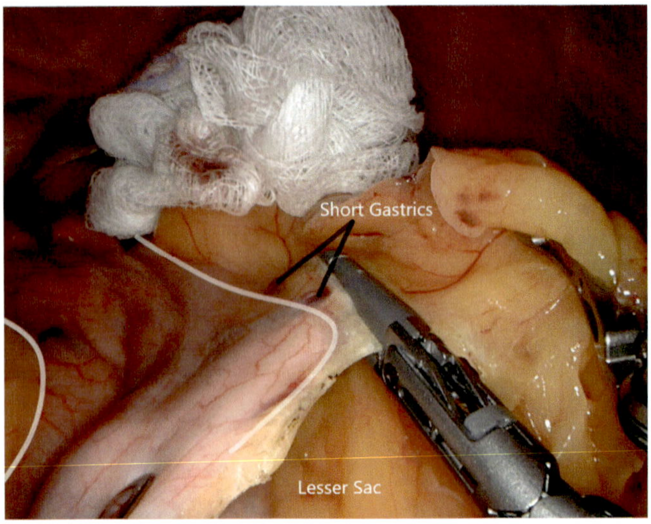

Fig. 21.15 Dissection continues along the greater curvature cephalad toward the fundus. Short gastric arteries are identified and ligated close to the stomach using the vessel sealer

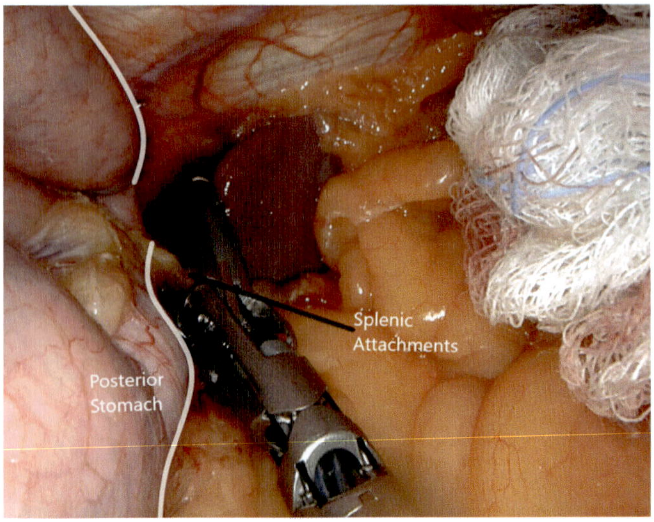

Fig. 21.17 Further splenic attachments are taken down. This exposure is enhanced by three-arm coordination, and an easy dissection plane is identified with good retraction on the stomach

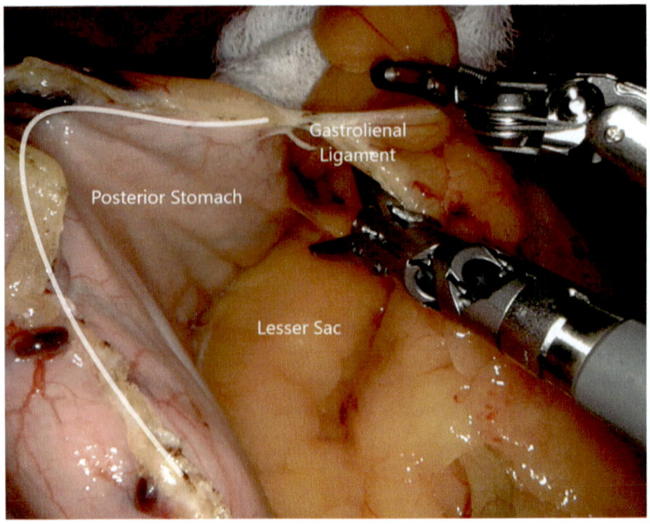

Fig. 21.16 The stomach is retracted anteriorly and inferiorly to expose the posterior wall. The gastrolienal and splenic attachments are dissected off the stomach

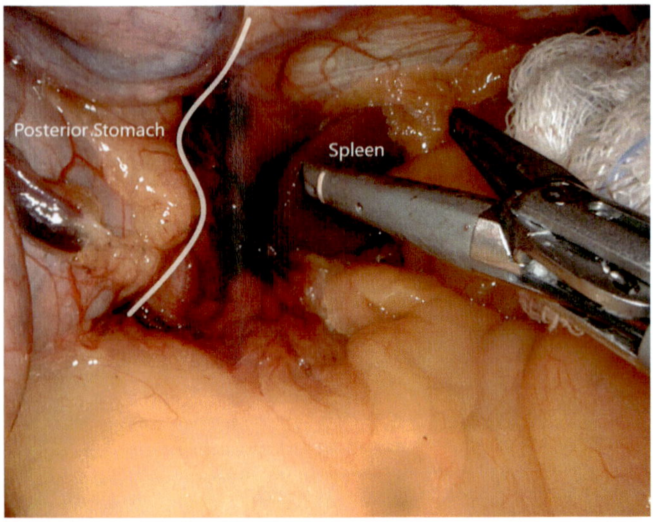

Fig. 21.18 The greater curvature and fundus are now nearly completely mobilized. The posterior stomach is further exposed to allow for dissection of the posterior attachments. Visualization of the left crus of the diaphragm is a good landmark for completed mobilization of the fundus

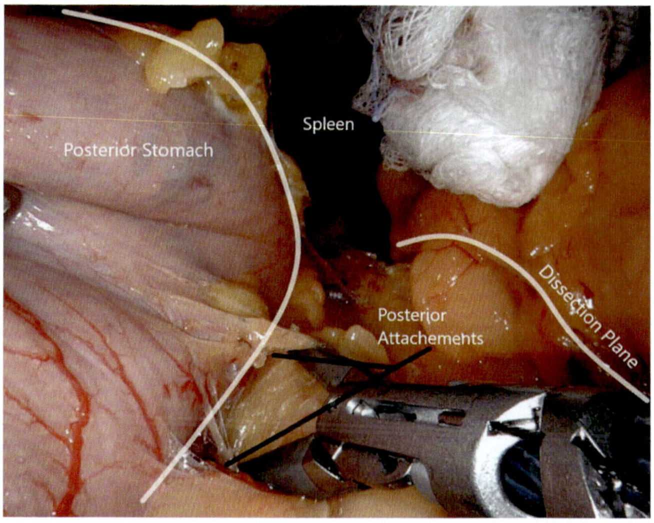

Fig. 21.19 Stomach mobilization continues with dissection of posterior stomach attachments. The dissection plan on the right side of the photo shows the now dissected gastrocolic ligament previously attached to the greater curvature

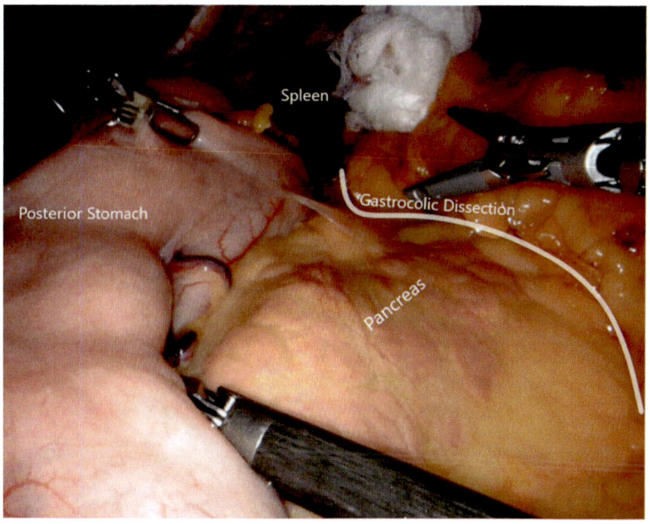

Fig. 21.21 Complete mobilization of the greater curvature and fundus. The posterior stomach is free for stapling

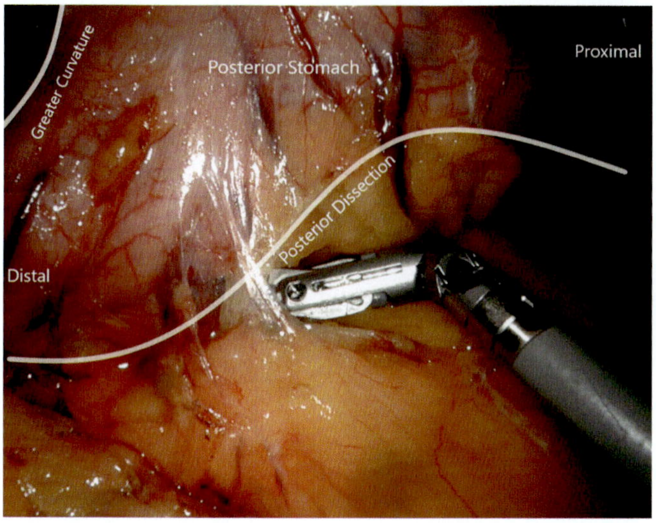

Fig. 21.20 Camera mobility and wrist articulation allows for easy dissection of the final posterior stomach attachments

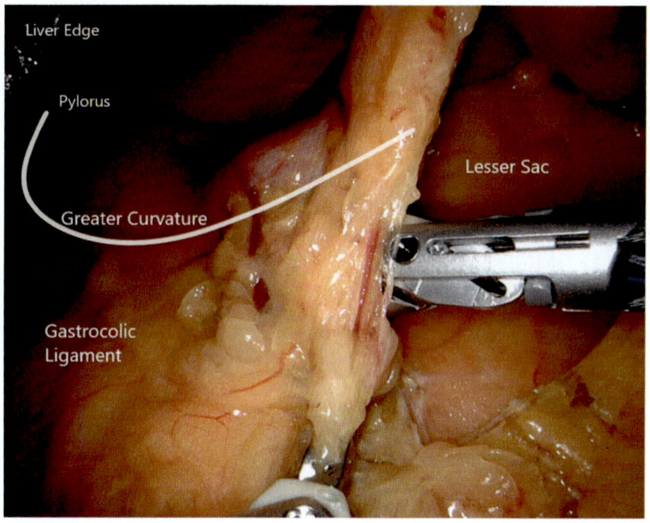

Fig. 21.22 The distal portion of the gastrocolic attachments are taken down to finish stomach mobilization

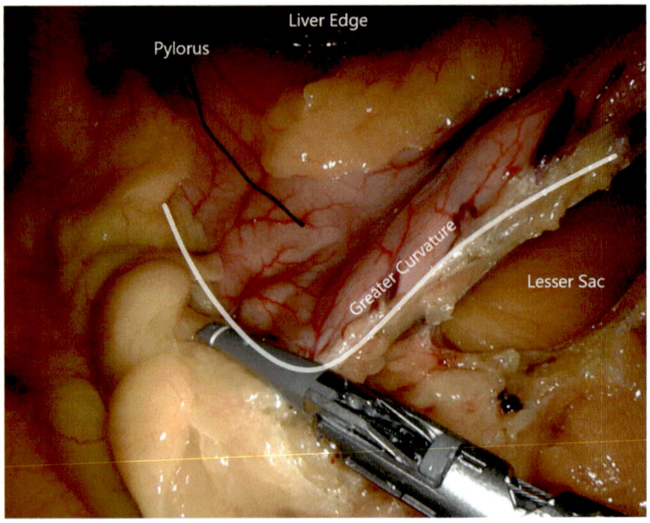

Fig. 21.23 Complete dissection of the distal gastrocolic ligament prior to stapling

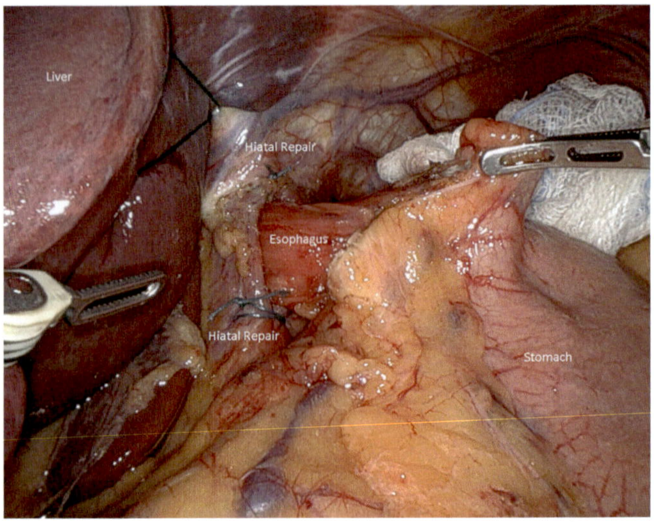

Fig. 21.25 Hiatal hernia repair is completed using a 0 Ethibond suture

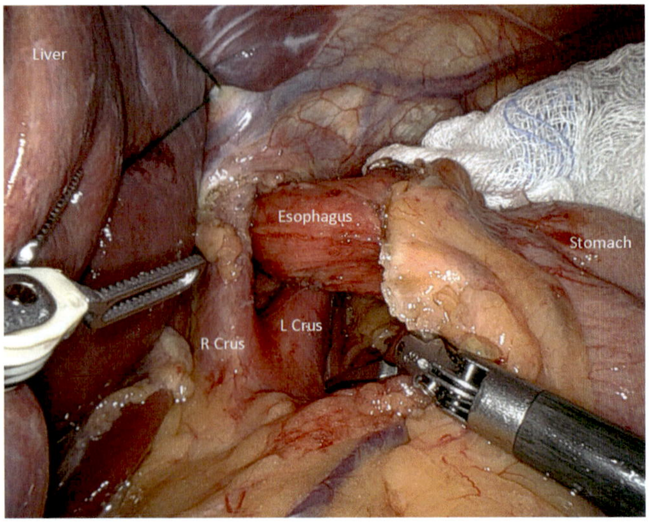

Fig. 21.24 Prior to stapling, attention is turned to the hiatus. The distal esophagus, diaphragmatic crura, and hiatal hernia are dissected and identified

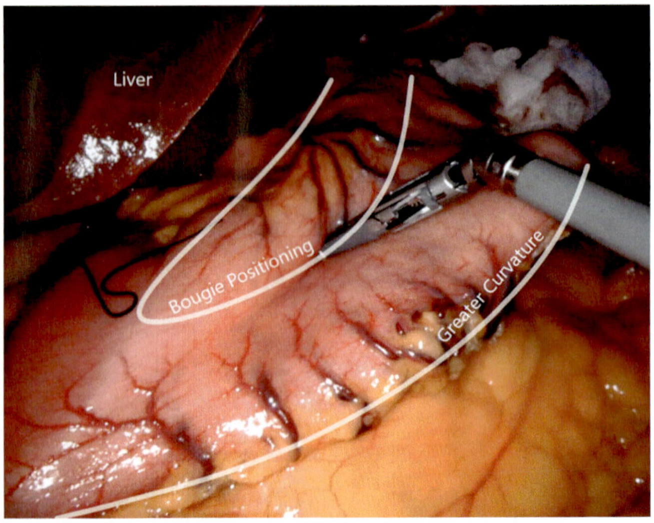

Fig. 21.26 A 38Fr bougie is placed intraluminal. Bougie positioning is adjusted to create the appropriate size and orientation for the gastric sleeve

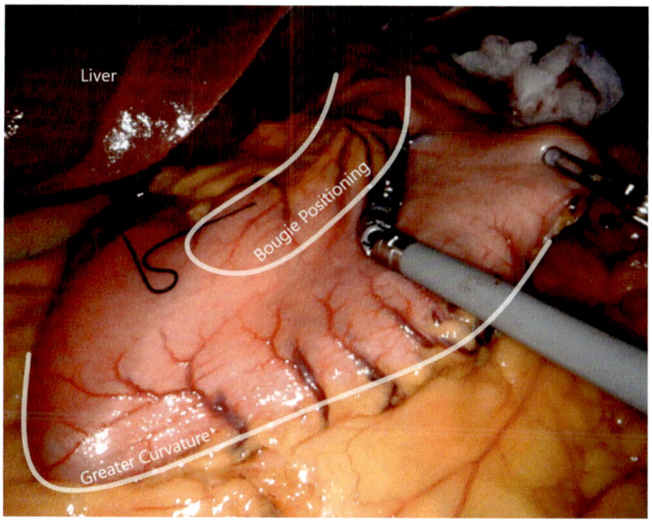

Fig. 21.27 Final positioning of the bougie prior to creation of sleeve gastrectomy. It is recommended to leave 3–5 mm of space adjacent to the bougie for optimal stapling and avoid excessive tension on the staple line

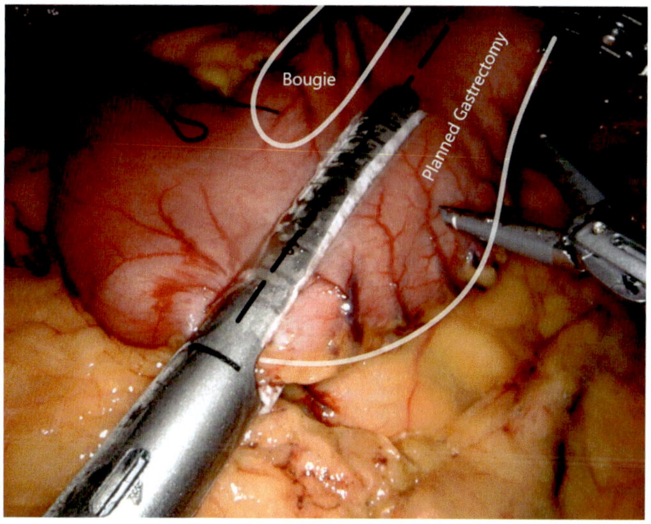

Fig. 21.29 The first staple fire is completed. After the first fire, it is appropriate to transition to the next staple height either green or blue load if the thickness of the tissue permits

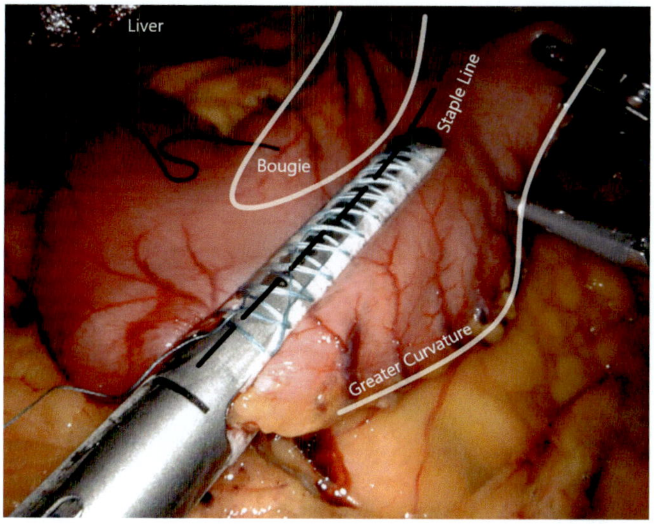

Fig. 21.28 With the bougie in appropriate positioning, the Robotic stapler is placed through the 1 port. Using a black load stapler for the first fire, division of the greater curvature begins at approximately 6 cm from the pylorus

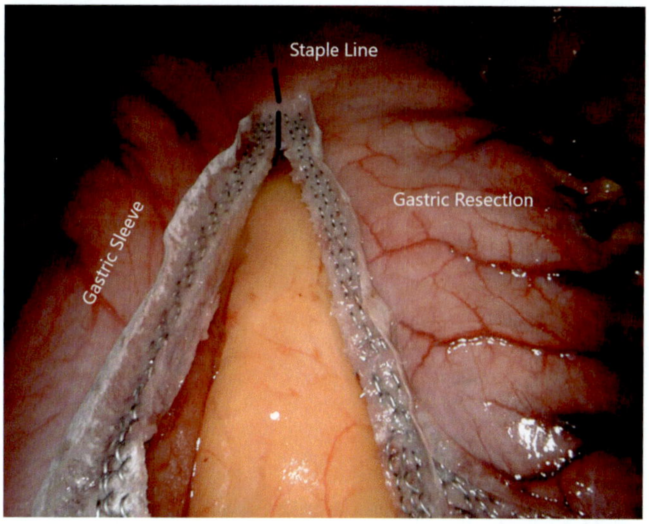

Fig. 21.30 The first staple line is inspected. Setup for the remaining staple fires is planned. The stapler is reloaded. Appropriate tension is kept on the gastric sleeve and gastric resection in order to keep the stomach flat and allow for a straight staple line

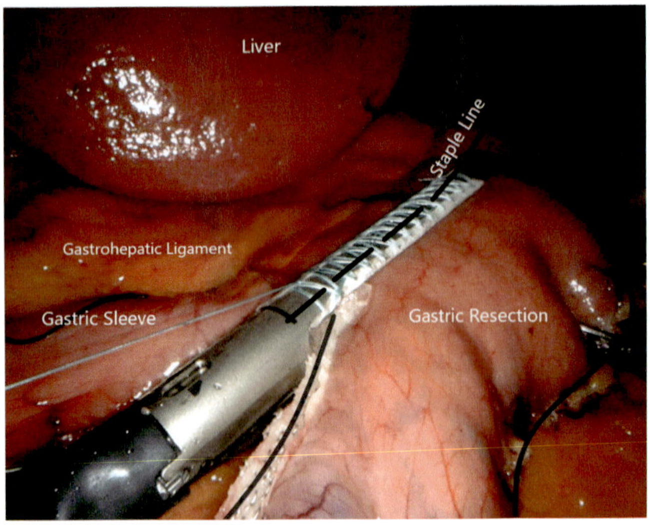

Fig. 21.31 Stapling continues. The bougie serves as a guide for stapling. Transition from the green load to the blue load is appropriate if the tissue permits

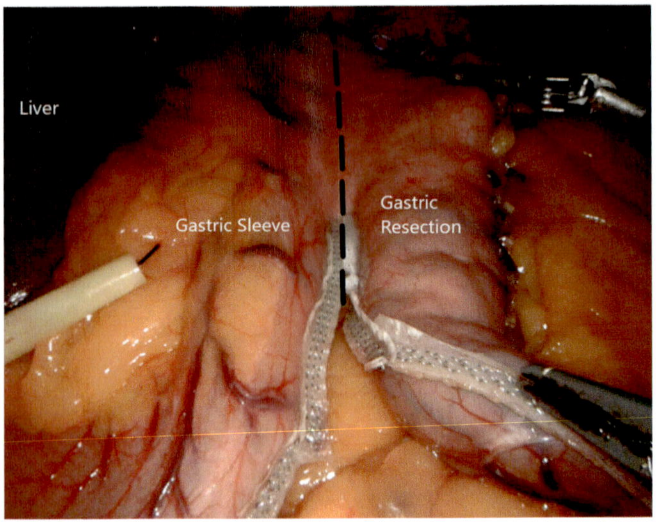

Fig. 21.33 Stapling becomes easier as it progresses toward the fundus. Tension is maintained on the greater curvature

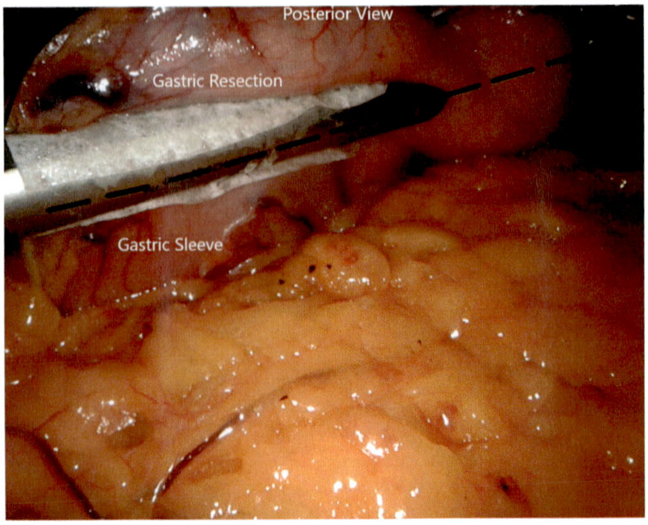

Fig. 21.32 Using the other arms to maintain adequate tension on the greater curvature keeps the stomach flat and staple line straight. An adequate posterior stomach dissection is necessary for stapling

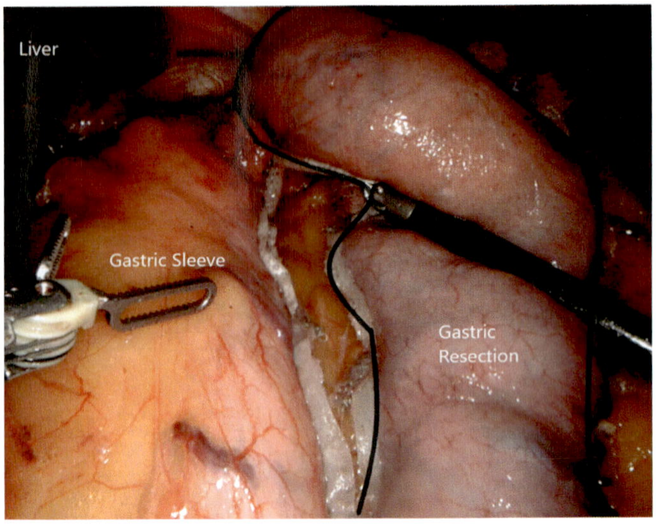

Fig. 21.34 Setting up for the final staple fire at the fundus

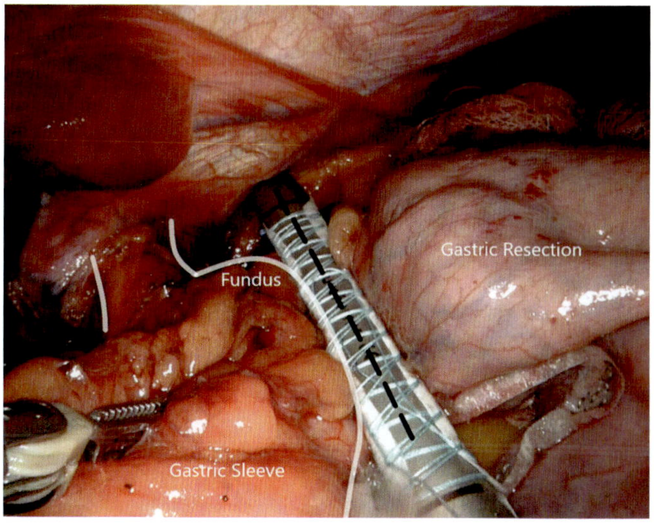

Fig. 21.35 Staple fire at the fundus. Complete the last staple fire leaving a small cuff of proximal stomach remaining – this should be approximately 5 mm next to the GE junction

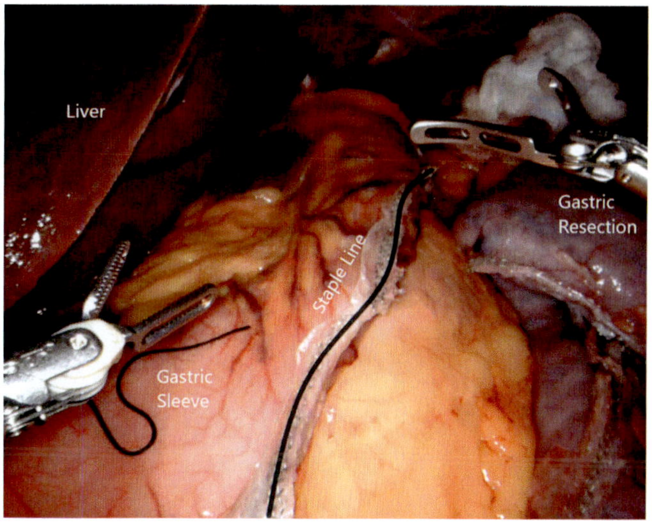

Fig. 21.37 The whole staple line is inspected

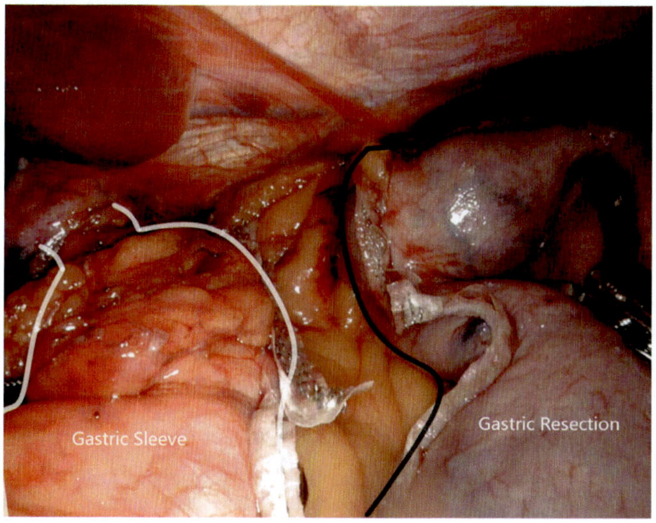

Fig. 21.36 Completion of the staple fire and creation of the sleeve gastrectomy

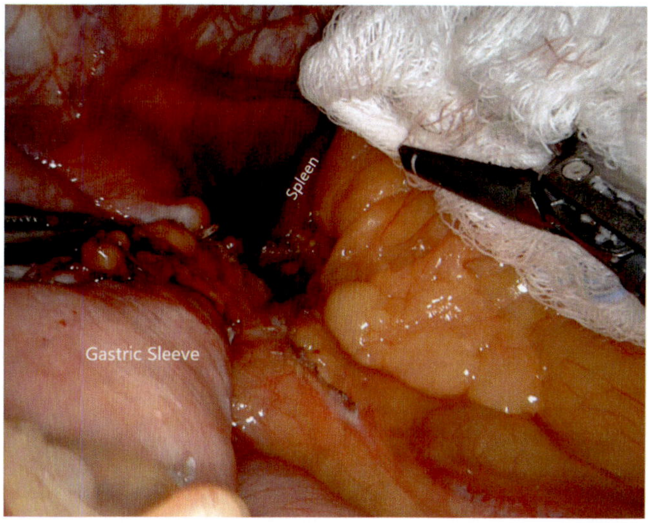

Fig. 21.38 The lesser sac, fundus, and splenic hilum are inspected for bleeding and injury post gastrectomy

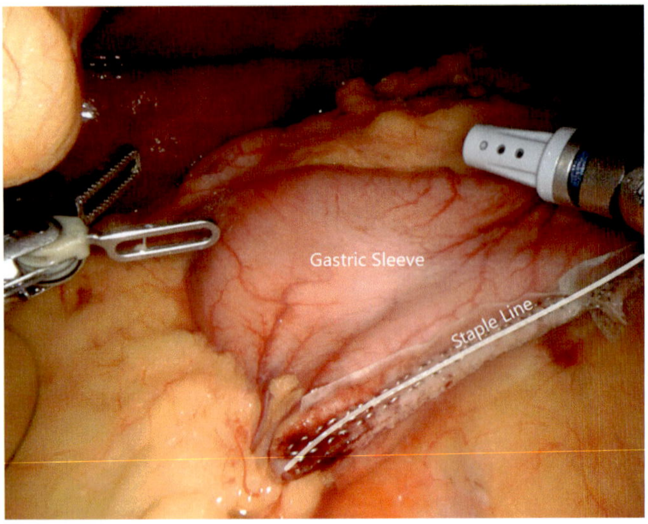

Fig. 21.39 Further inspection of the staple line and integrity of the gastric sleeve

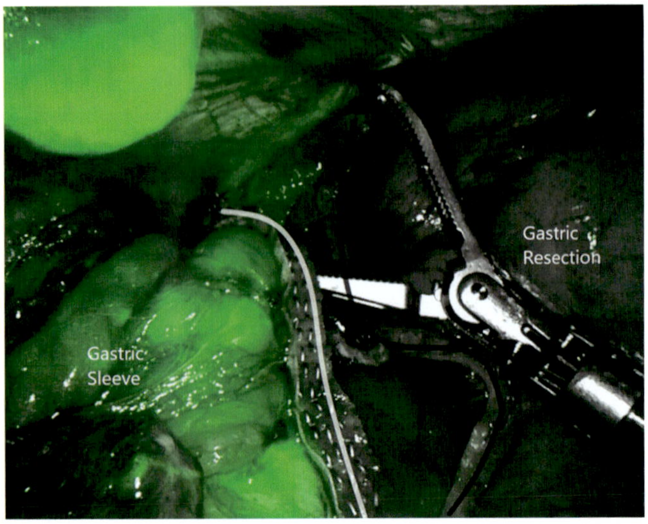

Fig. 21.40 7.5 mg of indocyanine green (ICG) is injected followed by a 10 cc flush. The camera lens is toggled which allows for perfusion visualization. The gastric sleeve perfusion is inspected

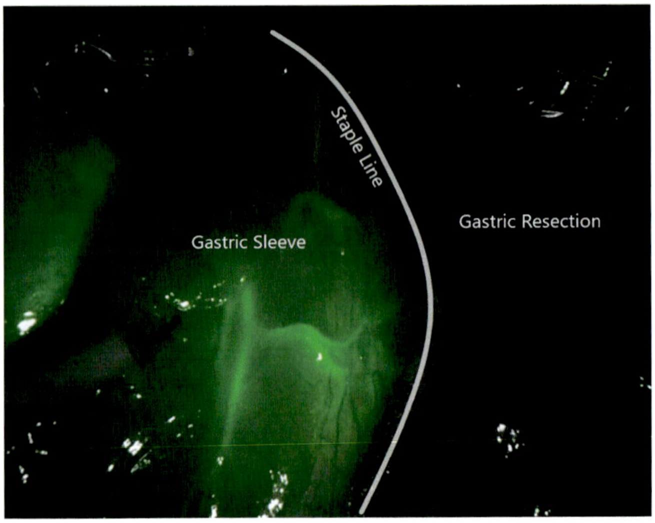

Fig. 21.41 Further inspection of the gastric sleeve perfusion. Take note of the contrast between the well-perfused sleeve and resected greater curvature

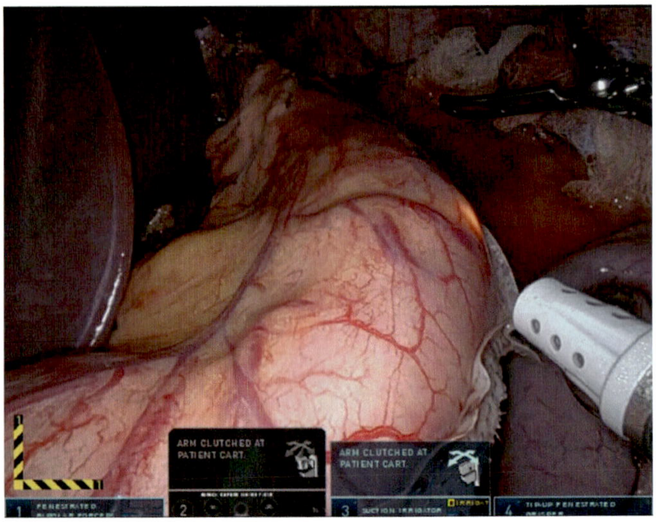

Fig. 21.42 We perform a routine intraoperative endoscopy at the end of the procedure to assess for any intraluminal bleeding and perform an air leak test

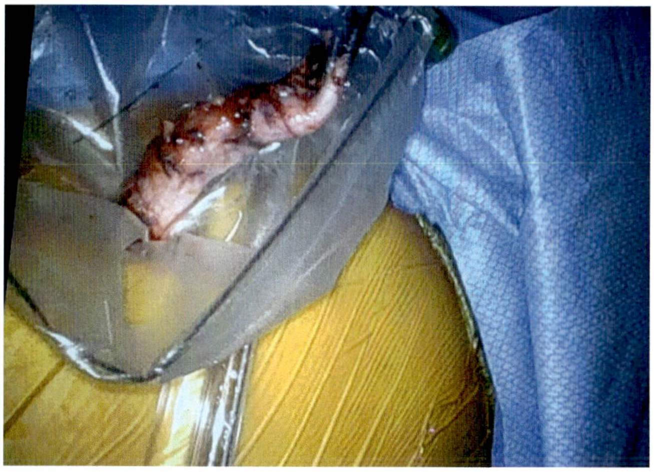

Fig. 21.43 Removal of the sleeve specimen through the right-sided 12 mm port with assistance of an Endo Catch bag

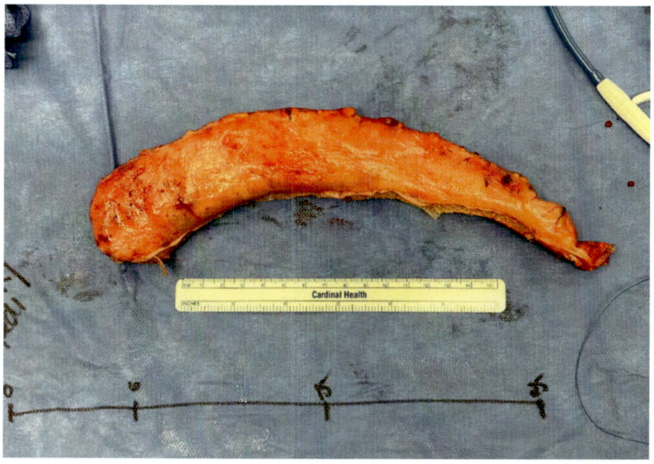

Fig. 21.44 Sleeve gastrectomy specimen

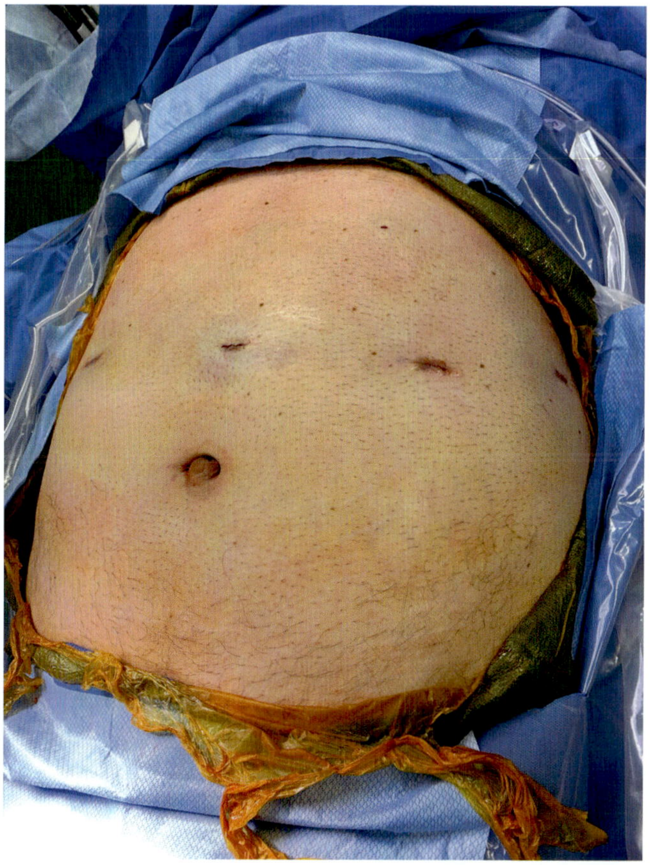

Fig. 21.45 Fascial layers and skin incisions are closed. Surgical glue is applied

References

1. Schneider B. Robotic bariatric surgery: a new weapon in the fight against obesity: digestive: nutrition: UT Southwestern Medical Center. Digestive|Nutrition|UT Southwestern Medical Center, 26 Sept. 2019, utswmed.org/medblog/robotic-bariatric-surgery-new-weapon-fight-against-obesity.
2. Fazl Alizadeh R, Li S, Inaba CS, Dinicu AI, Hinojosa MW, Smith BR, Stamos MJ, Nguyen NT. Robotic versus laparoscopic sleeve gastrectomy: a MBSAQIP analysis. Surg Endosc. 2019;33(3):917–22. https://doi.org/10.1007/s00464-018-6387-6.Epub 2018 Aug 20.
3. Altieri MS, Yang J, Telem DA, Chen H, Talamini M, Pryor A. Robotic-assisted outcomes are not tied to surgeon volume and experience. Surg Endosc. 2016;30:2825–33.

Robotic Gastric Bypass

22

Jan-Niclas Kersebaum and Jan Henrik Beckmann

Introduction

In recent years, surgery has evolved rapidly with the introduction of robotic-assisted systems. In bariatric surgery, too, robotics must first hold its own against highly standardized laparoscopy, which has few complications. With high acquisition, maintenance and material costs, as well as the lack of proof of cost efficiency, robotics is only slowly making inroads here. The advantages of using robotically assisted surgery in bariatrics are the decoupling between the nevertheless pronounced restoring forces of the abdominal wall of the obese patients and the surgeon and the 3D view combined with the fine preparation possibilities of the fine instruments in the sometimes exceedingly small surgical site. In international comparison, German patients have the highest BMI at the time of surgery (34.2 kg/m^2 in South Korea to 49.1 kg/m^2 in Germany) [1], which makes the use of robotic systems in this difficult cohort even more reasonable. The first robotic-assisted gastric bypass was performed in 2001 [2]. Since then, the system has been implemented internationally in the surgical care of obese patients [3].

Procedure: Illustrated Steps

Figures 22.1, 22.2, 22.3, 22.4, 22.5, 22.6, 22.7, 22.8, 22.9, 22.10, 22.11, 22.12, 22.13, 22.14, 22.15, 22.16, 22.17, 22.18, 22.19, 22.20, 22.21, 22.22, 22.23, 22.24, 22.25, 22.26, 22.27, 22.28, 22.29, 22.30, 22.31, 22.32, 22.33, 22.34, 22.35, 22.36, 22.37, 22.38, 22.39, 22.40, 22.41, 22.42, 22.43, 22.44, 22.45, 22.46, 22.47, 22.48, 22.49, 22.50, 22.51, 22.52, 22.53, 22.54, and 22.55 illustrate the technical aspects of robotic Roux-en-Y gastric bypass.

J.-N. Kersebaum · J. H. Beckmann (✉)
UKSH Department of General, Visceral-, Thoracic-, Transplantation-, and Pediatric Surgery, University Medical Center Schleswig-Holstein, Kiel, Germany
e-mail: jan.beckmann@uksh.de

O. Y. Kudsi, P. P. Grimminger (eds.), *Atlas of Robotic Upper Gastrointestinal Surgery*,
https://doi.org/10.1007/978-3-030-86578-8_22

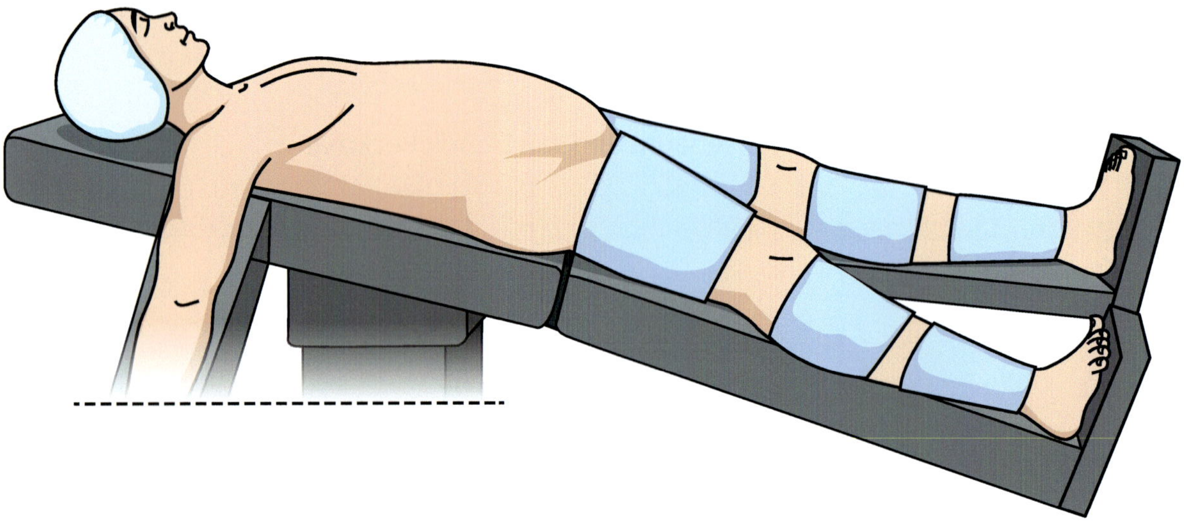

Fig. 22.1 The patient is positioned in the "French position" or 20° anti-Trendelenburg position with the legs spread, the left arm supported, and the right arm extended. In accordance with the in-house standard, all patients receive calf compression pumps. View from the side

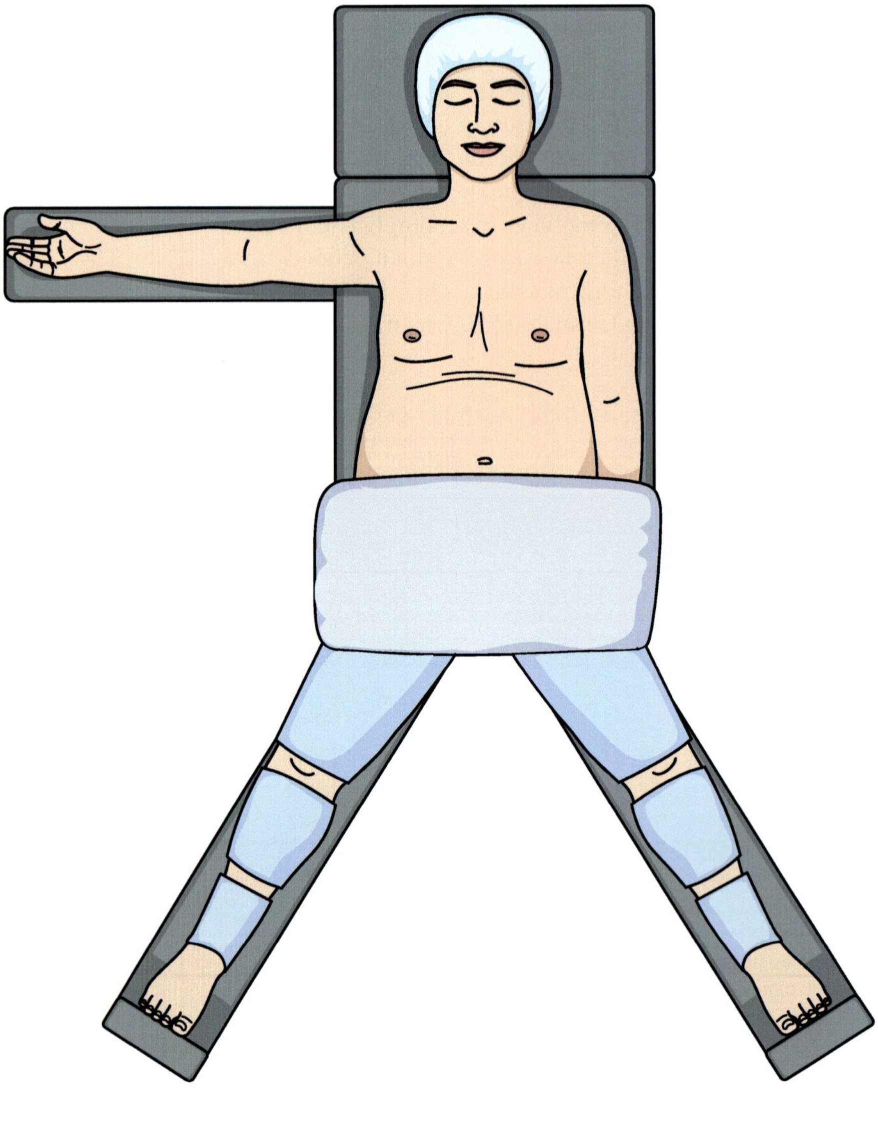

Fig. 22.2 View from the top

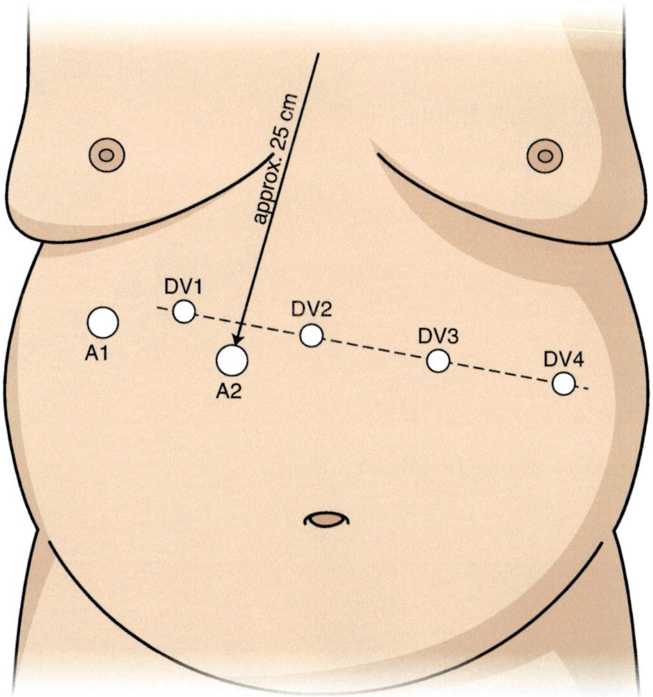

Fig. 22.3 Trocar placement. DV1 to DV 4 are Da Vinci Trocars; A1 and A2 are 12 mm laparoscopic assistance trocars

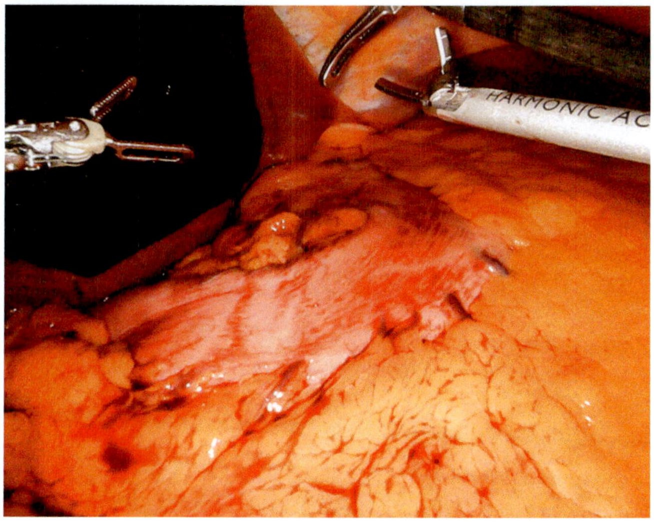

Fig. 22.4 In situ view of the surgical site with the uplifted left liver lobe

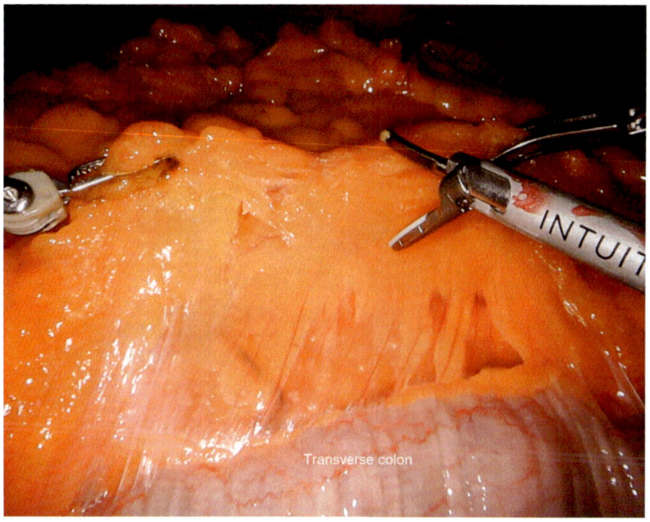

Fig. 22.5 Division of the greater omentum above the transverse colon

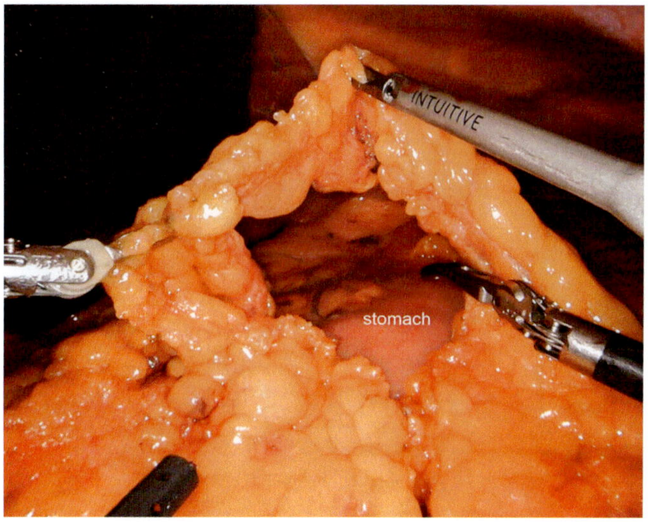

Fig. 22.6 Division of the greater omentum toward the stomach

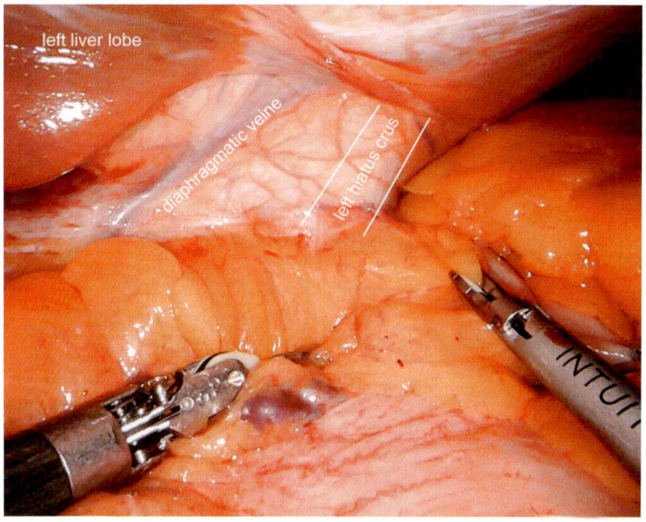

Fig. 22.7 Visualization of the left hiatus crus

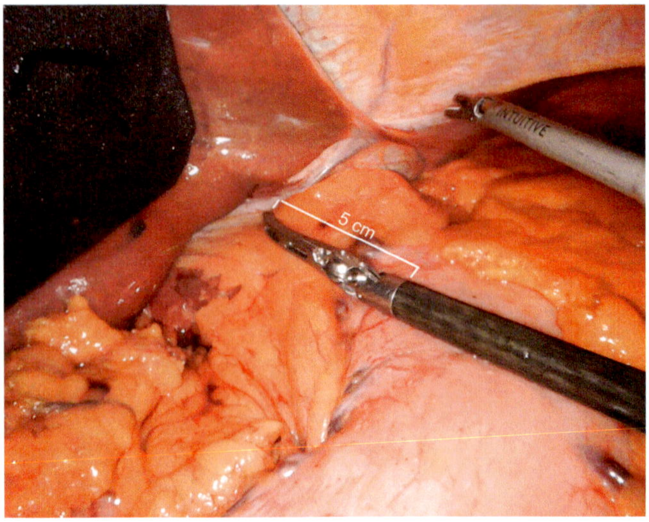

Fig. 22.8 Using the tip-up fenestrated grasper as a measurement tool

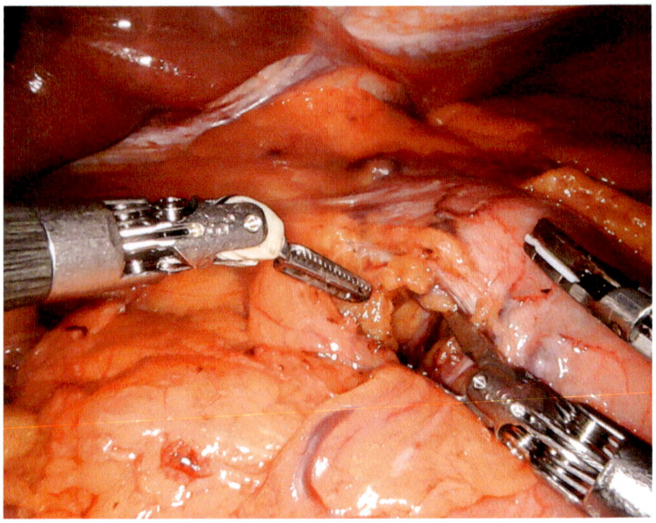

Fig. 22.10 Forming a retrogastric tunnel

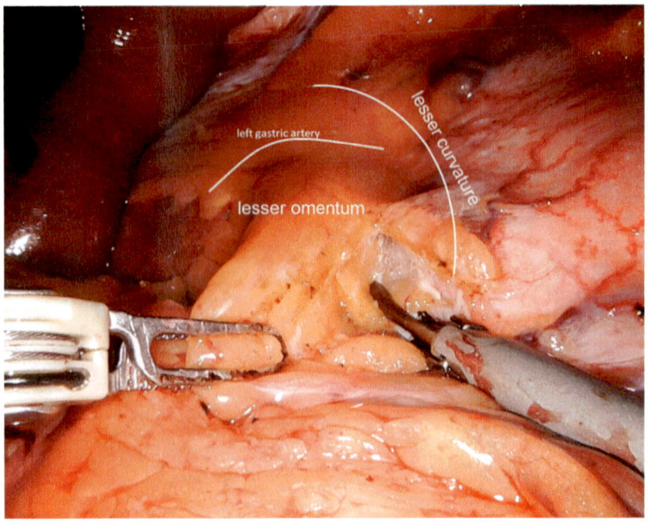

Fig. 22.9 Starting from the lesser curvature approximately 6 cm below the gastroesophageal junction, the lesser omentum is opened under preservation of the left gastric artery

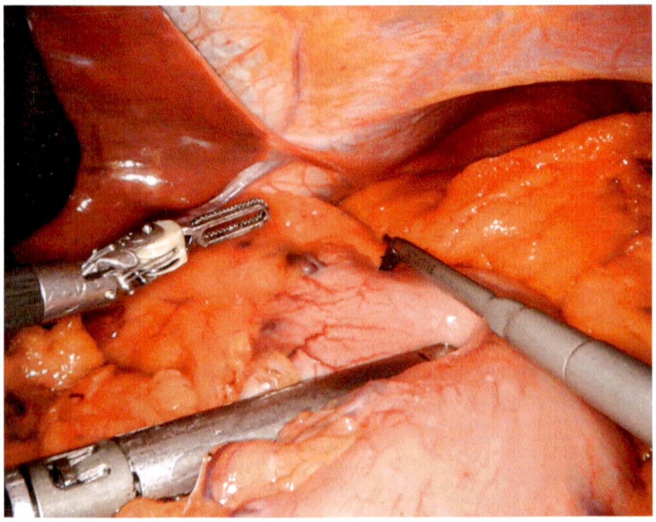

Fig. 22.11 Inserting a linear stapler into the prior formed retrogastric tunnel

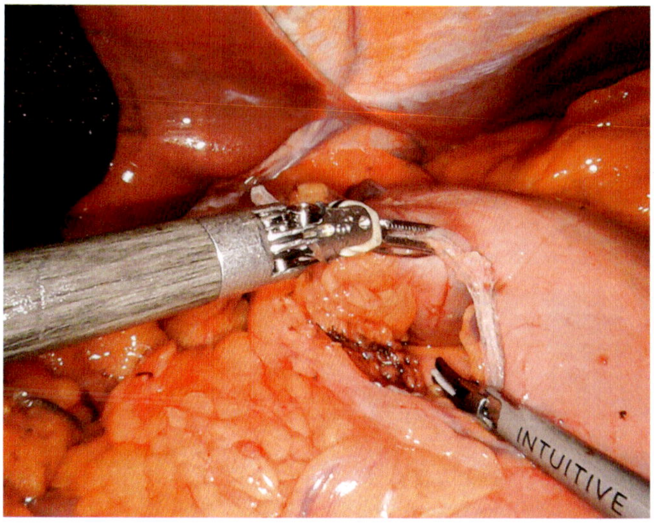

Fig. 22.12 Before the 40 Charrier Bougie is inserted, gastric adhesions are being severed

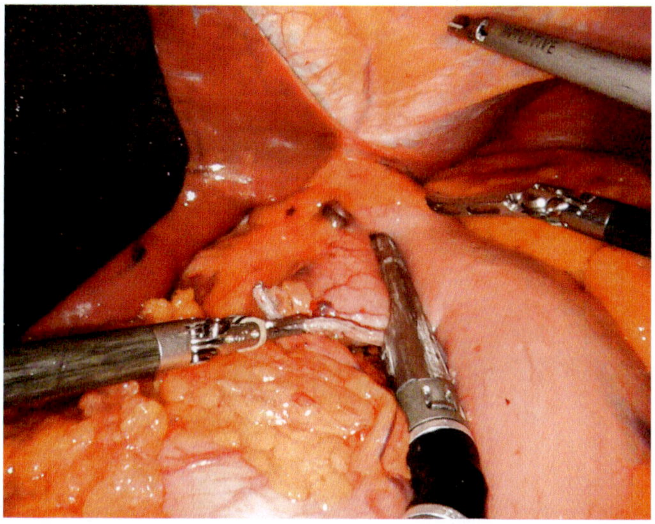

Fig. 22.13 Following the cross stapling, a second stapling device is inserted. The tip should aim toward the left hiatus' crus

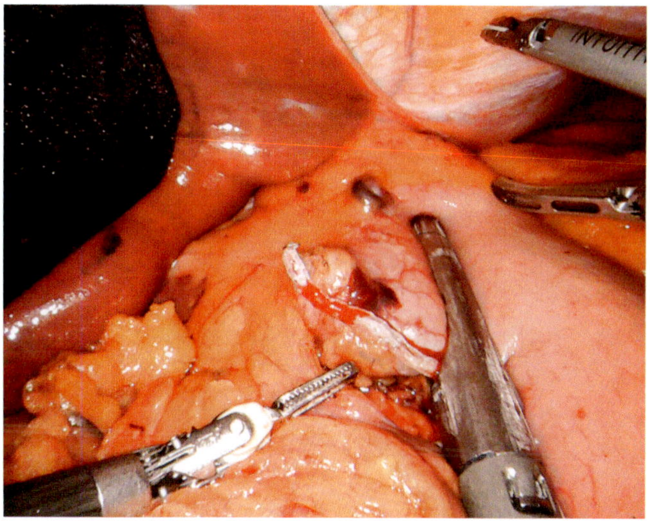

Fig. 22.14 After the bougie is inserted, the stapling device is repositioned toward the bougie to ensure a good pouch sized

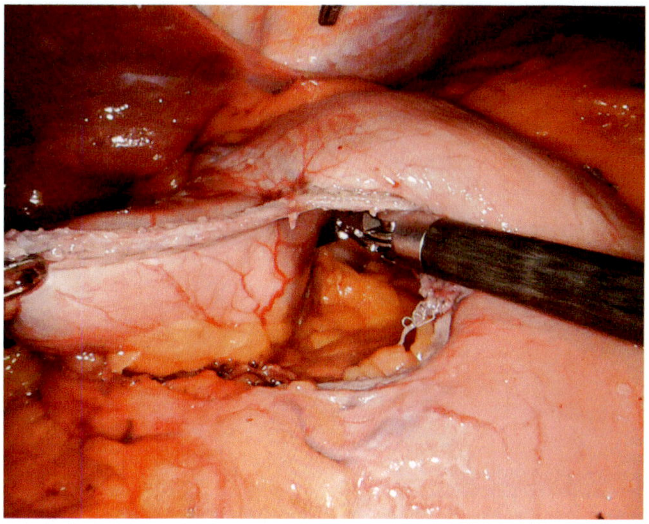

Fig. 22.15 View into the omental bursa. It is important to remove lose stapling brackets

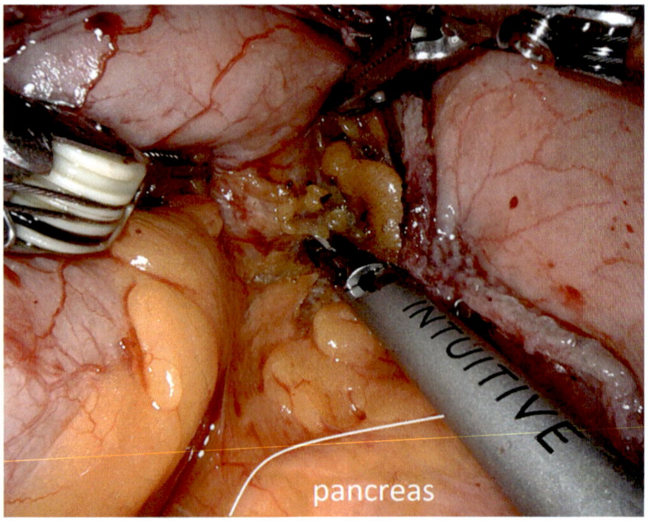

Fig. 22.16 Removal of the dorsal adhesions of the pouch

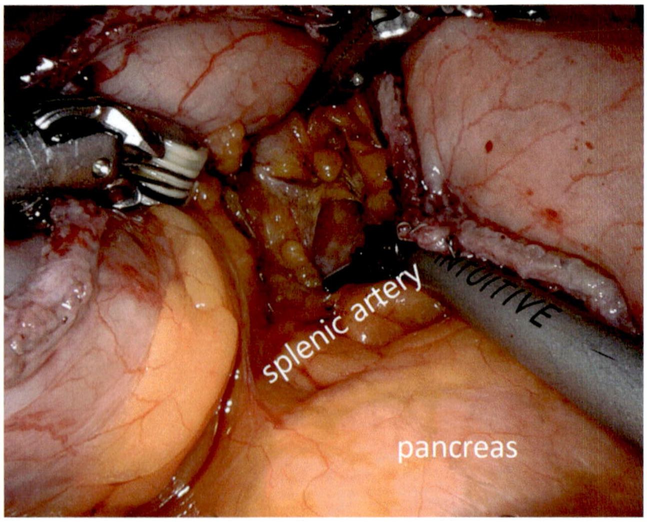

Fig. 22.17 Continuous removal of dorsal adhesions of the pouch

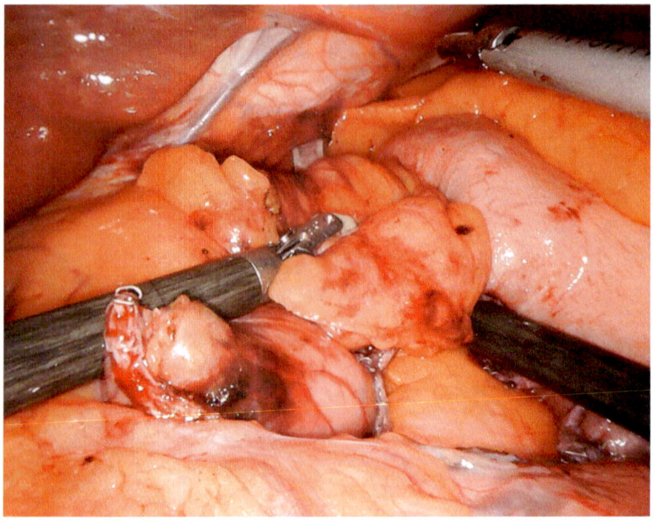

Fig. 22.18 For safety reasons, the tip-up fenestrated grasper is inserted in the omental bursa and its branches are opened. The fatty tissue is dissected with the energy device

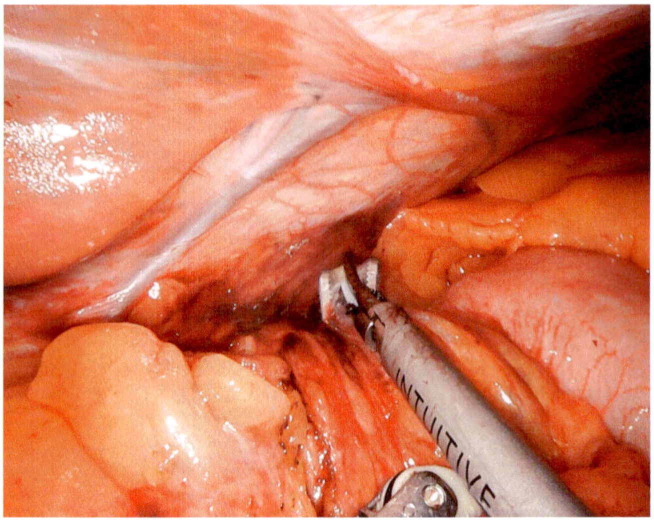

Fig. 22.19 The fatty tissue is dissected with the energy device

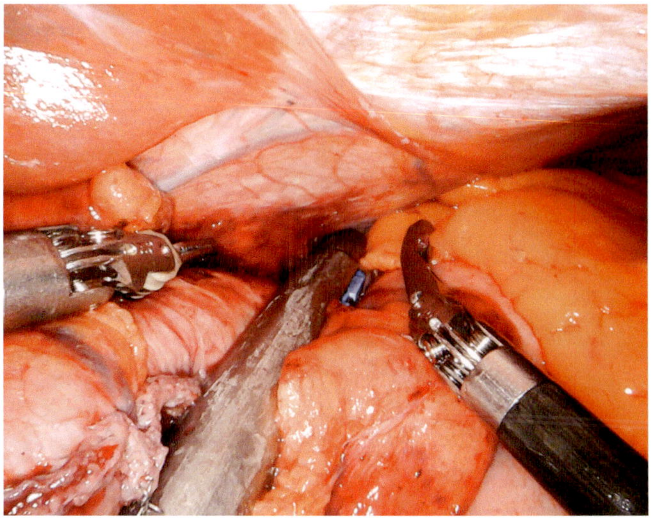

Fig. 22.20 After a successful dissection of the fatty tissue, the last stapler is inserted, and the gastric pouch is finished

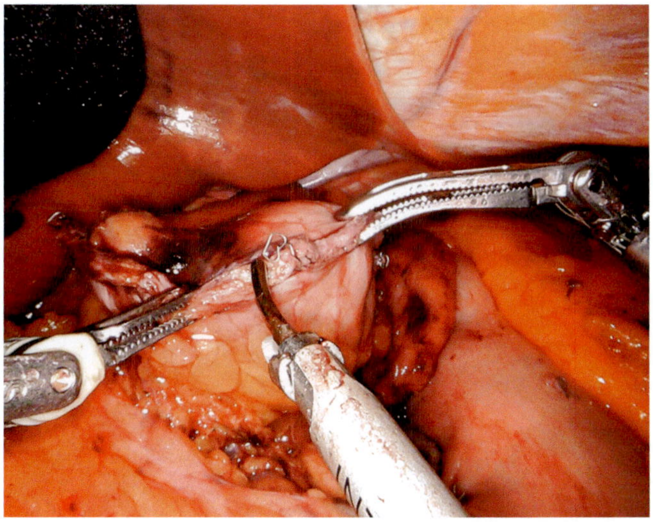

Fig. 22.21 The bougie is pulled back a bit, and the pouch is opened up at the conjunction of the two perpendicular staple lines

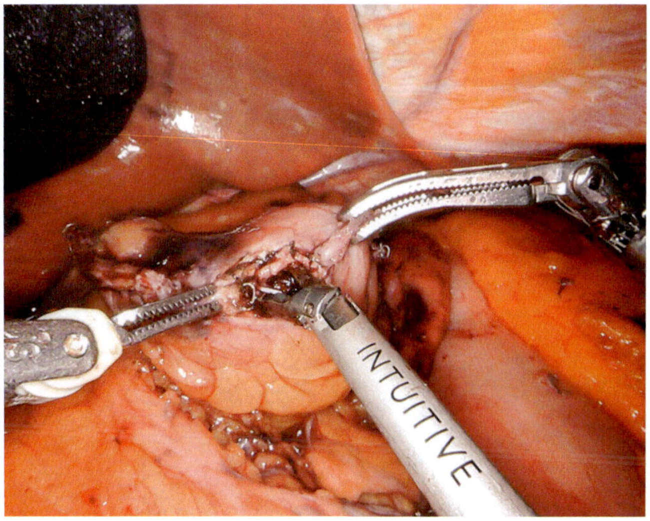

Fig. 22.22 To ensure a correct opening, the gastric mucosa must be visualized

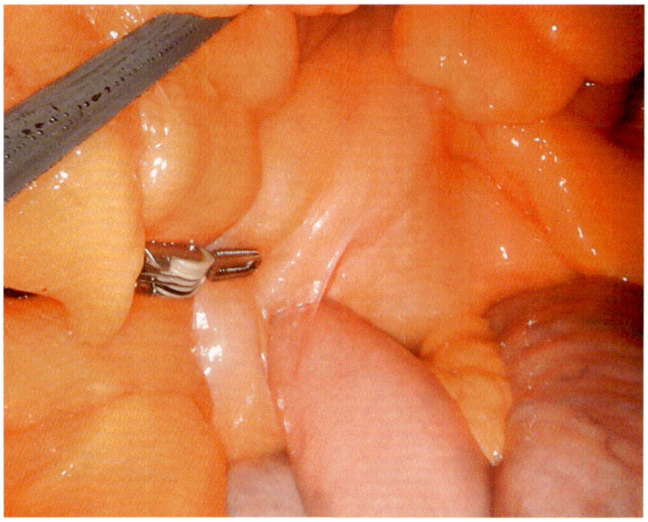

Fig. 22.23 The greater omentum is lifted toward the abdominal wall, and the ligament of Treitz is identified

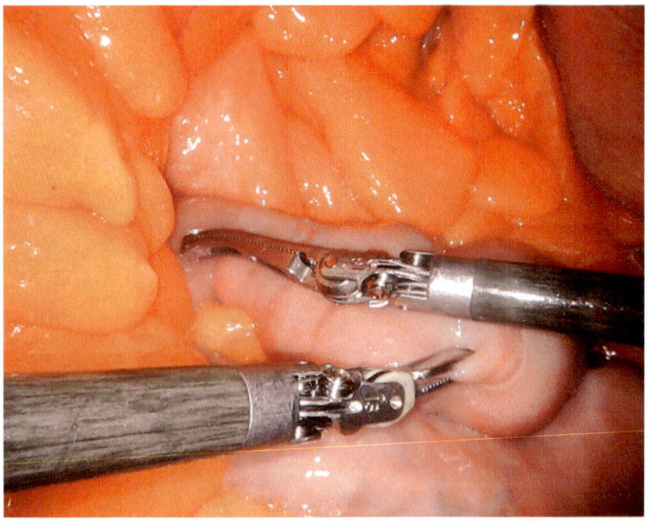

Fig. 22.24 Using the grasper as a ruler

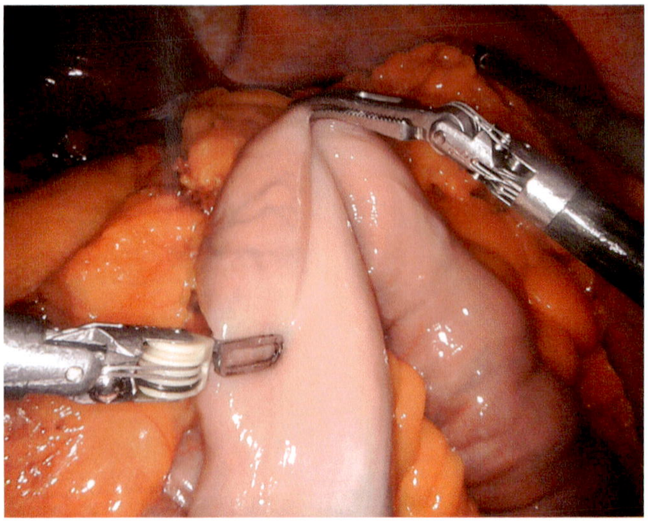

Fig. 22.25 Starting from the ligament of Treitz, the biliopancreatic limb is measured

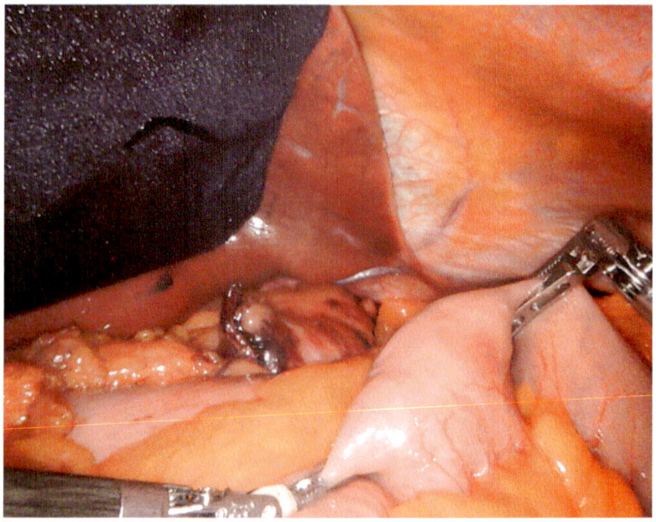

Fig. 22.26 100 cm aborally from the ligament of Treitz, the small bowel is grabbed and moved toward the gastric pouch to ensure a good positioning without tension

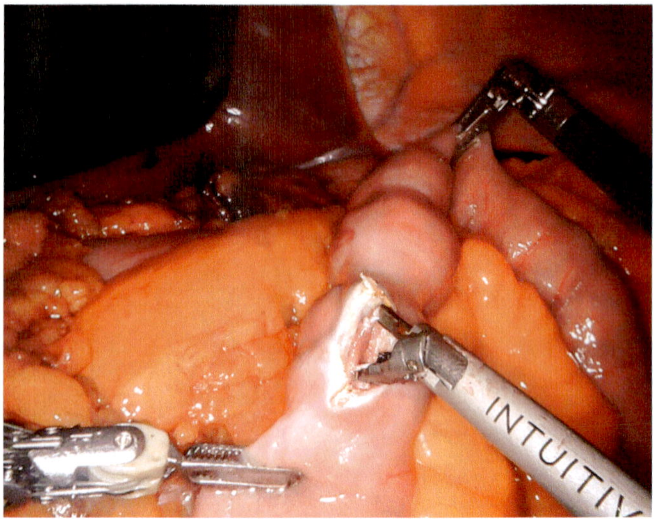

Fig. 22.27 The small bowel is opened up antimesenterically

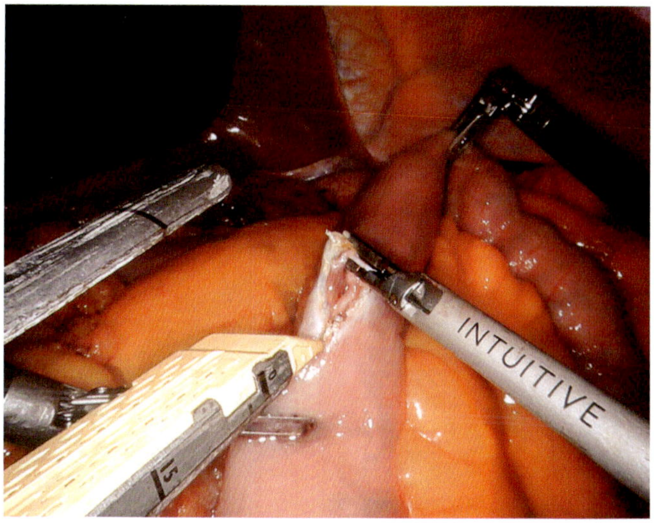

Fig. 22.28 Using all three arms, the small intestine is presented toward the stapler

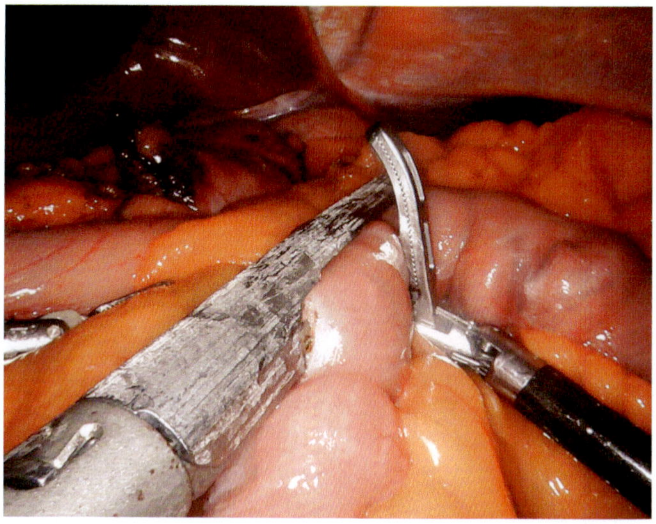

Fig. 22.29 The stapler is being inserted with the bigger side and slow oscillating movement to avoid mucosal stress and injuries

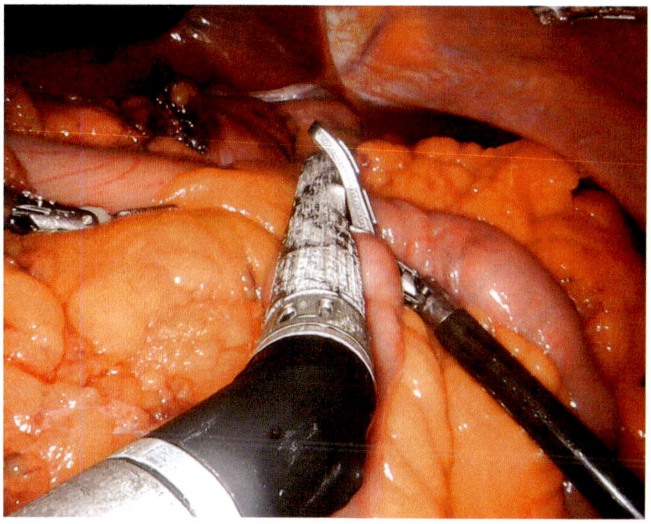

Fig. 22.30 Using the tip-up grasper as counter bearing, the stapler is bent

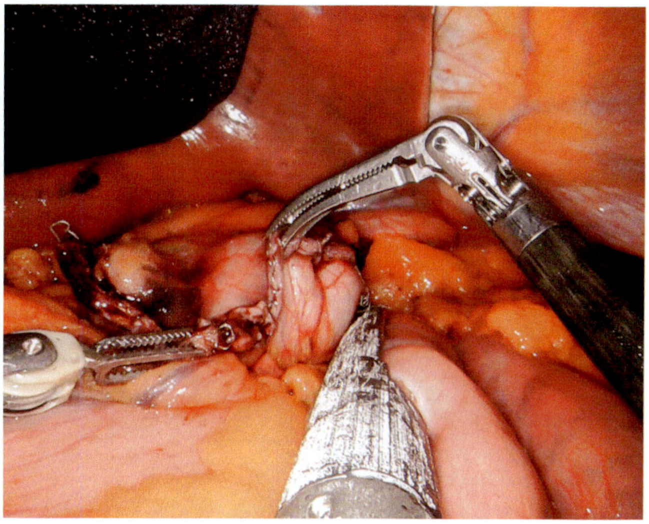

Fig. 22.31 The small intestine is approximated with the priorly formed gastric pouch via the inserted linear stapler

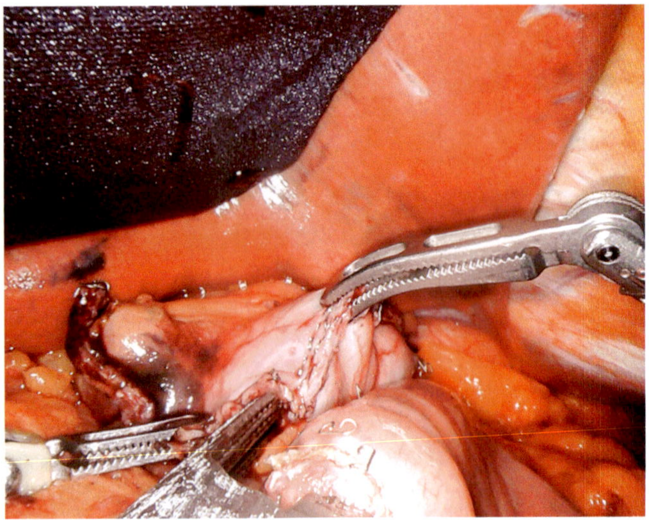

Fig. 22.32 The opening of the gastric pouch is visualized, and the small end of the stapler is carefully inserted to avoid a dissection of the gastric wall

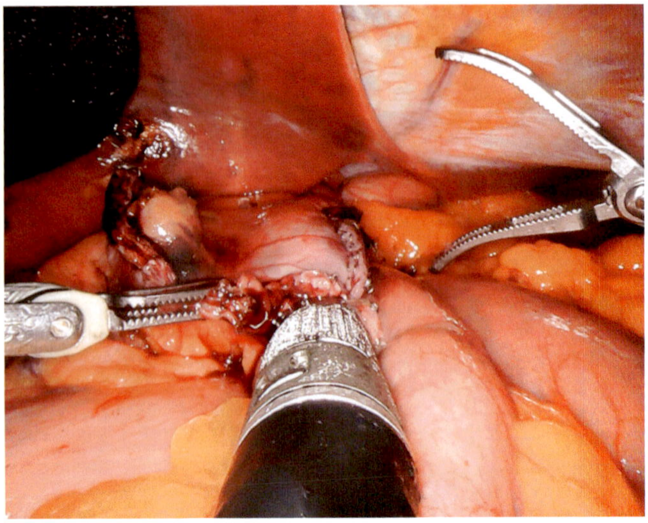

Fig. 22.33 Fashioning the gastrojejunostomy

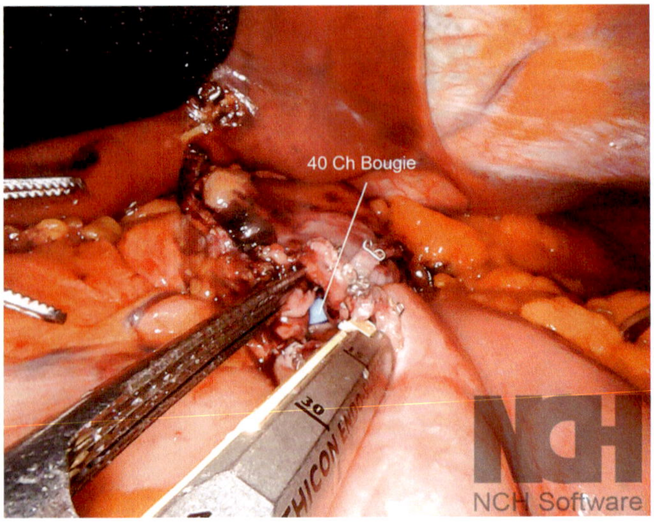

Fig. 22.34 On retraction, the stapler is only opened halfway to avoid stress on the anastomosis and a bigger enterostomy

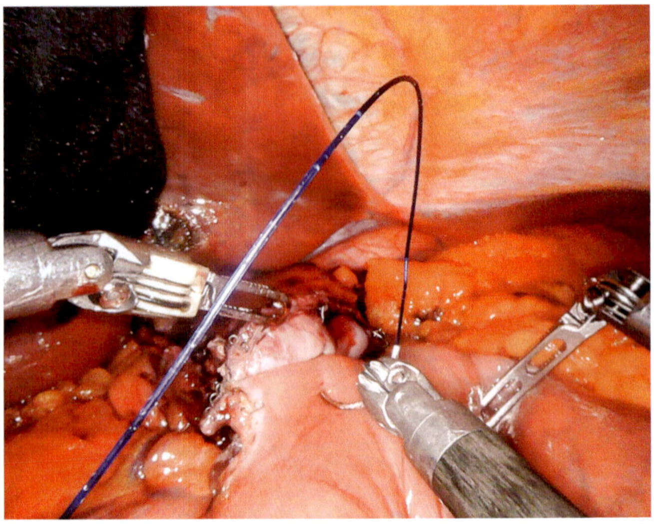

Fig. 22.35 Closing the enterostomy with a 15 cm, unidirectional 2–0 Stratafix (Ethicon, Johnson & Johnson, Cincinnati, OH, USA) thread beginning from the far left

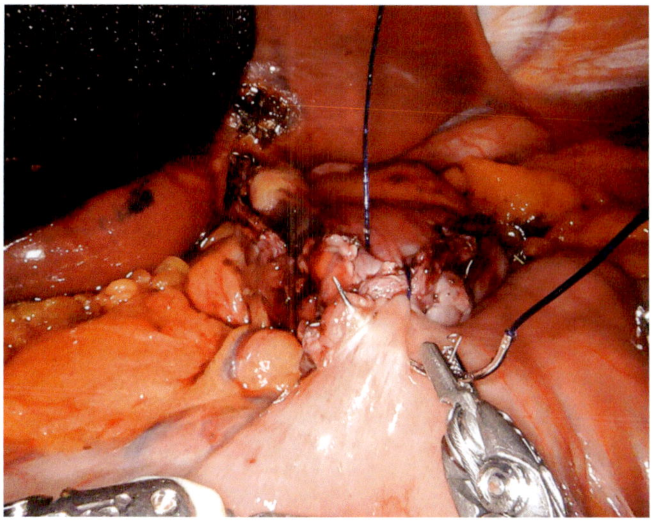

Fig. 22.36 We use continuous seromuscular stitches

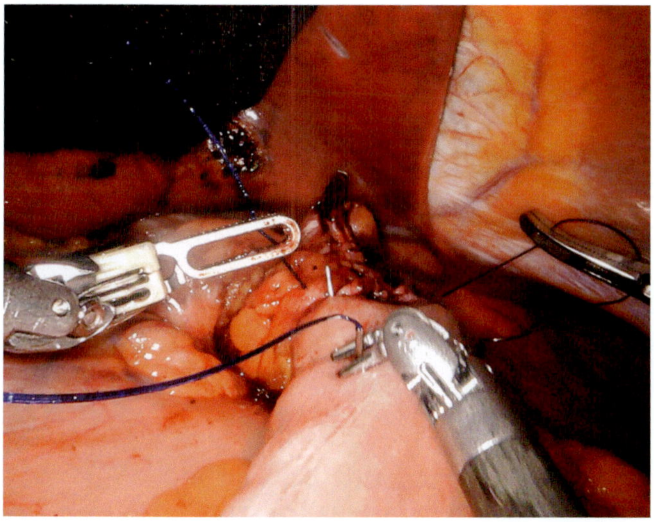

Fig. 22.37 After finishing half of the anastomosis, a second 15 cm, unidirectional 2–0 Stratafix (Ethicon, Johnson & Johnson, Cincinnati, OH, USA) thread is used closing up the enterostomy from the far right

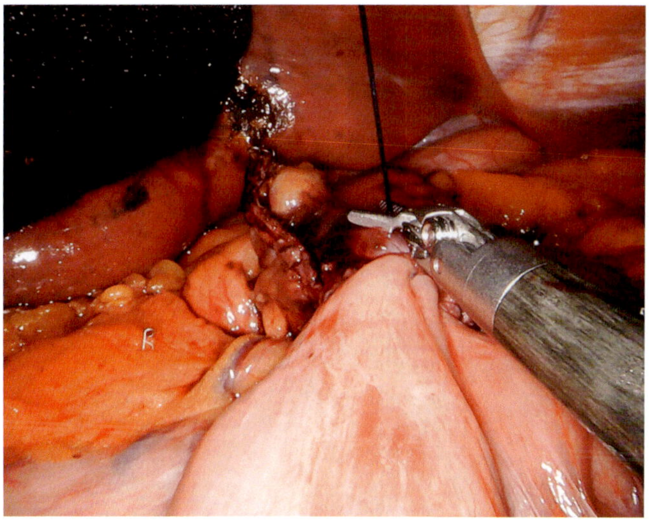

Fig. 22.38 Adjusting the tension using the needle driver as a bearing point

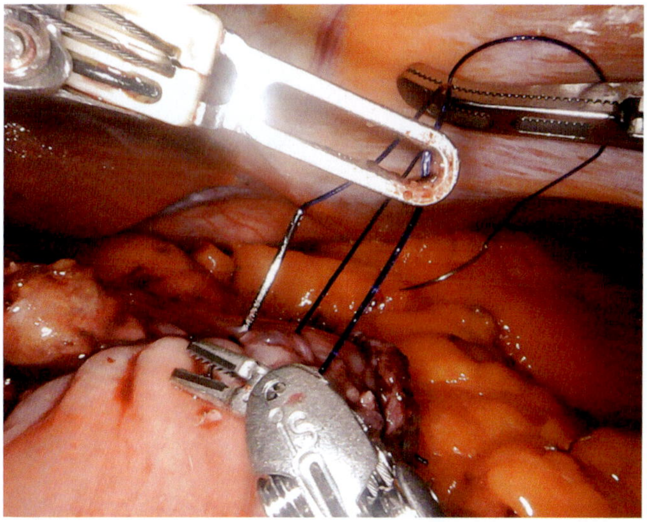

Fig. 22.39 The enterostomy is finished by two opposing stitches from each side

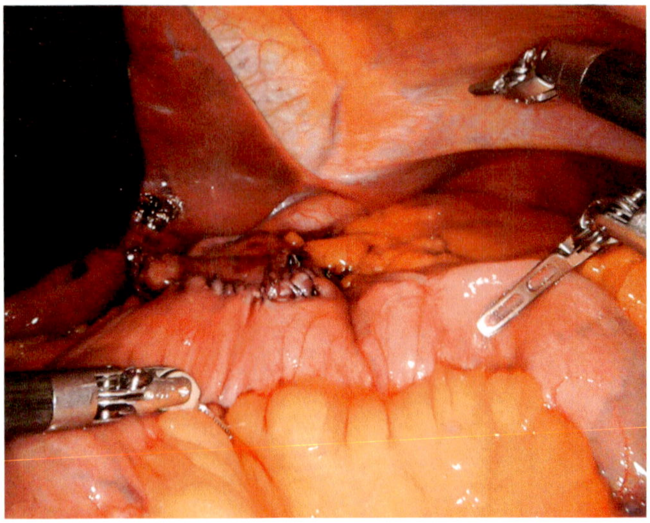

Fig. 22.40 Proximal to the anastomosis, the small bowel is positioned

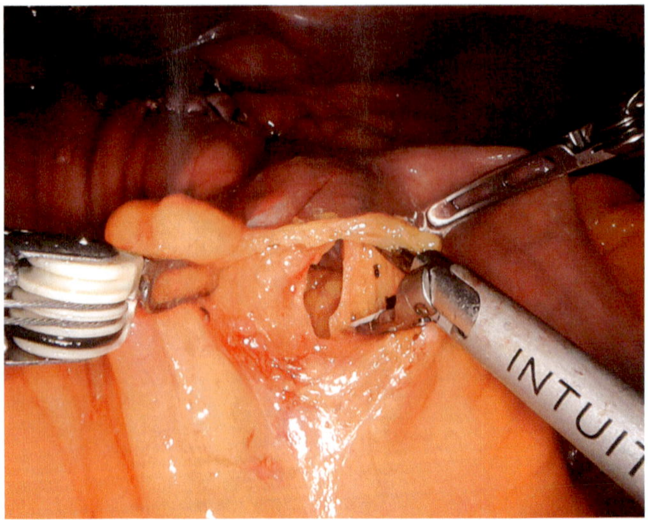

Fig. 22.41 The mesentery is opened with the energy device. This should neither be too close to the gastrojejunostomy to avoid a poor perfusion nor too long to avoid a blind loop

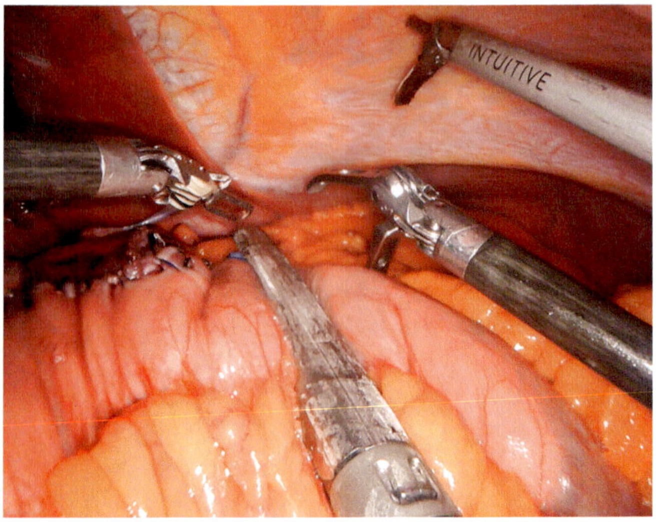

Fig. 22.42 Dissection of the small intestine proximal of the anastomosis with a linear stapler

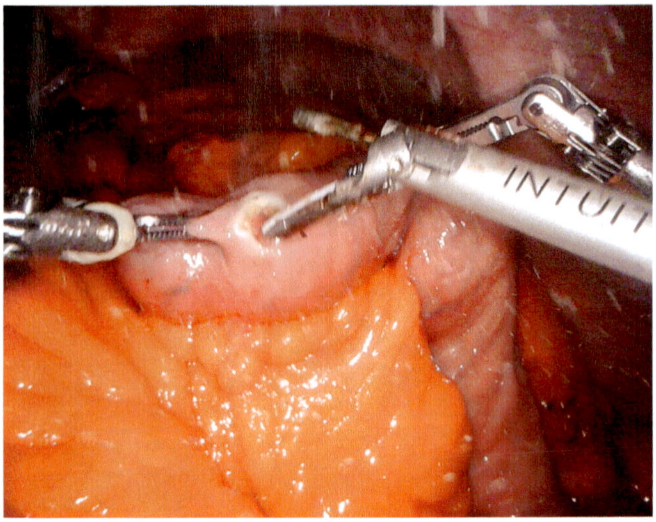

Fig. 22.43 Opening the small intestine for the anastomosis

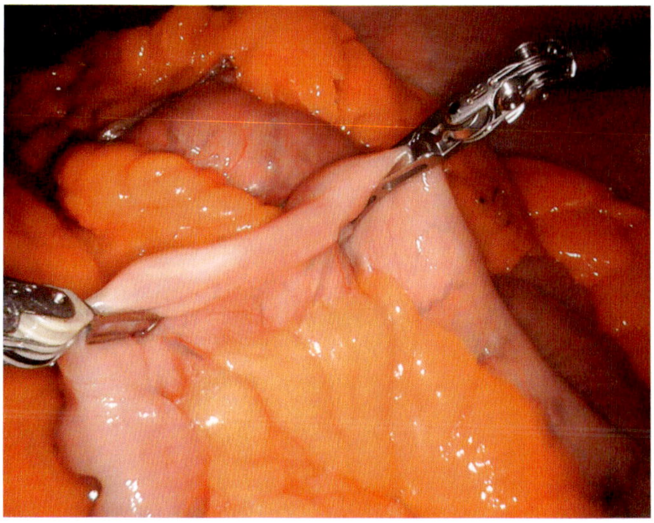

Fig. 22.44 Measurement of the Roux limb (150 cm)

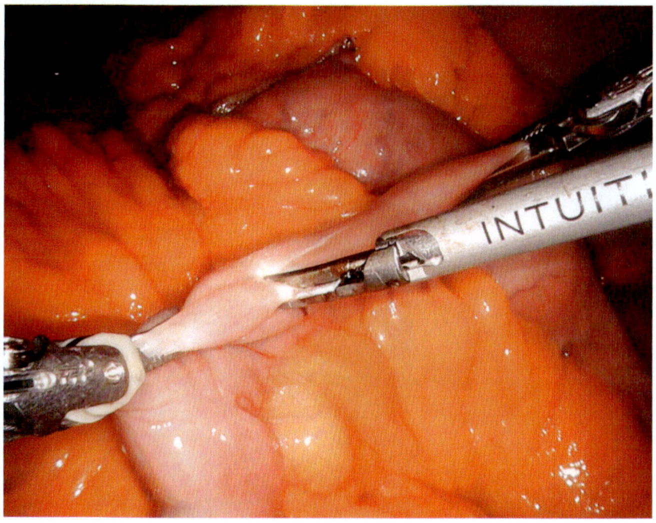

Fig. 22.45 Opening of the small intestine antimesenterically 150 cm aboral of the gastrojejunostomy

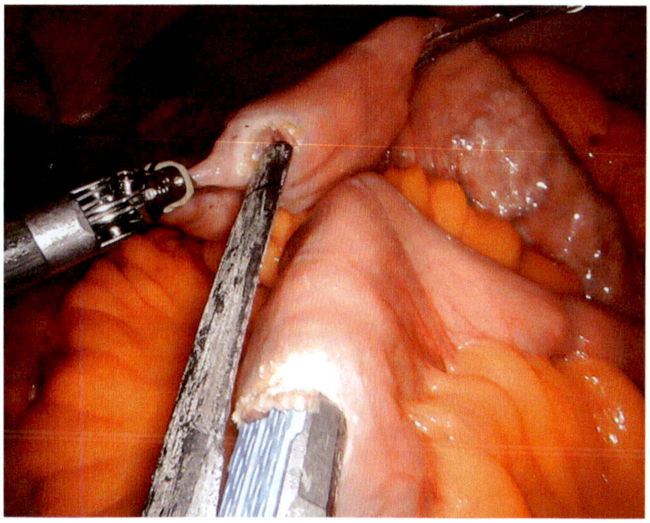

Fig. 22.46 After inserting the linear stapling device, the jejunal loop is approximated toward the dissected small intestine

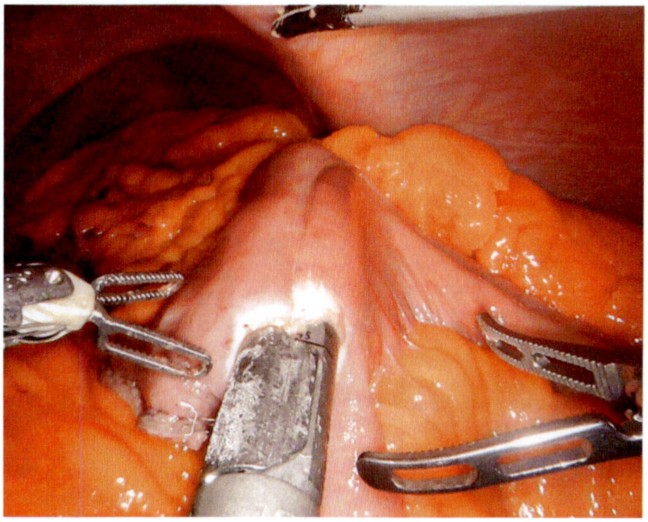

Fig. 22.47 Fashioning of the jejunojejunostomy with the linear stapler

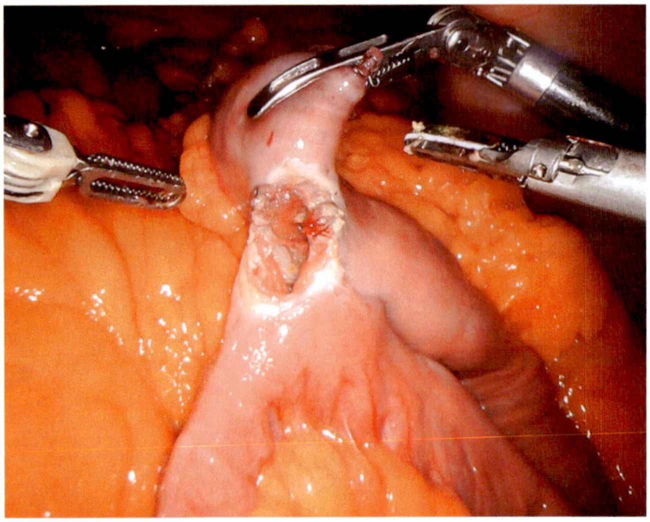

Fig. 22.48 To ensure low tension while stitching, the anastomosis is positioned as follows

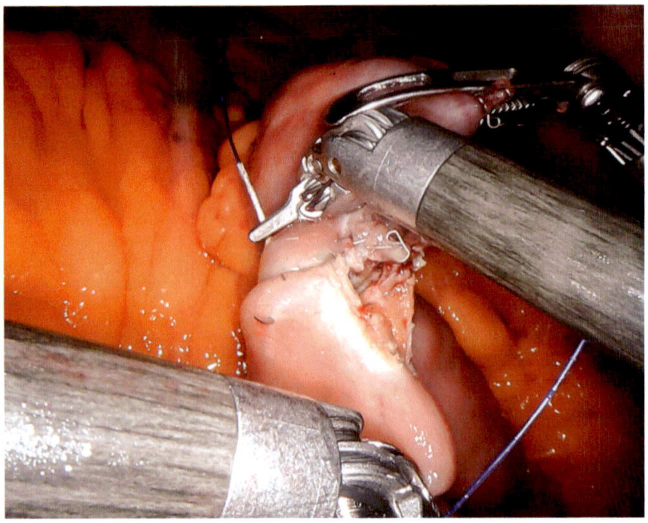

Fig. 22.49 Closure of the enterostomy using a 15 cm, unidirectional 3–0 Stratafix (Ethicon, Johnson & Johnson, Cincinnati, OH, USA) thread

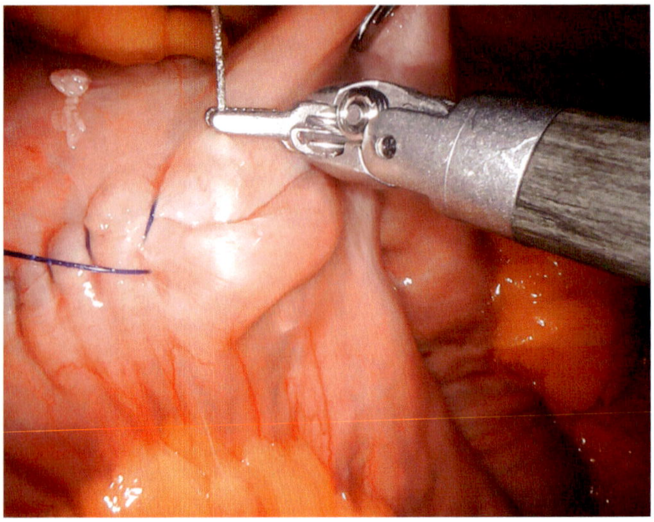

Fig. 22.50 Finished jejunojejunostomy

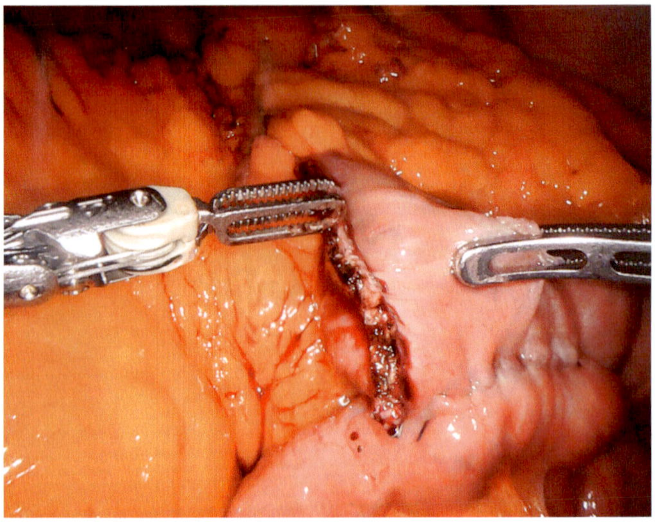

Fig. 22.51 Perform hemostasis if necessary. In this case with bipolar forceps

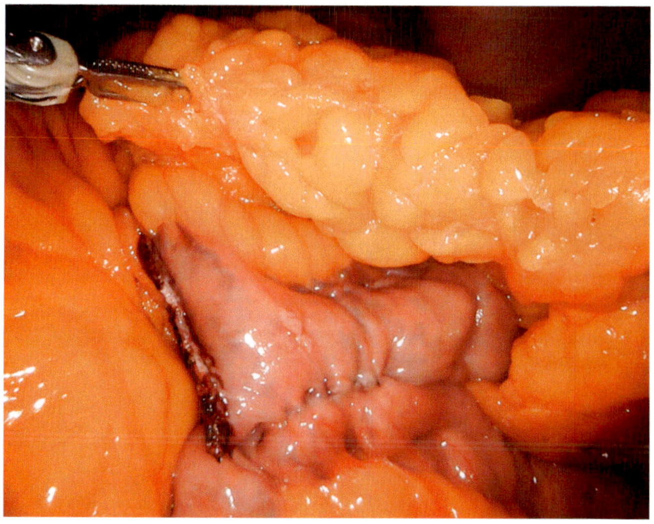

Fig. 22.52 Covering of the anastomosis with the omentum majus

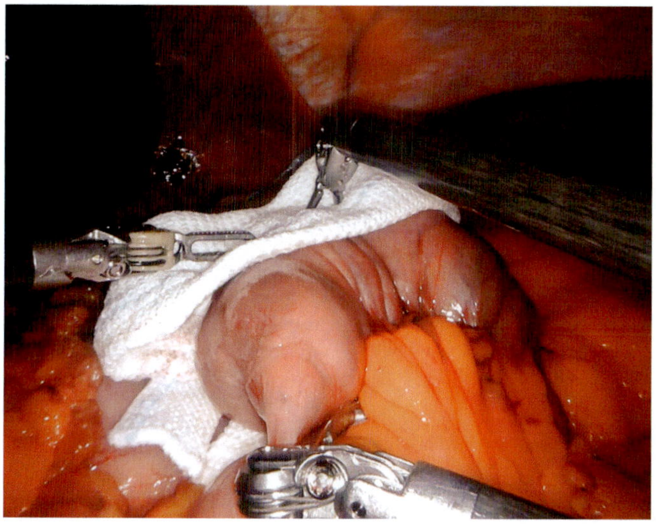

Fig. 22.53 Methylene blue test of the gastrojejunostomy via the 40 Charrier Bougie with an additional gastric tube

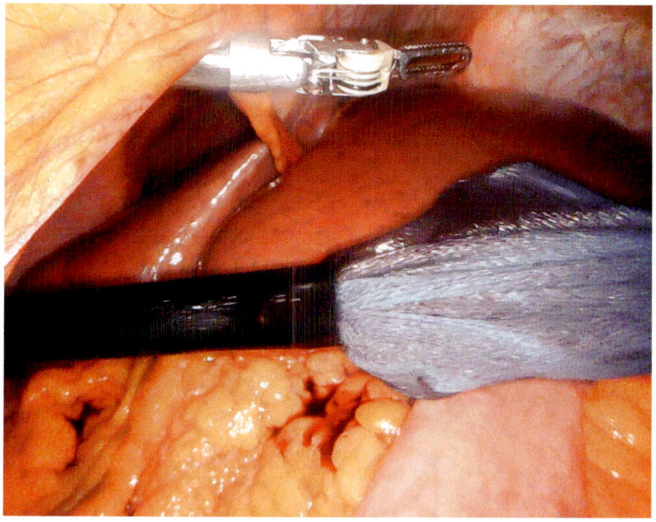

Fig. 22.54 Retracting the liver paddle in view to avoid tissue damage

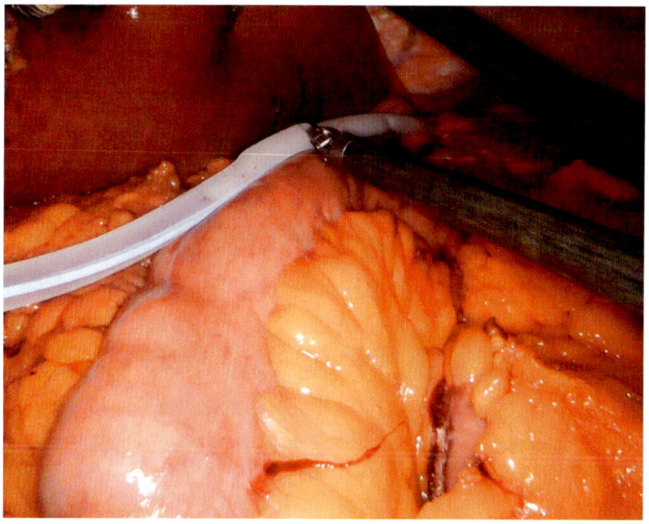

Fig. 22.55 Positioning of the drainage under the left liver lobe

References

1. Welbourn R, Hollyman M, Kinsman R, Dixon J, Liem R, Ottosson J, et al. Bariatric surgery worldwide: baseline demographic description and one-year outcomes from the fourth IFSO global registry report 2018. Obes Surg. 2019;29(3):782–95.
2. Horgan S, Vanuno D. Robots in laparoscopic surgery. J Laparoendosc Adv Surg Tech [Internet]. 2001 [cited 2019 Aug 11];11(6):415–9. Available from: http://www.ncbi.nlm.nih.gov/pubmed/11814134.
3. Szold A, Bergamaschi R, Broeders I, Dankelman J, Forgione A, Langø T, et al. European association of endoscopic surgeons (EAES) consensus statement on the use of robotics in general surgery. Surg Endosc [Internet]. 2015 [cited 2019 Aug 11];29(2):253–88. Available from: http://link.springer.com/10.1007/s00464-014-3916-9.

Robotic Duodenal Switch (rDS) and Robotic Single Anastomosis Duodenal-Ileal Bypass with Sleeve Gastrectomy (rSADI-S)

23

Curtis Peery

Successful long-term treatment of obesity has only been achieved with bariatric surgery. The sleeve gastrectomy (SG) and Roux-en-Y (RNY) gastric bypass are the most commonly performed bariatric surgeries in the United States. Very few biliopancreatic diversions with duodenal switch, commonly known as the duodenal switch (DS), are performed in comparison (0.9%). Several reasons may be responsible for this. First, management of these patients is complex with a higher risk for malnutrition and vitamin and mineral deficiencies. Second, historically the DS has had increased mortality and morbidity in comparison to the SG or RNY gastric bypass. Most DS have been performed either open or laparoscopically. It is well-known that open surgery increases surgical complications, and a laparoscopic DS is an overly complex procedure with safe results difficult to reproduce. As a result, surgical complications have been higher for the DS as compared to the gastric bypass and sleeve gastrectomy.

A modification of the DS has become increasingly popular and appears to have fewer metabolic and surgical complications. This modification is known by many different names: the single anastomosis DS, single anastomosis duodenal-ileal bypass with sleeve gastrectomy (SADI-S), loop DS, or stomach intestinal pylorus-sparing surgery (SIPS). The American Society for Metabolic and Bariatric Surgery (ASMBS) in 2020 came out with an endorsement of these procedures as an acceptable modification of the DS. To avoid confusion, we will refer to this modification as the SADI-S from here on out.

Because of the worsening obesity epidemic and increasing population of super-morbidly obese individuals, there has been a renewed interest in the DS and SADI-S. Also, robotic bariatric surgery is rapidly gaining acceptance, particularly for more complex surgeries such as bariatric procedures. When surgeons are adequately trained, the introduction of robotics into a bariatric surgeon's practice can be safe and increase the surgeon's ability to perform these more complex surgeries such as the DS, SADI-S, and revisions. This chapter discusses the utilization of the robotic platform as a tool to safely perform the DS and SADI-S (Figs. 23.1, 23.2, 23.3, 23.4, 23.5, 23.6, 23.7, 23.8, 23.9, 23.10, 23.11, 23.12, 23.13, 23.14, 23.15, 23.16, 23.17, 23.18, 23.19, 23.20, 23.21, 23.22, 23.23, 23.24, 23.25, 23.26, 23.27, 23.28, 23.29, 23.30, 23.31, 23.32, 23.33, 23.34, 23.35, 23.36, 23.37, 23.38, 23.39, 23.40, 23.41, 23.42, 23.43, and 23.44).

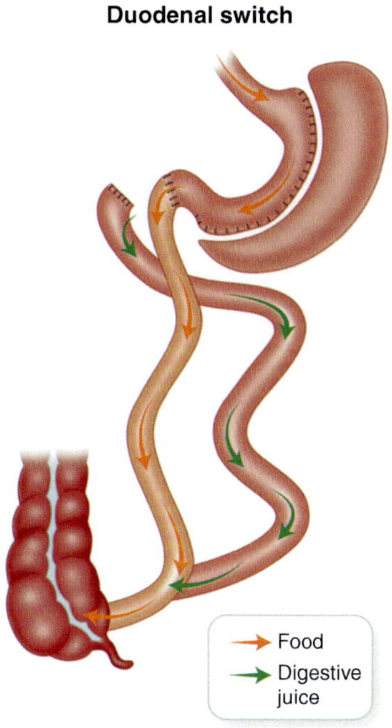

Fig. 23.1 This is an illustration of the essential components of the duodenal switch (DS). A sleeve gastrectomy has been created and the duodenum divided in the first portion. The small bowel is then reconfigured creating a Roux limb otherwise known as the alimentary limb. The biliopancreatic (BP) limb is anastomosed to the ileum leaving a common channel. In practice these limbs may vary in length, but the common channel is usually 100–200 cm long

C. Peery (✉)
Department of Surgery, Sanford School of Medicine University of South Dakota, Sioux Falls, SD, USA
e-mail: curtis.peery@sanfordhealth.org

O. Y. Kudsi, P. P. Grimminger (eds.), *Atlas of Robotic Upper Gastrointestinal Surgery*,
https://doi.org/10.1007/978-3-030-86578-8_23

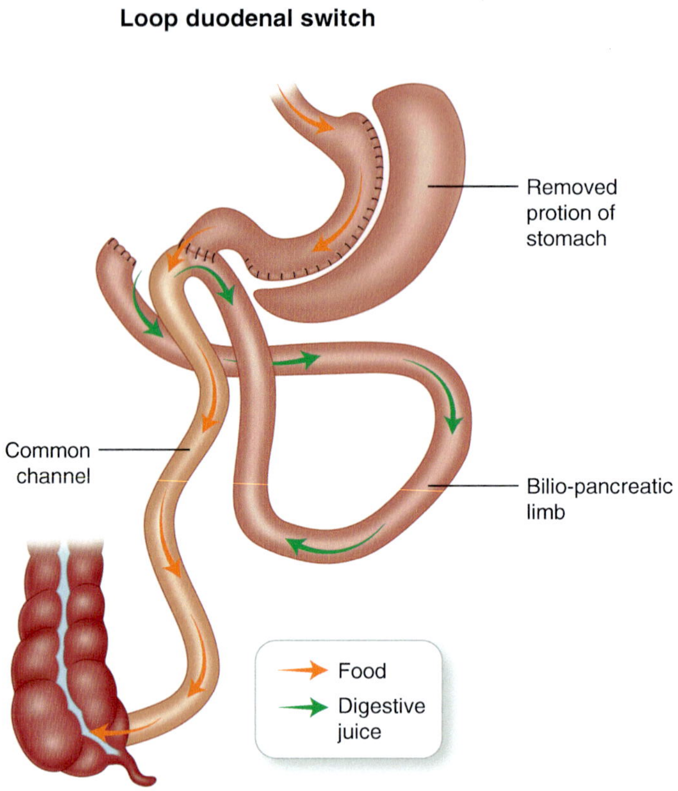

Fig. 23.2 A modification of the DS has been performed and called several different procedures and despite some minor differences is essentially the same. This procedure has been described as the single anastomosis DS (SADS), SIPS procedure (stomach intestine pylorus-preserving) Surgery, and loop duodenal switch (LDS) but is best described as the single anastomosis duodenal-ileal bypass with sleeve gastrectomy (SADI-S)

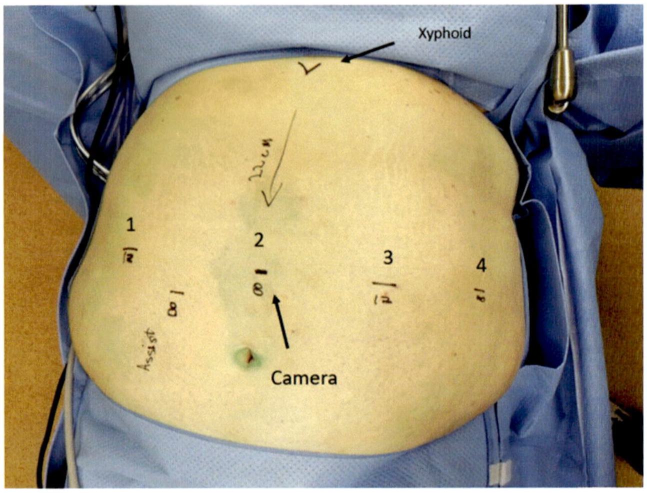

Fig. 23.3 Image of a patient with position of the planned trocar placement. Although differences in body habitus may influence changes in trocar placement, this is a typical schematic for the duodenal Switch and SADI-S. After measuring 22 cm down from the xiphoid, a camera trocar is placed near midline. With the camera in this position, the rest of the trocars are positioned in relation to it. Arms 1 and 3 are 12 mm to facilitate stapling. Arms 2 and 4 are 8 mm. The assistant trocar is 8 mm to facilitate needle introduction and removal. To keep external collision of the instruments to a minimum, I will optimize the distance between trocars. After the camera is placed, I will then place Arm 4 as far as reasonabl lateral to the left, and Arm 3 is then placed halfway between the camera and Arm 4. It is best to place the trocars after the patient is positioned in a 12-degree reverse Trendelenburg position

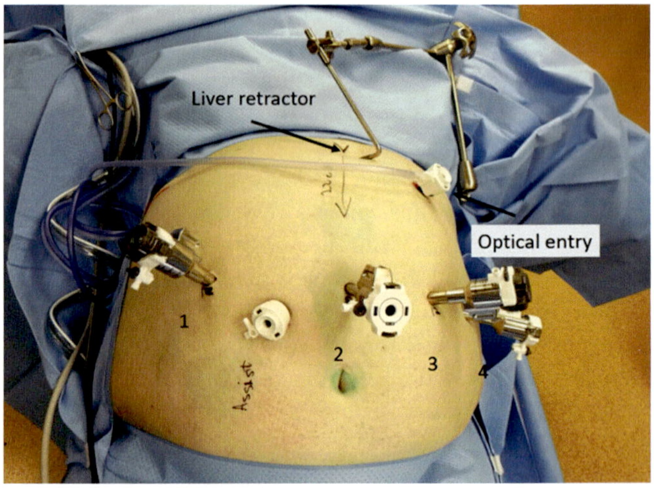

Fig. 23.4 In this photo the trocars have been placed. First an optical trocar is positioned at Palmer's point, and the abdomen is surveyed. This may influence the position of the trocars based on the surgeon's judgment. For example, a large liver may result in moving Arm 1 in a more inferior direction. Also, it is frequently beneficial to move Arm 4 in a more cephalad location. In this case an external liver retractor has been placed in the epigastrium. You can see the retraction device is also kept close to the patient to avoid colliding with the patient cart when it is brought into position. Normally the short robotic trocars are utilized rather than the bariatric length trocars

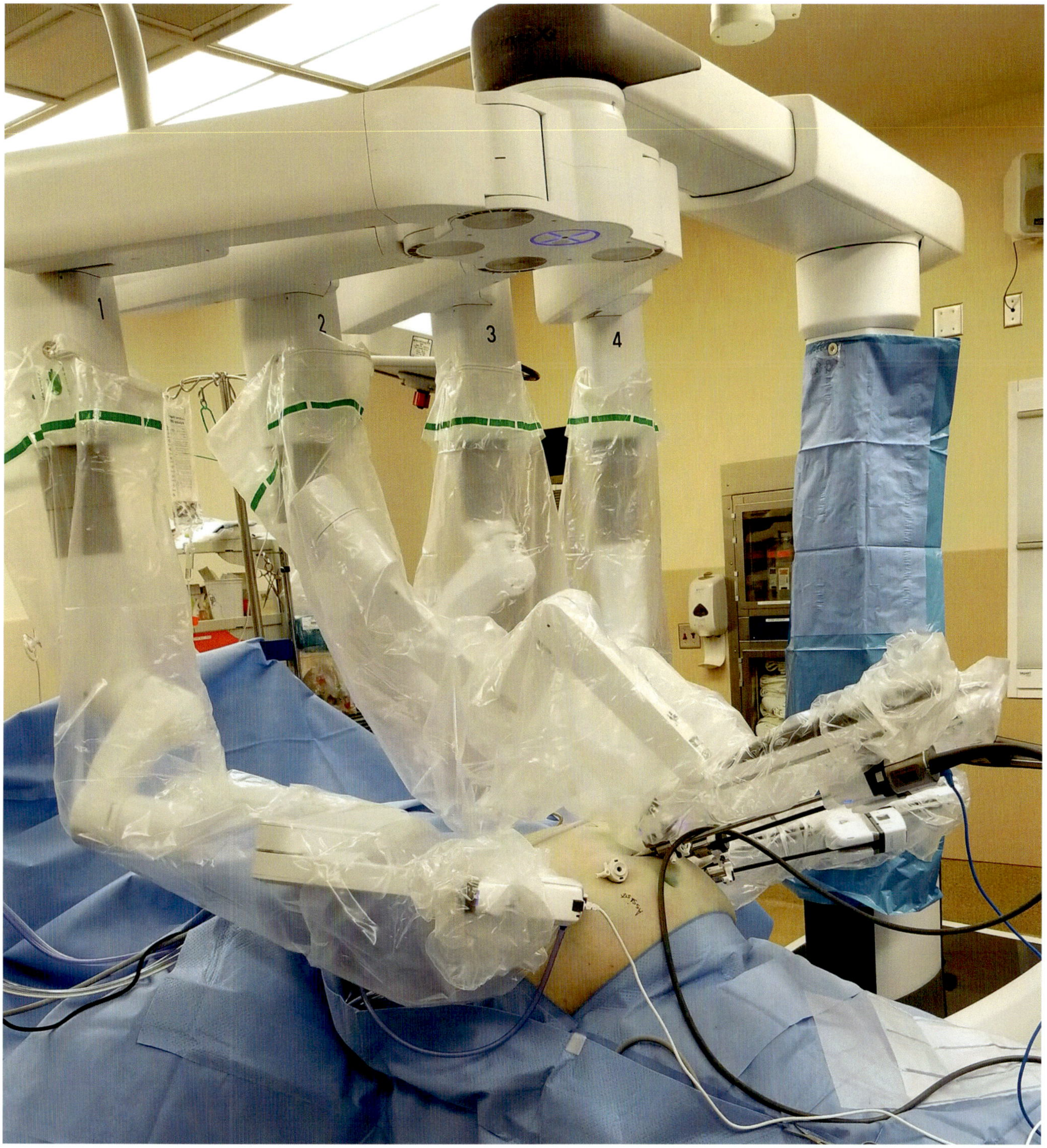

Fig. 23.5 This demonstrates appropriate surgical cart placement. It is well worth the time to go through the recommended steps of targeting the upper midline at the lower edge of the stomach and then dock the surgical arms. You can note that the Arm 2 is in line with the upper midline, and the remainder of the arm are positioned about 15–18 cm apart. This position optimizes the operative field for multi-quadrant surgery. If docking is done well, it will be unusual to need to dock more than once

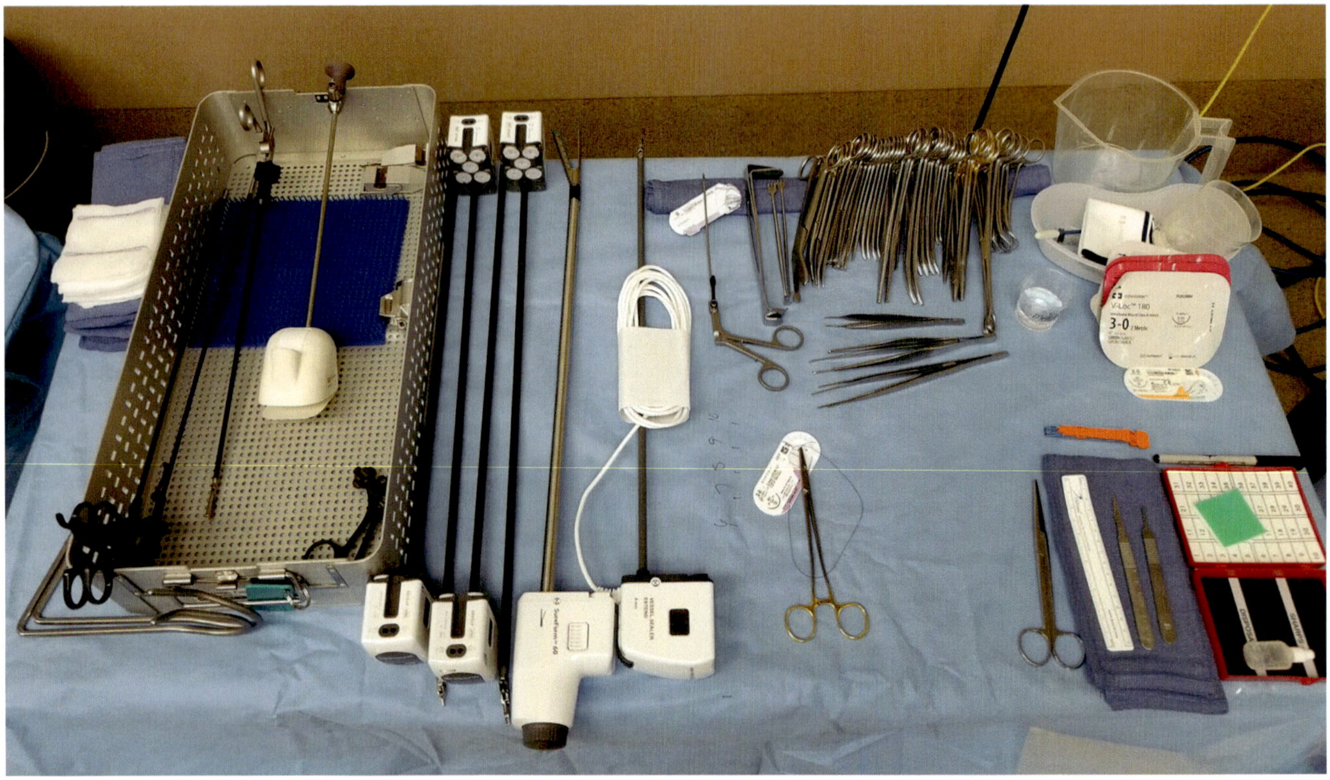

Fig. 23.6 This is the back table for the duodenal switch. Instruments utilized include the robotic stapler, robotic bipolar grasper, robotic bowel grasper, robotic vessel sealer, robotic needle driver, and robotic monopolar hook. Also needed are the liver retractor, a minor set, instrument to close the fascia at the 12 mm trocar sites, and laparoscopic scissors and grasper

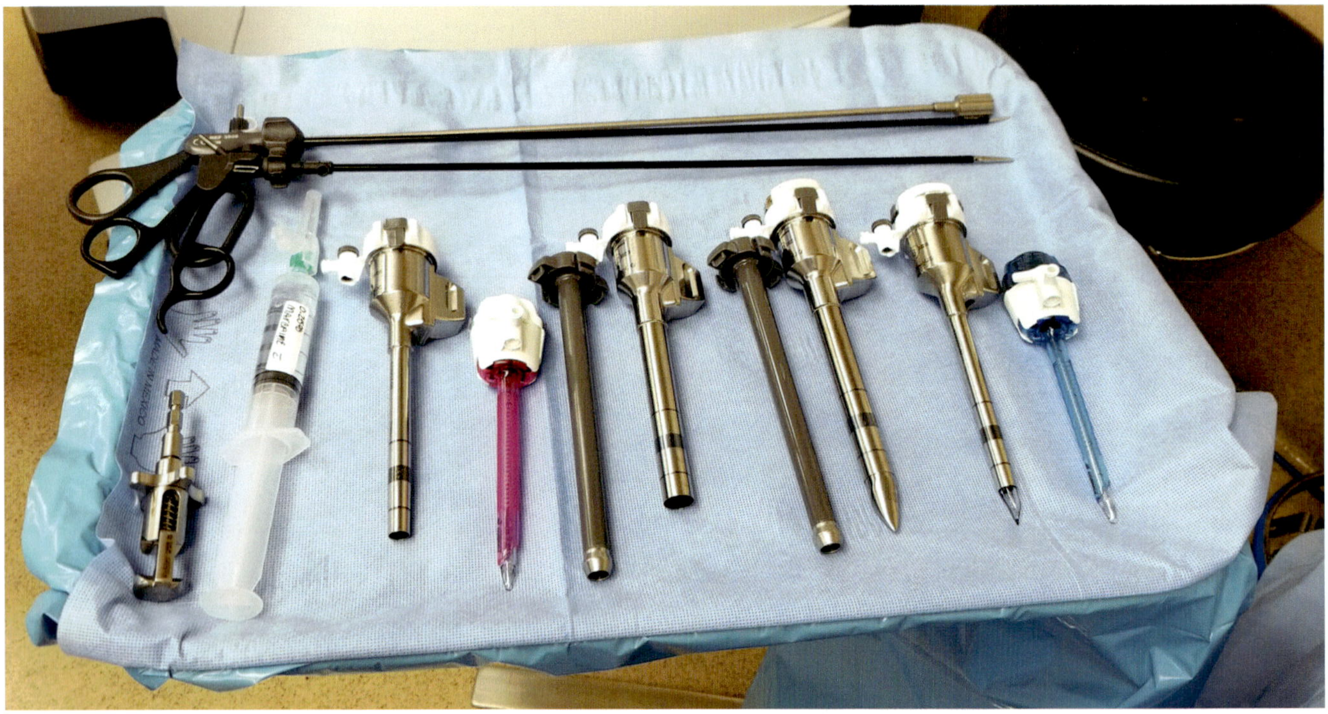

Fig. 23.7 This mayo stand shows the trocars used. Notice even in the super morbidly obese, it is unusual to need the bariatric length trocars

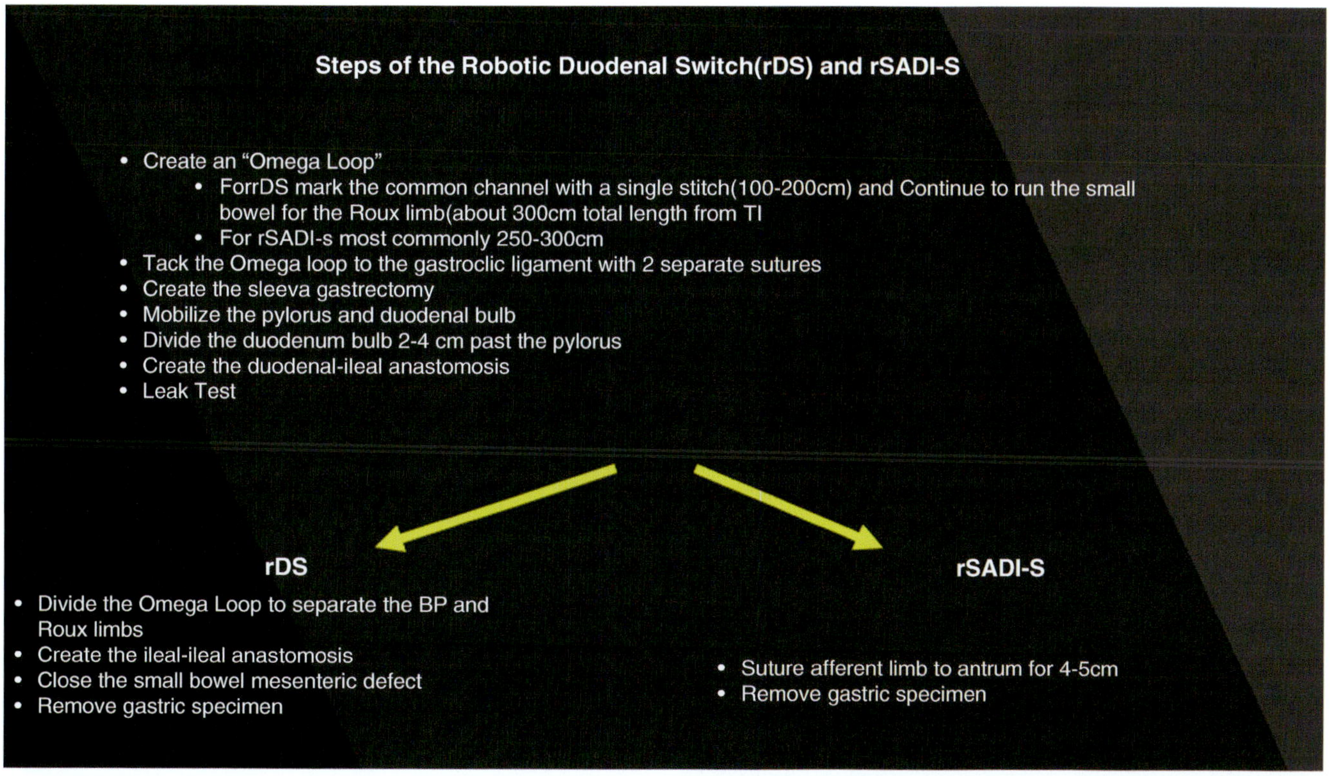

Fig. 23.8 Steps of the robotic single anastomosis duodenal-ileal bypass with sleeve gastrectomy (rSADI-S) and duodenal switch (rDS) are essentially the same, but in the rDS, the omega loop bypass of the small bowel which is preserved in the rSADI-S is then converted to a Roux-en-Y (RNY) configuration, and an ileal-ileal anastomosis (IIA) is created. The steps in this illustration are what I consider a best practice as it helps organize the case to flow smoothly without needing to dock the robotic cart more than once. By first creating the omega loop and duodenal-ileal anastomosis (DIA), the IIA for the rDS is fixed adjacent to the DIA making it feasible to perform the entire procedure with only one dock of the surgical cart

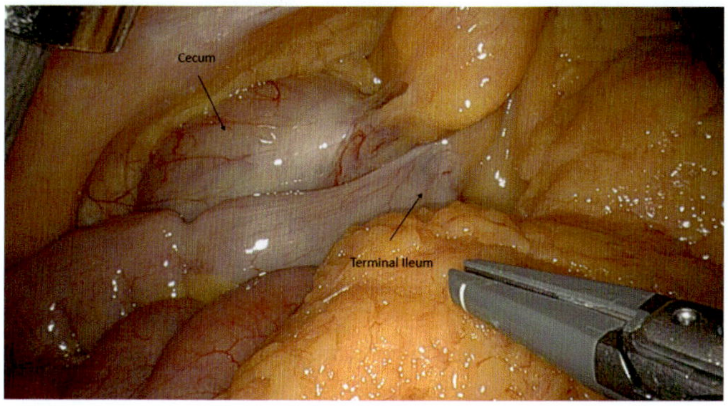

Fig. 23.9 It is best to begin the surgery by evaluating the small bowel. This step will be at the lower limit of the operative field, and arm interaction can be difficult. For that reason, it is essential to optimize port placement. Another alternative is to bring up the omega loop prior to docking the surgical cart. The patient is kept in a slight (12 degree) reverse Trendelenburg position throughout the entire case. Infrequently it is necessary to reposition the patient to find the cecum and terminal ileum (TI). The omentum is placed in a cephalad direction; next the cecum is found which leads the surgeon to the TI

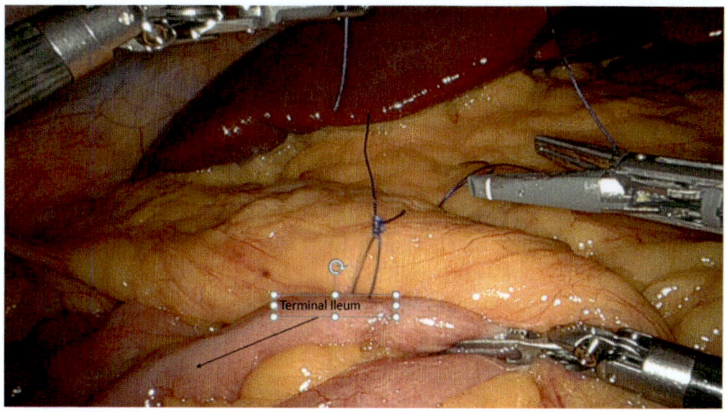

Fig. 23.10 The common channel is measured from the TI. The surgeon will determine the length (100–200 cm). Running the bowel in a proximal direction a single stich is used to mark this length. The bowel is kept oriented, so the distal small bowel is kept to the patient's right, and the proximal small bowel is kept to the left. This will be important to prevent a twist in the mesentery

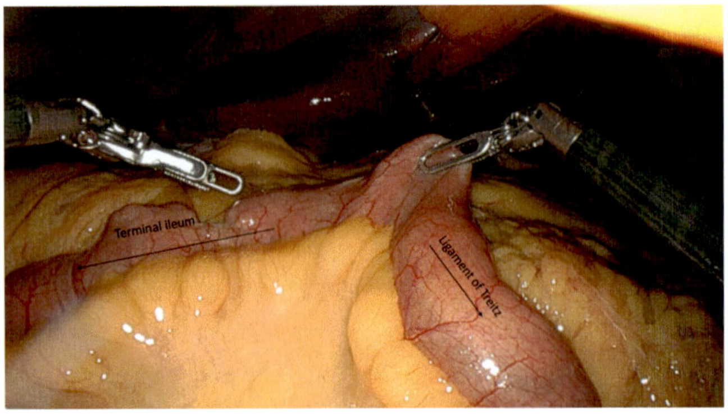

Fig. 23.11 This video illustrates how the orientation of the bowel is kept preventing any mesenteric twist. The bowel is not divided, and when it is brought into the upper abdomen, it is reminiscent of the Greek letter omega, therefore the name omega loop. The length of the limb on the patient's right is the length of the common change in the rSADI-S (250–300 cm) or in the case of the rDS the added length of the common channel (100–200 cm) and Roux limb (100–150 cm)

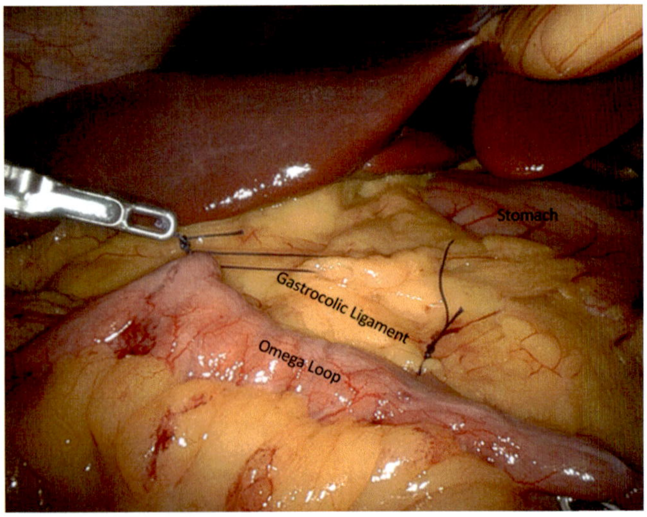

Fig. 23.12 To keep the omega loop orientated, two sutures are placed at the apex of the loop to the gastrocolic ligament. These two sutures will prevent the loop from twisting and later will be cut when the duodenal-ileal anastomosis is created

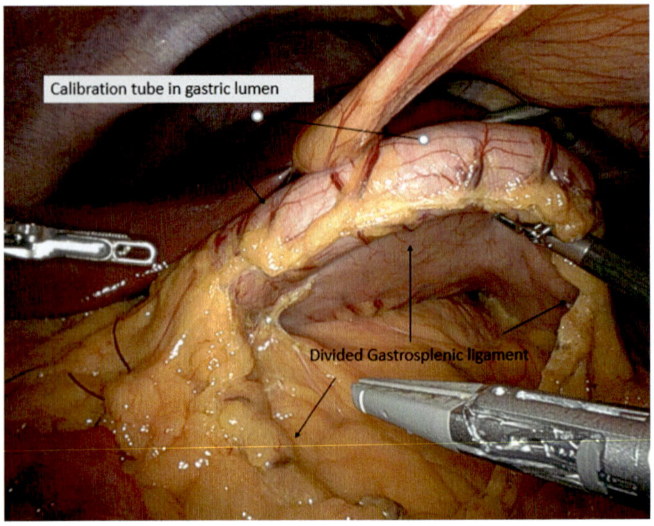

Fig. 23.13 After the omega loop has been created, the sleeve is started. A calibration tube is seen in the lumen of the stomach. This tube (40 French) was used to decompress the stomach and will next be used to calibrate the size of the sleeve. It can be advanced down into the stomach to distend the greater curve helping to expose the attachments to the greater curve and lesser sac

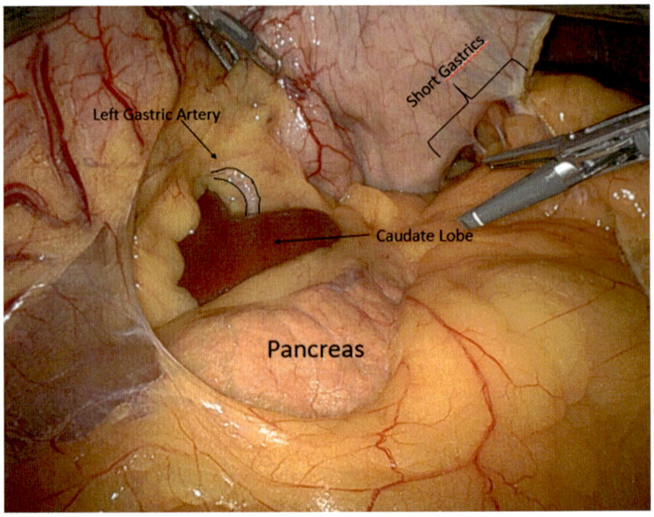

Fig. 23.14 In this photo the contents of the lesser curve are seen including the left gastric, caudate lobe, and pancreas. The attachments to the fundus have yet to be divided

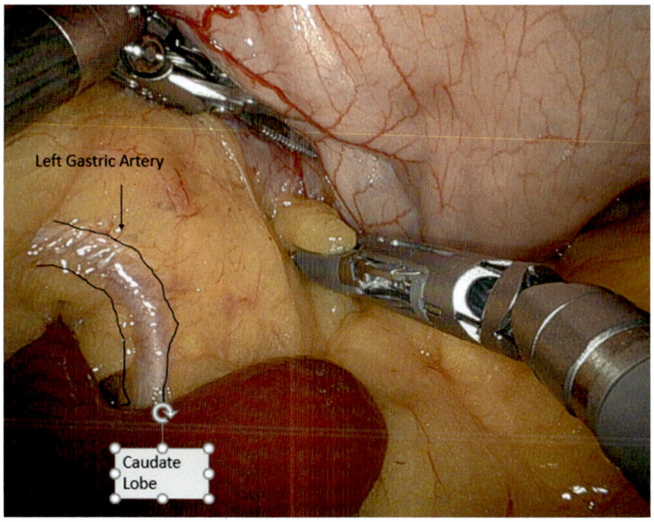

Fig. 23.15 Illustrated here is the left gastric artery. It is crucial to keep it protected as the attachments of the proximal stomach are taken down

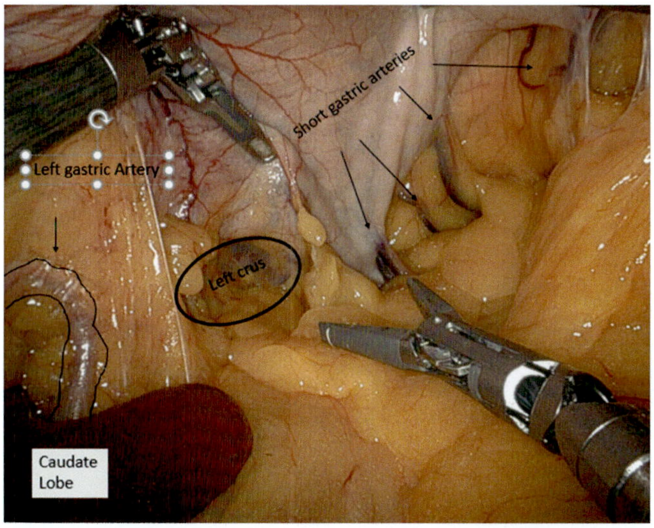

Fig. 23.16 This is a closer view showing the relationship of these structures to the left crus. The dissection is extended to expose the left side of the hiatus to assure no hiatal hernia is identified

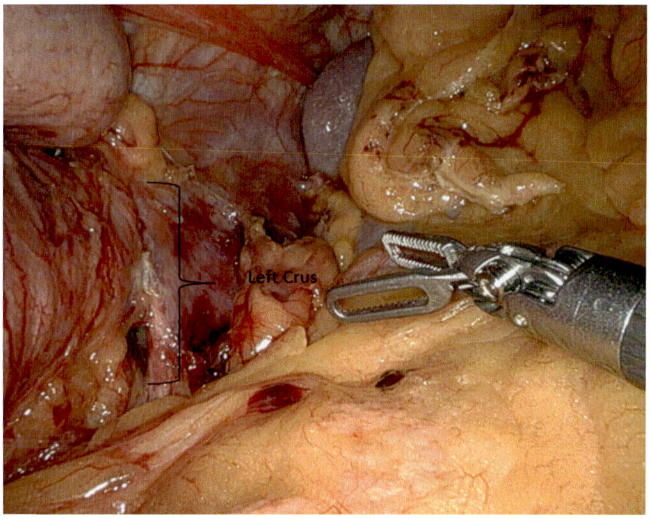

Fig. 23.17 The left crus has been exposed revealing a small defect posteriorly, which was closed to prevent slip of the sleeve into the chest causing gastroesophageal reflux or obstructive symptoms

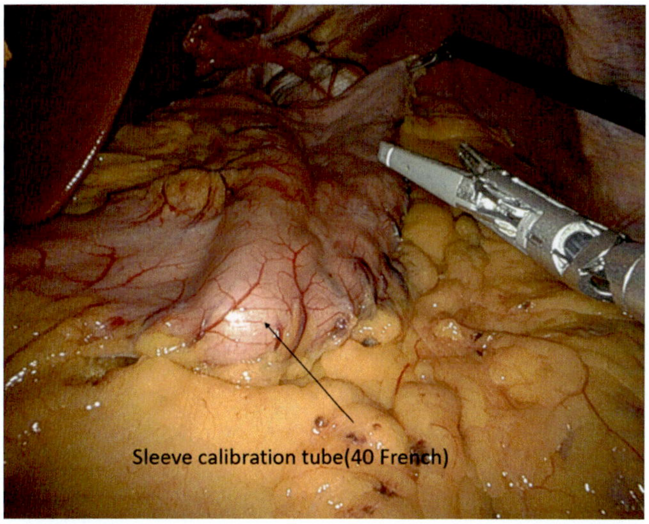

Fig. 23.18 The mobilized stomach is laid flat, and the calibration tube is positioned along the lesser curve of the stomach. Traditionally a 50 French dilator has been used. In this case a 40 French tube was used, and the sleeve formed loosely about the tube

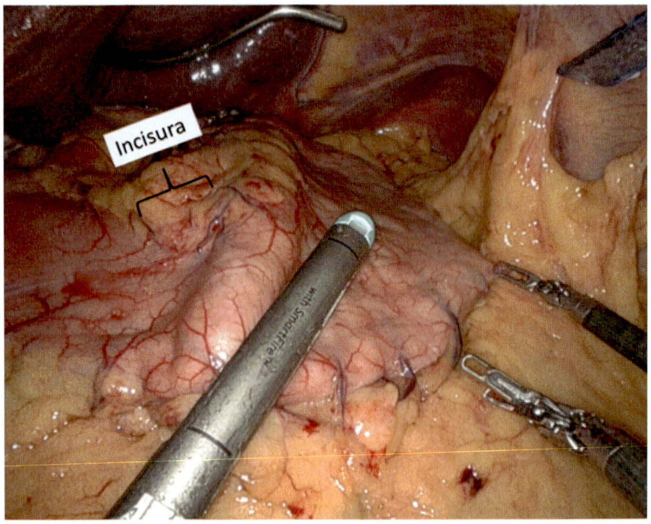

Fig. 23.19 The first staple fire is positioned to make sure it is wide about the incisura. The antrum is left mainly intact. Both Arms 1 and 3 are 12 mm and will accommodate the stapler. The first fire normally comes from Arm 1, and then the stapler is transitioned to Arm 3 after the first or second staple fire

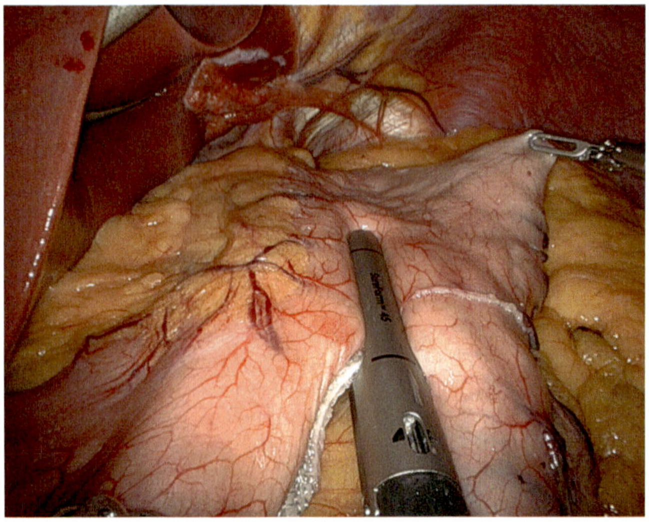

Fig. 23.20 This is the third staple fire coming from Arm 3. With the 60 mm robotic stapler, it will take 5–6 staple loads to complete the sleeve

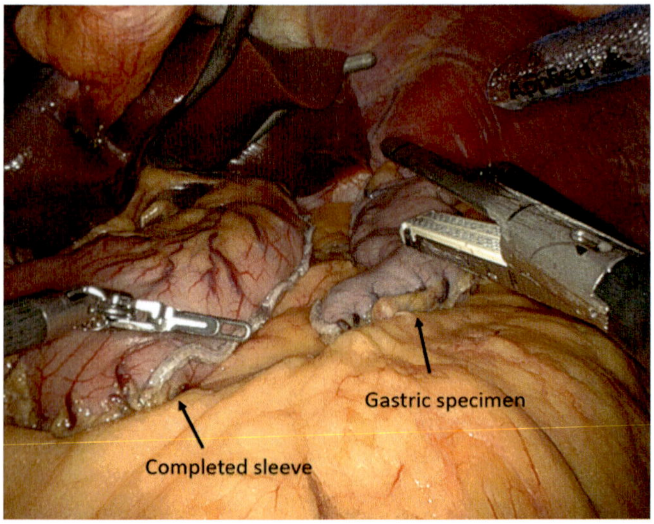

Fig. 23.21 The sleeve is completed. The excised stomach is removed at the end of the surgery

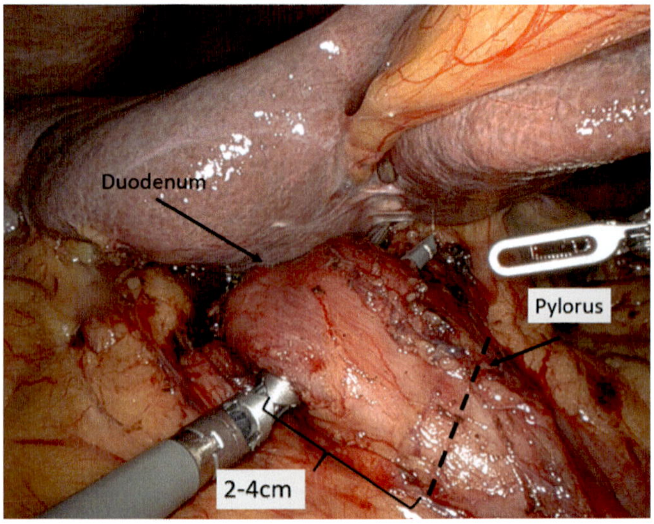

Fig. 23.22 The next step is to divide the duodenum 2–4 cm past the pylorus. Two variations of dissection can be utilized by the surgeon. In this image only a small tunnel has been created behind the duodenum in the area of desired transection. This minimizes the disruption of blood flow to the duodenum and has been favored by many surgeons. The downside is the anastomosis can be under an enlarged liver and the duodenal-ileal anastomosis may have more tension. Here the robotic instrument is in this tunnel

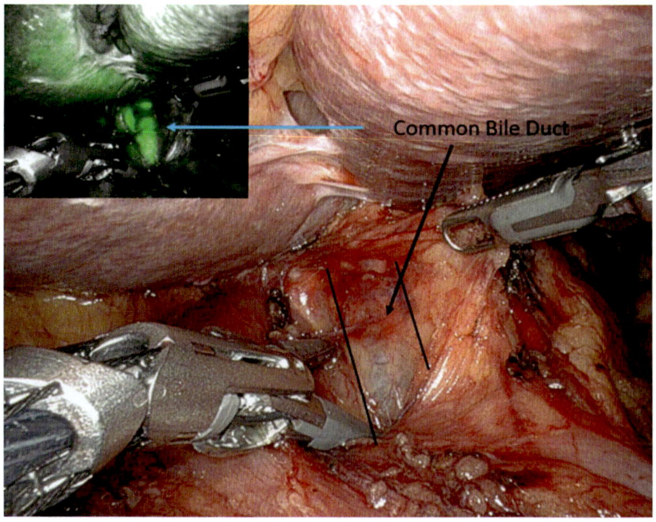

Fig. 23.23 This is the view of the superior dissection of the duodenum when tunneling. It is positioned over the CBD which is seen here in white light but also using near-infrared fluorescent imaging after giving indocyanine green intravenously (inset photo). The CBD is a nice landmark as it is easier to identify rather than the gastroduodenal artery

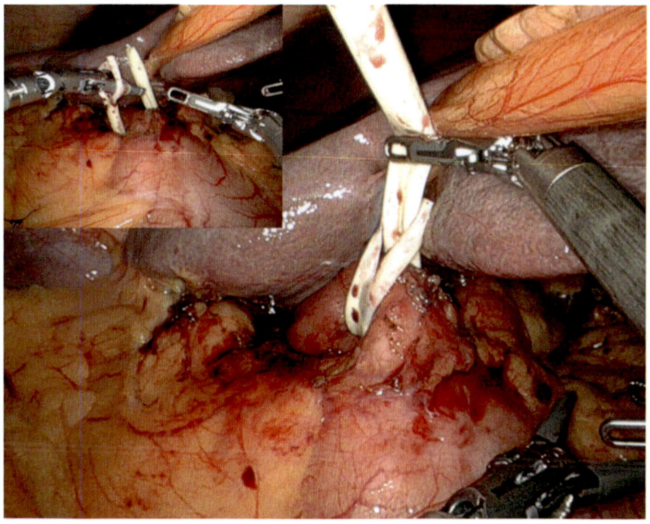

Fig. 23.24 A Penrose drain is used to help maintain access to this small tunnel as the stapler is being positioned. The inset picture shows placement of the Penrose drain

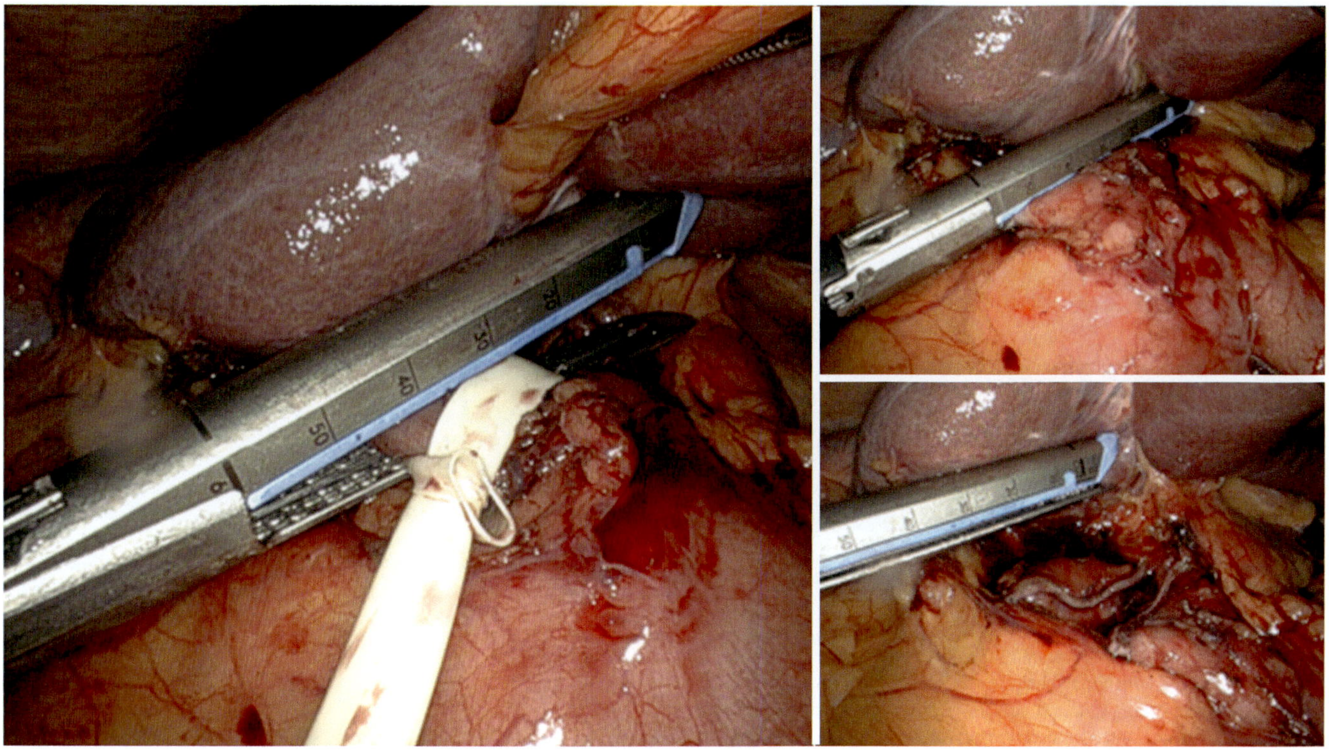

Fig. 23.25 The Penrose helps to facilitate placement of the stapler, but it needs to be removed prior to firing as you see in these photos

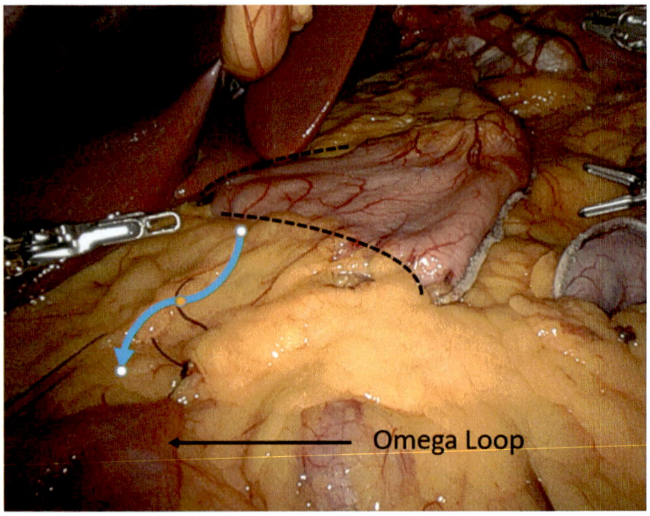

Fig. 23.26 The alternative to the limited dissection is to fully mobilize the distal stomach by releasing the attachments to the antrum and pylorus along the greater curve inferiorly and along the lesser curve superiorly including the right gastric artery or its branches. This photo shows the distal stomach, pylorus, and duodenum prior to this dissection but after the sleeve

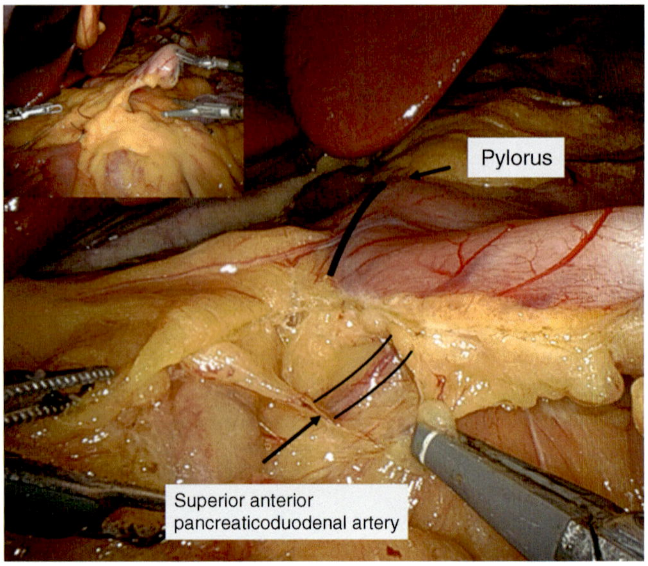

Fig. 23.27 This image illustrates the mobilization of the greater curve. A variety of robotic tools can be used to dissect this area including a robotic ultrasonic dissector, a robotic monopolar scissors, a robotic vessel sealer, and a robotic hook cautery. The author has performed this dissection mainly with the robotic vessel sealer. It is important to stay aware of the important vascular structures in the region. Here you can see a branch of the gastroduodenal artery, the superior anterior pancreaticoduodenal artery. A close dissection to the pylorus and duodenum helps to avoid injury to these deeper vascular structures

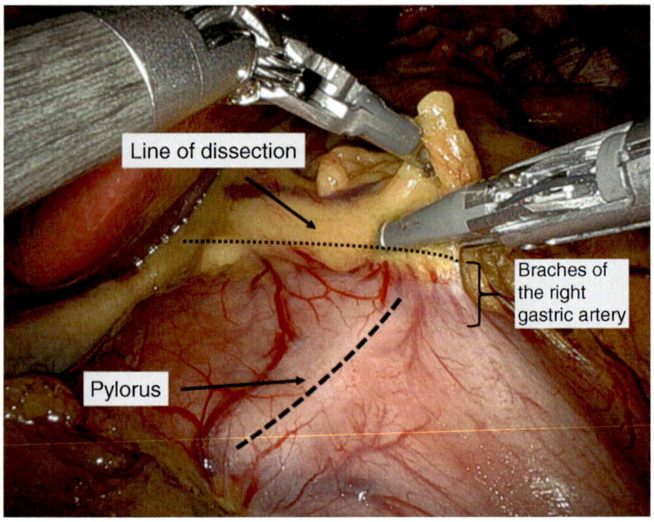

Fig. 23.28 The superior margin of dissection is seen here. With this wide dissection of the distal stomach, the right gastric artery and branches are divided. When completed this will allow the distal stomach to swing down to the omega loop. A wide dissection may give the appearance of ischemia, but perfusion is maintained through collateralization

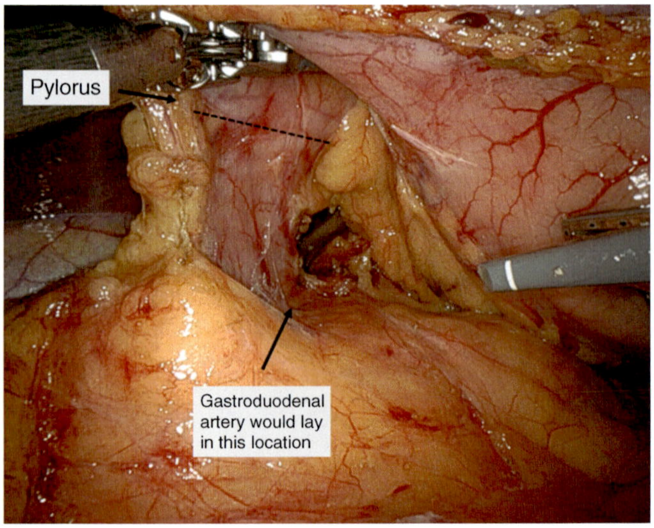

Fig. 23.29 Elevation of the stomach to see the posterior view facilitates the dissection. Visualized here is the nearly completed dissection as it is viewed from posteriorly. At times, the gastroduodenal artery is plain to see and at other times it is not

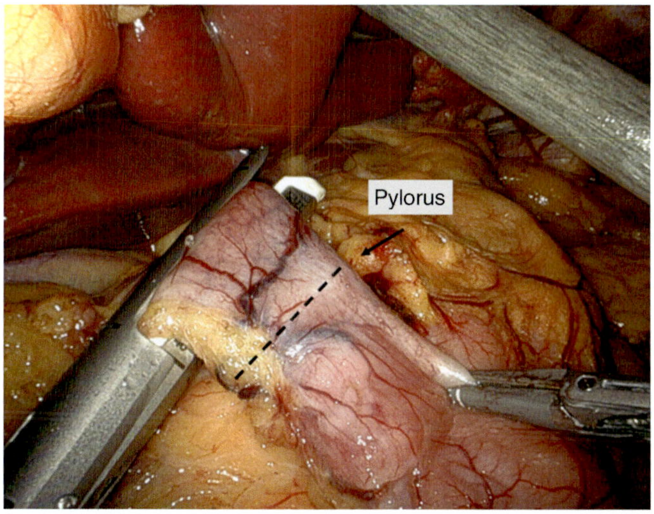

Fig. 23.30 The duodenum is divided 2–4 cm past the pylorus

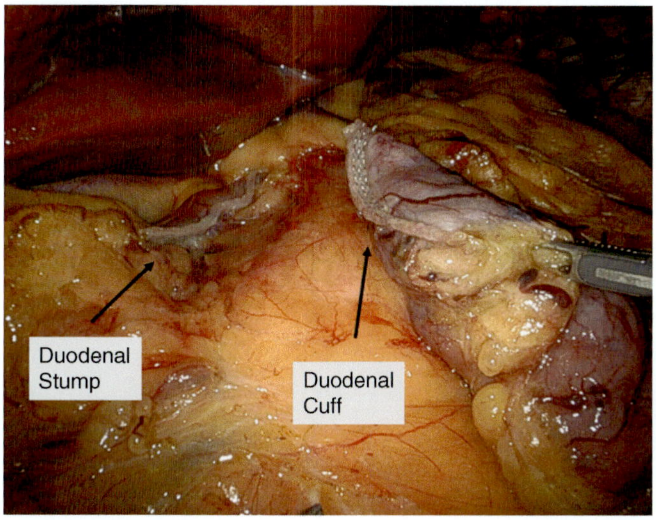

Fig. 23.31 The duodenal cuff staple line will be incorporated into the duodenal-ileal anastomosis. The duodenal stump is the blind end of the bypassed proximal bowel (biliopancreatic limb)

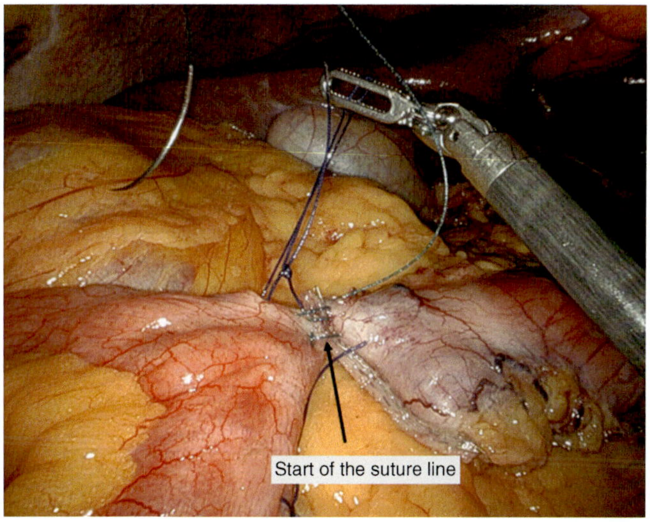

Fig. 23.32 The duodenal-ileal anastomosis (DIA) is created next. It is sewn in two layers. The staple line on the duodenal cuff is incorporated into the antimesenteric side of the ileum. To facilitate creation of the anastomosis, the posterior staple line is started on the upper corner. This allows the suture to be held, and the rest of the suturing is facilitated as it now faces the camera

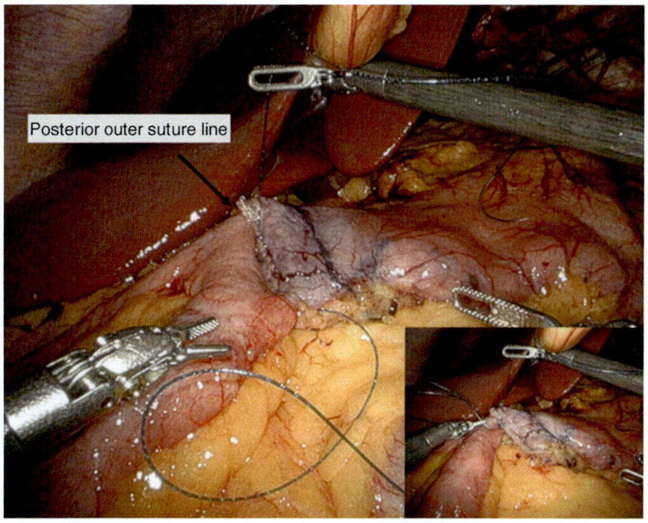

Fig. 23.33 The second barbed suture is started immediately adjacent to the first, as seen in the inset. This facilitates the remainder of the anastomosis creation. The second suture ends at the opposite corner of the staple line

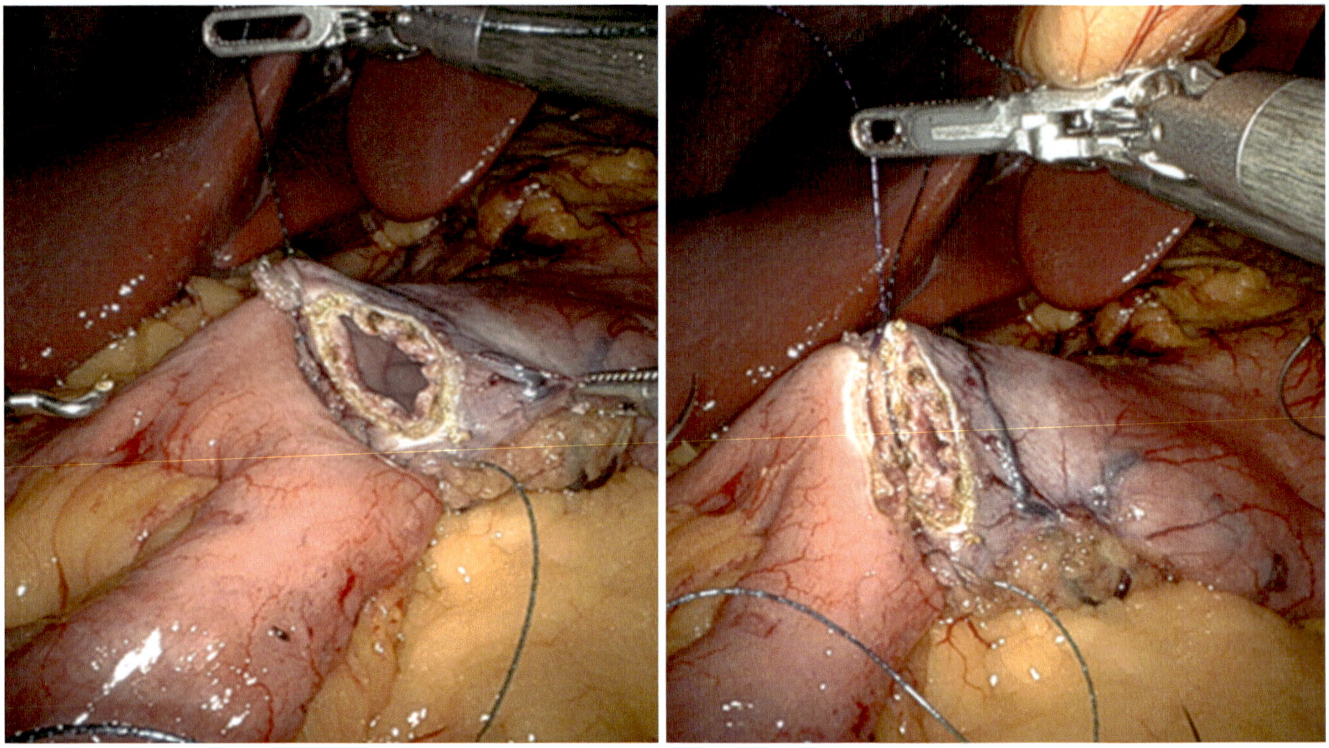

Fig. 23.34 Enterotomies are made adjacent to the suture line. Instruments which can be used include monopolar hook or scissors. Also, the bipolar vessel sealer can be utilized once the enterotomies are started

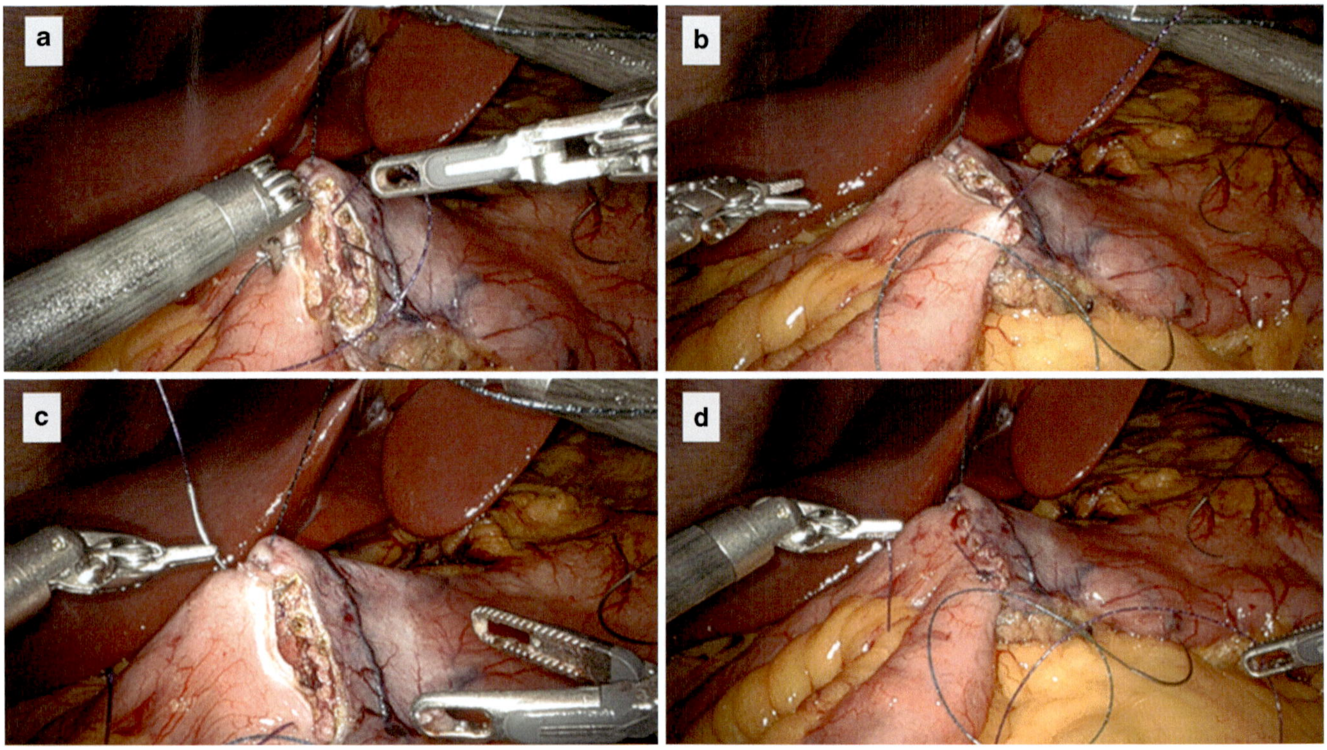

Fig. 23.35 The inner layer of the anastomosis is completed with two separate 6 inch 3–0 barbed sutures. It is convenient to have the out and the inner layer different colors as seen in this photo. To start the inner layer, the first suture is placed at the top corner of the enterotomies (**a**). It is carried to the bottom corner and brought around anteriorly (**b**). The second suture is started also at the top corner (**c**), but is carried anteriorly down to the previous suture on the bottom corner (**d**)

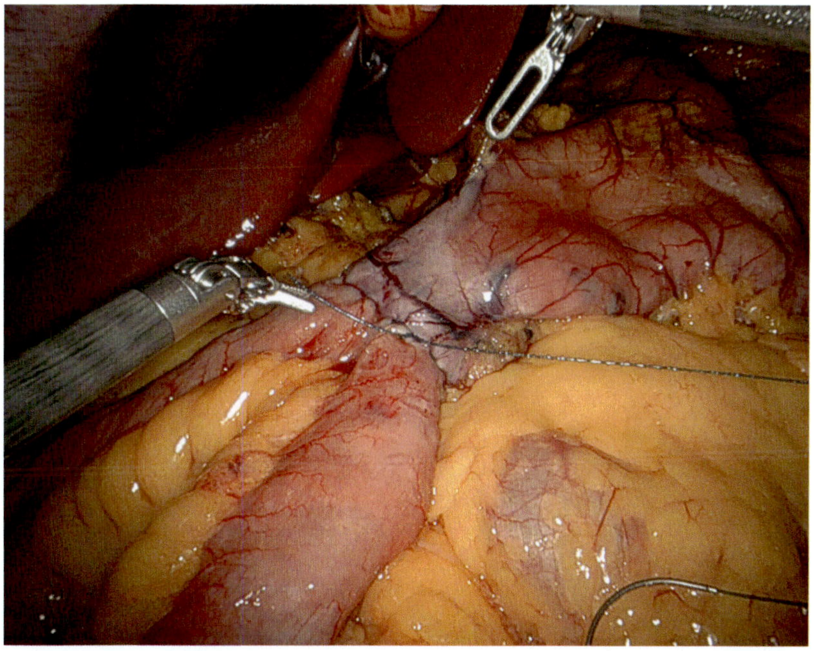

Fig. 23.36 The previously placed outer layer sutures seen on the corners are then brought from their posterior location and utilized to finish a second anterior layer. This completes the two-layer sewn DIA

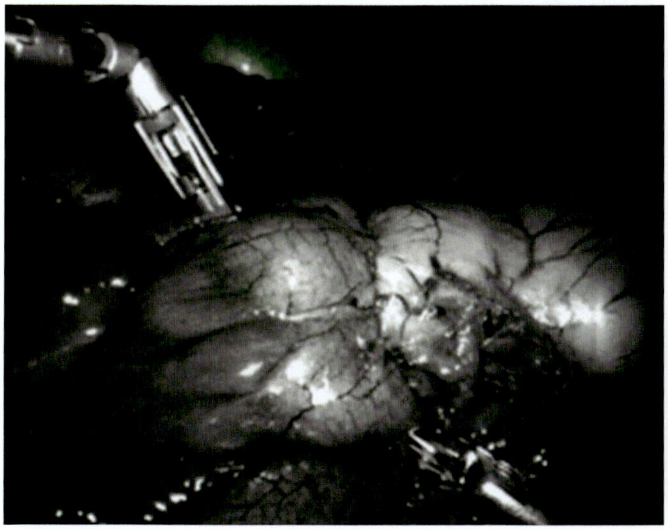

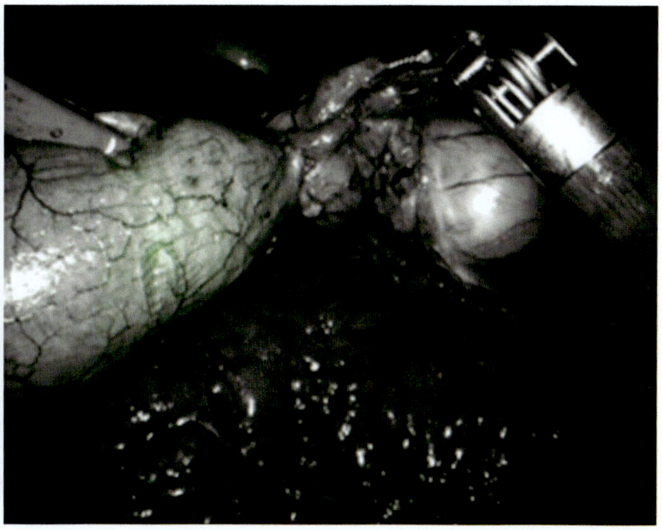

Fig. 23.37 A leak test is then performed of the DIA. Options include and air leak test with upper endoscopy or a nasogastric tube (NG). Also, via a NG a mixture of saline and methylene blue can be used. The author prefers to utilize a mixture of saline with indocyanine green and inspect the anastomosis under near-infrared imaging. In this image you see the leak test under fluorescent images. A leak would be an obvious spillage of green fluid. This technique results in a highly sensitive and specific test

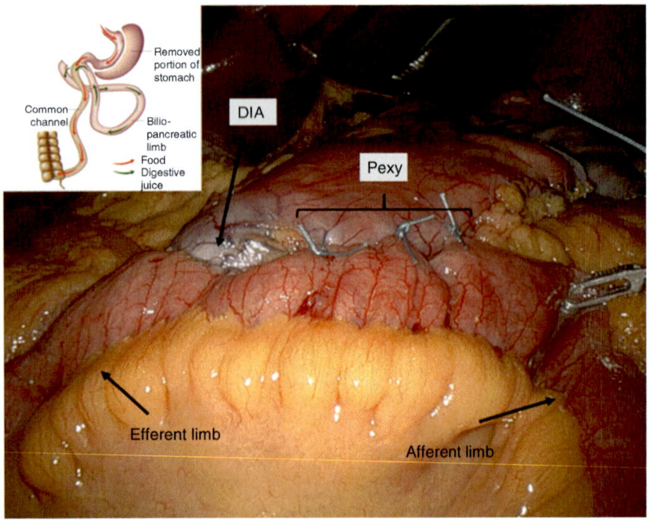

Fig. 23.38 With the completion of the DIA, there is only one more step and a rSADI-S is complete. But with the rDS, the omega loop would be converted to a Roux-en-Y configuration and an ileal-ileal anastomosis constructed. In this illustration you see how the afferent limb (biliopancreatic limb) of the omega loop is sutured to the inferior aspect of the antrum. This prevents afferent loop syndrome in which food would preferentially fill the afferent limb after a meal. In addition, it may prevent torsion in which the distal stomach twists along with the small bowel as this can be a narrow pedicle. Labeled is the efferent limb which correlates in a rSADI-S to the common channel

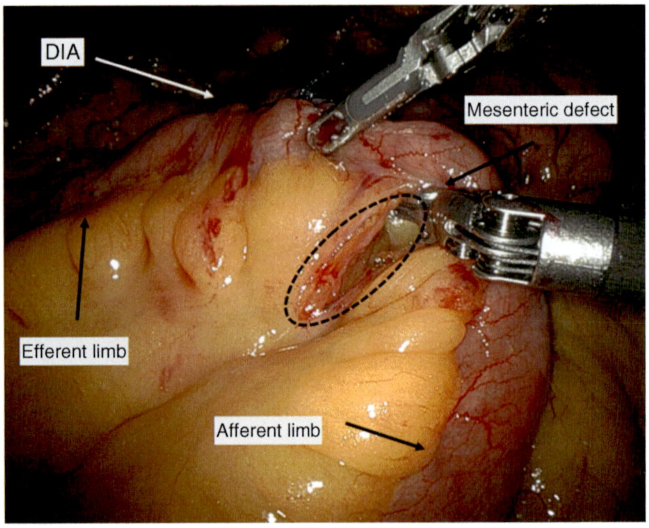

Fig. 23.39 The next step of the DS is to convert the loop bypass to a Roux-en-Y configuration. In this illustration a small mesenteric defect is created to the left of the DIA. This separates the afferent limb (BP limb) from the DIA and efferent limb. Only a small mesenteric defect is created so the ileal-ileal anastomosis (IIA) will stay readily in the operative field of the robotic system. The operative field is limited robotically at this point, so keeping it higher facilitates a robotic approach and creates efficiency. The bowel is then divided with a stapler

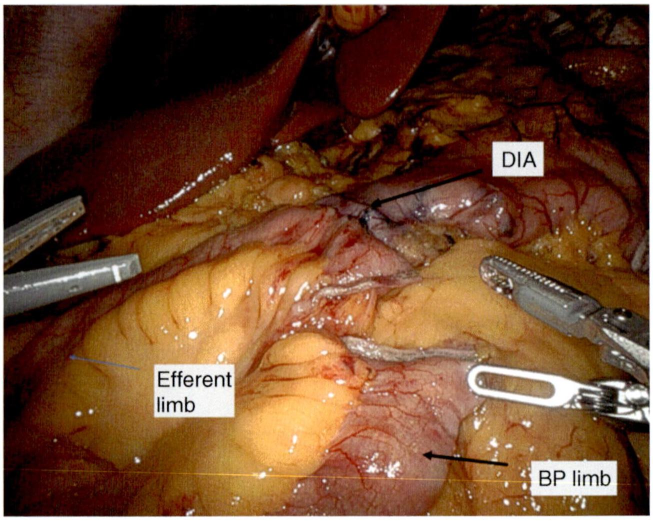

Fig. 23.40 Once the ileum is divided that has effectively separated the BP limb from the efferent limb, the efferent limb at this point is the combined length of the common channel and Roux limb

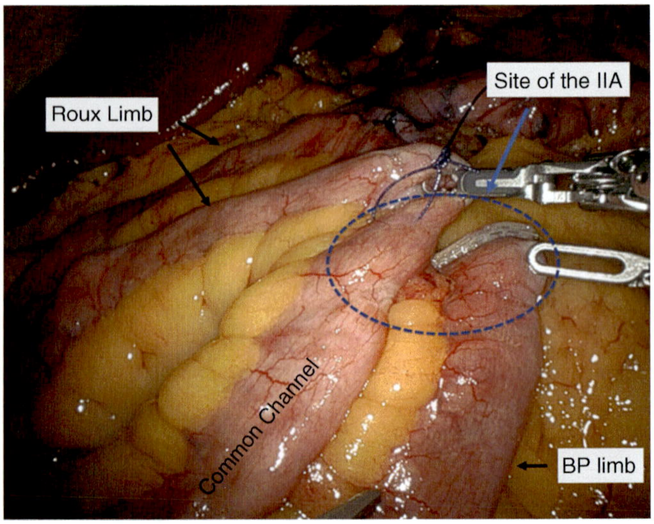

Fig. 23.41 After the omega loop is divided, the efferent limb is followed distally until the previously placed stich which marks the desired location to perform the ileal-ileal anastomosis (IIA). Care is taken to not twist the mesentery. The photo shows the relationship to the BP limb and the common channel as it is positioned to create the IIA. The surgeon has a choice of techniques to create the IIA anastomosis. If the robotic arms are still in good position to the surgical target, a side-to-side anastomosis can be created similar to the technique commonly used for the Jejuno-jejunal anastomosis for a RNY gastric bypass. At times, the surgical space is limited; therefore it can be beneficial to sew the anastomosis

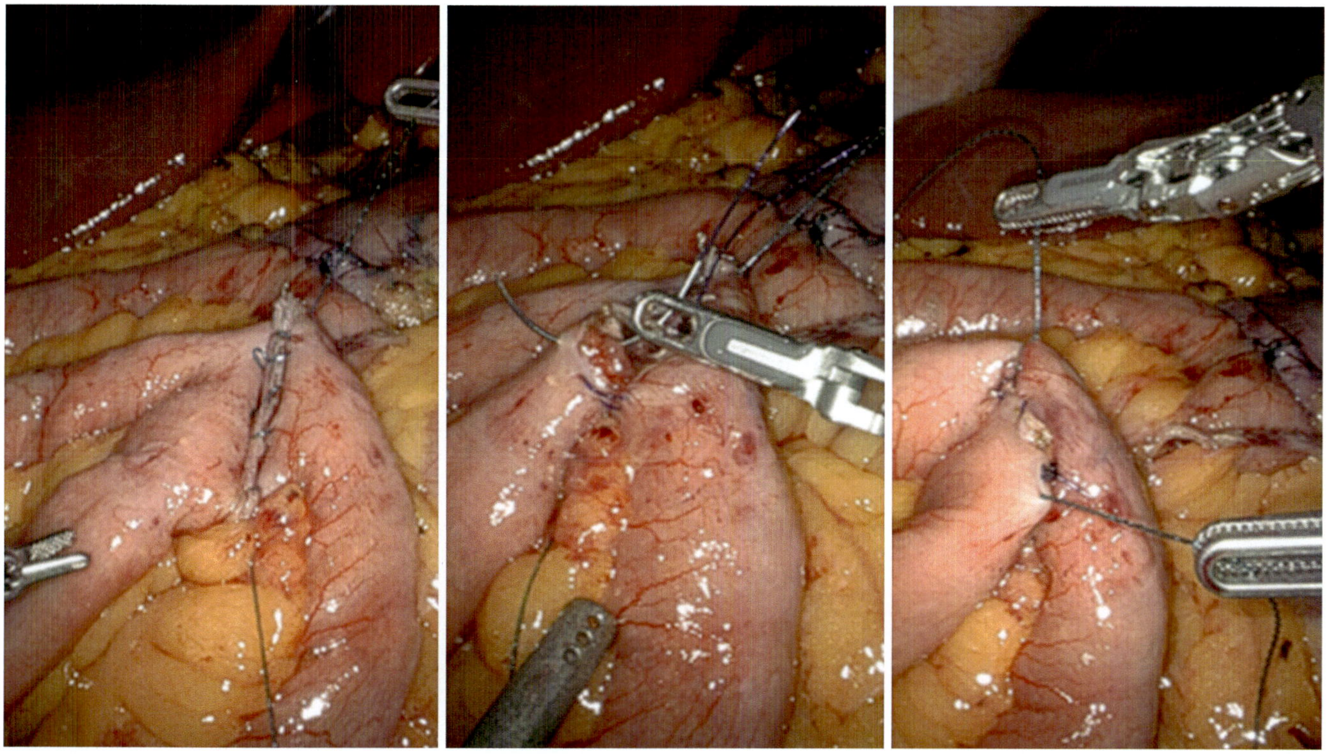

Fig. 23.42 The sewn IIA is created in a two-layer fashion by the author. It is preferred as introducing a stapler in this location can be challenging. Here you see the steps are similar to the sewn DIA. The distal BP limb staple line is sutured to the antimesenteric surface of the ileum creating the end-to side-anastomosis

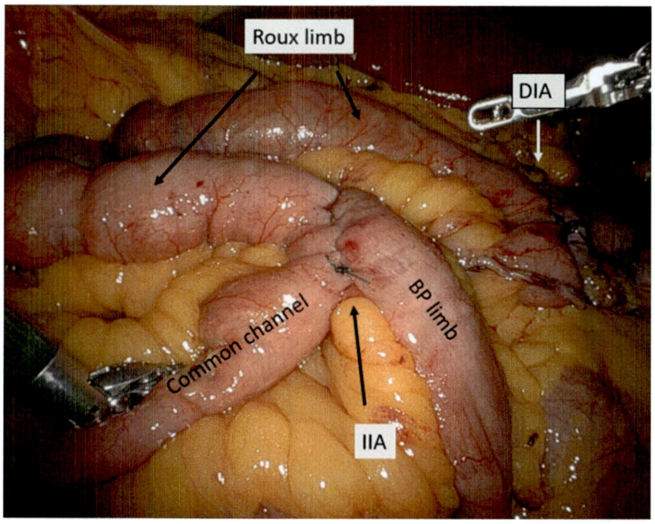

Fig. 23.43 With the creation of the IIA, the previous efferent limb now is formed into the Roux limb and the common channel. This is the final configuration of the robotic duodenal switch (rDS) with both the DIA and IIA clearly seen in relationship to the Roux limb, common channel, and BP limb. The last and final step is to close the loop defect which is created in the ileal mesentery alongside the IIA

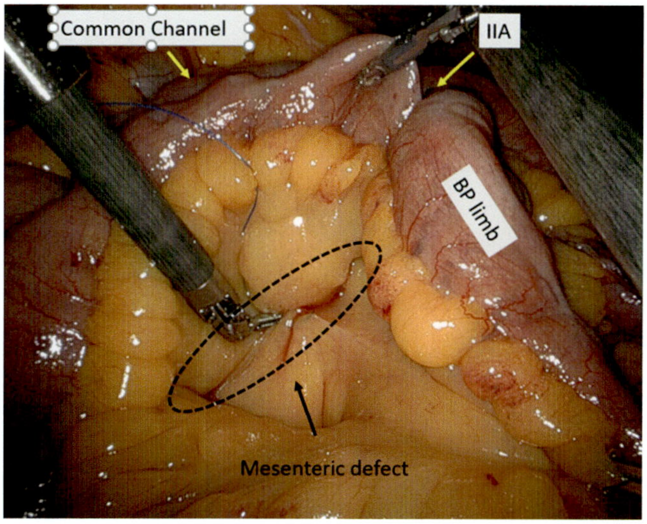

Fig. 23.44 A mesenteric loop defect is made adjacent to the IIA. This is a potential cause of an internal hernia. For that reason, the defect is closed by moving the common channel to the patient's right and the BP limb in a cephalad direction. A barbed permanent suture is used to close this defect in a running fashion. This completes the surgery with the exception of removing the gastric specimen

Suggested Reading

Kallies K, Rogers AM. American Society for Metabolic and Bariatric Surgery update statement on single-anastomosis duodenal switch. Surg Obes Rel Diseases. 2020:825–30. https://doi.org/10.1016/j.soard.2020.03.020.

Pastrana M, El Chaar M. Evolution of outcomes of robotic bariatric surgery: first report based on MBSAQIP database. Surg Obes Rel Diseases. 2020;16(7):916–22. https://doi.org/10.1016/j.soard.2020.01.006.

Sudan R, Podolsky E. Totally-assisted biliary pancreatic diversion with duodenal switch: single dock technique and technical outcomes. Surg Endo. 2015;29:55–60. https://doi.org/10.1007/s004-014-3653-0.

24 Robotic Revisional Bariatric Surgery

Danuel Laan and Carlos A. Galvani

Introduction

Revisional bariatric surgery accounts for up to 25% of bariatric procedures in the modern era and has increased 311% since 2011 [1].

The rate of revisional surgery varies with the index bariatric procedure. It could be as high as 40% after adjustable gastric band (AGB), 10–20% after Roux en Y gastric bypass (RYGB), and 5.5% after sleeve gastrectomy [2].There are two overarching reasons for revisional bariatric surgery: (1) complications after primary bariatric surgery, not including immediate postoperative complications, and (2) patients who have insufficient weight loss or weight regain after primary bariatric surgery.

Revisional bariatric procedures can also be classified as:

- Conversion: Procedures that change from an index procedure to a different type of procedure.
- Corrective: Procedures addressing complications or incomplete treatment effect of a previous bariatric operation.
- Reversal: Procedures that restore original anatomy.

The complication rate after laparoscopic revisional surgery is 15–31% and is highly dependent on the specific revisional procedure [3]. The application of robotics in primary bariatric surgery is emerging but not yet widespread. In primary surgeries, robotics has been shown to decrease anastomotic leaks, reoperations, and length of hospital stay when compared to laparoscopy [4, 5].

As it pertains to revisional bariatric surgery, some series have demonstrated its feasibility and safety, although recent advances in robotic technology can potentially improve upon those outcomes and demonstrate clear advantages favoring the routine use of robotics [6]. Herein we describe our evaluation and treatment of patients requiring reoperative bariatric surgery and the potential benefits of robotic-assisted surgery.

The decision to perform revisional surgery should be based on the index procedure (Fig. 24.1):

1. Complications after primary bariatric surgery, not including immediate postoperative complications:
   (a) Laparoscopic Adjustable Gastric Band (LAGB): Postoperative complications after LAGB are band slippage, erosion, stenosis, band intolerance, esophageal dilation, severe GERD, and port-related problems.
   (b) Nonadjustable Gastric Band (NAGB): Most complications post NAGB are nausea, vomiting, severe

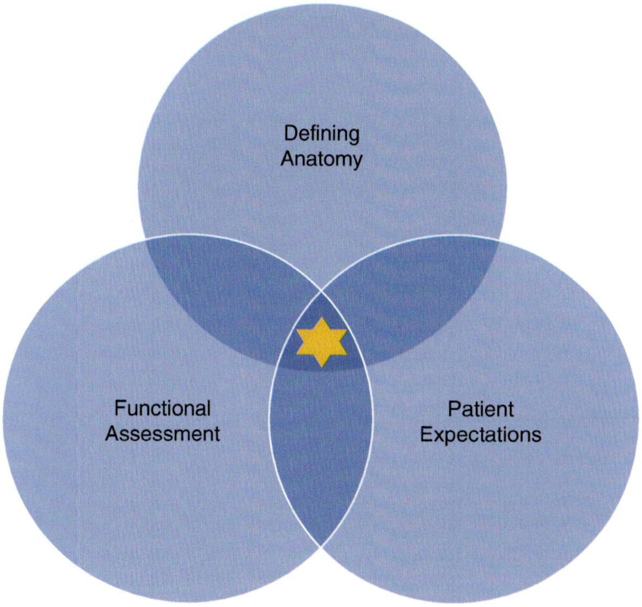

Fig. 24.1 Decisional flowchart according to the index procedure and the indication for robotic revisional bariatric surgery

D. Laan · C. A. Galvani (✉)
Division of Minimally Invasive Surgery. Department of Surgery, Tulane University School of Medicine, New Orleans, LA, USA
e-mail: cgalvani@tulane.edu

O. Y. Kudsi, P. P. Grimminger (eds.), *Atlas of Robotic Upper Gastrointestinal Surgery*,
https://doi.org/10.1007/978-3-030-86578-8_24

GERD, malnutrition, band erosion, and esophageal dilation.
   - (c) Roux-en-Y Gastric Bypass (RYGB): Marginal ulcer, bleeding, anastomotic stricture, dilated gastric pouch, and gastro-gastric fistula are common after RYGB.
   - (d) Laparoscopic Sleeve Gastrectomy (LSG): Severe GERD is the most common cause for revisional surgery after sleeve gastrectomy. Patients can also suffer from sleeve dilation and strictures.
   - (e) Duodenal Switch (DS): Malnutrition is one of the most common complications of DS. Because of the SG associated with the DS, GERD is a possible complication of the DS.
   - (f) Vertical Banded Gastroplasty: Patients with VBG most common complains are severe GERD, band erosion, stricture, dysphagia, and disruption of the staple line.
2. Patients who have insufficient weight loss, weight regain, or recurrence of obesity-related medical conditions after primary bariatric surgery. Prior to any revisional surgery, all patients with weight regain or insufficient weight loss should go for consultation with the program psychologist and dietician to determine the reason for the lack of weight loss or weight regain.

Preoperative Assessment (Fig. 24.2)

Defining Anatomy

- Performing history and physical: Dietary habits, percentage of initial weight loss and subsequent weight regain, symptoms such as dysphagia, reflux, food regurgitation, and postprandial abdominal pain. These symptoms could be sign of anatomical issues such as stenosis at the anastomosis, hiatal hernia, marginal ulcer, pouch dilation, gastro-gastric fistula in patients with history of gastric bypass, or inadequate removal of gastric fundus in initial sleeve gastrectomy.
- Reviewing prior operative reports: Retrocolic or antecolic Roux limb in RYGB, mesenteric defect closure in RYGB, Bougie size in sleeve gastrectomy, concurrent hiatal hernia repair, and use of silastic or any other type of nonadjustable band.
- Obtaining imaging: We choose upper gastrointestinal (UGI) series as our initial investigation as this also provides some functional assessment of reflux. Timed barium swallow along with marshmallows swallow is also indicated in selected cases within the preoperative workup.
- Performing upper endoscopy: Endoscopy is vitally important to detect sequelae of GERD such as esophagitis, stricture and Barrett's esophagus, as well as hiatal hernia, marginal ulcer, anastomotic stenosis, stomal stenosis, bleeding, and gastro-gastric fistula, band erosions, dilated sleeve, or neo-fundus. We believe it's important for the operating surgeons to perform the EGD themselves in preparation for these cases to define the surgical anatomy and sometimes to define the indication for surgery.

Defining Function

- Timed Barium Swallow/Marshmallow Swallow: Helpful to define either esophageal/gastric/pouch emptying.
- Esophageal Manometry: Especially useful in patients with dysphagia without obvious mechanical reasons, patients with previous history of a restrictive procedure (LAGB, VBG, Sleeve, etc.)
- Gastric Emptying Study: Patients with history of poor oral tolerance, nausea, and vomiting may benefit from GES (e.g., sleeve gastrectomy).

Patient Education

- Managing Expectations:
  - Postoperative complications (Reoperations, Leaks, Bleeding, Pulmonary embolism, Death, etc.).
  - Postoperative diet: Retraining of the patient is needed since many of these patients had remote history of their index procedure.
  - Psychological evaluation is an important aspect of the preoperative workup of patients undergoing reoperative bariatric surgery.

Operating Room Setup

A large operating room is preferable when performing robotic surgery (Fig. 24.3). Larger operating rooms allow the robot components to be stored in the room and allow the operating room personnel to move freely around the room. The room should also facilitate docking of the system depending of the type of surgery to be performed. Preferably, the room will be a dedicated room with an integration system to allow for flat panel monitors which are mounted from the ceiling, CO2 gas is piped directly into the room for insufflation, and ceiling mounted equipment booms can house insufflators, electrosurgical units, laparoscopic camera equipment, and light sources. The operating table is placed directly under the room lights. Anesthesia equipment is located at the head of the operating table. The advent of the new da Vinci Xi offers some advantages with respect to the da Vinci Si providing streamlined setup and port placement.

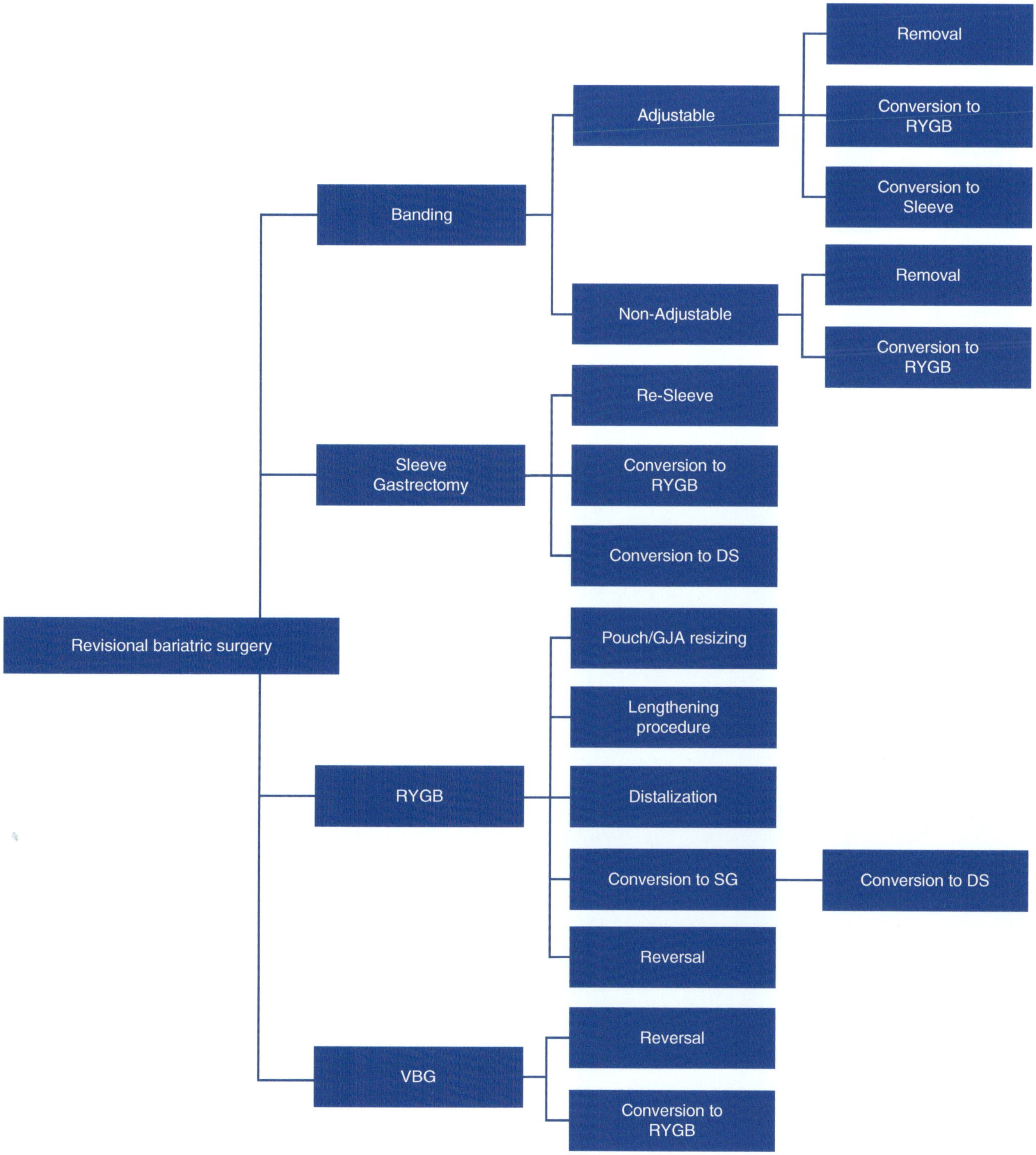

Fig. 24.2 Preoperative assessment

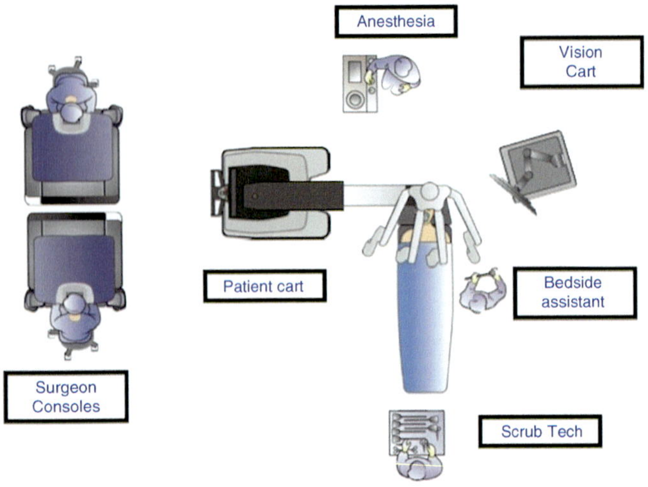

Fig. 24.3 Operating room setup

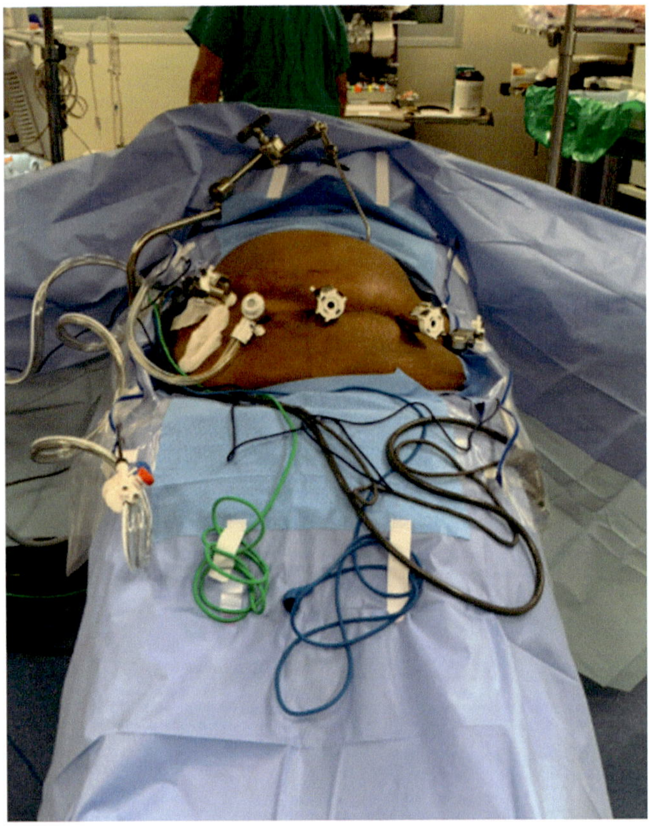

Fig. 24.4 Patient positioning

Patient Positioning

The use of a specialized OR table that can accommodate the needs of bariatric patients is mandatory (Fig. 24.4). The table must have the capacity to support super-obese patients, by providing steep Trendelenburg and the best working height as required for exposure of the operative field. In addition, a transfer mat should be used for repositioning and lateral transfer of the patient.

The patient is placed in a supine position with the arms tucked and properly padded if extensive laparoscopic adhesiolysis is anticipated. The patient is then secured to the bed around the legs using a safety strap. Pneumatic compression devices are placed on the lower legs prior to induction of anesthesia. Following successful endotracheal intubation, an orogastric tube (ViSiGi) is placed in order to decompress the stomach. This tube is also used for sizing of the stomach and stenting of anastomosis. Preoperative antibiotics are given prior to making an incision. An upper body Bair Hugger® (Arizant Inc., Eden Prairie, MN) is then placed above the nipples. Once the patient is positioned, a face protection donut is used to protect the patient's face and endotracheal tube from inadvertent damage or dislodgement during movement of the robotic endoscope. Once this is established, the abdomen and lower chest are prepped widely with iodine and then sterile drapes.

Access/Port Placement

The port placement described is specific for the da Vinci Xi System (Fig. 24.5). Entry into the abdominal cavity is obtained through a gasless optical technique in the periumbilical area, just to the left of the midline, using a 8-mm robotic optical trocar. However, if there is a history of open surgery, the entry to the abdominal cavity will migrate to the left upper quadrant, right upper quadrant, and sometimes periumbilical using a Hasson technique. If gasless technique is used, a 5-mm 0/30 degrees laparoscope is used for access and port placement. The first port is placed in the left mid-abdomen two fingerbreadths lateral to the umbilicus and one palm width inferior to the left costal margin. This port is used for the robotic camera (Arm #2). If there is previous open surgery, the first entry port is placed left subcostal.

Insufflation is started to 15 mmHg. Two 8-mm trocars and one 12-mm trocar are then placed at the same level of the camera port: 12-mm port on the right midclavicular line (Arm #1), one on the left midclavicular line (Arm #3), and one in the left anterior axillary line (Arm #4). A 5-mm sub-xiphoid incision is used for the placement of the Nathanson liver retractor. Finally, an assistant port (8 mm) is inserted in between arms #2 and #3 or between #1 and #2 . The robotic surgical cart is then approximated into position, and the arms are attached to the four specific trocars. The da Vinci Xi Surgical system can be docked from the patient's right or left side.

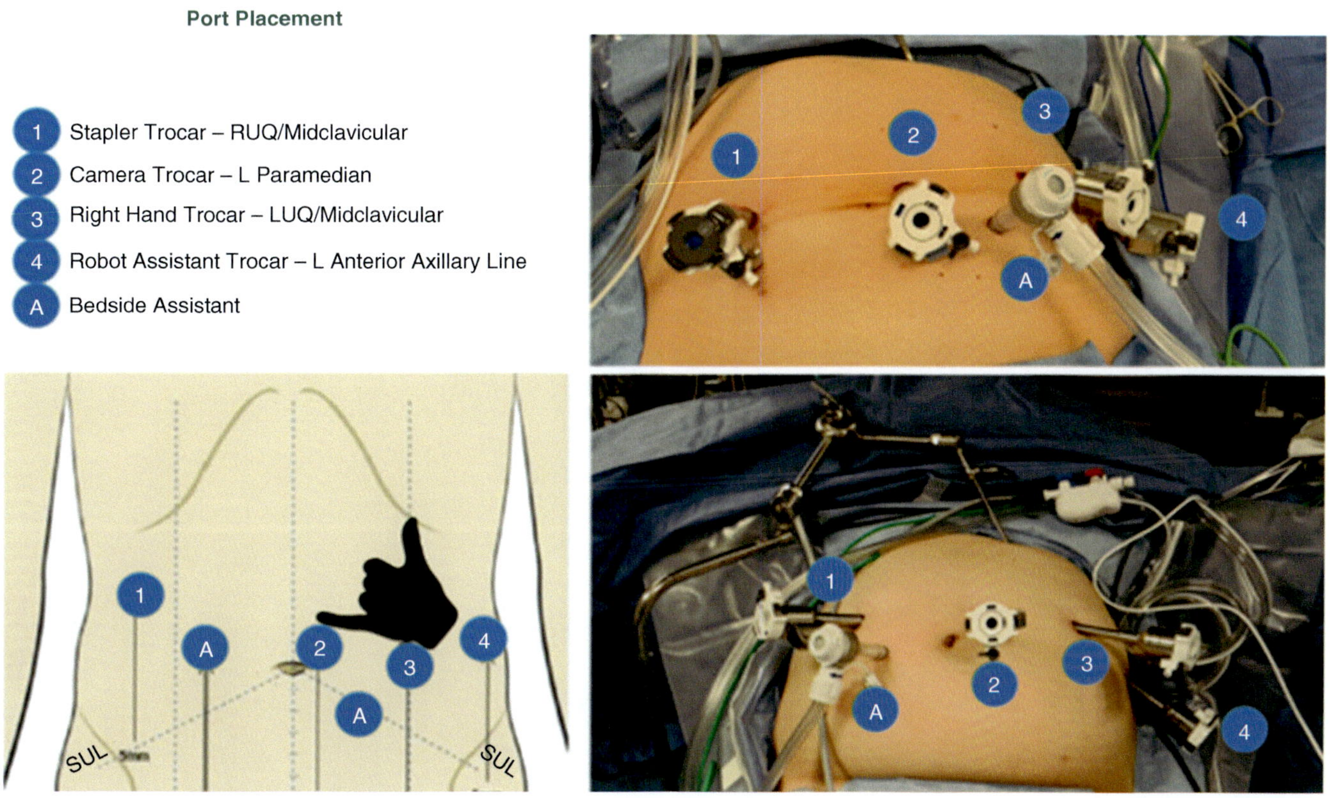

Fig. 24.5 Access/port placement

Adhesiolysis

One of the most challenging aspects of revisional bariatric surgery is adhesiolysis (Fig. 24.6). Previous open surgery lends itself toward midline adhesions. Some degree adhesions are almost always present between the liver and stomach.

Other common areas for adhesions are at the angle of His and retrogastric to the pancreas. Adhesiolysis can be started laparoscopically in order to create space for the insertion of the robotic trocars. However, we endeavor to dock the robot as early as possible to facilitate the adhesiolysis and shorten operative time. Sometimes this can represent starting with two working arms.

- Adhesiolysis then continues with monopolar scissors in Arm #3 and a fenestrated bipolar in Arm #1. The main advantages of the robotic system are self-assisting, better exposure/visualization of structures, and the articulated energy device. These benefits decrease the incidence of iatrogenic perforations and bleeding. While separating the left lobe of the liver from the stomach, the identification of the right crus is our anatomic landmark and will facilitate delineation of the hiatus and identification of hiatal hernias and prevent injuries to vascular structures, namely, the inferior vena cava (IVC). This portion of the procedure could be relatively bloody, and for that reason, the utilization of two energy sources (Arms #1/#3) is a significant progress from laparoscopic surgery. The fourth robotic arm gives the console surgeon greater independence from the assistant by facilitating retraction and dissection.
- The purpose of the bedside assistant is to provide suction, retraction, exchange of robotic instruments, and insertion of and removal of sponges/sutures.

Hiatal Hernia Repair

Utilizing a combination of blunt dissection and the vessel sealer, the right crus is dissected from the esophagus starting at the right side of the phrenoesophageal membrane, working anterior to posterior, until it is fully exposed (Fig. 24.7). A retroesophageal window is then created and extended exposing the confluence of the crura. A Penrose drain is passed behind the esophagus and used to encircle the esophagus and vagus nerves. Then attention is focused on the left crura. Typically the dissection starts from posterior to anterior and is continued counterclockwise around the rim of the hiatus with complete exposure of the left crus and takedown

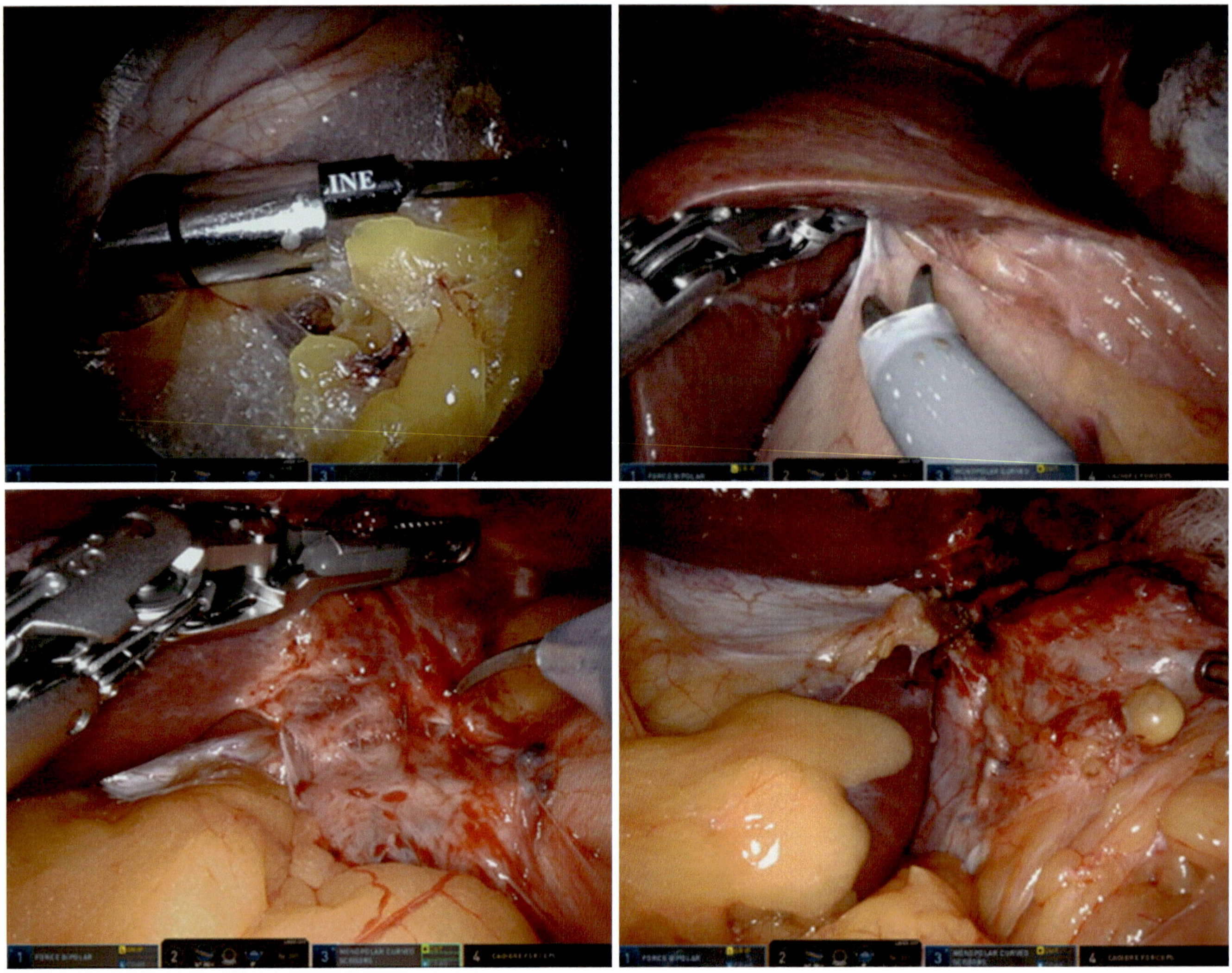

Fig. 24.6 Adhesiolysis

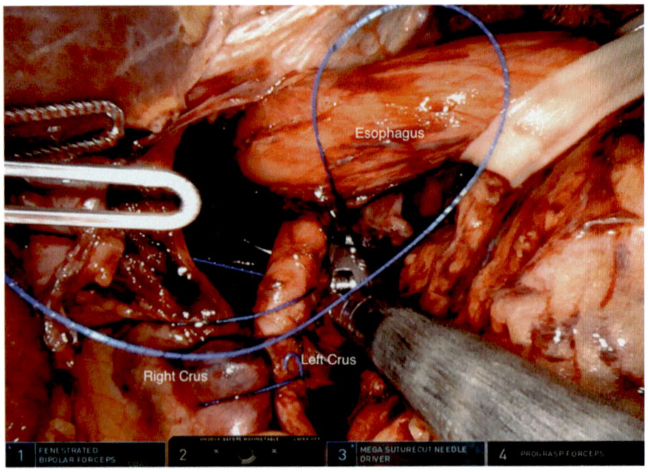

Fig. 24.7 Hiatal hernia repair

of the phrenoesophageal membrane. Transhiatal dissection of the esophagus is continued in cephalad. The articulated vessel sealer device and the fenestrated bipolar grasper are used for the circumferential dissection of the esophagus. Mobilization of the esophagus can typically be accomplished using blunt dissection of relatively thin alveolar tissue with traction/countertraction and always dissecting away from the esophagus. Esophageal mobilization is completed only after 3 cm of tension-free, intraabdominal esophagus is observed. The esophagus is retracted anteriorly and to the left by Arm #4. Closure of the diaphragmatic defect is started at the junction of the right and left crus to decrease tension on every stitch and is carried out anteriorly. The closure is performed using running non-absorbable barbed suture. We utilize a "shoelacing technique" in order to decrease tension.

- The incidence of hiatal hernias during reoperative surgery is much higher than reported for primary bariatric surgery. Simultaneous repair of hiatal hernias during reoperative surgery is warranted.

Identification of the Surgical Anatomy (Upper Endoscopy/TilePro)

Upper endoscopy is utilized at any point during the procedure if anatomy is unclear (Fig. 24.8). The TilePro TM feature is used to project intraoperative endoscopic images onto the console screen. The upper endoscopy can be performed by the bedside assistant.

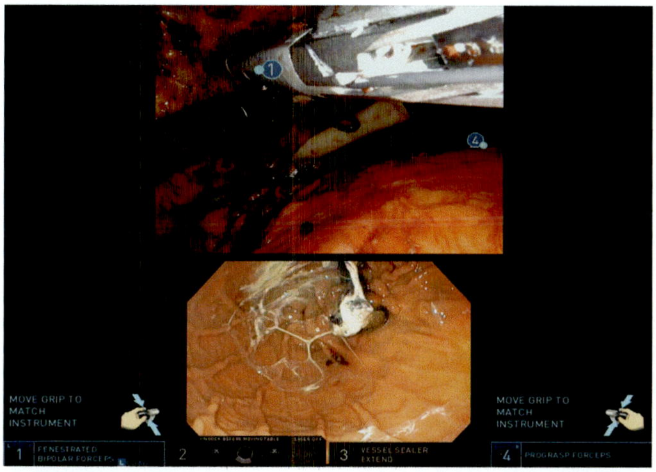

Fig. 24.8 Identification of the surgical anatomy (upper endoscopy/TilePro)

- TilePro is a multi-image video display mode of the da Vinci Xi that allows the surgeon to simultaneously view up to two additional images, such as intraoperative endoscopy, as a picture-on-picture on the three-dimensional console screen and assistant monitors.

Anatomy Takedown/Reconstruction/Use of Firefly

After the adhesiolysis is completed and anatomy of the previous surgery is outlined, the previous anatomy is taken down according to the surgical plan (Fig. 24.9). The risk of leak after revisional surgery is higher than primary surgery likely due to the less predictable tissue thickness. For that reason, when using staplers for resection of previous anastomosis, distal stomach, first portion of the duodenum, devascularized stomach, or thickened small bowel one should use a staple load with proper height due to chronic inflammation and edema scarring. This point deserves special consideration when using staple line reinforcement. It is also important to

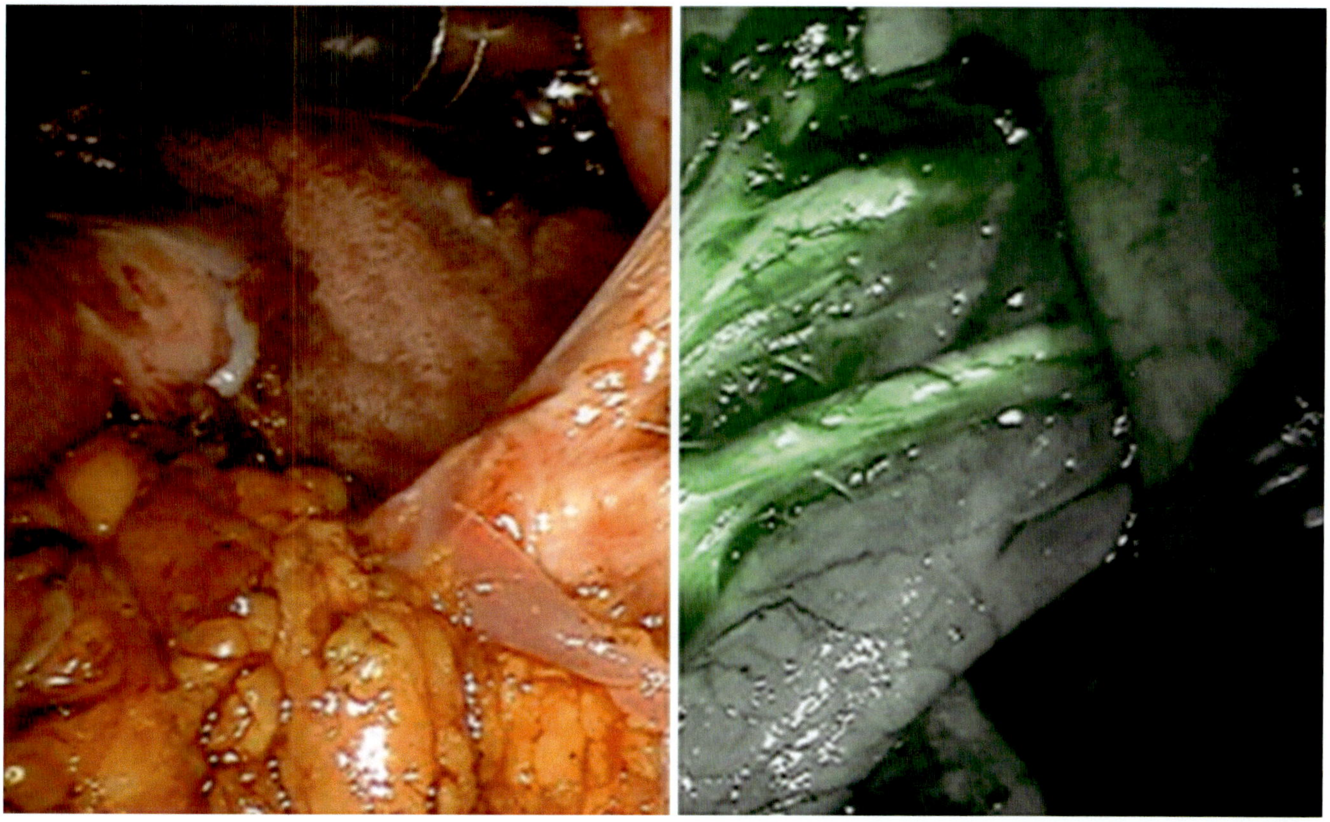

Fig. 24.9 Anatomy takedown /reconstruction/use of Firefly

be cognizant of previous staple lines, suture materials, clips, and silastic/mesh banding which could cause the stapler to jam and cause a misfire and damage the tissue. Irrespective of the index procedure, it is critical to identify and preserve in the left gastric artery. The Firefly feature of the robotic system can facilitate the identification of the vascular supply.

We use robotic linear stapler (SureForm60 TM) with stapler line reinforcement to decrease bleeding and potentially leaks. The stapler comes with white (2.5 mm staple height), blue (3.5 mm staple height), green (4.3 mm staple height), and black (4.6 mm staple height) reloads that can be selected according to the tissue thickness. This stapler also offers a 120 degrees cone of articulation that allows for less tissue pulling and improved tissue transection. In addition, the increased articulation of the stapler could decrease the need for two 12 mm trocars in the field.

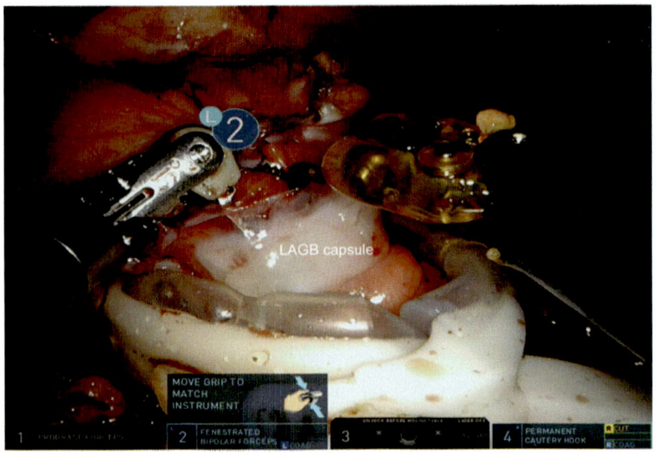

Fig. 24.11 LAGB

NAGB

Extensive lysis of adhesions is usually required during this case since these cases were routinely performed in an open fashion (Fig. 24.10). Finding and removing the band from the perigastric position is an essential step of the procedure. If the band cannot be removed due to adhesions, then excision of the stomach proximal and distal of the band should be performed. Alternatively, if the band is eroded into the gastric lumen, transgastric removal of the band can be attempted.

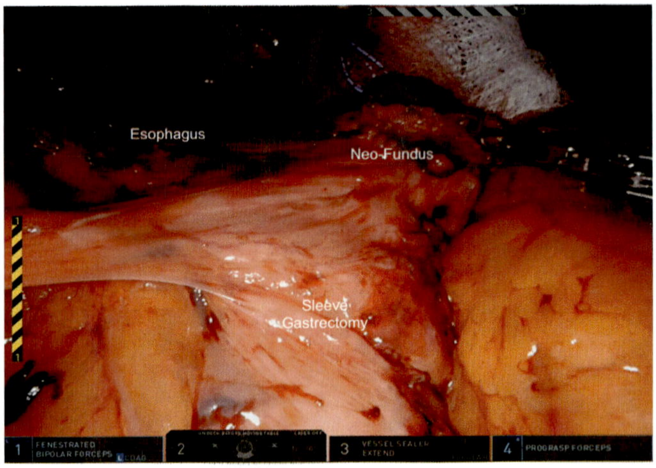

Fig. 24.12 Sleeve gastrectomy conversion to gastric bypass

LAGB

Excision of the perigastric capsule created by the band is essential to prevent staple misfiring. Common conversion procedures post LAGB removal are sleeve gastrectomy and gastric bypass (Fig. 24.11). Usual stapler reloads for either gastric bypass or sleeve conversion are blue, green, or black depending on tissue thickness.

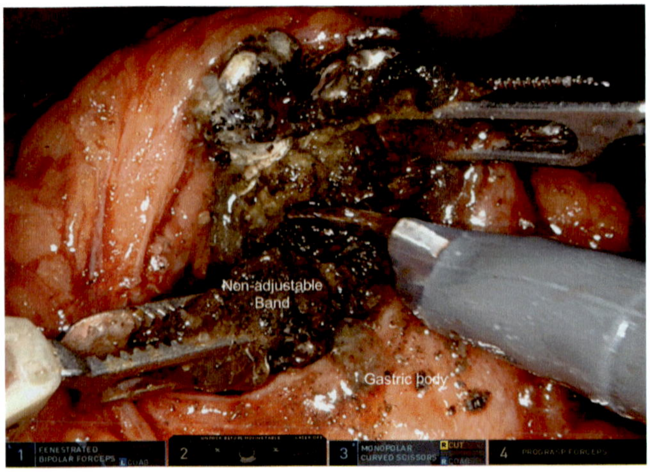

Fig. 24.10 NAGB

Sleeve Gastrectomy Conversion to Gastric Bypass

Adhesiolysis is performed from the antrum of the stomach progressing in a cephalad direction until the angle of His (Fig. 24.12). If a neofundus is present, it should be complete freed and excised during the creation of the gastric pouch. Usual stapler reloads for pouch creation are either blue or green. Care must be taken to identify clips on the staple line from the index procedure. If the intention is to preserve the sleeve and conversion to duodenal switch, dissection of the inferior aspect of the sleeve is performed until the first portion of the duodenum (2–3 cm distal to the pylorus). In patients with chronic sleeve fistulas, conversion to esophagojejunostomy must be considered.

VBG

Conversion to gastric bypass: the gastric pouch must be created proximal to the ostoma and medial to the gastro-gastric staple line of the VBG (Fig. 24.13). It is our practice to excise the fundus and most of the body of the stomach that includes the previous staple line. For this purpose, the short gastric vessels are taken down with vessel sealer. Stapler reloads for the gastric resection are usually black or green.

RYGB

It is crucial to delineate the anatomy of the gastric bypass at the beginning of the procedure (Fig. 24.14). The remnant stomach is dissected off the gastric pouch with robotic monopolar scissors. Then the posterior aspect of the GJA and the proximal alimentary limb are also dissected off. If the gastric bypass reconstruction was done retrocolic/retrogastric, further dissection may be necessary to be able to perform the reconstruction with no tension. Also, if a banded bypass was performed, the previous nonadjustable band must be removed. Once the anastomosis is freed, the gastric pouch is transected proximal to the GJA with linear stapler with either blue or green reload. The proximal jejunum is also transected with a white reload along with the mesentery of the small bowel. There are multiple options for revision of a gastric bypass including revision of the GJA anastomosis, pouch trimming, distalization, lengthening procedure, conversion to duodenal switch, and reversal.

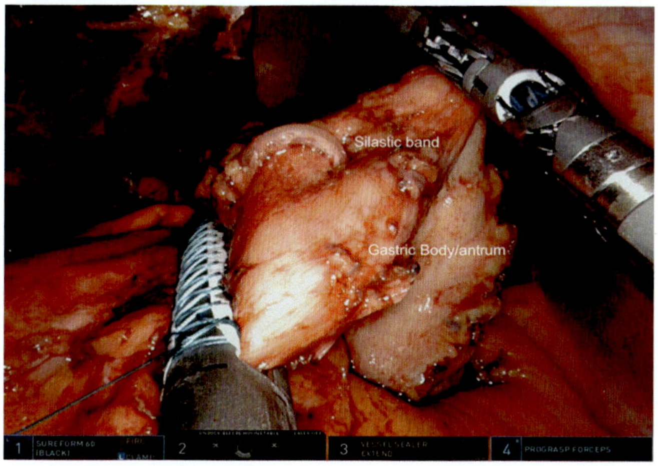

Fig. 24.13 VBG conversion to gastric bypass

Hand-Sewn Gastrojejunostomy Anastomosis

Hand-sewn gastrojejunostomy anastomosis, commonly the gastrointestinal reconstruction, is carried out in the form of gastric bypass (gastrojejunostomy) (Fig. 24.15). However, a hand sewn anastomosis (HSA) can be performed during reversal/conversion procedures as a gastro-gastrostomy, duodeno-ileostomy, or esophagojejunostomy.

For GJA, a gastrotomy and jejunotomy are created with monopolar scissors. To create the gastrotomy, the anesthesia team will advance the bougie slowly to create tenting of the anterior wall of the stomach; at this time the gastrotomy is carried out with cautery against the bougie. Then a 1.5–2 cm gastrojejunostomy was "hand-sewn" in two layers using two needle drivers and absorbable 6-inch barbed sutures (×3). Starting from lateral to medial, an inner posterior layer of running 3–0 absorbable barbed suture is created with full-thickness bites between the stomach and jejunum.

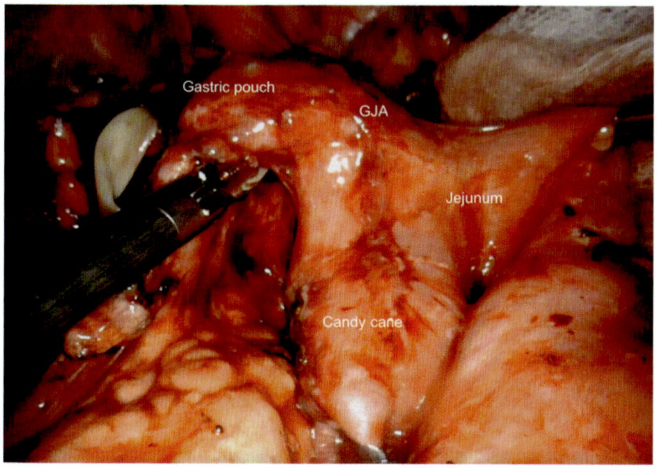

Fig. 24.14 RYGB

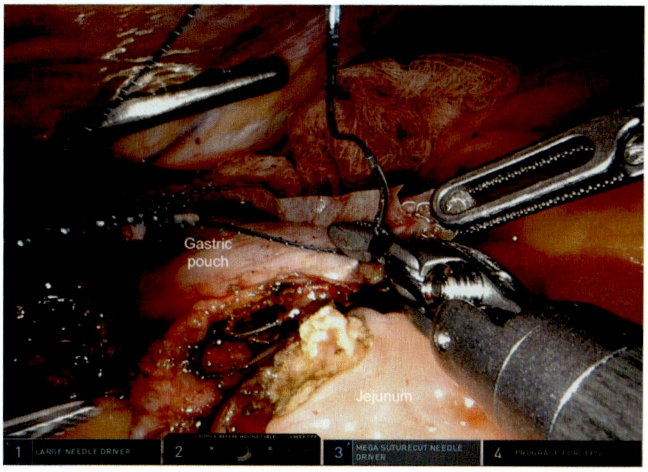

Fig. 24.15 Hand-sewn gastrojejunostomy anastomosis

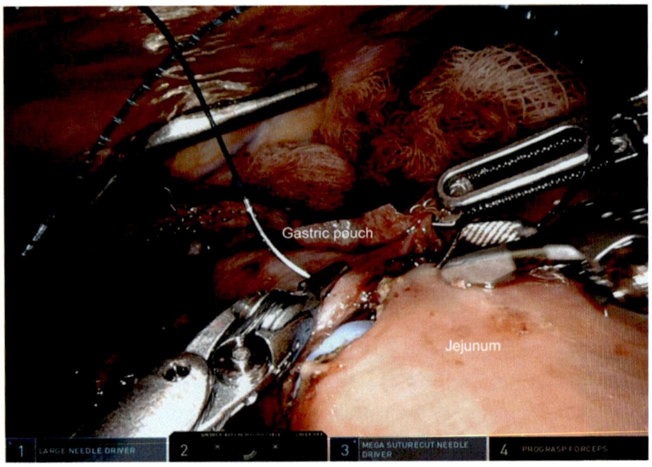

Fig. 24.16 Anterior layer of GJA

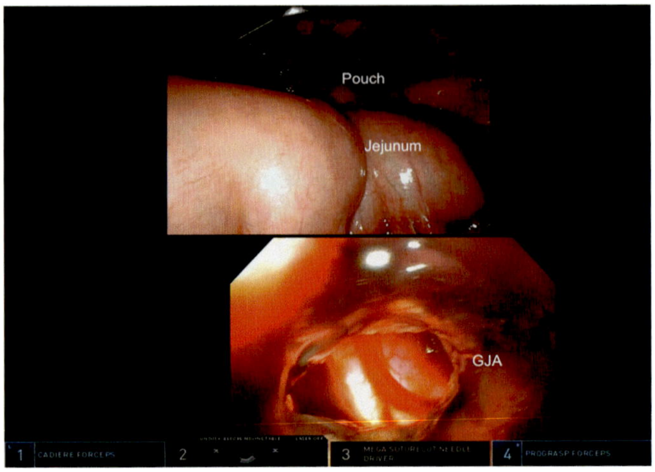

Fig. 24.17 Leak test

Anterior Layer of GJA

Once the posterior layer is completed, the bougie is advanced into the jejunum to stent the anastomosis (Fig. 24.16). Finally, two anterior layers of running seromuscular (Lembert sutures) absorbable 6-inch 3–0 barbed sutures are used.

Leak Test

Once this is completed, the alimentary limb is clamped distally, and the upper abdomen was filled with water to perform an air leak test (Fig. 24.17). The robotic image is switched to TilePro™ that enables the endoscopic view to be incorporated into the surgical field of view within the console. The gastroscope is inserted into the patient's esophagus insufflating along the way. The gastric pouch is entered, and the anastomosis is transverses. If no air leak is observed, the procedure is completed.

A. The HSA has the advantages of allowing for direct examination of the anastomosis, reducing the risk of bleeding, and can be used in situations where the use of stapler would be contraindicated like such us poor quality tissue or thicker. In addition, it has decreased long-term complications such as strictures.

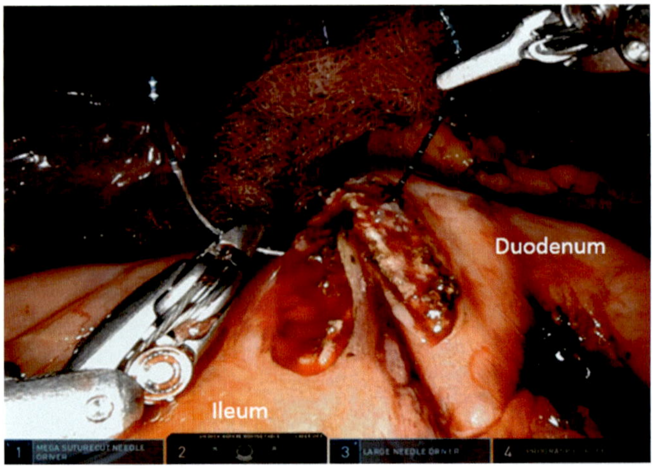

Fig. 24.18 Duodeno-ileostomy

B. The most notable advantages of the use of robotics for the HSA are the surgeon's autonomy, decreased variability, and reproducibility that lead to better quality anastomosis.
C. Similar technique is applied to other GI anastomosis (gastro-gastrostomy, duodeno-ileostomy [Fig. 24.18], or esophagojejunostomy [Fig. 24.19]) during the reconstruction.

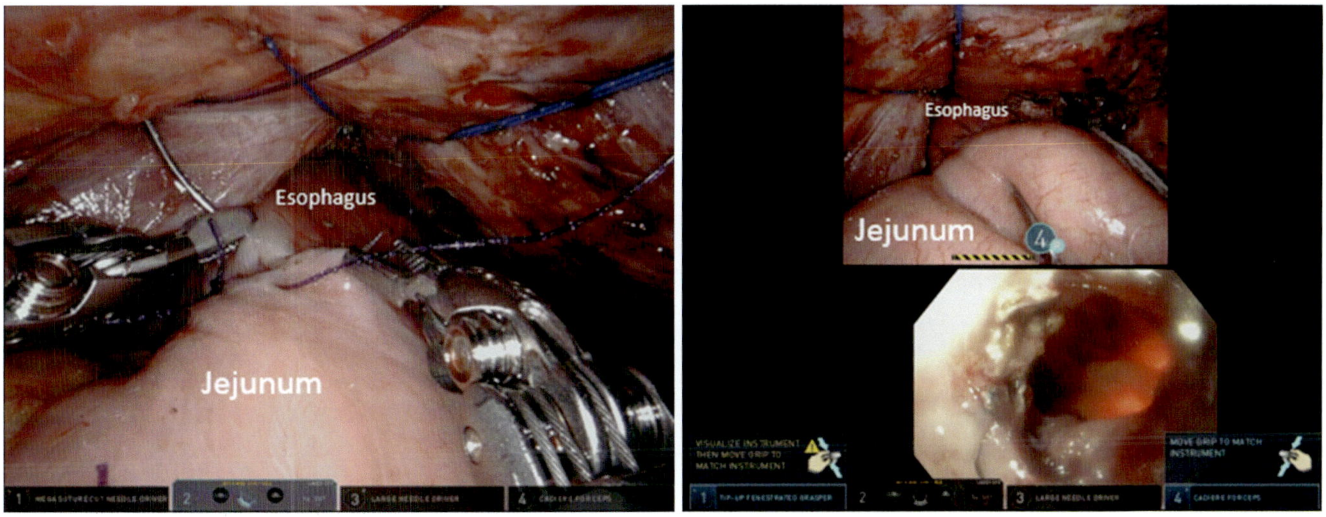

Fig. 24.19 Esophagojejunostomy

References

1. English WJ, DeMaria EJ, Brethauer SA, Mattar SG, Rosenthal RJ, Morton JM. American Society for Metabolic and Bariatric Surgery estimation of metabolic and bariatric procedures performed in the United States in 2016. Surg Obes Relat Dis. 2018;14(3):259–63. https://doi.org/10.1016/j.soard.2017.12.013.
2. Park JY, Kim YJ. Revisional bariatric surgery. In: Bariatric and metabolic surgery. Berlin Heidelberg: Springer; 2014. p. 87–96.
3. Snyder B, Wilson T, Woodruff V, Wilson E. Robotically assisted revision of bariatric surgeries is safe and effective to achieve further weight loss. World J Surg. 2013;37(11):2569–73. https://doi.org/10.1007/s00268-013-1968-y.
4. Economopoulos KP, Theocharidis V, McKenzie TJ, Sergentanis TN, Psaltopoulou T. Robotic vs. laparoscopic Roux-En-Y gastric bypass: a systematic review and meta-analysis. Obes Surg. 20`15;25(11):2180–9. Springer New York LLC,. https://doi.org/10.1007/s11695-015-1870-9.
5. El Chaar M, King K, Pastrana M, Galvez A, Stoltzfus J. Outcomes of robotic surgery in revisional bariatric cases: a propensity score-matched analysis of the MBSAQIP registry. J Robot Surg. 2020; https://doi.org/10.1007/s11701-020-01098-z.
6. Cheng YL, Elli EF. Role of robotic surgery in complex revisional bariatric procedures. Obes Surg. 2021; https://doi.org/10.1007/s11695-021-05272-6.

Index

O. Y. Kudsi, P. P. Grimminger (eds.), *Atlas of Robotic Upper Gastrointestinal Surgery*,
https://doi.org/10.1007/978-3-030-86578-8